PHOTO ATLAS
of NURSING PROCEDURES

THIRD EDITION

Pamela L. Swearingen, RN
Special Projects Editor

Cheri A. Howard, RN, MSN
Unit Director, Indiana University Medical Center

in association with

Indiana University School of Nursing
Department of Nursing Services
Indiana University Medical Center

and the

Physical Therapy Program
Respiratory Therapy Department
Division of Allied Health Sciences
Indiana University School of Medicine
Indianapolis, Indiana

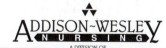

ADDISON-WESLEY
NURSING
A DIVISION OF
THE BENJAMIN/CUMMINGS PUBLISHING COMPANY, INC.

Menlo Park, California • Reading, Massachusetts • New York
Don Mills, Ontario • Wokingham, UK • Amsterdam • Bonn • Paris
Milan • Madrid • Sydney • Singapore • Tokyo • Seoul • Taipei
Mexico City • San Juan, Puerto Rico

Executive Editor: *Patricia L. Cleary*
Acquisitions Editor: *Erin Mulligan*
Project Editor: *Grace Wong*
Managing Editor: *Wendy Earl*
Production Coordinator: *Bradley Burch*
Text and Cover Designer: *Gary Head*
Text Photographer: *Jeffry Collins*
Artist: *Nea Hanscomb*
Copy Editor: *John Hammett*
Proofreader: *Kristin Barendsen*
Indexer: *Karen Hollister*
Compositor: *Greene Design*
Prepress: *GTS Graphics*
Senior Manufacturing Supervisor: *Merry Free Osborn*
Text Printer and Binder: *Courier Kendallville*

Swearingen, Pamela L.
    Photo atlas of nursing procedures / Pamela L. Swearingen, Cheri A. Howard; in association with Indiana University School of Nursing [and the] Department of Nursing Services, Indiana University Medical Center and the Physical Therapy Program, Division of Allied Health Sciences, Indiana University School of Medicine, Indianapolis, Indiana. — 3rd ed.
        p. cm.
    Includes bibliographical references and index.
    ISBN 0-8053-8789-7
    1. Nursing—Pictorial works. I. Howard, Cheri A. II. Indiana University. School of Nursing. III. Indiana University. Dept. of. Nursing Services. IV. Indiana University. Physical Therapy Program. V. Title.
    [DNLM: 1. Nursing—atlases. 2. Home Care Services—atlases. WY 17 S974a 1996]
RT41.S96 1996
610.73'022'2—dc20
DNLM/DLC
for Library of Congress   95-40797
                                                                CIP

ISBN 0-8053-8789-7

2 3 4 5 6 7 8 9 10—CRK—99 98 97

Addison-Wesley Nursing
A Division of The Benjamin/Cummings Publishing Company, Inc.
2725 Sand Hill Road
Menlo Park, California 94025

Preface

Do you remember the anxiety that surrounded your first performance of a new procedure in the hospital—an injection, a catheterization, suctioning an airway? Most nurses never forget.

Mastering the procedures—the psychomotor skills that underlie day-to-day nursing care—is one of the most important and most difficult educational experiences in nursing. Performed correctly, as part of the overall plan of nursing care, these procedures help promote comfort and recovery for clients. Performed less than competently, some procedures can be life-threatening.

Procedures usually are learned by watching a skilled demonstration and then performing a return demonstration. Because one on-site performance is seldom enough practice, methods and guidelines are needed to repeat the demonstrations until skills are mastered. The *Photo Atlas of Nursing Procedures, Third Edition,* offers you that extra assistance.

This single volume provides convenient access to realistic and detailed demonstrations of the procedures most frequently required of general duty staff nurses. It focuses on procedures directly involving a client; thus, such skills as bedmaking are not included. Critical care procedures are not included nor are those procedures that require a hands-on inservice demonstration to ensure safe client care. Because cardiopulmonary resuscitation is a basic technique taught to all hospital personnel, it is not included here.

Audience

Faculty, students, and practitioners alike will find this two-color atlas a highly effective supplemental text for use in teaching, learning, or practice. New graduates, staff nurses, and nurses returning to practice will welcome its comprehensive reference value. This new atlas uses more than 1400 black-and-white photographs taken in a clinical setting to graphically present the more than 325 guidelines and procedures. It

assumes the reader's understanding of basic sciences and nursing fundamentals.

Organization and Approach

The *Photo Atlas of Nursing Procedures, Third Edition,* is organized in two units: Unit One includes procedures basic to all nursing care; Unit Two includes procedures related to disorders of individual body systems. Since these are procedures that can be depicted by photography, psychosocial skills are not included.

Each body-system chapter begins with a review of anatomy and physiology, followed by a nursing assessment guideline for that system. Where appropriate, variations of care throughout the life cycle are included in the narrative.

Every attempt has been made to include the necessary detail and rationale for each procedure while making each step easy to understand. The steps are within the nursing process framework, thus helping ensure optimal care of the client. The clear, professional tone of the presentation and the inclusion of rationale help establish an ideal climate for client teaching.

There are often several "correct" ways to perform a procedure based on agency practice and/or personal preference. This atlas depicts generic procedures that can be adapted to materials and equipment available and to the method the reader has used successfully. Occasional use of identifiable commercial products in the photographs is not intended as product endorsement.

The photographs in this book represent the variety of nursing attire currently worn in hospitals and other health care settings around the nation. Thus, nurses are shown wearing many different styles of professional attire. For simplicity and to avoid referring to clients as he or she, we have chosen instead to refer only to the gender of the client in each photograph.

Additions to the Third Edition

An exciting addition to the third edition is "Home Health Care Considerations." These boxed guidelines are found throughout the book and pertain to procedural variations for clients in the home setting. We have not added guidelines if the home procedure remains virtually the same. This edition also focuses on the use of sheathed needles or needleless systems for preventing needlestick when accessing the peripheral vascular system. Many different systems are employed throughout hospitals to avoid needlestick and it would be outside the scope of this book to show all such systems.

In addition, we have added new procedures to this edition including irrigating a wound, managing alternating pressure therapy, understanding peripherally inserted central venous catheters (PICCs) and midline catheters (MLCs), repairing a multi-lumen central venous catheter, understanding percutaneous endoscopic gastrostomy (PEG) tubes, replacing a disposable inner cannula for tracheostomy, monitoring oxygen saturation using pulse oximetry, applying pneumatic sequential compression devices, using a foot pump, caring for clients undergoing dialysis, and managing the client undergoing cryotherapy via a knee compression dressing.

All procedures reflect 1995 Standard- and Transmission-Based Precautions from the CDC and 1991 ruling from OSHA for exposure to bloodborne pathogens. Because one of the primary audiences for this book is the student, who may be performing injections for the first time, we have shown the injection procedures with gloves.

The *Photo Atlas of Nursing Procedures, Third Edition,* was created and developed to assist nurses at every level of practice as they learn, relearn, review, and update their hands-on skills in client care. Ultimately, this will enhance the quality of that care—a goal we all share.

Acknowledgments

The journey from idea to bound book is never solitary. On a project of this magnitude, the author requires assistance, encouragement, and support from many. We are fortunate to have found an abundance of all three requisites at every step.

The *Photo Atlas of Nursing Procedures, Third Edition,* had its inception at one of the great teaching centers in nursing—Indiana University School of Nursing at Indianapolis. We are grateful to Dean Angela McBride for granting us permission to use the Learning Resources Laboratory once again and to Dr. Diane Billings, Professor and Assistant Dean of Learning Resources and Lynn Dial, Learning Resources Coordinator, all of Indiana University School of Nursing, who were wonderful and went out of their way to make sure our work there went smoothly. Sonna Ehrlich, Associate Director of Hospitals for Nursing at Indiana University Medical Center, graciously granted us access to Indiana University Medical Center and enabled us to work with the many excellent and knowledgeable nurses.

As in the first two editions, we enjoyed working with Dr. Rebecca Porter, Director and Associate Professor of the Graduate Program in Physical Therapy, School of Medicine, Indiana University, and Chuck Christoph, Clinical Instructor, Respiratory Therapy Program, Indiana University Medical Center. For this edition we had the pleasure of working with the following individuals who made our work a lot easier because of their contributions: Deana Edenburn, Assistant Program Director, Indiana University Medical Center, who gave us valuable and timely information regarding care of clients with central venous access devices and who also graciously allowed us to photograph the care of their lines; and Grace Schoonveld, Infusion Clinical Coordinator, Indiana University Medical Center Homecare, who helped us develop the Home Health Care Considerations. A special thanks goes to Kristine McClary, who stepped in at the eleventh hour to save one of our shoots.

We are especially appreciative of our friend Jeffry Collins, one the country's best medical photographers, who has been with us from the first edition, helping make the long hours of shooting as pleasant as possible. Marguerite Jackson, Administrative Director of Medical Center Epidemiology Unit and Assistant Clinical Professor of Family and Preventative Medicine at University of California, San Diego, always has made herself available to us as advisor to the many infection control issues that nurses face daily. Her practical, no-nonsense approach to infection control eliminates the "ritual and magic" that historically have been a part of techniques and fundamental books and promotes, instead, understanding of why and when nurses use gloves and other barrier devices to prevent the spread of infection. You are all dear and valued friends.

Careful and thoughtful critiques from the following experts helped ensure the accuracy and clarity of the procedures depicted: Jacqueline Jones Barrows, Manager of Clinical Research of Haemonetics Corporation in Braintree, Massachusetts; Brian Holmes, Senior Territory Manager of B. Brian Medical, Inc.; Ray Ellen Johnson, Territory Manager of KCI Medical

Services; and Mary Quinn, Sales Specialist, Vascular Therapy Division, of Kendall Healthcare Products Company.

The following reviewers helped us plan the revision with the needs of the student in mind:

Patricia A. Dennis, RN, MSN, Ohio Valley Hospital School of Nursing

Bonnie Fae Fador, BSN, MSN, Belmont Technical College

Barbara Goodkin, RN, MS, Washtenaw Community College

Claudia Landberg, RN, BSN, Monroe County Community College

Kathleen V. Van Etten, RN, BSN, Monroe County Community College

Marguerite Jackson, RN, MS, CIC, FAAN, University of California, San Diego Medical Center

These individuals reviewed the final product with care and precision:

Patricia Graham, RN, MN, Medical College of Georgia

Catherine Hrycyk, RN, MSCN, DeAnza College

Marguerite Jackson, RN, MS, CIC, FAAN, University of California, San Diego Medical Center

Marian K. Yoder, RN, EdD, San Jose State University

Thank you all for your critical and creative insights.

P.L.S.
C.A.H.

First Edition On-Site Advisory Board

Brief Contents

UNIT I
PERFORMING BASIC CARE PROCEDURES 1

CHAPTER 1
Employing Techniques for Infection Prevention and Control 3

CHAPTER 2
Using Proper Positioning, Mobilization, and Transferring Techniques 33

CHAPTER 3
Administering Medications and Monitoring Fluids 81

UNIT II
PERFORMING SPECIALIZED NURSING PROCEDURES 179

CHAPTER 4
Managing Female Reproductive Procedures and Immediate Care of the Newborn 181

CHAPTER 5
Managing Gastrointestinal Procedures 235

CHAPTER 6
Managing Respiratory Procedures 311

CHAPTER 7
Managing Cardiovascular Procedures 385

CHAPTER 8
Managing Renal-Urinary Procedures 429

CHAPTER 9
Managing Musculoskeletal Procedures 493

CHAPTER 10
Managing Neurosensory Procedures 583

Index 629

Home Health Care Considerations

1

Employing Techniques for Infection
Prevention and Control 6, 28

2

Using Proper Positioning, Mobilization,
and Transferring Techniques 55, 63

3

Administering Medications
and Monitoring Fluids 90, 99, 162

5

Managing Gastrointestinal
Procedures 248, 266, 285

6

Managing Respiratory
Procedures 333, 337, 342

8

Managing Renal-Urinary
Procedures 443, 448

Detailed Contents

UNIT I
PERFORMING BASIC CARE PROCEDURES   1

CHAPTER 1

Employing Techniques for Infection Prevention and Control   3

APPLYING BASIC INFECTION CONTROL MEASURES   4

Protocols for Handwashing and Cleansing Agents   4

Handwashing   4

Cleansing Agent   4

Reviewing Basic Handwashing   6

Implementing Standard and Transmission-Based Precautions   7

Isolation Precautions for Clients with Pulmonary or Laryngeal Tuberculosis (TB)   7

Using Protective Barriers   12

Applying a Fluid-Resistive Gown   12

Applying a Fluid-Resistive Mask   13

Applying Gloves   13

Removing Protective Barriers   14

Managing Intravascular Devices to Reduce Infection Risk   15

PREPARING FOR A STERILE PROCEDURE   16

Applying Sterile Gloves   16

Establishing a Sterile Field   18

Opening a Sterile Pack   18

Dropping Sterile Supplies onto a Sterile Field   19

Placing a Sterile Bowl onto the Sterile Field   20

Pouring Sterile Solutions   20

Putting on Sterile Attire (Including the Closed-Glove Technique)   21

PERFORMING OTHER PROCEDURES   24

Obtaining a Throat Culture   24

Performing Wound Care   25

Packing a Wound (Using Wet to Damp Dressing)   25

Irrigating a Wound   29

CHAPTER 2

Using Proper Positioning, Mobilization, and Transferring Techniques   33

ASSISTING THE CLIENT WITH POSITIONING AND MOBILIZATION   34

Performing Passive Range of Motion Exercises   34

Performing Traditional ROM Exercises   34

Exercising the Neck   35

Exercising the Shoulders   37

Exercising the Elbows 40

Exercising the Wrists and Fingers 41

Exercising the Hips and Knees 44

Exercising the Ankles and Toes 47

Performing Proprioceptive Neuromuscular
Facilitation Exercises 49

Exercising the Neck 49

Exercising the Upper Extremities 50

Exercising the Lower Extremities 52

*Nursing Guidelines: Using Pressure-Relief
Mattresses and Pads 53*

Nursing Guidelines: Proper Client Positioning 56

Assisting the Client with Crutches,
Canes, and Walkers 61

Checking for Correct Crutch Height 61

Guarding the Client 61

Assisting the Client with Crutches to Sit in a Chair 63

TRANSFERRING MOBILE
AND IMMOBILE CLIENTS 64

Nursing Guidelines: Lifting and Transferring Clients 64

Moving the Client Up in Bed 65

Assisting the Mobile Client 65

Lifting the Immobile Client 66

Dangling the Client's Extremities
on the Side of the Bed 67

Assisting the Mobile Client 67

Moving the Immobile Client 68

Moving the Client from the Stretcher to the Bed 69

Teaching the Segmental Transfer Technique 69

Transferring the Immobile Client 72

Logrolling the Immobile Client 74

Assisting the Client from the Wheelchair (or Chair) to the Bed 76

Using a Mechanical Lifting Device 78

CHAPTER 3

*Administering Medications and
Monitoring Fluids 81*

ADMINISTERING TOPICAL MEDICATIONS 83

Giving Ophthalmic Medications 83

Instilling Ointment 83

Instilling Drops 84

Instilling Ear Drops 84

Instilling Nose Drops 85

Giving Inhalant Medications 86

Using a Metered-Dose Inhaler 86

Using a Nebulizer 87

Giving Nitroglycerin 88

Applying Nitroglycerin Ointment 88

Applying a Nitroglycerin Disk 89

Administering Medications Through a Nasogastric Tube 90

Performing a Vaginal Irrigation (Douche) 92

Giving Rectal Medications 94

Inserting a Suppository 94

Instilling Ointment 94

ADMINISTERING INJECTABLE MEDICATIONS 95

Giving Intradermal Injections 95

Locating the Site 95

Injecting the Medication 96

Giving Subcutaneous Injections 97

Locating the Site 97

Injecting the Medication 98

Administering Heparin 100

Giving Intramuscular (IM) Injections 101

Mapping Muscle Sites for IM Injections 101

Providing an Air Lock 106

Injecting the Medication 107

Performing the Z-Track Technique 108

Disposing of Needles and Sharp Instruments 110

Nursing Guidelines: Managing Insulin Pumps 110

ADMINISTERING INTRAVENOUS FLUIDS AND MEDICATIONS 113

Preparing the Solution and Infusion Set 113

Inspecting the Container 113

Assembling the Infusion Set 114

Spiking the Container 115

Priming the Infusion Set 116

Labeling the Tubing and Container 116

Inserting a Peripheral Vascular Access Device 117

Assembling the Materials 117

Choosing a Venipuncture Site 118

Dilating the Vein 119

Preparing the Site 119

Inserting a Wing-Tipped Needle 120

Taping the Wing-Tipped Needle 121

Inserting an Over-the-Needle Catheter 121

Taping the Over-the-Needle Catheter 124

Applying Antimicrobial Ointment and a Gauze Dressing 126

Immobilizing the Extremity 127

Using an Armboard or Splint 127

Applying a Commercial Wrist Restraint 128

Applying a Gauze Restraint 129

Administering Intravenous (IV) Medications 130

Injecting Medications into Hanging IV Containers 130

Giving Medications by IV Bolus 132

Inserting a Saline/Heparin Lock for Intermittent Infusion Therapy 134

Giving Medications via a Partial-Fill (Piggyback) Container 136

Assembling a Volume-Control IV Set 138

COLLECTING, MONITORING, AND ADMINISTERING BLOOD 140

Collecting a Blood Sample with a Vacuum Collection System 140

Teaching the Diabetic Client Self-Monitoring of Blood Glucose 142

Initiating and Monitoring Blood Transfusions 144

Nursing Guidelines: Safe Administration of Blood 144

Administering Blood or Blood Components 145

Initiating Patient-Controlled Analgesia 149

Managing Venous Access Devices (VADs) 154

Nursing Guidelines: Managing Chronic (Long-Term) Central Venous Catheters 154

Nursing Guidelines: Managing Acute (Short-Term) and Intermediate (Medium-Term) Multilumen Central Venous Catheters 155

Nursing Guidelines: Managing Peripherally Inserted Central Venous Catheters (PICCs) 156

Nursing Guidelines: Managing Midline Catheters (MLCs) 157

Nursing Guidelines: Managing Implantable Subcutaneous Ports 158

Changing the Exit Site Dressing for a Chronic Central Venous Catheter 159

Drawing Blood from a Chronic (Hickman®-Type) Central Venous Catheter and Flushing the Catheter Following Blood Withdrawal 163

Performing a Routine Irrigation of a Chronic Central Venous Catheter 166

Changing the IV Solution and Tubing for a Chronic (Hickman®-Type) Central Venous Catheter 167

Repairing a Multilumen Central Venous Catheter 168

Accessing the Implantable Subcutaneous Port 170

Withdrawing Blood from an Implantable Subcutaneous Port 173

Establishing a Heparin Lock in an Implantable Subcutaneous Port 175

Assessing and Intervening for an Air Embolism 176

UNIT II
PERFORMING SPECIALIZED NURSING PROCEDURES 179

CHAPTER 4

Managing Female Reproductive Procedures and Immediate Care of the Newborn 181

PERFORMING ROUTINE GYNECOLOGIC TECHNIQUES 182

The Female Reproductive System 182
Nursing Assessment Guidelines 182
Teaching Breast Self-Examination 183
Assisting the Client with Postsurgical Mastectomy Exercises 187

Providing Perineal Care 190
Using a Squeeze Bottle 190
Preparing a Sitz Bath 191
Using a Surgi-Gator 192
Providing Care for Clients with Cervical-Uterine Radiation Implants 193

PERFORMING PRENATAL TECHNIQUES 194

Assessing the Prenatal Abdomen 194
Measuring Fundal Height 194
Inspecting and Palpating Fetal Parts 194
Auscultating Fetal Heart Tones 196
Using Ultrasonic (Doppler) Auscultation 197
Performing External Electronic Fetal Monitoring 198

Assessing for Amniotic Fluid 201

Providing Comfort Measures 202
Applying Counterpressure to Relieve Leg Cramps 202
Applying Pressure to Relieve Back Pain 202

PERFORMING POSTPARTUM TECHNIQUES 203

Assessing the Mother 203
Inspecting and Palpating the Breasts 204
Palpating the Fundus and Bladder 205
Evaluating the Lochia 206
Inspecting the Perineum 207

Assisting with Infant Feeding 207
Positioning the Infant 208
Burping the Infant 210
Massaging the Breasts for Manual Expression of Breast Milk 211

Using Breast Pumps 212
Managing Hand Pumps 212
Assisting with Electric Breast Pumps 213

CARING FOR THE NEWBORN 215

Admitting the Neonate to the Hospital 215
Obtaining Footprints 215
Instilling Ophthalmic Erythromycin 216
Administering a Vitamin K Injection 217
Obtaining a Blood Sample 218
Obtaining a Urine Specimen 219

Assessing the Neonate 220
Performing a General Inspection 220
Auscultating 221
Taking an Axillary Temperature 222
Palpating 222
Measuring and Weighing the Infant 229
Taking an Arterial Blood Pressure 230

Providing Neonatal Care 231
Giving Umbilical Cord Care 231
Suctioning (Bulb) 231
Suctioning (Mechanical) 232
Using Phototherapy 233

CHAPTER 5

Managing Gastrointestinal Procedures 235

ASSESSING THE GASTROINTESTINAL SYSTEM 236

The Gastrointestinal System 236
Nursing Assessment Guidelines 237

Examining the Oral Cavity 238
Inspecting the Mouth 238
Inspecting the Tongue and Pharynx 238

Examining the Abdomen 239
Inspecting the Abdomen 239
Auscultating the Abdomen 240
Percussing the Abdomen 241
Palpating the Abdomen 241
Measuring Abdominal Girth 242

Examining the Rectum 243
Inspecting the Rectum 243
Palpating the Rectum 243

MANAGING GASTRIC TUBES 244
Nursing Guidelines: Managing Gastric Tubes 244
 Single-Lumen Tube 244
 Double-Lumen Tube 245
 Triple-Lumen Esophageal-Nasogastric (Blakemore) Tube 246
 Four-Lumen (Minnesota Sump) Tube 247
 Gastrostomy Tube 248
 Percutaneous Endoscopic Gastrostomy (PEG) Tube 249
 Gastrostomy Button 250
Inserting a Nasogastric Tube 252
Inserting a Small-Bore Feeding Tube 258
Inserting an Orogastric Tube 260
Removing a Nasogastric Tube 261
Irrigating a Nasogastric Tube 262

Administering Nasogastric Tube Feedings 264
Giving an Intermittent Tube Feeding 264
Giving a Continuous-Drip Tube Feeding 267
Giving Gastrostomy Tube Feedings 268
Administering Gastric Lavage 271
Aspirating Stomach Contents for Gastric Analysis 273

MANAGING INTESTINAL TUBES 274
Nursing Guidelines: Managing Intestinal Tubes 274
 Single-Lumen Tube 274
 Double-Lumen Tube 275
 Jejunostomy Tube 276

MANAGING RECTAL ELIMINATION AND DISTENTION 277
Administering a Nonretention Enema 277
Administering a Retention Enema 280
Inserting a Rectal Tube 283
Testing Stool for Occult Blood 285

MANAGING STOMA CARE 286
Nursing Guidelines: Managing Ostomies 286
 Ascending Colostomy 286
 Transverse Colostomies 287
 Descending or Sigmoid Colostomy 291
 Ileostomy 292
 Continent Ileostomy 294
 Ileoanal Reservoir 295
Patch Testing the Client's Skin 296
Applying a Drainable Pouch 297
Dilating a Stoma 302
Irrigating a Colostomy 304
Draining a Continent Ileostomy 307

CHAPTER 6

Managing Respiratory Procedures 311

ASSESSING THE RESPIRATORY SYSTEM 312

The Respiratory System 312
Nursing Assessment Guidelines 313

Examining the Thorax 314
Inspecting 314
Palpating for Thoracic Expansion 316
Palpating for Fremitus and Crepitation (Subcutaneous Emphysema) 316
Percussing 317
Auscultating 317

MAINTAINING PATENT AIRWAYS 320
Nursing Guidelines: Artificial Airways 320
    Oropharyngeal Tube 320
    Nasopharyngeal Tube 321
    Endotracheal Tube 322
    Tracheostomy Tube 323
    Tracheostomy Button 324

Inserting Artificial Airways 325
Inserting an Oropharyngeal Airway 325
Inserting a Nasopharyngeal Airway 327
Performing Mouth-to-Mask Ventilation 329

Managing Routine Tracheostomy Care 330
Suctioning the Client with a Tracheostomy 330
Managing Tracheostomy Cuffs 335
Providing Tracheostomy Hygiene 337
Replacing a Disposable Inner Cannula 341

MANAGING RESPIRATORY THERAPY 342

Administering Oxygen, Humidity, and Aerosol Therapy 342
Nursing Guidelines: Devices Used in the Delivery of Oxygen, Humidity, and Aerosols 342

Simple Face Mask (Low-Flow System) 342
Nasal Cannula (Low-Flow System) 343
Partial Rebreathing Mask (Low-Flow System) 344
Nonrebreathing Mask (Low-Flow/High-Flow System) 345
Venturi (Air Entrainment) Mask (High-Flow System) 346
CPAP Mask 347
Oxygen Hood 348
Incubator (Isolette) 349
Oxygen Analyzer 350
Aerosol Face Mask 351
Tracheostomy Collar 352
T-Piece 353
Monitoring Oxygen Saturation Using Pulse Oximetry 354
Converting a Nonrebreathing Mask to a Partial Rebreathing Mask 355
Assembling a Venturi Delivery System 356
Setting Up an Oxygen System with Humidification 358
Delivering Heated Humidity 360
Assembling a Nebulizer 361

Employing Techniques for Lung Inflation 362
Instructing Clients in Deep-Breathing Exercises 362
Assisting with Coughing 364
Using Incentive Spirometers 365
Assisting with IPPB 366

Performing Chest Physiotherapy 368
Percussing, Vibrating, and Draining the Adult 368
Percussing, Vibrating, and Draining the Infant or Small Child 374

MANAGING THE CLIENT WITH A CHEST TUBE 377
Nursing Guidelines: Disposable Closed Chest Drainage System 377

Suction Control 377
Water Seal Chamber 378
Collection Chamber 378
Monitoring the Client with a Chest Tube 379
Assisting with the Removal of a Chest Tube 382

CHAPTER 7

Managing Cardiovascular Procedures 385

ASSESSING THE CARDIOVASCULAR SYSTEM 386

The Cardiovascular System 386
Nursing Assessment Guidelines 387

Examining the Cardiac Area (Precordium) 388

Inspecting and Palpating 389

Auscultating 390

Palpating Arterial Pulses 394

MONITORING THE CARDIOVASCULAR SYSTEM 396

Inspecting the Jugular Veins 396

Measuring Blood Pressure 397

Obtaining the Ankle-Brachial Pressure Ratio (A/B Ratio) 401

Measuring Paradoxical Pulse 403

Nursing Guidelines: Identifying Common Telemetry Lead Sites 404

Applying Disposable Electrodes for Telemetry Monitoring 405

Positioning Electrodes for a 12-Lead EKG 409

Assessing the Postcardiac Catheterization Client 411

Measuring Central Venous Pressure (CVP) 414

CARING FOR CLIENTS WITH VASCULAR DISORDERS 417

Applying Elastic (Antiembolic) Stockings 417

Applying Pneumatic Sequential Compression Devices 420

Using a Foot Pump 423

Employing Buerger-Allen Exercises 425

CHAPTER 8

Managing Renal-Urinary Procedures 429

ASSESSING THE RENAL-URINARY SYSTEM 430

The Renal-Urinary System 430
Nursing Assessment Guidelines 432

Assessing the Bladder 433

Inspecting 433

Palpating 433

Percussing 434

Palpating the Kidneys 435

Assessing Skin Turgor 435

Weighing the Client on a Bed Scale 436

Collecting a Timed Urine Specimen 436

CATHETERIZING AND MANAGING CATHETER CARE 437

Performing Intermittent Catheterization 437

Inserting a Robinson (Straight) Catheter into a Female 437

Inserting a Robinson (Straight) Catheter into a Male 444

Managing a Foley Catheter 446

Performing a Catheterization with a Foley (Indwelling) Catheter 446

Nursing Guidelines: Foley Catheter Management 449

Making a Catheter Strap 450

Obtaining a Urine Specimen 452

Emptying the Drainage Bag 454

Using a Urine Meter 455

Irrigating the Catheter 457

Removing a Foley Catheter 460

CARING FOR CLIENTS WITH RENAL-URINARY DISORDERS 461

Applying an External Urinary Device (with a Leg Drainage System) 461

Monitoring the Client Receiving Continuous
Bladder Irrigation (CBI) 465

Establishing CBI 465

Nursing Guidelines: Care of the Client with CBI 466

*Nursing Guidelines: Care of the Client with a
Suprapubic Catheter 467*

*Nursing Guidelines: Care of the Client with a
Nephrostomy Tube and Ureteral Stents 468*

Administering a Sodium Polystyrene Sulfonate (Kayexalate) Enema 470

Performing Credé's Maneuver 473

CARING FOR CLIENTS UNDERGOING DIALYSIS 474

*Nursing Guidelines: Quinton and Permcath
Dialysis Accesses 474*

**Administering an Exchange for a Client
with Chronic Ambulatory Peritoneal Dialysis 475**

*CARING FOR CLIENTS WITH URINARY
DIVERSIONS 478*

*Nursing Guidelines: Common Types of
Urinary Diversions 478*

    Ileal Conduit 478

    Cutaneous Ureterostomy 480

    Continent Urinary Diversion 482

Performing a Postoperative Assessment 484

Managing Appliance Care 486

Applying a Postoperative (Disposable) Pouch 486

Picture Framing the Pouch 490

Connecting the Pouch to a Urinary Drainage System 491

CHAPTER 9

*Managing Musculoskeletal
Procedures 493*

ASSESSING THE MUSCULOSKELETAL SYSTEM 494

The Musculoskeletal System 494

Nursing Assessment Guidelines 495

Performing a General Assessment of the
Musculoskeletal System 496

Inspecting 496

Palpating the Spine 498

Evaluating Joint Range of Motion (ROM) and Muscular Strength 500

Measuring Muscle Girth 505

Evaluating Activities of Daily Living 506

Performing Neurovascular Assessments 506

Evaluating Neurovascular Integrity 506

Assessing Nerve Function 508

USING IMMOBILIZATION AND COMFORT DEVICES 511

*Nursing Guidelines: Care of Clients in
Immobilization Devices 511*

    Soft Cervical Collar 511

    Hard Cervical Collar 512

    Clavicle Splint 513

    Arm/Shoulder Immobilizer 514

    Wrist/Forearm Splint 515

    Abduction Pillow 516

    Knee Immobilizer 517

    Hinged Brace 518

    Denis-Browne Splint 519

Applying Elastic Bandages 520

Wrapping a Long, Cylindrical Body Part 520

Wrapping a Joint 521

Wrapping a Residual Limb (Stump) 522

Managing Routine Cast Care 524

Assisting with Cast Application 524

Performing Routine Assessments and Interventions for Clients in Casts 529

Nursing Guidelines: Care of Clients in Casts 531

Petaling a Cast 532

MANAGING ROUTINE TRACTION CARE 533

Making a Bowline Traction Knot 533

Nursing Guidelines: Care of Clients in Traction 534

Caring for Clients in Skin Traction 535

Applying Cervical Traction 535

Applying a Pelvic Belt 539

Applying a Buck's Boot for Extension Traction 543

Caring for Children in Bryant's Traction 547

Caring for Clients in Skeletal Traction 551

Performing Routine Care of Clients in Skeletal Traction 551

Performing Routine Care and Assessments for Clients in Halo Vests 554

Providing Pin Care 560

PROVIDING SPECIAL CARE FOR CLIENTS WITH MUSCULOSKELETAL DISORDERS 561

Making a Traction Bed 561

Maintaining a Portable Wound-Drainage System 563

Applying a Hydroculator Pack (Moist Heat) to Arthritic Joints 565

Managing the Client with a Blood Reinfusion System 567

Monitoring the Client Undergoing Continuous Passive Motion (CPM) 570

Managing the Client Undergoing Cryotherapy via a Knee Compression Dressing 571

Transferring the Client with a Total Hip Replacement 572

CHAPTER 10

Managing Neurosensory Procedures 583

ASSESSING THE NEUROLOGIC SYSTEM 584

The Neurologic System 584

Nursing Assessment Guidelines 585

Monitoring the Status of a Neurologically Impaired Client 586

Performing a Neurologic Check 586

Testing Cerebellar and Motor Function 597

Assessing Sensory Function Using a Dermatome Chart 598

Evaluating Deep Tendon Reflexes 600

Assessing Cranial Drainage for the Presence of Cerebrospinal Fluid 602

CARING FOR CLIENTS WITH NEUROLOGIC DISORDERS 603

Assisting the Client with a Transcutaneous Electrical Nerve Stimulator Device 603

Providing Care During a Seizure 605

Using a Hyperthermia or Hypothermia System 606

Assessing Clients with Subarachnoid Drains 610

Nursing Guidelines: Care of Clients on Special Beds and Frames 612

    Roto Rest Kinetic Treatment Table 612

    Clinitron Air Fluidized Therapy 616

    Therapulse Pulsating Air Suspension Therapy 620

CARING FOR CLIENTS WITH DISORDERS OF THE SENSORY SYSTEM 623

Assessing Auditory Function 623

Performing the Watch Test 623

Performing the Weber and Rinne Tests 623

Irrigating the External Auditory Canal 625

Irrigating the Eye 627

Index 629

UNIT I

PERFORMING BASIC CARE PROCEDURES

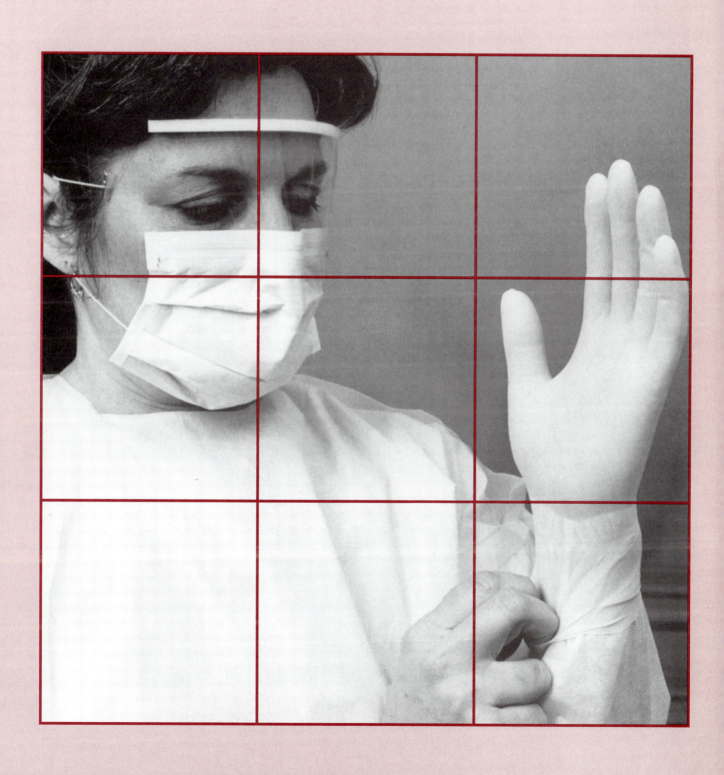

CHAPTER 1

Employing Techniques for Infection Prevention and Control

CHAPTER OUTLINE

APPLYING BASIC INFECTION CONTROL MEASURES

Protocols for Handwashing and Cleansing Agents

Handwashing

Cleansing Agent

Reviewing Basic Handwashing

Implementing Standard and Transmission-Based Precautions

Isolation Precautions for Clients with Pulmonary or Laryngeal Tuberculosis (TB)

Using Protective Barriers

Applying a Fluid-Resistive Gown

Applying a Fluid-Resistive Mask

Applying Gloves

Removing Protective Barriers

Managing Intravascular Devices to Reduce Infection Risk

PREPARING FOR A STERILE PROCEDURE

Applying Sterile Gloves

Establishing a Sterile Field

Opening a Sterile Pack

Dropping Sterile Supplies onto a Sterile Field

Placing a Sterile Bowl onto the Sterile Field

Pouring Sterile Solutions

Putting on Sterile Attire (Including the Closed-Glove Technique)

PERFORMING OTHER PROCEDURES

Obtaining a Throat Culture

Performing Wound Care

Packing a Wound (Using Wet to Damp Dressing)

Irrigating a Wound

Applying Basic Infection Control Measures

PROTOCOLS FOR HANDWASHING AND CLEANSING AGENTS

Handwashing

Handwashing is the single most important procedure for preventing transmission of organisms among clients and health care workers. According to the Centers for Disease Control and Prevention (CDC), in clinical situations in which superficial contact has been made with a client, handwashing generally is not required. Superficial contact includes handshaking, measuring blood pressure, and handing medications or food to the individual. However, you should wash your hands when you have had prolonged and intense client contact. Wash your hands before performing invasive procedures; before caring for susceptible individuals, such as newborns, individuals in intensive care units, or individuals who are immunocompromised; before and after touching wounds; and every time you remove your gloves. In addition, wash your hands after situations in which microbial contamination of the hands is likely to have occurred, even if you were wearing gloves. These situations include contact with mucous membranes, blood, body fluids, secretions, and excretions as well as contact with inanimate objects likely to be contaminated (eg, urine measuring device). You should also wash your hands between procedures for the same client (eg, after touching the urinary drainage container and before changing a wound dressing). Finally, wash your hands any time you are in doubt about its necessity!

Cleansing Agent

Absolute indications for handwashing with plain soaps and detergents versus handwashing with products containing antimicrobial agents are unknown. However, for most routine client care activities, the use of plain soap appears to be sufficient because the friction used with the soap allows most transient microorganisms to be washed off. Antimicrobial handwashing agents are used before caring for clients in high-risk areas, including newborns and severely immunocompromised individuals. Hands are also washed with antimicrobial agents between clients in high-risk areas. For more information, see Table 1.1.

Table 1.1   Recommended Agents for Preparing Hands and Cleaning Skin Before Nonsurgical and Surgical Procedures*

Procedure	Example	Handwashing	Gloves†	Preparation of Patient's Skin	Comment
Nonsurgical					
Instruments used in procedure will come in contact with intact mucous membranes.	Bronchoscopy, gastrointestinal endoscopy, and tracheal suction.	Soap and water.	Recommended.	In general, none is required.	
	Cystoscopy, urinary tract catheterization.	Soap and water.	Sterile.	Antiseptics should be used to prepare urethral meatus.	

*Hands should be washed after all procedures in which microbial contamination of the operator is likely to occur, especially those involving contact with mucous membranes, whether or not gloves are worn. Soap and water are usually adequate for such handwashing.

From Centers for Disease Control and Prevention. *Guideline for Handwashing and Hospital Environmental Control.* Atlanta, GA: U.S. Department of Health and Human Services, 1985.

Centers for Disease Control and Prevention. Update: Universal precautions for prevention of transmission of human immunodeficiency virus and other bloodborne pathogens in health care settings. *MMWR* (June 24) 1988;37:377–388.

Source: Department of Labor, Occupational Safety and Health Administration: Occupational exposure to bloodborne pathogens; final rule 29 CFR part 1910: 1030. *Federal Register* 56:64003–64182, December 6, 1991.

† Gloves protect the patient and operator from potentially infectious microorganisms.

Table 1.1 Recommended Agents for Preparing Hands and Cleaning Skin *(continued)*

Procedure	Example	Handwashing	Gloves†	Preparation of Patient's Skin	Comment
Insertion of peripheral intravenous or arterial cannula.	Intravenous therapy, arterial pressure monitoring.	Soap and water or antiseptic.	Clean.	Antiseptics should be used; a fast-acting one is desirable. Tincture of iodine is preferred, but alcohol is adequate if it is applied liberally and allowed to act for 30 seconds.	Most epidemics of infection associated with arterial pressure-monitoring devices appear to be caused by hospital-associated contamination of components external to the skin, such as transducer heads or domes.
Percutaneous insertion of a central catheter or wire.	Hyperalimentation, central venous and capillary wedge pressure monitoring, angiography, cardiac pacemaker insertion.	Antiseptic.	Sterile.	Antiseptics should be used; a fast-acting one is desirable. Tincture of iodine is preferred. "Defatting" agents, such as acetone, are not recommended.	"Defatting" agents do not appear to decrease infections but can cause skin irritation.
Insertion (and prompt removal) of a sterile needle in deep tissues or body fluids, usually to obtain specimens or instill therapeutic agent.	Spinal tap, thoracentesis, abdominal paracentesis.	Soap and water or antiseptic.	Sterile.	Antiseptics should be used; a fast-acting one is desirable. Tincture of iodine is preferred.	
Surgical					
Insertion of a sterile tube or device through tissue into normally sterile tissue or fluid.	Chest tube insertion, culdoscopy, laparoscopy, peritoneal catheter insertion.	Antiseptic.	Sterile.	Antiseptics should be used. Hair should be clipped with scissors if hair removal is considered necessary.	Shaving hair can cause microabrasions, which predispose the client to infection.
Minor skin surgery.	Skin biopsy, suturing of small cuts, lancing boils, mole removal.	Soap and water.	Sterile.	Antiseptics should be used.	Gloves are usually worn for a short time and thus antiseptic handwashing is not usually necessary to suppress resident flora for these superficial procedures.
Other procedures (major and minor surgery) that enter tissue below skin.	Hysterectomy, cholecystectomy, herniorrhaphy.	Antiseptic.	Sterile.	Antiseptics should be used after the site has been scrubbed with a detergent. The patient can be shaved immediately before the procedure, although clipping hair or using a depilatory is preferred.	Handwashing before surgical procedures that enter deep tissue is usually prolonged to ensure that all areas that harbor bacteria are adequately cleaned.

† Gloves protect the patient and operator from potentially infectious microorganisms.

REVIEWING BASIC HANDWASHING

According to the CDC, frequent handwashing is the single most important procedure for reducing the transmission of potentially infectious agents.

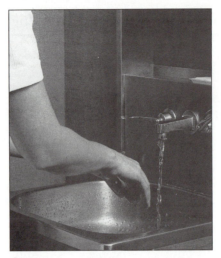

1 Before washing your hands, remove the rings from your fingers to facilitate thorough cleansing and drying. If your watch has an expansion band, slide it above your wrist. Adjust the water to a warm temperature, and rinse your hands.

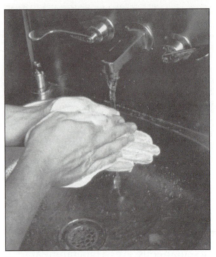

2 Apply cleansing agent and lather your hands thoroughly. The friction from rubbing your hands together removes potentially infectious organisms from the skin. A 10-second vigorous handwashing will remove most transient flora adequately.

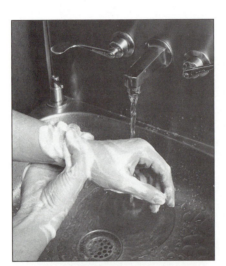

3 Wash each wrist by vigorously sliding the opposite hand around its surface area.

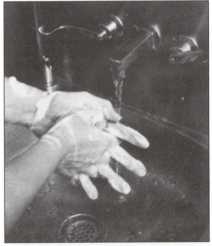

4 Interlace your fingers and thumbs, and slide them back and forth. Clean under your nails and around the nailbeds with the fingertips and nails of the opposite hand.

HOME HEALTH CARE CONSIDERATIONS

- For clients without running water, ensure access to a waterless handwashing product.

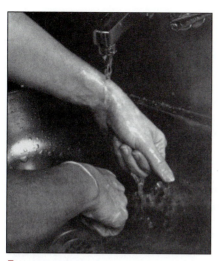

5 Thoroughly rinse each hand from the wrist down. If your hands were grossly soiled, repeat steps 2–5.

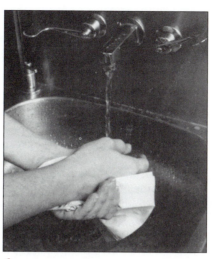

6 Dry your hands with disposable towels.

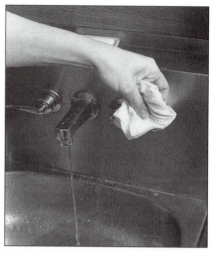

7 To protect your hands from the contaminated surface of the faucet handle, turn off the faucet by placing a dry section of your used towel over the handle.

IMPLEMENTING STANDARD AND TRANSMISSION-BASED PRECAUTIONS

The CDC recommends using *Standard Precautions* in caring for all clients regardless of their diagnosis or presumed infection status. These precautions pertain to (1) blood; (2) all body fluids, secretions, and excretions, except sweat, regardless of whether or not they contain visible blood; (3) nonintact skin; and (4) mucous membranes. Standard Precautions synthesize Universal Precautions and Body Substance Isolation and were designed to reduce the risk of transmitting microorganisms from recognized and unrecognized sources of infection. Standard Precautions include handwashing and use of gloves, masks, eye protectors, and gowns, as appropriate, for client contact in which splashing or soiling is likely to occur.

Transmission-Based Precautions are used in caring for clients documented as or suspected of being infected or colonized with organisms that are transmitted via the airborne route, droplets, and organisms that are epidemiologically important. These precautions replace the category-specific and disease-specific systems of isolation precautions from 1983. Table 1.2 discusses implementation of Standard and Transmission-Based Precautions.

CDC gives hospitals the option of modifying these recommendations according to need and circumstance and as directed by federal, state, or local regulations. The bloodborne pathogens standard (1991) from the Occupational Safety and Health Administration (OSHA) is still operable and incorporated into the Standard Precautions.

Isolation Precautions for Clients with Pulmonary or Laryngeal Tuberculosis (TB)

Because of an increasing incidence of pulmonary TB in the United States, the CDC published guidelines for prevention of the transmission of TB in the health care setting in 1990, and these guidelines were revised in 1994. Airborne precautions is one component of these guidelines, and it was designed for individuals diagnosed with or suspected of having pulmonary or laryngeal TB that can be transmitted via the airborne route. Early identification and treatment is the main focus of these guidelines. In addition, CDC requires rooms with special ventilation and masks (called particulate respirators [PRs]) that provide a tighter fit and better filtration than standard surgical masks.

Table 1.2 Recommendations for Isolation Precautions in Hospitals (CDC, 1996)*

	Standard Precautions	Transmission-Based Precautions: Airborne	Transmission-Based Precautions: Droplet	Transmission-Based Precautions: Contact
When to use	All patients	Use in addition to Standard Precautions for patients known to be or suspected of being infected with microorganisms transmitted by airborne droplet nuclei (≤ 5 microns) of evaporated droplets containing microorganisms that can remain suspended in the air and can be widely dispersed by air currents.	Use in addition to Standard Precautions for patients known to be or suspected of being infected with microorganisms transmitted by droplets (> 5 microns) that can be generated during coughing, sneezing, talking, or performance of procedures.	Use in addition to Standard Precautions for specified patients known to be or suspected of being infected or colonized with epidemiologically important microorganisms that can be transmitted by direct contact with patient, such as occurs during patient care activities, or by indirect contact, such as touching surfaces or equipment in patient's environment.
Handwashing	Wash hands after touching blood, body fluids, secretions, excretions, and contaminated items, regardless of whether gloves are worn; wash hands immediately after gloves are removed, between patient contacts, and to prevent transfer of microorganisms to other patients or environments. Use plain (nonantimicrobial) soap for routine handwashing.			Wash hands with antimicrobial agent or waterless antiseptic agent.
Gloves	Wear nonsterile gloves when touching blood, body fluids, secretions, excretions, and contaminated items; put on clean gloves just before touching mucous membranes and nonintact skin; remove gloves promptly after use, and before touching noncontaminated items, environmental surfaces, and going to another patient; wash hands immediately to avoid transfer of microorganisms to other patients or environment.			In addition to glove use as described in Standard Precautions, wear gloves when entering the room. During patient care, change gloves after contact with infective material (e.g., fecal or wound drainage). After glove removal and handwashing, do not touch items in room.

* Table based on CDC Guideline for isolation precautions in hospitals: Infect Control *Hosp Epidemiol* 17:53–80, 1996.

Source: Mosby/Year Book. From Jackson, MM: Infection prevention and control. Swearingen, PL and Keen, JH (editors): *Manual of Critical Care Nursing*, ed 3, St. Louis: Mosby–Year Book, 1995.

Table 1.2   Recommendations for Isolation Precautions in Hospitals *(continued)*

	Standard Precautions	**Transmission-Based Precautions: Airborne**	**Transmission-Based Precautions: Droplet**	**Transmission-Based Precautions: Contact**
Mask, eye protection, face shield	Wear mask and eye protection or face shield to protect mucous membranes of eyes, nose, and mouth during procedures and patient care activities likely to generate splashes or sprays.	Wear respiratory protection when entering room of patient known to have or suspected of having tuberculosis (a type of particulate respirator is recommended). Do not enter room of patient known to have or suspected of having measles (rubeola) or varicella (chickenpox) if susceptible to these infections.	Wear a mask when working within 3 ft of patient.	
Gown	Wear clean, nonsterile gown to protect skin and prevent soiling of clothing during procedures and patient care activities likely to generate splashes or sprays of blood, body fluids, secretions, or excretions, or to cause soiling of clothing; remove gown promptly when tasks are completed; wash hands.			Wear clean, nonsterile gown when entering room if substantial contact is anticipated with patient, surfaces, or items in environment; wear gown when entering room if patient is incontinent, has diarrhea, an ileostomy, colostomy, or uncontained wound drainage; remove gown carefully when tasks are completed; wash hands.
Patient care equipment	Handle used patient care equipment in manner that prevents skin and mucous membrane exposures, contamination of clothing, and environmental soiling.			When possible, dedicate use of noncritical patient care equipment to a single patient to avoid sharing between patients; if common equipment or items must be shared, adequately clean and disinfect them between uses.
Linen	Handle, transport, and process used linen in manner that prevents skin and mucous membrane exposure, contamination of clothing, and environmental soiling.			

Table 1.2   Recommendations for Isolation Precautions *(continued)*

	Standard Precautions	Transmission-Based Precautions: Airborne	Transmission-Based Precautions: Droplet	Transmission-Based Precautions: Contact
Patient placement	Place patient who contaminates environment or who does not (or cannot) assist in maintaining appropriate hygiene or environmental control in private room, if possible; consult infection control professionals for other alternatives.	Place patient in private room that has (1) monitored negative air pressure in relation to surrounding areas, (2) six to twelve air exchanges per hour, and (3) appropriate discharge of air outdoors or monitored high-efficiency filtration of room air before air is circulated to other areas of the hospital; keep room door closed when patient is in room. When a private room is not available, patient may be placed in room with another patient who has an active infection with the same microorganism; consult infection control professionals for alternatives.	Place patient in private room; when a private room is not available, cohort infected patients or maintain spatial separation of at least 3 ft between infected patient and other patients and visitors; consult infection control professionals for other alternatives.	Place patient in private room; when a private room is not available, cohort infected patients; consult infection control professionals for selection of suitable roommates or other alternatives.
Patient transport		Limit movement and transport of patient from room to essential purposes only; if transport or movement is necessary, minimize patient dispersal of droplet nuclei by placing surgical mask on patient, if possible.	Limit movement and transport of patient from room to essential purposes only; if transport or movement is necessary, minimize patient dispersal of droplets by masking patient, if possible.	Limit movement and transport of patient from room to essential purposes only; if transport is necessary, ensure that precautions are maintained to minimize contamination of environmental surfaces or equipment.
Environmental control	Ensure that hospital has adequate procedures for routine care, cleaning, and disinfection of environment and items therein.			Ensure that patient care items, bedside equipment, and frequently touched surfaces receive daily cleaning.

Table 1.2   Recommendations for Isolation Precautions *(continued)*

	Standard Precautions	Transmission-Based Precautions: Airborne	Transmission-Based Precautions: Droplet	Transmission-Based Precautions: Contact
Occupational Safety and Health Administration (OSHA) blood-borne pathogens standard (1991)	Take care to prevent injuries when using needles, scalpels, and other sharp instruments or devices; when handling sharp instruments after procedures; when cleaning used instruments; and when disposing of used needles. Never recap used needles or otherwise manipulate them using both hands, or use any other technique that involves directing the point of a needle toward any part of the body. Use either one-handed "scoop" technique or mechanical device designed for holding needle sheath if recapping is required by procedure. Do not remove used needles from disposable syringes by hand; do not bend, break, or manipulate used needles by hand. Place used sharps in appropriate puncture-resistant containers located as close as practical to location of use. Use mouthpieces, resuscitation bags, or other ventilation devices as an alternative to mouth-to-mouth resuscitation methods in areas where need is predictable.			

Cohorting: Term used when patients share a room if infected by the same microorganism, provided they are not infected with other potentially transmisable microorganisms and the likelihood of reinfection with the same organism is minimal.

USING PROTECTIVE BARRIERS

Protective barriers include the following: fluid-resistive gowns (or plastic aprons), masks with eye shields (or mask and goggles or mask and glasses with side shields), gloves, and appropriate roommate and caregiver selection. Roommate and caregiver selection involves avoiding roomsharing when one individual extensively soils articles with body substances, thereby placing the roommate at risk of contacting the soiled articles. Another example is avoiding roomsharing or client care for individuals whose infections are spread by the airborne route (eg, chickenpox [herpes zoster]) by individuals who are not immune to these diseases; for example, a client with chickenpox or shingles should not be cared for by someone who has not had chickenpox.*

---

*Chickenpox is the clinical presentation for primary infection with the herpes zoster (varicella) virus. Once an individual has had chickenpox, the virus remains latent in the dorsal root ganglia of the spinal cord. Sometimes the virus becomes active, travels down the ganglion, and produces eruptions that are called shingles. In some clients, the virus disseminates and causes a clinical syndrome similar to primary chickenpox. Transmission of the virus from isolated shingles lesions is by contact; disseminated herpes zoster is also believed to be transmitted by the airborne route. Health care workers who have not had chickenpox can be infected with the herpes zoster virus from clients with either chickenpox or shingles.

APPLYING A FLUID-RESISTIVE GOWN

Gowns or plastic aprons are worn to prevent soilage of clothing when caring for clients. You should wear them when caring for any client if clothing is likely to be soiled with secretions or excretions, for example, when changing the bed of an incontinent client.

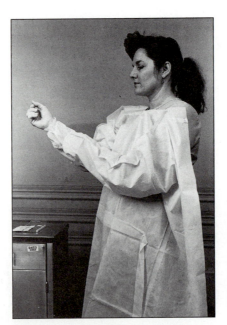

1 To put on a gown, slip your arms into the sleeves and then secure the back of the neck.

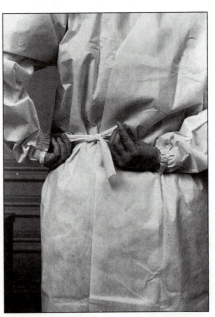

2 Overlap the gown in the back so that it covers the back of your clothing, and tie the strings at the waistline.

APPLYING A FLUID-RESISTIVE MASK

Masks with eye protectors are needed when it is likely that the caregiver's oral and nasal mucous membranes will become splattered with the client's moist body substances or when the caregiver is working directly over large open skin lesions, such as an open wound or burn injury. ***Note:*** *Traditionally, masks have been worn while caring for clients with airborne communicable diseases, but there is no evidence that masks protect caregivers who are susceptible to chickenpox or measles and minimal or no evidence that they protect the individual from tuberculosis. CDC recommends special respiratory protection against exposure to tuberculosis organisms (see page 7).*

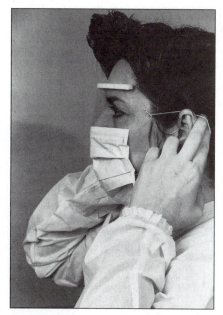

1 To apply the mask, position the elastic straps securely around your ears. If you wear glasses in lieu of eye shields or goggles, be sure the sides of the glasses are protected with shields (see page 21).

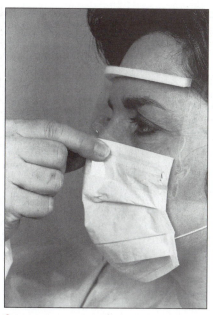

2 To minimize the gap between the mask and your nose, pinch the nose clip, as shown.

APPLYING GLOVES

Gloves are worn for three reasons. First, they protect the wearer from contact with the client's microorganisms. Second, they minimize the potential for the wearer to transmit his or her own resident microbial flora to the client; and third, they minimize the risk of cross-contamination from one client to another. Wear gloves when touching blood, secretions, excretions, or body fluids.

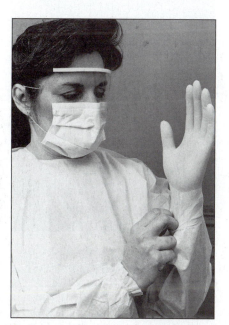

1 Put on the gloves, making sure they cover the wrist cuffs of the gown if the gown is also worn.

REMOVING PROTECTIVE BARRIERS

When you have completed the care for your client, remove your contaminated attire before leaving the room.

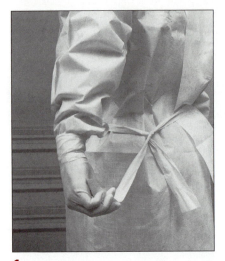

1 If you are wearing a gown, untie its waist strings.

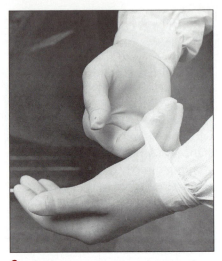

2 Remove your gloves: With your dominant hand, make a cuff by hooking gloved fingers into the lower outside edge of the other glove. Pull the glove inside out as you remove it and either discard it or hold the glove in your gloved hand.

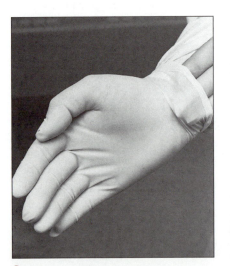

3 Tuck your ungloved fingers into the inside edge of the remaining glove. Remove that glove by pulling it inside out and encase the other glove as you do if you haven't already discarded it. Discard the gloves into the designated waste container. If you are wearing a gown, untie the neck strings next or detach the adhesive tab.

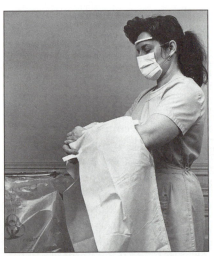

4 After untying the neck strings, remove the gown by turning it inside out during the process.

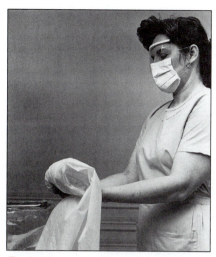

5 Hold the gown away from your body, and roll it up so that the contaminated side is innermost.

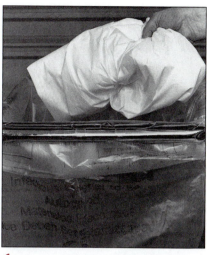

6 Place the gown in a laundry container or the appropriate waste container if the gown is disposable.

MANAGING INTRAVASCULAR DEVICES TO REDUCE INFECTION RISK

In addition to using barriers as described in the previous section, other procedures and devices can be used to reduce the risk of nosocomial infection. Rotating the access site for intravascular (IV) therapy at designated intervals and using the newer catheter materials that are less traumatic to the tissues are examples of a procedure and device that are known to reduce infection risk for clients. In addition, using the needleless IV devices that access line ports once an IV catheter already has entered the vascular system has been shown to reduce the risk of infection to both the client and health care worker, whose risk of puncture injury is reduced when working with these devices. Needleless or needle-free IV access devices are discussed and illustrated in Chapter 3.

7 Finally, remove the mask by grasping it by the elastic straps and pulling it off. Dispose of it in the waste container, and wash your hands before leaving the room.

Preparing for a Sterile Procedure

APPLYING STERILE GLOVES

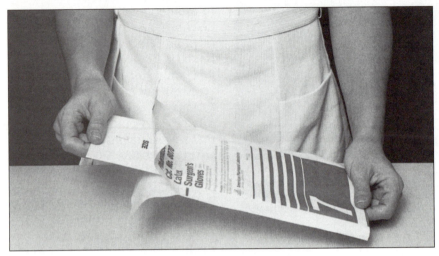

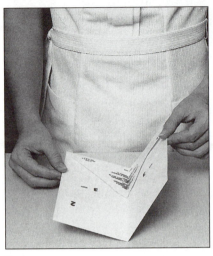

1 After washing your hands, open the outer wrap of the sterile glove pack and remove the inner wrap.

Place the inner wrap on a clean, dry surface.

2 Carefully unfold the inner wrap, touching only the outside edges.

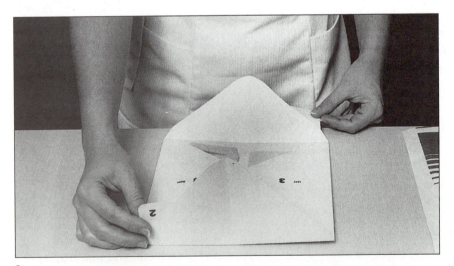

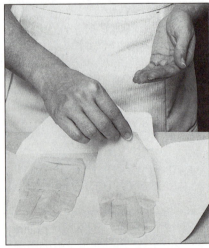

3 If the inner wrap has numbered flaps (as shown), open them numerically. Be sure to touch only the folded tabs. If the wrap is unnumbered, open the gloves by following the steps for opening a sterile pack on page 18.

4 With your dominant hand, grasp the opposite glove at the inner edge of the folded cuff.

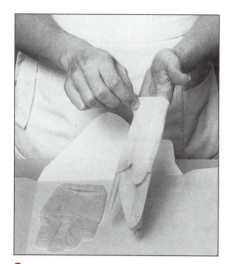

5 Carefully slip your hand into the glove.

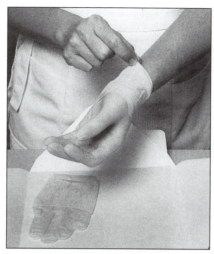

6 While still grasping the inner edge of the folded cuff, pull the glove over your hand.

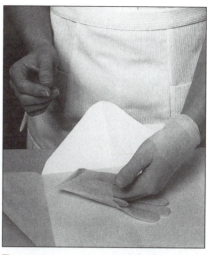

7 With your sterile gloved hand, slip your fingers into the folded cuff of the remaining glove.

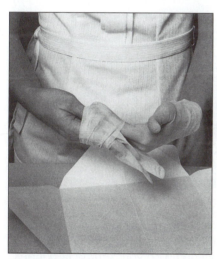

8 Carefully slip the glove over your fingers. Keep the sterile thumb out of the way when pulling on the second glove.

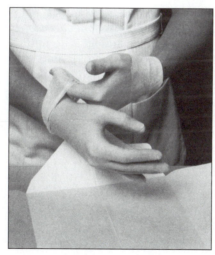

9 Pull the glove over your hand.

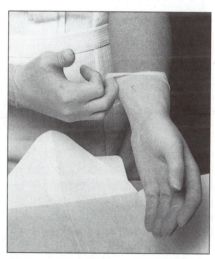

10 Adjust each glove to ensure a snug fit over your hands and fingers. Carefully slide your fingers under each cuff and pull it up.

ESTABLISHING A STERILE FIELD

OPENING A STERILE PACK

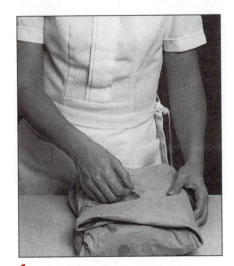

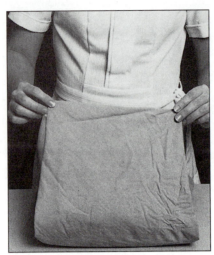

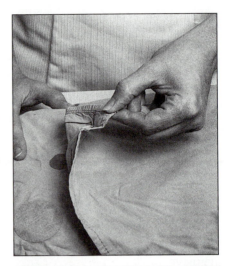

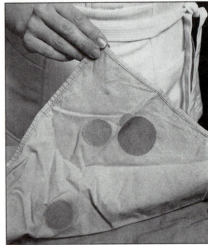

1 Wash your hands with an antimicrobial soap before opening the sterile pack. A sterile pack must be opened on a clean, dry surface. The outer wrap of commercially wrapped sterile packs should be inspected both for tears and for the sterility expiration date. Follow agency policy for returning outdated supplies. If the pack is agency-wrapped (as shown), ensure its sterility by inspecting the chemical indicator tape both for the integrity of its seal with the pack and for a change of color, indicating it has been properly sterilized. Also check the sterility expiration date, which is written on the tape. Remove the indicator tape by pulling it from the center toward the outer edge of the pack.

2 Position the pack so that its outermost flap faces away from you and will not hang over the edge of the table when it is opened. With your thumbs and index fingers, grasp the flap by small sections of its folded crease and lift it up and away from you. Hold your arms at the sides of the pack to avoid reaching over the sterile area.

3 Open the side flaps (top). Grasp the folded corner of the uppermost flap by touching a small section with your thumb and index finger; lay the flap to the side. Do the same with the opposite flap. Lift the remaining flap toward you (bottom), stepping back 12.5–25 cm (5–10 in) as you do, so that you do not contaminate the wrap with your clothing. If the pack has an inner wrap, repeat the above procedure to open it.

DROPPING STERILE SUPPLIES ONTO A STERILE FIELD

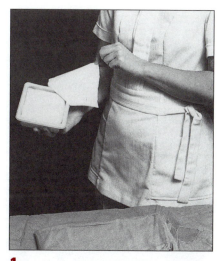

1 If your commercially wrapped sterile package is a peelback container (as shown), grasp the flap by its unsealed corner and pull the flap toward you. Position the pack so that its open end will face the sterile field.

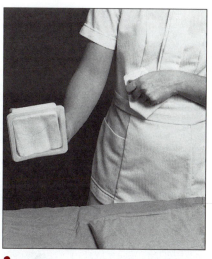

2 To prevent the container from contaminating the field, hold the opened pack approximately 15 cm (6 in) above the sterile field, and allow the contents to drop well within the sterile area. Remember that the 2.5 cm (1 in) border along the edge of the field is considered to be contaminated.

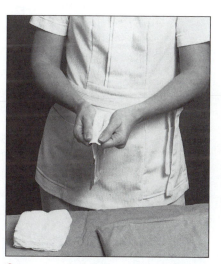

3 To open other types of commercially wrapped peelback containers such as glove packs or syringes (as shown), grasp both sides of the pack's unsealed edge and gently pull them apart.

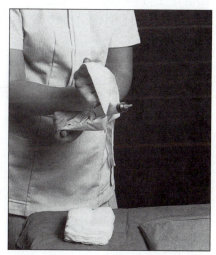

4 Hold the package so that its opened end is positioned away from your body and facing the sterile field. Carefully fold the sides back so that the outside wrap covers your hands and protects the contents. With the contents protected in this manner, drop them onto the sterile field.

PLACING A STERILE BOWL ONTO THE STERILE FIELD

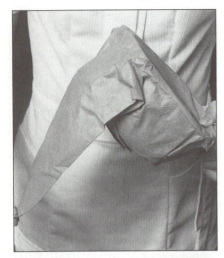

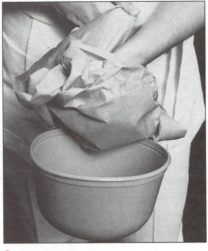

2 In the same manner, bring all the ends up to the rim; hold them in place with your thumb and index finger, confining the ends to a small area at the rim.

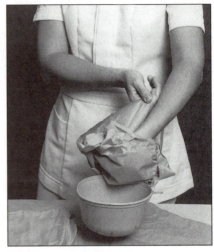

3 Place the bowl onto the sterile field. If it will be used to contain sterile solutions, place it near the edge of the field. This will enable you to pour the solution without reaching over a large section of the sterile area.

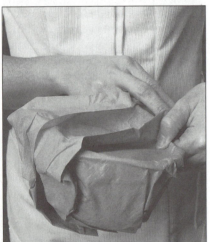

1 Hold a wrapped bowl at the rim with your thumb and index finger. Detach one of the corners (top) and bring it up and over the rim (bottom). Then hold the detached corner in place with your thumb and index finger.

POURING STERILE SOLUTIONS

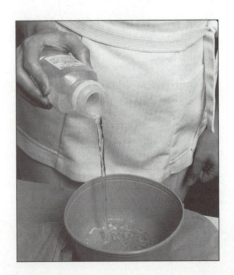

Because the sterility of a solution cannot be ensured once its container has been opened, try to obtain a container with an amount of solution appropriate to the procedure. As you pour the solution, hold the container to the side of, and at an angle to, the sterile field so that your hand and arm do not reach over the sterile area. To minimize the risk of contamination, hold the container approximately 10–15 cm (4–6 in) above the bowl; pour slowly to avoid splashing the sterile drape and contaminating the sterile field.

PUTTING ON STERILE ATTIRE (INCLUDING THE CLOSED-GLOVE TECHNIQUE)

1 When you are required to wear sterile attire for procedures in which surgical asepsis is necessary, you must first wash your hands, put on a hair cover and face mask, and then open the sterile pack containing the sterile gown. (See steps on p 18.) If splashing is anticipated during the procedure, you will also need to put on goggles or glasses with side shields (as shown).

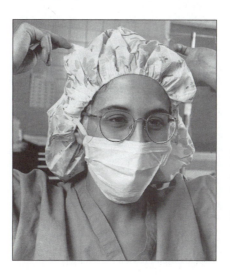

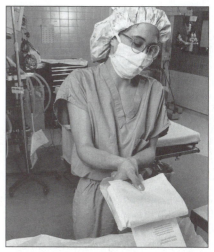

2 Remove the sterile gloves from their outer wrap and drop the inner wrap onto the sterile pack (as shown). Wash your hands with an antimicrobial soap and dry them thoroughly with the towel provided in the gown pack.

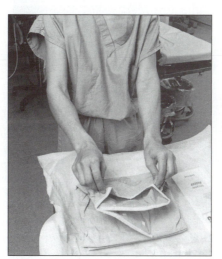

3 Grasp the sterile gown by its uppermost folded crease near the neckline.

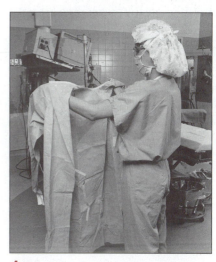

4 Step into an area in which you will have space to open the gown without contaminating it, and hold it away from you to allow the gown to unfold. Place your hands inside the gown and work your arms through the shoulders, being certain to touch the inside of the gown only.

➤

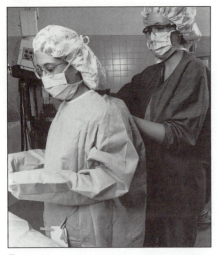

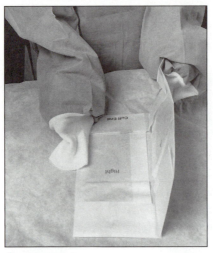

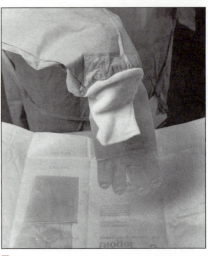

5 If you perform the closed-glove technique, advance your hands only as far as the proximal edge of the cuff (as shown). However, if you apply sterile gloves using the usual aseptic (open-glove) technique, extend your hands through the cuff, but do not touch the outside of the gown. Regardless of the gloving technique you use, a coworker will be needed for assistance. The coworker should first put on a mask and hair cover and then grasp the neckline area at the back of your gown and pull the gown up to cover the neckline of the front of your uniform. She will then secure the gown at the neck and tie the ties inside the back of the gown without touching the exterior of your gown.

6 Unfold the inner wrap of the sterile gloves. If you are using the closed-glove technique, do this with your covered hands (as shown). Otherwise, follow the guidelines for applying sterile gloves using the technique described on pp 16–17 and proceed to step 14.

7 Grasp the first glove by manipulating your thumb and index finger through the fabric of the sleeve or cuff.

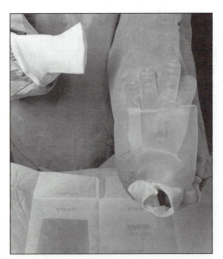

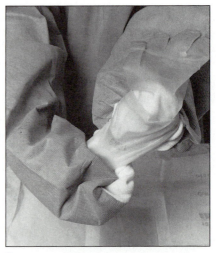

8 Place the glove palm down onto the cuff of your sterile gown. The fingers of the glove should point toward your elbow, and the thumb of the glove should be directly over the thumb of your hand.

9 Manipulate your fingers within the cuff to anchor the glove. With your other covered hand, stretch the glove over the entire cuff.

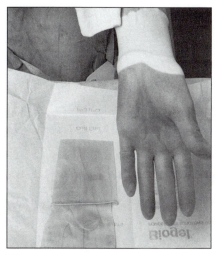

10 When the glove has been pulled successfully over the cuff, extend your fingers into the glove.

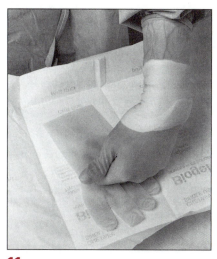

11 Place your gloved fingers within the folded cuff of the remaining glove.

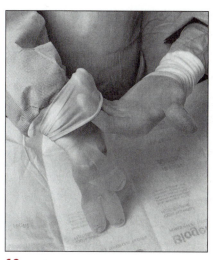

12 Position the glove over the closed cuff.

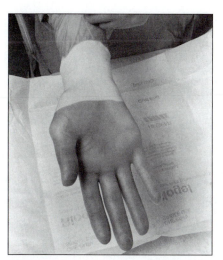

13 Pull the glove up over the gown's cuff as you extend your fingers through the glove. Adjust the glove to fit your fingers. Make sure both gloves cover the cuffs of the gown.

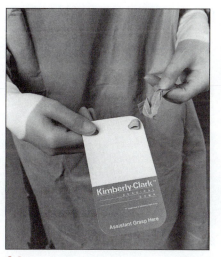

14 Pull the front tie away from the card to which it is attached.

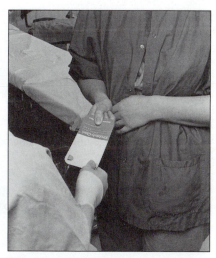

15 Hand the card to a coworker and instruct her to touch only the card and not your gloved hand.

➤

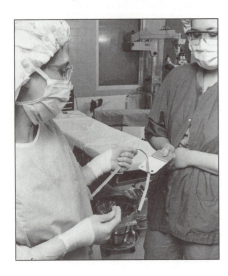

16 Make a three-quarter turn; then pull the tie from the card and tie the gown at the front. *Note: If you prefer, your coworker may instead put on a sterile glove and grasp the tie with her gloved hand while you make a three-quarter turn.*

←

Note: For nondisposable sterile gowns you may instead place the back tie of the gown's waistband into the crease of the glove wrapper card (as shown). Close the wrapper. Proceed as shown in steps 15 and 16.

→

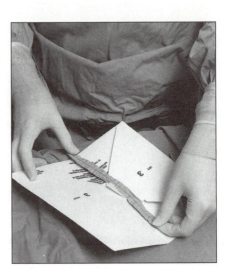

Performing Other Procedures

OBTAINING A THROAT CULTURE

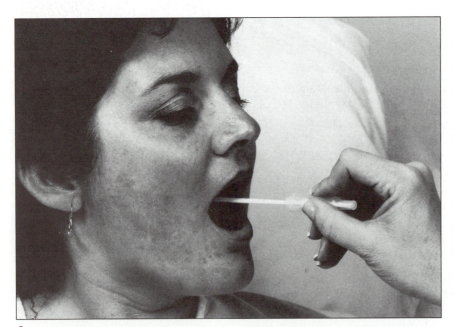

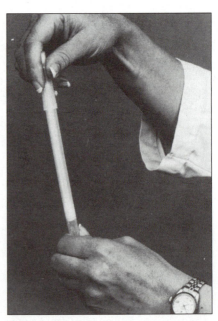

1 If a throat culture has been prescribed, obtain the culture tube and applicator stick. Wash your hands and remove the applicator stick from the culture tube. With the client in Fowler's position, place her so that natural light or a treatment light provides adequate visualization. Ask the client to open her mouth. Swab the back of her throat along the tonsillar area, using a tongue blade, if necessary, to depress her tongue.

2 After obtaining the specimen, replace the applicator stick in the culture tube, pushing the stick firmly until it punctures the compartment containing the culture medium. Label the culture tube and send it to the laboratory. Wash your hands.

PERFORMING WOUND CARE

PACKING A WOUND (USING WET TO DAMP DRESSINGS)

Assessing and Planning

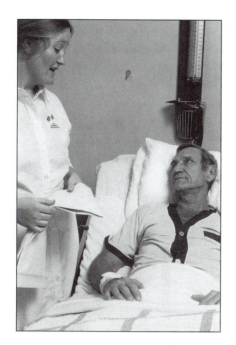

1 Check the client's chart and care plan or nursing Kardex for wound care information.

Explain the dressing change procedure to your client. Assess the client's level of comfort; if a pain medication has been prescribed, ask him whether he will need one for the procedure. If you do administer the medication, delay the procedure for 20 minutes until the medication takes effect. Position the bed at an optimal working height, provide privacy for the client, and place a bed-saver pad under the area of the wound to protect the bed linen. Inspect the dressing site and determine the approximate number of gauze pads you will need for the packing and outer dressing, as well as the need for either tape, fresh Montgomery straps, gauze roll, or surgical netting. Be sure to employ Standard Precautions throughout the procedure (see pages 7-11).

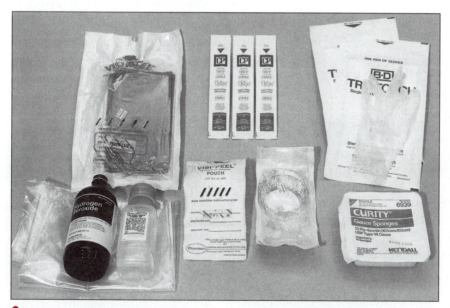

2 Assemble the following materials:

☐ sterile barrier

☐ prescribed cleansing/debriding and wetting solutions (hydrogen peroxide and normal saline are being used for this procedure)

☐ sterile basins

☐ sterile cotton swabs

☐ one pair of clean gloves

☐ two pairs of sterile gloves

☐ sterile gauze pads*

☐ impervious plastic bag for disposal of used supplies

☐ supplies for adhering the dressing if Montgomery straps are not used, eg, paper or plastic tape, gauze roll or surgical netting if the wound is on an extremity

---

* It is important that the gauze pads be unfilled and made of a fine mesh. A filled gauze pad has cotton fiber filling that can get left behind in the wound, and fine mesh is necessary for optimal wound debridement because larger mesh gauze may remove the healing granulation tissue.

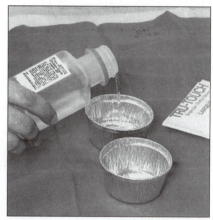

3 Place the impervious plastic bag in a convenient place that is away from the dressing change site. Adjust the client's gown or remove it, and provide warmth and privacy. Wash your hands and prepare the sterile field at this time, following the steps on pages 18–20. Carefully pour the prescribed solutions into the sterile basins (see page 20). For this procedure, the nurse will use one basin for the cleansing and debriding solution (equal parts of normal saline and hydrogen peroxide) and the other basin for the wetting solution (normal saline).

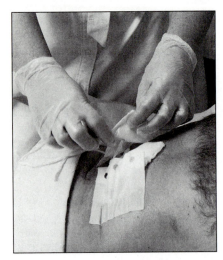

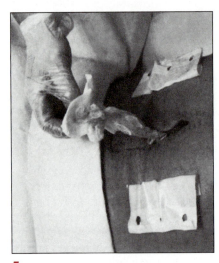

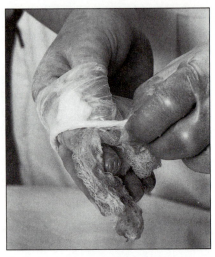

4 Put on the clean gloves and untie the Montgomery straps, move the netting away from the area of the wound, or remove the tape and outer cover dressing.

5 Grasp the gauze packing by securing it with the outer dressing that covers it. Pull gently to remove all the packing.

Caution: Use a sterile glove when removing the packing from a deeper wound.

6 Inspect the contaminated dressing to assess the amount and color of debris and drainage; note if it has an odor, which may be indicative of an infection. Encase the dressing in your gloves as you remove them, and dispose of both in the impervious plastic bag.

Implementing

7 Put on a pair of sterile gloves and soak a gauze pad in the cleansing solution. At this time, designate one hand contaminated for cleaning and rinsing and the other sterile for contact with the sterile field. Before cleaning the site, inspect the wound and assess for swelling, size color, odor, and drainage. Estimate the amount of healing granulation tissue. Saturate the wound from top to bottom with the cleansing solution, and dispose of the contaminated pad.

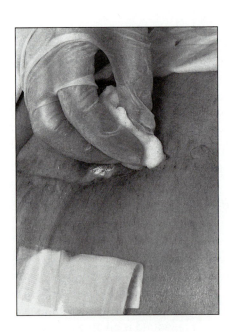

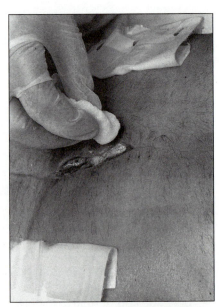

8 Soak another gauze pad in the cleansing solution and clean the area around the wound, beginning at the wound edge and working away from it in a circular motion.

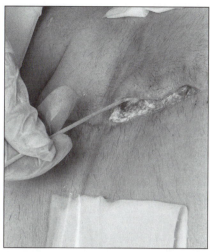

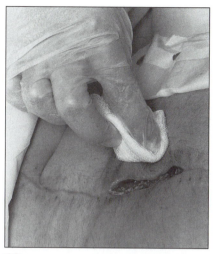

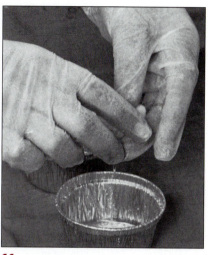

9 Moisten a cotton swab in the cleansing solution and clean the crevices of the wound. You may also use a fresh cotton swab to assess the depth of the crevice. This information will be important later when you pack the wound. Then, rinse the wound and surrounding area with the normal saline or designated wetting solution, following steps 7 and 8.

10 Use a dry gauze pad to blot the skin surrounding the wound. Remove your gloves and dispose of them along with the contaminated gauze and cotton swabs.

11 Apply a fresh pair of sterile gloves and prepare to pack the wound by moistening a gauze pad in the wetting solution. Be certain to wring out the excess moisture because packing that is too wet will not debride the wound effectively. In addition, saturated packing could moisten the outer dressing and draw potentially infectious organisms into the wound.

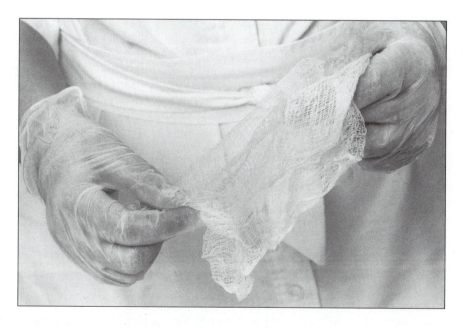

12 Unfold the moistened gauze pad to expand its surface area into a single layer.

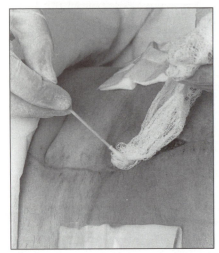

13 Hold the gauze in your non-dominant hand to prevent it from touching your client's skin and, thus, potentially introducing contaminants into the wound. Use a sterile cotton swab to pack the gauze into the crevices of the wound.

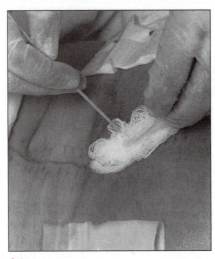

14 Completely fill the wound, adding more gauze as necessary. Pack loosely and do not overpack.

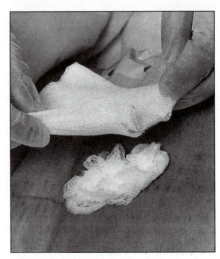

15 Cover the wet gauze with a dry dressing.

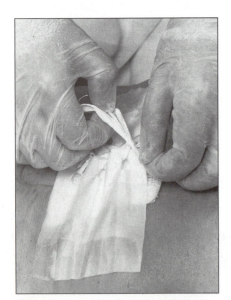

16 Tape the dressing in place. If the wound is on an extremity, wrap the dressing with a strip of gauze roll to secure it. If Montgomery straps are used, change them if they are soiled, and then tie them securely (as shown). If surgical netting is used, roll it back into place. Replace it if it is soiled. Then remove your gloves and place them in the bag with the dressing waste.

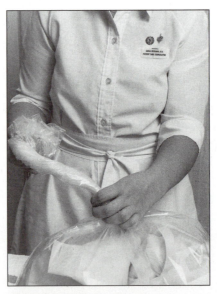

Evaluating

17 Return the client to a position of comfort and assist him with his gown if he is unable to do it himself. Securely tie off the impervious plastic bag, remove it from the bedside, and dispose of it according to agency policy. Then, wash your hands. Finally, record the procedure in your nurse's notes. Document the appearance, size, and odor (if present) of the wound and describe the amount and quality of the drainage. Note the amount and appearance of the granulation tissue as well.

HOME HEALTH CARE CONSIDERATIONS

- Teach client to use sterile or clean gloves, depending on agency protocol.
- Wrap contaminated trash securely and follow agency, municipal, or county protocol for disposal.
- Launder contaminated linens and clothing separately and in hot soapy water.

IRRIGATING A WOUND

Assessing and Planning

1 Assemble the following supplies:

☐ clean gloves

☐ sterile gloves

☐ sterile irrigation kit or sterile basin with sterile 60 mL irrigating syringe

☐ prescribed irrigation solution (be sure to let it warm to room temperature if it has been refrigerated)

☐ appropriate dressing materials including tape

☐ bed-saver pad

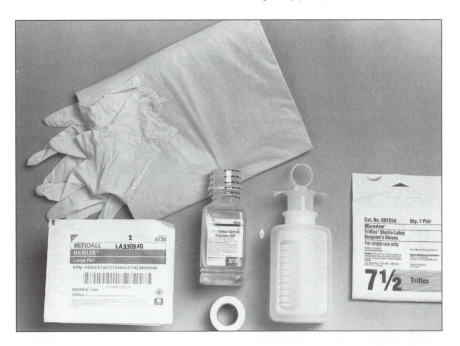

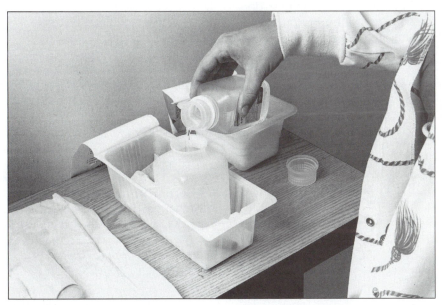

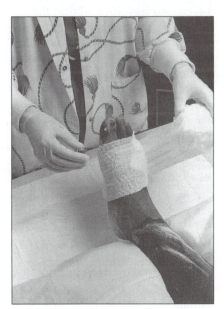

2 Establish a sterile field with the glove pack, placing the basin and syringe on the field (see page 19 for placing an object on the sterile field). Using aseptic technique, pour the irrigant (here we are using saline) into the irrigation container.

3 Put on clean gloves. Place a bed-saver pad under the area that is to be irrigated. Remove the soiled dressing and discard according to agency policy (see procedure on page 26). Inspect the dressing and wound, noting color, odor, and any other characteristics of the wound and drainage.

Implementing

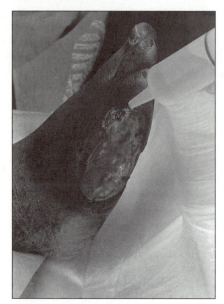 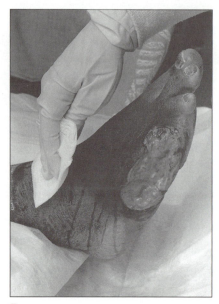 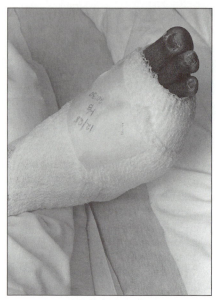

4 Position the client so that the wound to be irrigated is dependent and the solution will flow away from the wound, thereby carrying contaminated tissue and exudate away from clean tissue. Put on sterile gloves. Fill the syringe with the irrigating solution. Without touching the tip of the syringe to the wound, flush the wound using gentle force on the piston of the syringe. Refill the syringe and continue the procedure until the wound is clean.

Note: If the wound is deep, consider inserting a soft-tipped rubber catheter into the wound and connecting the syringe to the catheter to facilitate irrigation.

5 Using no-touch technique, dry the skin around the wound to prevent breakdown.

6 Dress the wound as prescribed, using sterile technique. Remove and discard gloves. Discard used supplies according to agency policy for infection control. Position the patient for comfort. Label a piece of tape with the date and time of dressing change, and adhere it to the dressing.

Evaluating

7 Document characteristics and any changes in the wound and the client's tolerance to the procedure.

Note: Also see "Home Health Care Considerations," page 28.

REFERENCES

Bennett JV, Brachman PS, eds: *Hospital Infections,* ed 4. Boston: Little, Brown, 1996.

Centers for Disease Control and Prevention: Guidelines for preventing the transmission of *Mycobacterium tuberculosis* in health care facilities. *MMWR* 1994;43(*No. Rr-13):1–133.

Centers for Disease Control and Prevention: Guideline for isolation precautions in hospitals: *Infect Control Hosp. Epidemiol* 17:53–80, 1996.

Centers for Disease Control and Prevention: Guidelines for preventing the transmission of tuberculosis in health-care settings, with special focus on HIV-related issues. *MMWR* 39(RR 1–17), 1990.

Centers for Disease Control and Prevention: Update: Universal precautions for prevention of transmission of human immunodeficiency virus and other bloodborne pathogens in healthcare settings. *MMWR* 37:377–388, 1988.

Centers for Disease Control and Prevention: Recommendations for prevention of HIV transmission in health care settings. *MMWR* 36(suppl 2):1–18, 1987.

Centers for Disease Control and Prevention: Guideline for isolation precautions in hospitals. *Infection Control* 4:245–325, 1983.

Department of Labor, Occupational Safety and Health Administration: Occupational exposure to bloodborne pathogens, final rule, 29 CFR part 1910:1030. Federal Register 56:64003–64182, December 6, 1991.

Jackson MM: Infection prevention and control. *Crit Care Nurs Clin North Am* 4(3):401–409, 1992.

Jackson MM: Infection prevention and control. In Swearingen PL and Keen JH (eds): *Manual of Critical Care Nursing,* ed 3. St. Louis: Mosby–Year Book, 1995.

Jackson MM, Lynch P: Development of a numeric Health Care Worker Risk Assessment Scale to evaluate potential for bloodborne pathogen exposure. *Am J Infect Control* 23:13–21, 1995.

Jackson MM, Lynch P: An attempt to make an issue less murky: A comparison of four systems for infection precautions. *Infect Control Hosp Epidemiol* 12:448–450, 1991.

Jackson MM, Lynch P: In search of a rational approach. *Am J Nurs* 90(10):65–73, 1990.

Jackson MM, Lynch P: Infection control: Too much or too little? *Am J Nurs* 84:208–210, 1984.

Jackson MM, et al: Why not treat all body substances as infectious? *Am J Nurs* 87:1137–1139, 1987.

Lynch P, et al: Rethinking the role of isolation practices in the prevention of nosocomial infections. *Ann Intern Med* 107:243–246, 1987.

Lynch P, et al: Implementing and evaluating a system of generic infection precautions: body substance isolation. *Am J Infect Control* 18:1–12, 1990.

Martone WJ, Garner JS, eds: Proceedings of the Third Decennial International Conference on Nosocomial Infections. *Am J Med* 91(3B):1–333, 1991.

Mayhall CG (ed): *Hospital Epidemiology and Infection Control,* Baltimore, Williams & Wilkins, 1996.

Pugliese G, Lynch P, Jackson MM, eds: *Universal Precautions: Policies, procedures, and resources.* Chicago: American Hospital Publishing, 1990.

Wenzel RP: *Prevention and Control of Nosocomial Infections,* ed 2. Baltimore: Williams & Wilkins, 1993.

CHAPTER 2

Using Proper Positioning, Mobilization, and Transferring Techniques

CHAPTER OUTLINE

ASSISTING THE CLIENT WITH POSITIONING AND MOBILIZATION

Performing Passive Range of Motion Exercises

Performing Traditional ROM Exercises

Exercising the Neck

Exercising the Shoulders

Exercising the Elbows

Exercising the Wrists and Fingers

Exercising the Hips and Knees

Exercising the Ankles and Toes

Performing Proprioceptive Neuromuscular Facilitation Exercises

Exercising the Neck

Exercising the Upper Extremities

Exercising the Lower Extremities

Nursing Guidelines: Using Pressure-Relief Mattresses and Pads

Nursing Guidelines: Proper Client Positioning

Assisting the Client with Crutches, Canes, and Walkers

Checking for Correct Crutch Height

Guarding the Client

Assisting the Client with Crutches to Sit in a Chair

TRANSFERRING MOBILE AND IMMOBILE CLIENTS

Nursing Guidelines: Lifting and Transferring Clients

Moving the Client Up in Bed

Assisting the Mobile Client

Lifting the Immobile Client

Dangling the Client's Extremities on the Side of the Bed

Assisting the Mobile Client

Moving the Immobile Client

Moving the Client from the Stretcher to the Bed

Teaching the Segmental Transfer Technique

Transferring the Immobile Client

Logrolling the Immobile Client

Assisting the Client from the Wheelchair (or Chair) to the Bed

Using a Mechanical Lifting Device

Assisting the Client with Positioning and Mobilization

PERFORMING PASSIVE RANGE OF MOTION EXERCISES

To prevent disuse syndrome caused by contractures (the shortening of soft tissues/muscles, ligaments, joint capsules, or fasciae) and anky-losis (the abnormal consolidation of a joint), nurses must ensure that range of motion (ROM) exercises are performed every day for all immobilized clients with normal joints. At particular risk are those individuals who are debilitated and those who cannot move independently (eg, clients with peripheral nerve injury). Modification may be necessary if the client has decreased tone (flaccidity), which is seen initially following spinal cord injury or cerebrovascular accident; if ROM is done incorrectly, the potential for subluxation increases. In addition, if the client has increased tone (spasticity), which may develop as the recovery sequence progresses in either of the above disorders, the use of routine exercise positions may actually enhance spasticity. If you lack experience with these disorders, consult with the educational staff, physician, physical therapist, or occupational therapist to assist you in modifying the exercise plan for these clients. ROM is contraindi-cated during the inflammatory phase of rheumatologic diseases and for joints that are dislocated or fractured. However, after assess-ment of the client, the need for initiation of ROM is an indepen-dent nursing judgment, and it should be incorporated into the daily care plan of the immobilized client. You can perform many of the movement patterns concurrent with position changes and bed baths. In addition, you can apply the principles of ROM when getting a client on and off the bedpan or while changing the hospital gown.

Before initiating ROM, familiar-ize yourself with the following terms:

- *Passive Range of Motion:* These exercises are performed by the nurse, therapist, or significant other to help the client maintain full joint movement and to pre-vent contractures. Because the client's muscles are not used to perform the exercise, muscle strength is neither maintained nor augmented.

- *Active Range of Motion:* These exercises are performed by the client, helping to maintain full joint movement. They also assist in the maintenance of muscle strength.

- *Assisted Range of Motion:* The client moves the part through some portion of the range of motion, with the nurse, thera-pist, or significant other assisting in completing the movement. The degree of the client's partici-pation in the exercise will deter-mine the degree to which muscle strength will be maintained.

- *Abduction:* Moving a limb away from the body's midline.

- *Adduction:* Moving a limb toward the body's midline.

- *Extension:* Straightening of a bent part (increasing the angle between two bones at a joint).

- *Flexion:* Bending (decreasing the angle of two bones at a joint).

- *Hyperextension:* Moving a body part beyond the plane of the body.

- *Opposition:* Combination of abduction, rotation, and flexion of the thumb so that the tip of the thumb can touch the fingers.

- *Radial Deviation:* Moving the hand toward the radial (thumb) side of the wrist while the hand and forearm stay in the same plane.

- *Ulnar Deviation:* Moving the hand toward the ulnar (fifth-finger) side of the wrist while the hand and forearm stay in the same plane.

- *Rotation:* Turning of a body part on its vertical axis.

Performing Traditional ROM Exercises

The exercises in the following pro-cedures are passive and employed when the client is unable to move the specified body part. Adapt these exercises for situations in which the client has partial body movement and requires assisted ROM. When active ROM is desired, you can teach these exercises to the client. You may also teach these exercises to clients who are capable of exercising their paralyzed sides with the assistance of their stronger sides. Remember to include family members and significant others so that they, too, can help exercise the client.

Before starting the exercises, explain them to the client, and obtain a sheet or bath blanket for warmth and privacy. Remove the pillow to allow full movement of the client's head and shoulders.

Unless it is contraindicated, assist the client into a supine posi-tion. Perform the exercises from head to toe, completing them on one side of the body before moving to the other side of the body. Then assist the client into a prone posi-tion and perform the exercises that are indicated for that position. Never push a movement beyond the point at which the client complains of discomfort or at which you feel resistance to the movement. Always support the areas above and below the joint, or cup the joint in your palm. If possible, consult with a physical therapist or occupational therapist to assist you with modifying the exercise on a joint in which you have elicited pain, tremors, or spasms. To avoid straining your back, elevate the bed to an optimal working level; move the client to the right side of the bed before exercising the right side of the body (and vice versa). Be sure to allow room at the head of the bed for the neck and arm movements. To assist you with proper hand positioning, we have shown the neutral (start) position for the exercises. For convenience, all the exercises have been demonstrated on the right side of the client's body. Be certain that you practice correct body mechanics when performing all exercises. Repeat each exercise at least three to five times.

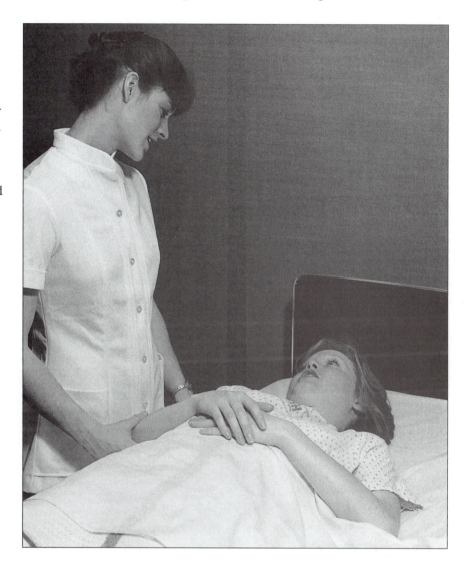

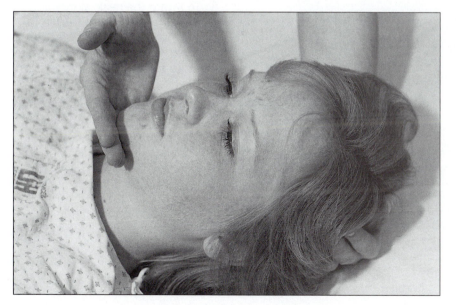

EXERCISING THE NECK

1 To begin the neck exercises, cup the client's chin with your right hand and support the back of the head with your left hand. Be sure to position your right hand high enough on the chin to avoid putting pressure on the trachea during the flexion exercises. ***Caution:*** *Do not force any of the neck movements.*

→

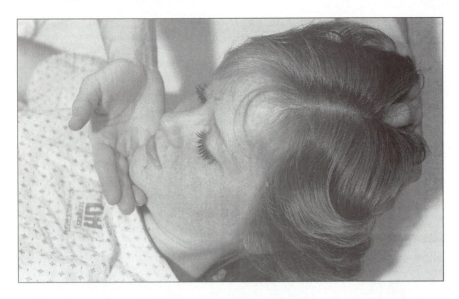

2 To flex the neck, gently tilt the back of the head forward and move the chin toward the chest, touching it if possible.

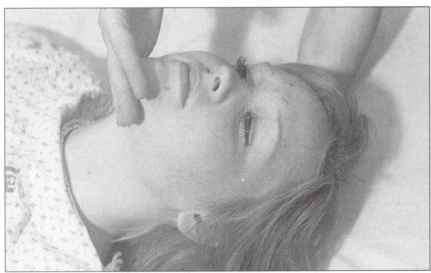

3 Extend the neck by gently tilting the chin upward and moving the head back as far as it will comfortably go without forcing the movement. Return to the neutral position.

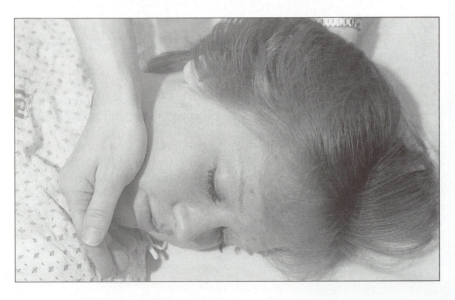

4 To rotate the neck, slowly and gently turn the head to the left (as shown), and touch the left ear to the mattress if possible. Then rotate the neck to the right in the same manner.

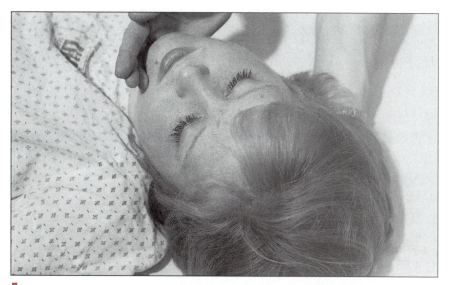 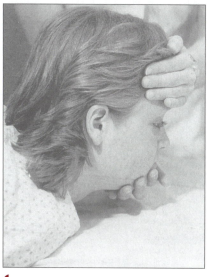

5 To flex the neck laterally, gently guide the ear toward the left shoulder, keeping the client's nose pointing toward the ceiling (as shown); then guide the ear toward the right shoulder.

6 When the client is prone, you may extend the neck by supporting the chin with your right hand and gently pushing back on the forehead with your left hand. Move the back of the head toward the spine as far as it will comfortably go without forcing the movement.

EXERCISING THE SHOULDERS

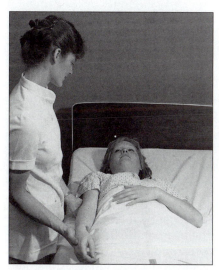 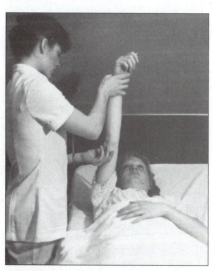 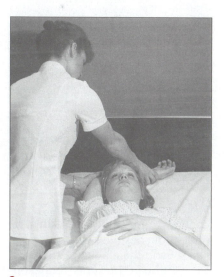

1 To achieve the neutral position for flexing and extending the shoulders, support the elbow with your left hand and the wrist and hand with your right hand. The arm should be in alignment with the body and flat on the bed.

2 As you elevate the arm, maintain the extension of the elbow. Move the arm toward the head of the bed.

3 At the point at which the arm touches the client's ear, allow the elbow to bend so the movement can be completed without hitting the headboard. From this flexed position, return the arm to the neutral position to extend the shoulder and elbow.

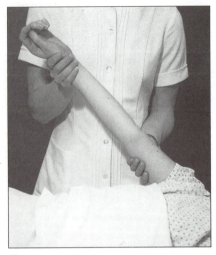

4 When the client is prone, you may extend the shoulder beyond the plane of the body (hyperextension) by supporting the upper arm above the elbow and lifting gently on the forearm. *Caution: Do not force the anterior aspect of the shoulder down into the bed.*

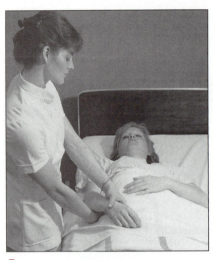

5 To achieve the neutral position for shoulder abduction, support the wrist with your left hand and the elbow with your right hand.

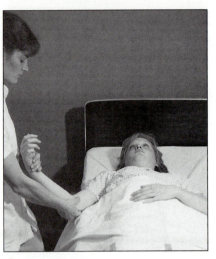

6 As you abduct the arm, step back (as shown) and ensure that the humerus remains level with the bed. Note that the humerus must externally rotate as the nurse abducts the arm.

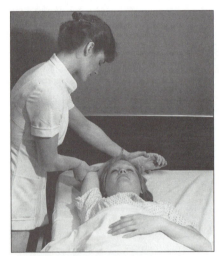

7 To complete the abduction, continue to move the arm laterally until it touches the side of her head. Bend the elbow (as shown) if the headboard prevents abduction with the elbow extended. To adduct the arm, return to the neutral position while maintaining support of the wrist and elbow.

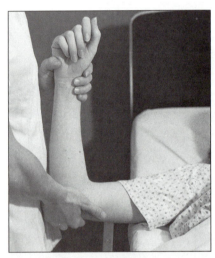

8 To achieve the neutral position for internal and external shoulder rotation, abduct the arm to shoulder level at a 90-degree angle to the body. The humerus should be level with the bed. Flex the elbow to a 90-degree angle to the body. Support the wrist with your left hand and the upper arm with your right hand.

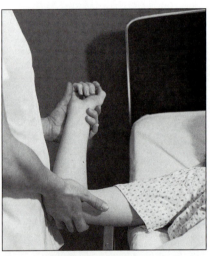

9 To rotate the shoulder externally, gently rotate the arm toward the head of the bed so that the forearm is moving toward the plane of the bed surface. Continue the movement as far as it will comfortably go without raising the client's back from the bed's surface. Return to the neutral position.

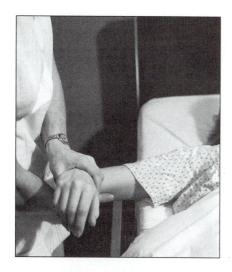

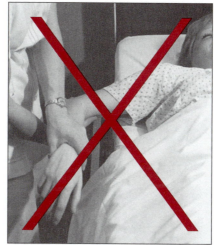

10 Internally rotate the shoulder by moving the forearm toward the foot of the bed as far as it will comfortably go (left). *Note: A common mistake with internal rotation is to force the rotation beyond the range of the shoulder joint (right). Notice how the proximal aspect of the humerus moves off its supporting surface.*

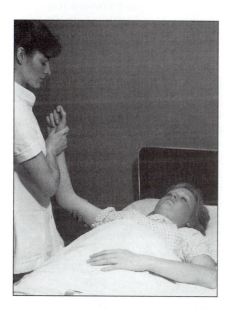

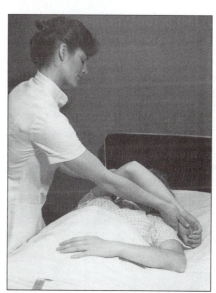

11 To achieve the neutral position for horizontal shoulder adduction, support the upper arm with your left hand and the hand and wrist with your right hand (left). Hold the arm with the elbow flexed at a 45–90-degree angle to the body. Slowly guide the arm across the body toward the left side of the bed (right).

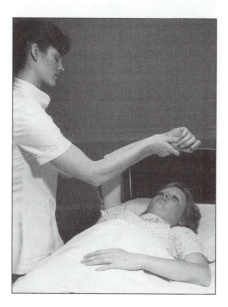

12 To complete the horizontal adduction, move the arm as far across the body as possible. Allow the elbow to extend slightly so that the contact of the hand with the bed does not block the motion of the humerus.

EXERCISING THE ELBOWS

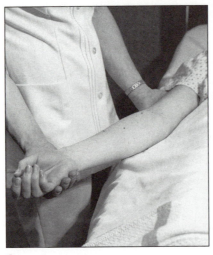

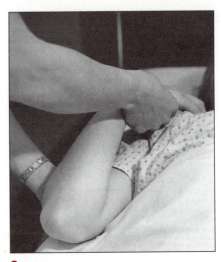

1 To achieve the neutral position for flexing the elbow with the forearm in supination, support the wrist with your right hand and the upper arm with your left hand. The arm should be slightly abducted from the body with the elbow extended and the palm turned up.

2 Guide the palm toward the shoulder. The degree of elbow flexion will be determined by the amount of upper arm musculature. (The greater the musculature, the less the degree of flexion.) Return to the neutral position while maintaining support of the upper arm and wrist.

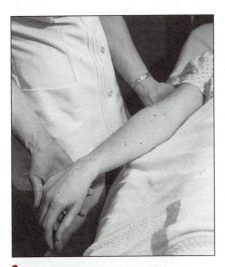

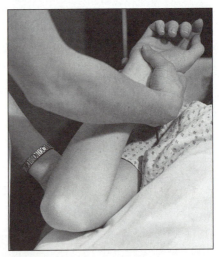

3 To achieve the neutral position for flexing the elbow with the forearm in pronation, support the wrist with your right hand and the upper arm with your left hand. The arm should be slightly abducted from the body with the elbow extended and the palm turned down.

4 Flex the elbow and guide the dorsum of the hand toward the shoulder. Again, the degree of elbow flexion will be determined by the amount of upper arm musculature. Return to the neutral position. Alternating flexion with supination and flexion with pronation allows you to perform the elbow and forearm movements simultaneously.

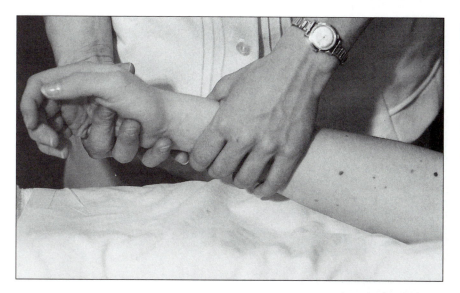

EXERCISING THE WRISTS AND FINGERS

1 To achieve the neutral position for wrist flexion and extension, support the forearm proximal to the wrist with your left hand. Support the hand distal to the wrist with your right hand.

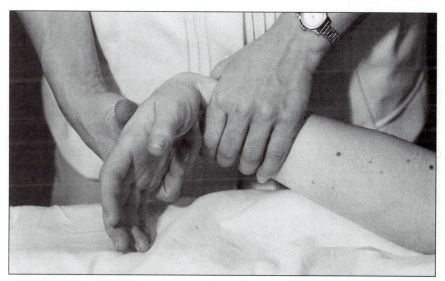

2 To flex the wrist (palmar flexion), gently push down on the dorsum of the hand.

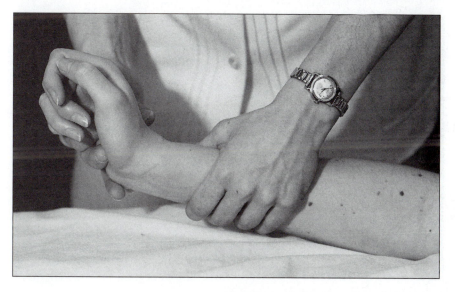

3 Extend the wrist (dorsiflexion) by gently pushing up on the palmar surface of the hand.

➤

4 To achieve the neutral position for radial and ulnar deviation, support the hand with your right hand and the wrist with your left hand. The hand and wrist should be in the same plane.

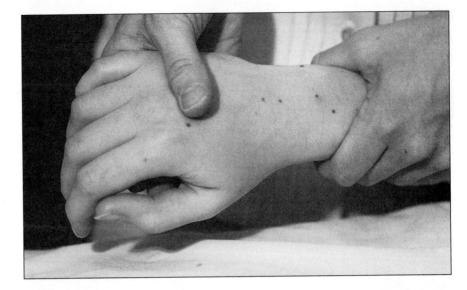

5 For radial deviation, gently guide the thumb side of the hand toward the wrist.

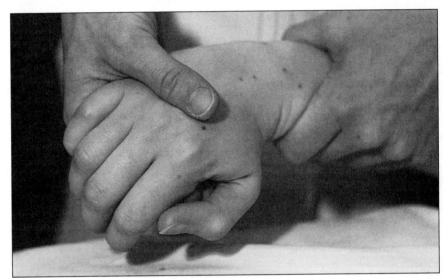

6 Gently guide the fifth-finger side of the hand toward the wrist for ulnar deviation.

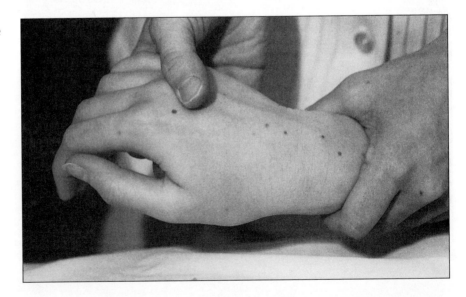

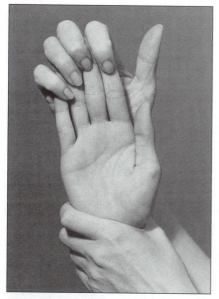

7 Extend the fingers by gently straightening them with your right hand while you support the wrist with your left hand. Do not pull the fingers beyond the plane of the hand.

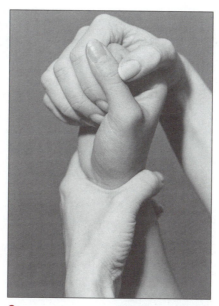

8 Flex the fingers by gently curling them with your fingers.

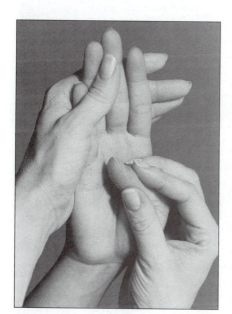

9 With the fingers extended, oppose the thumb to the base of the fifth finger.

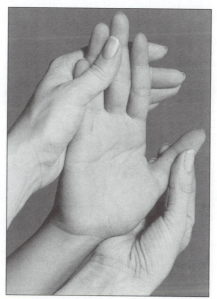

10 Extend the thumb.

EXERCISING THE HIPS AND KNEES

1 To achieve the neutral position for hip and knee flexion and extension, place your left hand under the knee and your right hand under the ankle (top). Lift the leg so that it bends at the hip and knee, and move the thigh as close to the trunk as possible (bottom). Do not allow the thigh to drift to the outside of the trunk (into hip abduction). To avoid blocking the flexion at the knee, place your left hand on top of the knee as you complete the movement.

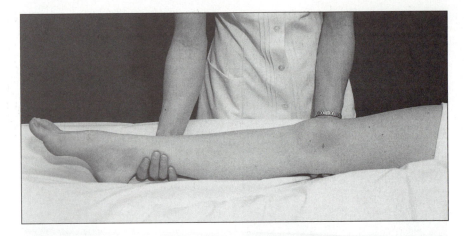

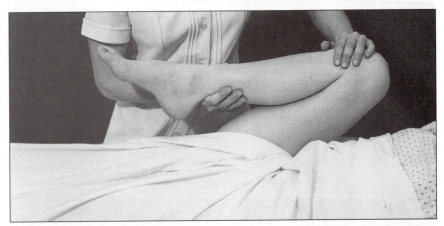

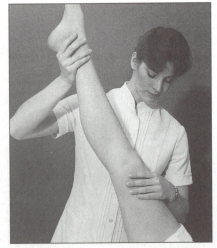

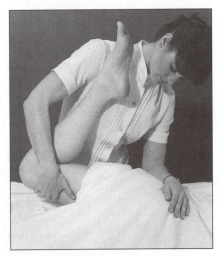

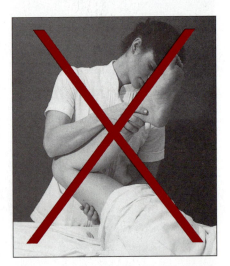

2 To flex the hip with the knee extended, return to the neutral position. Then gently lift up on the ankle with your right hand while keeping the knee straight with your left hand. You have reached the client's full range when you feel the knee begin to bend or when the client complains of a pulling sensation in the back of the knee.

3 When the client is prone, you may extend the hip while flexing the knee. To do this, stabilize the pelvis with your left hand and support the anterior thigh with your right hand. Lift gently on the anterior thigh, no more than 7.5–12 cm (3–5 in), depending on the client's range.

Note: This photo depicts incorrect hip extension. The movement is occurring in the lumbar joints because the nurse is lifting the thigh too high.

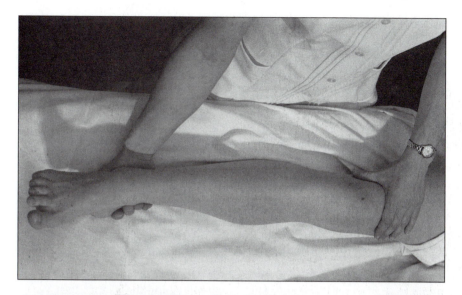

4 To achieve the neutral position for internal and external rotation of the hip with the hip and knee extended, support the ankle with your right hand and place your left hand proximal to the knee. The knee should point toward the ceiling.

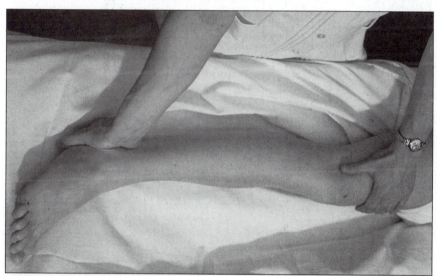

5 To rotate the hip internally, gently turn the leg toward the midline of the client's body.

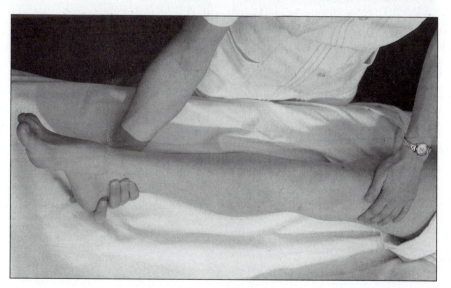

6 Turn the leg toward yourself (laterally) for external rotation.

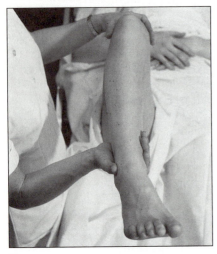

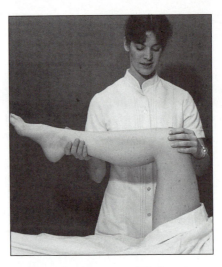

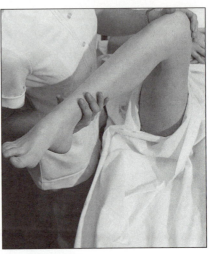

7 These photos depict the neutral position for internal and external rotation of the hip with the hip and knee flexed. Position the femur at a 90-degree angle to the body.

and flex the knee at a 90-degree angle to the femur. Place your left hand on the knee, and support the ankle with your right hand.

8 To rotate the hip externally, gently guide the client's foot toward yourself. Remember to keep the knee and dorsum of the foot pointing toward the ceiling to ensure that you do not change the vertical position of the femur.

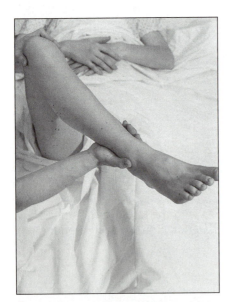

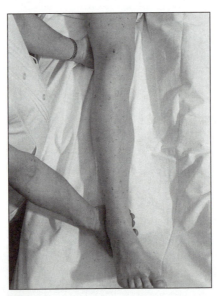

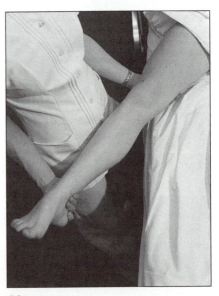

9 To rotate the hip internally, guide the foot toward the client's midline.

10 This photo depicts the neutral position for hip abduction and adduction. Position your left hand under the knee and your right hand under the ankle.

11 To abduct the hip, simultaneously move the leg off the bed as you step back with your right foot and pivot onto your left foot. Keep the client's toes and knee pointing toward the ceiling as you move the leg. Then, adduct the hip by returning the leg to the midline.

EXERCISING THE ANKLES AND TOES

1 To achieve the neutral position for ankle dorsiflexion, place your left hand under the knee and cradle the foot with your right hand and forearm.

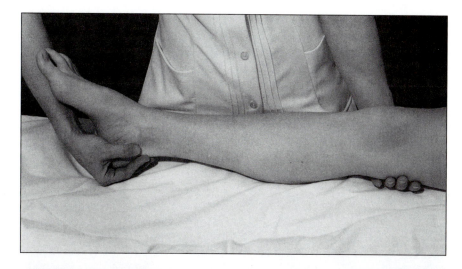

2 To dorsiflex the ankle, shift your weight onto your left leg and push against the ball of the client's foot with your right forearm. As you do this, pull the heel in the opposite direction with your right hand in order to stretch the gastrocnemius-soleus muscle group.

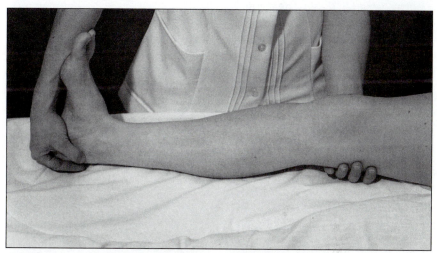

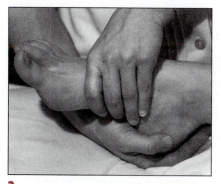

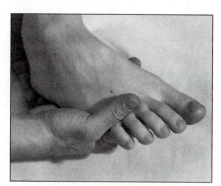

3 It is seldom necessary to plantar-flex the ankles because in bed, feet posture naturally in this position. However, if the client can pull the toes up but cannot push them down, you must also plantarflex the ankles. To do this, cradle the heel with your right hand and press gently on the dorsum of the foot with your right hand.

4 To invert the ankle, turn the client's foot toward the midline without changing the position of the heel.

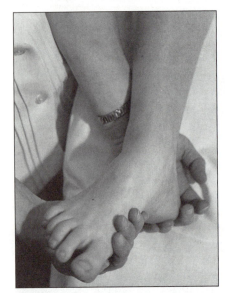

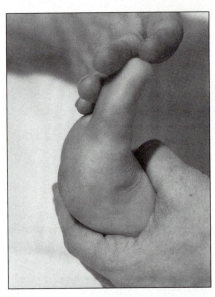

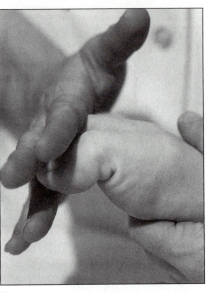

5 Evert the ankle by turning the foot laterally toward yourself. Normally, your client will have more range with inversion than with eversion.

6 To extend the toes, support the forefoot with your left hand and gently guide the toes toward the dorsum of the foot with your right hand.

7 Flex the toes by bending them toward the sole of the foot with your opened fingers.

PERFORMING PROPRIOCEPTIVE NEUROMUSCULAR FACILITATION EXERCISES

The movement patterns described below provide an alternative to the traditional passive ROM exercises. Their advantage over the latter is that they combine movements at several joints simultaneously, thereby reducing the amount of time necessary to complete the series. To achieve this end, each exercise is performed on the diagonal. For example, one movement pattern (diagonal) for the upper extremities combines components of flexion, abduction, and external rotation of the shoulder. To help you understand both the movement components occurring at each joint and the correct hand positioning for the involved joints, review the steps for the traditional ROM exercises (see pages 35–48). Consult with your agency's educational staff or occupational or physical therapist for added information if these exercises are new to you.

Explain the exercises to your client, and provide a drape for warmth and privacy. Elevate the bed to an optimal working level, remove the pillow (if your client can tolerate it), and position her so that she is flat on her back. If you will exercise her right side first, move her to the right side of the bed. Never push the movement beyond the client's range; and modify the exercise on a joint in which you elicit pain, spasms, or tremors. Remember to use proper body mechanics. Repeat each movement three to five times.

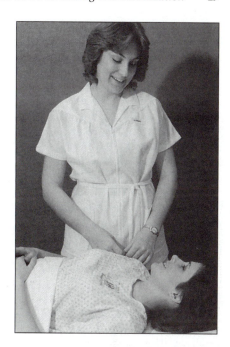

EXERCISING THE NECK

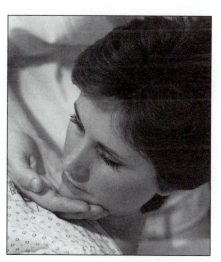

1 For the first diagonal movement, position the client's head so that her neck is flexed and rotated to the left as if she were looking down at her left elbow.

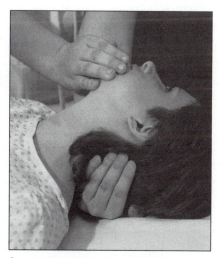

2 Extend the neck while you rotate it to the right so that she is looking up and over her right shoulder. The second diagonal is the direct opposite of the first. Position the client so that the neck is flexed and rotated to the right as if she were looking at her right elbow. Extend her neck while rotating it to the left so that she is looking up and over her left shoulder.

EXERCISING THE UPPER EXTREMITIES

1 To perform Diagonal-One (D-1) movements, start with the arm extended, abducted, and internally rotated at the shoulder so that the client's thumb points toward the floor. If you are exercising the right upper extremity, your right hand will guide the movement of the client's hand while your left hand will support and guide the movement of the humerus.

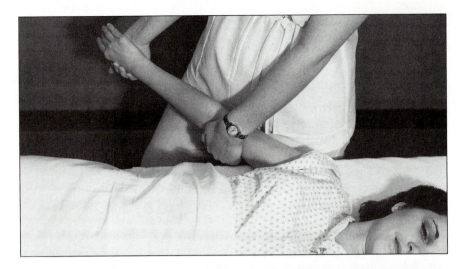

2 Move the arm diagonally up and across her nose as if she were reaching for the opposite corner of the bed. This movement results in shoulder flexion, adduction, and external rotation with the elbow extended.

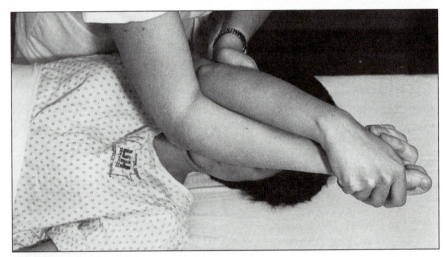

3 Return to the start position for D-1, and perform the same shoulder movements, but allow the elbow to flex as the shoulder flexes.

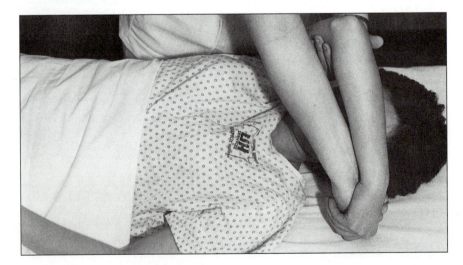

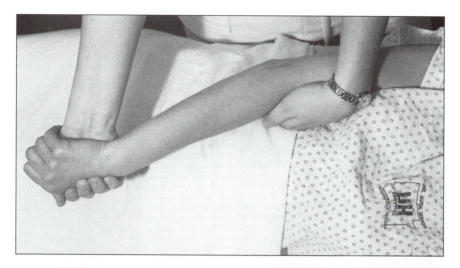

4 For Diagonal-Two (D-2) movements, start with the arm extended, adducted, and internally rotated at the shoulder. The client's thumb should be resting against her left anterior iliac crest.

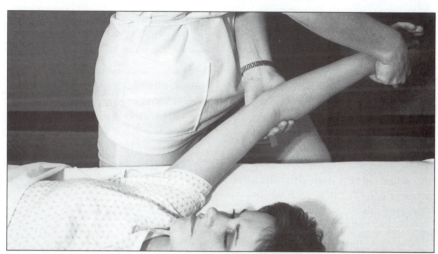

5 Lift the arm up and across the client's body so that her hand points toward the opposite corner of the room and the thumb points downward. This movement flexes, abducts, and externally rotates the shoulder with the elbow extended.

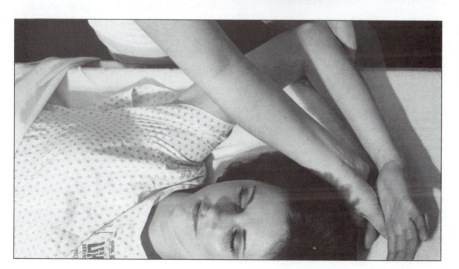

6 Return to the start position for D-2 and perform the same shoulder movements, but this time allow the elbow to flex as you flex the shoulder.

EXERCISING THE LOWER EXTREMITIES

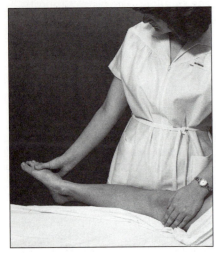

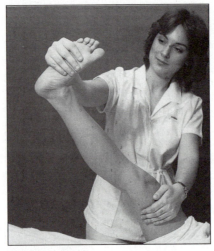

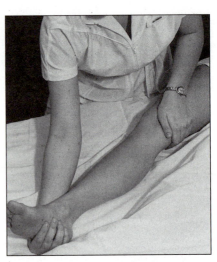

1 To perform D-1 movements, start with the hip extended, abducted, and internally rotated. The knee should be extended and the ankle plantarflexed (as shown). Your right hand will support and guide the movement of the lower leg while your left hand will guide the movement of the thigh.

2 Lift up on the leg and move it along the diagonal into a position of hip flexion, adduction, and external rotation with the ankle moving into dorsiflexion and inversion. The completed diagonal is similar to a soccer kick in which the ball is kicked with the inner aspect of the foot. Return to the start position.

3 For D-2 movements, start with the client's hip extended, adducted, and externally rotated with the knee extended and the foot plantarflexed.

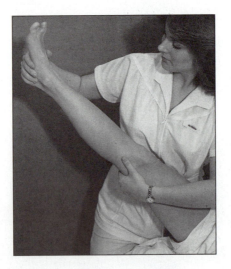

4 Move into a position in which the client's hip is flexed, abducted, and internally rotated with the knee extended and the foot moving into dorsiflexion. This diagonal can be compared to kicking a ball with the outer aspect of the foot. Return to the start position. Now assist the client to the left side of the bed and perform the exercises on her left side. *Note: Knee flexion also can be performed along with the hip flexion patterns, or it can be done separately.*

NURSING GUIDELINES: USING PRESSURE-RELIEF MATTRESSES AND PADS

Sheepskin

Use

The cushionlike fibers pad the body to distribute pressure around the bony prominences and minimize the potential for skin breakdown. The sheepskin also improves air circulation and enhances the drying of perspiration to prevent skin maceration, potentially caused by continued exposure to moisture.

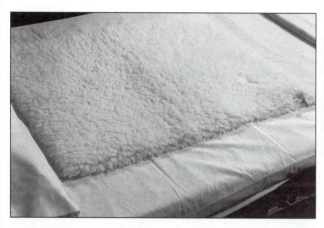

Nursing Considerations

- Change the pad whenever it becomes wet or soiled. Larger pads are impractical for the incontinent client. For incontinent clients, consider the use of smaller pads placed under heels or shoulders.

- Because the client buys the sheepskin, make sure it is properly labeled prior to each laundering.

- Pads made from synthetic fabrics launder better than natural sheepskin.

- Place the pad on top of the bottom sheet so that it has immediate contact with the client's skin.

Eggcrate Mattress

Use

The corrugated surface minimizes the pressure points under the bony prominences. In addition, it promotes better air circulation to help prevent skin breakdown.

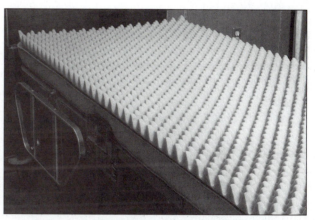

Nursing Considerations

- To keep the bottom sheet taut and wrinkle-free, knot each corner (see below).

- If the client is diaphoretic, consider using a thin bath blanket rather than a bottom sheet.

- If the mattress becomes soiled, wash the soiled area with soap and water. Let the mattress dry thoroughly before replacing it on the client's bed.

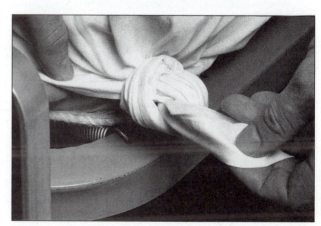

Nursing Guidelines: Using Pressure-Relief Mattresses and Pads (continued)

Flotation Pad

Use

The gel-like inner substance molds to the client's body to help minimize pressure over the bony prominences. The smaller pad (as shown) fits in a chair or wheelchair.

Nursing Considerations

- Keep pins, needles, and other sharp objects away from the pad.
- Cover the pad with nothing thicker than a sheet or pillowcase so that you do not diminish its effectiveness.
- The pad's plastic outer surface may promote increased perspiration that could lead to skin maceration. Inspect the client's skin frequently.

Air Mattress

Use

This mattress overlay is designed to suspend the client on a low air loss surface, thereby providing pressure relief over bony prominences. The covering on the overlay provided by the manufacturer is a smooth, low-friction fabric that reduces shearing effect.

Nursing Considerations

- To ensure adequate mattress inflation, slide your hand between the client and the mattress. Adjust the pressure so that you are able to depress 2–3 fingers' width (1½ in) under the client and into the mattress. Remember that underinflation can promote hip flexion contractures and protraction

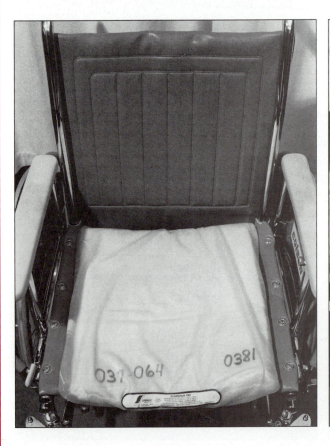

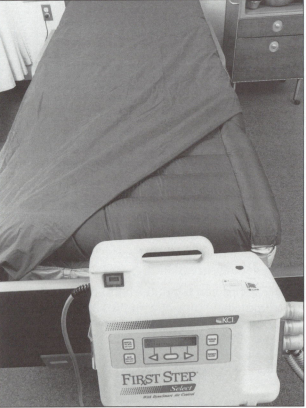

NURSING GUIDELINES: USING PRESSURE-RELIEF MATTRESSES AND PADS (continued)

of the shoulder girdle, and overinflation can cause excessive pressure on the bony prominences.

- When bathing the client using this type of air mattress, use the "Instaflate" feature to firm up the mattress support. Remember to turn off this feature when you are finished to return the mattress to the appropriate pressure-relieving status.

- Use only the dry flow underpad or the overlay covering provided by the manufacturer between the client and mattress surface so as not to impede the low air loss feature.

- To perform CPR, disconnect the hoses between the mattress and the blower, and follow agency protocol for CPR initiation. Many beds have a CPR switch that immediately deflates the mattress.

- Even though immobilized clients on these mattresses may require fewer position changes, it is important to continue ROM exercises to prevent contractures and ankylosis.

- Monitor client's skin for erythema or irritation at least every 4 hours.

HOME HEALTH CARE CONSIDERATIONS

- Properly grounded three-prong plugs are necessary for preventing fire and electric shock.

- Extension cords and multiple-outlet adaptor's should not be used for the same reason as above.

Alternating Pressure Therapy

Use

The mattress overlay changes its pressure points over the body every 5 minutes and rapidly circulates air in a wavelike fashion throughout the mattress. These features prevent pressure ulcers and stimulate peripheral circulation.

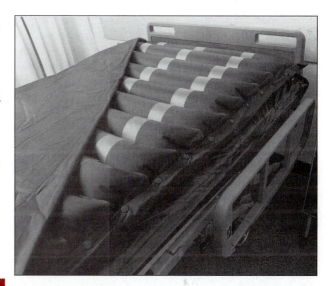

Nursing Considerations

- Confirm that the tamper-proof mechanism on the coverlet is intact to ensure that the coverlet cannot be removed from the air mattress during client use. This will minimize the risk of cross-contamination between clients.

- The coverlet is fluid resistant and washable. The client may be placed directly on the coverlet, or regular sheets may be used on the mattress overlay.

- To perform CPR, pull the rapid deflation cap to deflate the mattress. The blower can be turned off later.

- To transport the client in the bed, kink the hose connecting the mattress to the blower; disconnect the hoses and cap the ends.

NURSING GUIDELINES: PROPER CLIENT POSITIONING

Supine

Lower Body

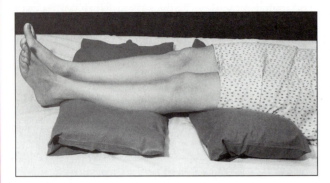

In addition to ROM exercises, meticulous skin care, and frequent turning, the immobilized client also requires carefully planned positioning to prevent the complications of prolonged bed rest. Proper positioning will minimize pressure to the bony prominences, maintain correct body alignment to reduce stress and strain to the joints, ensure maximal chest expansion for proper breathing, and prevent the formation of contractures. Any time the client moves or is moved on the bed linen, shearing forces may damage the skin. Skin abrasions are more likely to occur in clients who are debilitated or in those with poor circulation or poor nutritional status. Use care to avoid abrasions.

For most clients a good rule for positioning in bed is to try to achieve the proper standing alignment. The head should be neutral or slightly flexed on the neck, the hips extended, the knees extended or minimally flexed, and the feet at 90-degree angles to the legs. If pillows are unavailable for maintaining your client's position, consider substituting blankets, towels, or spreads. Review the following general procedures to assist you in positioning immobile clients.

- To take pressure off the lower back, slightly flex the client's hips by placing a thin pillow under the thighs. The pillow should not extend into the popliteal area, nor should it be placed directly under the knees because it could occlude the popliteal arteries.

- If the client experiences increased pressure or pain in the lower back, positioning the knees in slight flexion (≤ 30 degrees) usually alleviates the complaint.

- To prevent hip flexion contractures, ensure that the client is side-lying or prone with the hips extended for the approximate amount of time she is supine.

- Placing a pillow under the thighs is contraindicated for clients with inflammatory joint diseases because they have a tendency to posture in flexion due to pain. It is important that you attempt to move their hips and knees through their full extension range with every position change.

- Place a thin pillow under the client's ankles and lower legs to keep the heels off the bed's surface, thereby preventing pressure. As an alternative, use sheepskin or heel protectors; or, if possible, use a pressure-relief mattress or pad.

NURSING GUIDELINES: PROPER CLIENT POSITIONING *(continued)*

Supine *(continued)*

Upper Body

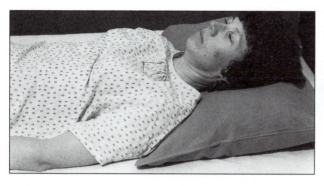

Unless a flat position is required (for example, for neck pain or neck injury), support the client's head and shoulders with a small pillow or foam wedge so that the head is neutral or slightly flexed on the neck. Position the pillow carefully so that it does not cause protraction (forward rounding) of the shoulders.

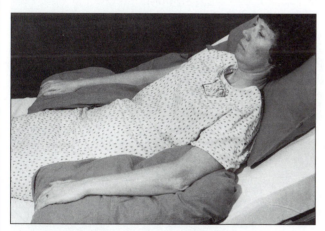

Semi-Fowler's Position (30-Degree Head Elevation)
When the head must be elevated, extend the shoulders and support the arms on each side of the body with pillows. Allow the fingertips to extend over the edge of the pillows to maintain the normal arching of the hands. Because this position places the client in hip flexion, ensure that alternate positions, with the client's hips in extension, are also used.

Side-Lying

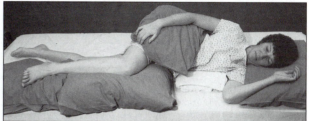

- Ensure that the client's spinal column is in straight alignment from the head to the coccyx.

- Place a pillow under the head to maintain its normal alignment with the body. The pillow should be just thick enough to accommodate the space between the bed and the head.

- For curvaceous clients, a pad positioned between the iliac crest and axilla will help to maintain proper spine alignment. It should be thick enough to prevent the vertebral column from sagging into the bed and wide enough so that the pressure it may potentially produce in the soft tissues can be evenly distributed over the entire rib cage.

- Place a pillow under the upper arm to prevent shoulder adduction and internal rotation. To ensure optimal chest expansion for proper breathing, the weight of the upper arm and pillow should be centered over the pelvis rather than over the rib cage.

- The upper leg should be flexed at the hip and knee and supported by a thick pillow to prevent both internal rotation and adduction of the hip and pressure to the patella. Ensure that the thigh is well supported and that the pillow does not touch the lower leg.

- If necessary, place a second pillow under the upper foot to prevent its inversion and to maintain its alignment with the rest of the leg. This is an optimal time to position the lower leg in extension from the hip. You may slightly flex the knee for the client's comfort.

- It may be necessary to support the client's position by placing a pillow behind the back.

NURSING GUIDELINES: PROPER CLIENT POSITIONING (continued)

Prone

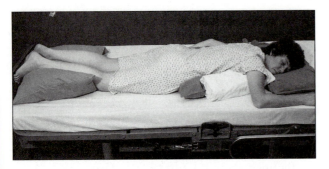

Caution: This position is contraindicated for clients with tracheostomies, cervical injuries, or breathing difficulties.

- Turn the client's head to the side and place a flat pillow under the head and shoulders to prevent hyperextension of the neck.

- Place thin pads under the angles of the axillae and the lateral aspects of the clavicles. This will prevent internal rotation of the shoulders, maintain the anatomic position of the shoulder girdle, and promote optimal chest expansion for breathing.

- Position one arm so that it is flexed at the shoulder and elbow and the other arm so that it is extended from the shoulder with the palm flat on the bed. Periodically reposition the arms to prevent joint stiffness.

- Place a flat pillow (the darker pillow in the photo) under the waistline so that it cushions the anterior superior iliac spines and prevents pressure to the area. It will also minimize strain to the lower back, promote chest expansion, allow room for breast tissue, and prevent a lordotic position (swayback).

- To flex the knees minimally, position a thin pillow under the lower legs. This will minimize pressure to the patellas and keep the toes off the mattress as well. Be certain that the toes clear the pillow.

- To prevent plantarflexion and hip rotation and to prevent injury to the toes and heels, move the client to the end of the bed to allow her feet to recline between the edge of the mattress and the footboard. Position the feet so that they are as close to a 90-degree angle from the legs as possible.

Positioning Aids

Trochanter Rolls

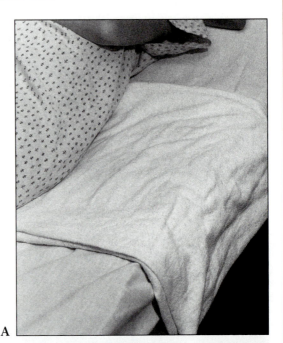

A

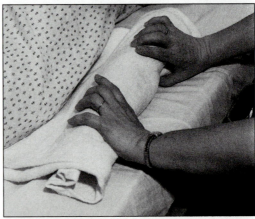

B

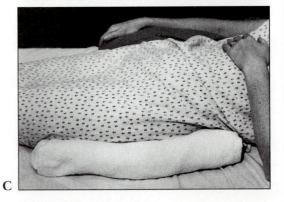

C

NURSING GUIDELINES: PROPER CLIENT POSITIONING (continued)

Foot Supports

To prevent abduction and external rotation of the hip, position the client on a large towel or bath blanket that has been folded so that it extends from the client's waist to the midthigh (see A on page 58). The material should drape equally on either side of the body. Turn the fabric as the nurse is doing in the photo (B) so that the roll is undermost. Commercially made rolls and wedges also are available.

   Tuck the roll tightly against the client's hips, and do the same on the opposite side (C). Ensure that the lower legs and feet internally rotate.

Sandbags

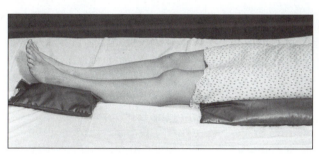

Sandbags are positioning aids that prevent abduction and external rotation of the hips. Although smaller clients might be properly supported by placing only the larger sandbags at the hip area, bigger or more flaccid clients requiring added support will benefit from two sets of sandbags (as shown). Place the larger bags from the waist to the midthighs and the smaller bags along the lower legs. The bags are positioned correctly if the legs and feet are rotated internally toward the midline. For client comfort, wrap the sandbags with pillowcases or towels.

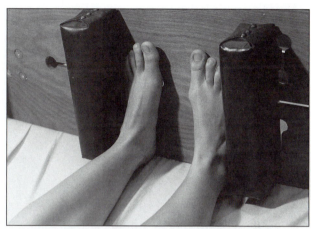

Caution: Foot supports might be contraindicated for clients who are hypertonic (spastic), for example, those with head injuries, multiple sclerosis, or in the spastic recovery phase of a cerebrovascular accident. Experts contend that the contact of the foot's surface on the board may actually trigger spasticity and hence reinforce plantarflexion.

   Your spastic clients might benefit instead from foot cradles, which keep bed linen off their feet, or from more frequent ROM exercises. Another option is to cut off a pair of high-top tennis shoes so that each shoe ends just proximal to the head of the client's metatarsals. These shoes will maintain dorsiflexion, yet prevent contact of the balls of the feet with a hard surface. However, clients without spasticity usually are helped with foot supports, such as the device in the photo. This foot support not only prevents plantarflexion, but prevents external rotation of the hips as well. Pad these devices with fleece, a blanket, or a towel to prevent the formation of pressure ulcers on the soles of the feet.

NURSING GUIDELINES: PROPER CLIENT POSITIONING (continued)

Positioning Aids *(continued)*

Hand Rolls, Cones, and Splints

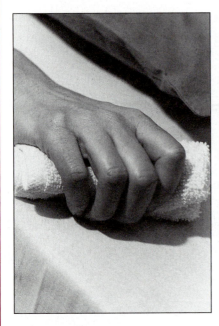
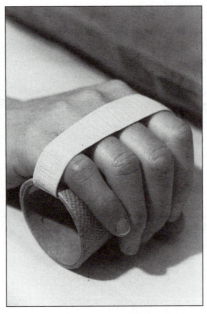
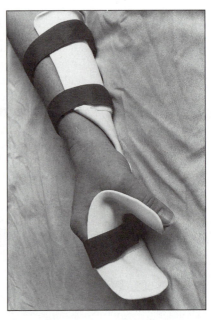

Hypotonic (flaccid) clients (for example, those with spinal cord injuries) may benefit from positioning devices such as a rolled washcloth (left) placed within their grasp. This will place the hand, wrist, and fingers in a position that maintains a functional grasp. The thumb is positioned so that it opposes the tip of the index finger. Spastic clients, on the other hand, may require the firm surface of a cone (center) or a splint (right). The hard surface of these devices presses on the muscle to inhibit spasticity. In addition, the elastic bands that secure them to the hand stimulate the extensor muscles, thus encouraging finger extension.

ASSISTING THE CLIENT WITH CRUTCHES, CANES, AND WALKERS

Checking for Correct Crutch Height

Before assisting your client with crutch walking, it is important to ensure that the crutches are the correct height. With the client's elbows flexed 20–30 degrees, the shoulders in a relaxed position, and the crutches placed approximately 15 cm (6 in) anterolateral from the toes, you should be able to place two fingers comfortably between the axillae and the axillary bars (as shown). Adjust the crutches if you find either too much or too little space at the axillary area. Advise the client never to rest the axillae on the axillary bars because this could injure the brachial plexus (the nerves in the shoulder that supply the arm and shoulder area). Terminate ambulation and recheck the crutch height if the client complains of numbness or tingling in the hands or arms.

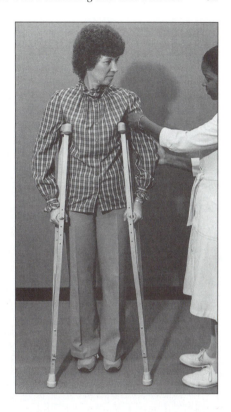

Guarding the Client

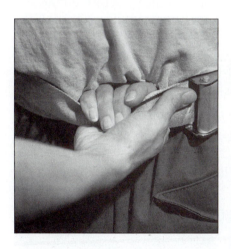

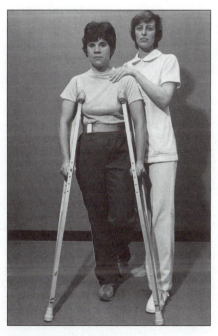

Crutches: When walking with clients who are using crutches, stand on the affected side and grasp the security belt in the mid-spine area at the small of the back (left). Position your free hand at the shoulder area so that you can pull the client toward you in the event that there is a forward fall (right). Make sure, however, that you do not obstruct the movement of the humerus. Instruct the client to look up and outward toward her destination rather than at her feet. ***Caution:*** *For your client's safety, always inspect the rubber tips of the assistive device to make sure they are not worn; also ensure that the client wears appropriate shoes with nonslip soles.*

➡

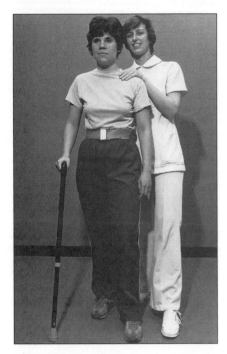

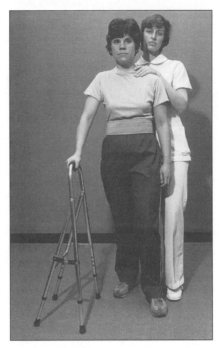

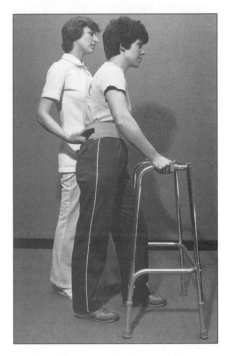

Canes: If your client is walking with a cane, stand at the affected side and guard her by grasping the security belt and positioning your free hand at the shoulder area. This is the same stance used in crutch walking. Remind the client to place the cane on the unaffected side so that the cane and the weaker leg can work together with each step. The top of the cane should reach the level of the greater trochanter of the client's femur.

Hemi or Quad Canes: Hemi canes are used for clients who have the use of only one upper extremity, and they give more security than a quad cane (below) can provide. Both canes give the client greater stability than a single-tipped cane. Either is positioned at the client's unaffected side, with the straight, nonangled side adjacent to the body. The canes should be positioned approximately 15 cm (6 in) from the client's side, with the handgrips level with the greater trochanter of the femur. Guard the client as you would if she were using a single-tipped cane.

Walkers: If your client is using a walker, guard her as you would a client using a cane or crutches, and stand adjacent to her affected side. Instruct the client to put all four points of the walker flat on the floor before putting weight on the hand pieces. This will prevent stress cracks in the walker and help ensure the client's safety. Instruct her to move the walker forward and walk into it and then repeat the movement.

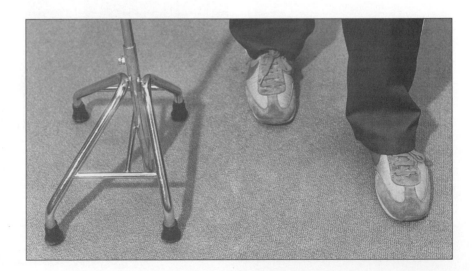

ASSISTING THE CLIENT WITH CRUTCHES TO SIT IN A CHAIR

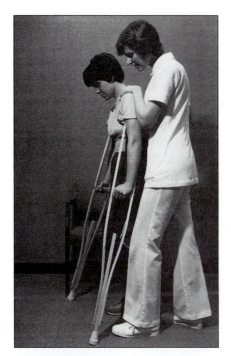

1 Before the client sits in a chair, you must first secure the chair by bracing it against a wall. Then instruct her to walk toward the chair and when she reaches it to begin her turn (as shown) so that ultimately the chair will be directly behind her.

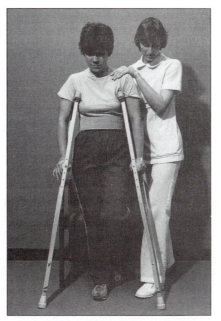

2 She should place her unaffected leg against the front of the chair.

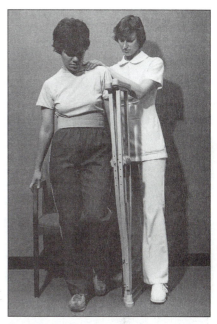

3 Instruct the client to move the crutches to her affected side and to grasp the chair's arm with the hand on the unaffected side.

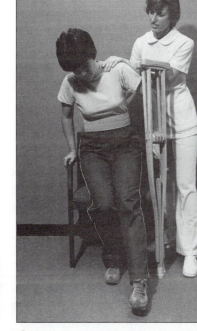

4 Tell her to flex the knee of her unaffected leg to lower herself into the chair. Advise the client to place her affected leg straight out in front of her to ensure that it remains nonweight bearing, if this is appropriate.

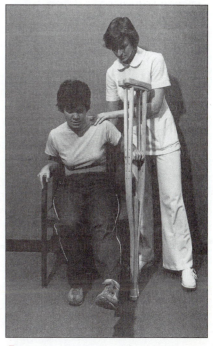

5 Once she has been seated, she should slide back into the chair so that she is in a good sitting posture. Place a support under the foot if the knee must remain extended while the client is sitting. Reverse these steps to assist her to stand from a sitting position.

Transferring Mobile and Immobile Clients

NURSING GUIDELINES: LIFTING AND TRANSFERRING CLIENTS

- To promote your clients' independence and to help maintain their muscular strength, always encourage them to move themselves or to participate in the move as much as possible.

- Whenever possible, use mechanical lifting devices to transfer immobile clients, especially those who are obese.

- Always adjust the height of the bed to a level that enables you to maintain a vertical back while lifting and transferring.

- To avoid bending your back or stretching across the bed, position yourself as close to the client as possible.

- Instead of using the muscles in your upper body for lifting, flex your knees and use your larger leg and hip muscles; straighten your knees as you lift.

- Before initiating a lift or transfer, spread your feet apart to provide a wide base of support. One foot should be positioned slightly in front of the other.

- As you move the client from one position to another, shift your weight in the direction of the move.

MOVING THE CLIENT UP IN BED

ASSISTING THE MOBILE CLIENT

If your client is strong enough to lift up with her arms and push down on her feet, teach her how to move herself up in the bed. This is important because it will promote independence, help to maintain her physical strength, and minimize the strain on your own back as well.

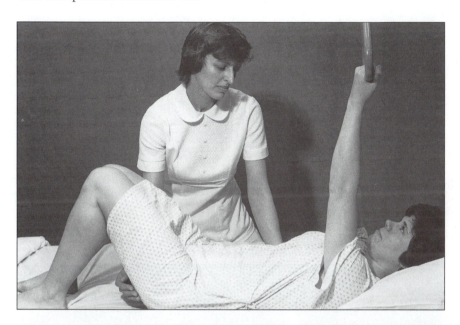

1 Flatten the bed, and adjust its height to an optimal working level. Instruct the client to bend her knees and to reach up and grasp the trapeze. (In most agencies, it is not necessary to obtain a prescription for a trapeze for the adult client.) Place your right hand under her buttocks so that you can guide her during the move.

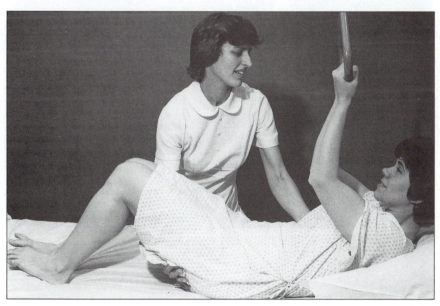

2 Instruct her to push down on her feet and to lift her upper body with her arms. As you guide her, face the direction of the move; shift your weight to the leg that is closer to the head of the bed.

LIFTING THE IMMOBILE CLIENT

1 If your client is immobile, ask one or more helpers to assist you with the lift. Position her on a draw sheet that extends from her head to her midthighs. Cross her arms across her chest to prevent them from dragging across the bed; then roll the draw sheet close to her body. With two movers, each would stand on opposite sides of the bed and grasp the sheet at the head and buttocks area. With three movers (as shown) the nurses on the same side will cross their adjacent arms to distribute the client's weight more evenly between them. If one is available, a fourth mover can be positioned at the foot of the bed to support the client's legs during the move. If a fourth mover is unavailable, be sure that the draw sheet extends beyond the client's knees, and that her heels are not bumped during the transfer.

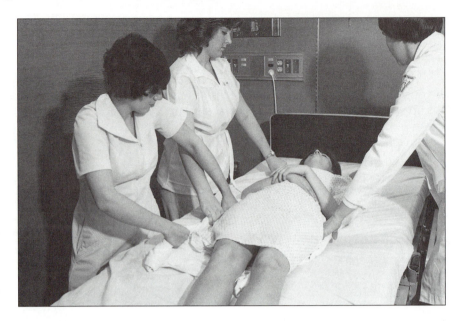

2 On a predetermined signal, shift your weight back and away from the client as if you were pulling the sheet apart. In this way, the taut sheet will elevate the client just enough to make the move to the head of the bed easier. To avoid injuring your back, it is important that you keep the natural curve in your back and avoid extending it as you pull back. As soon as the client has been elevated, shift your weight to the foot closer to the head of the bed and move the client forward. *Note: When the movers are of different heights, all will not be at an optimal working height with the bed.*

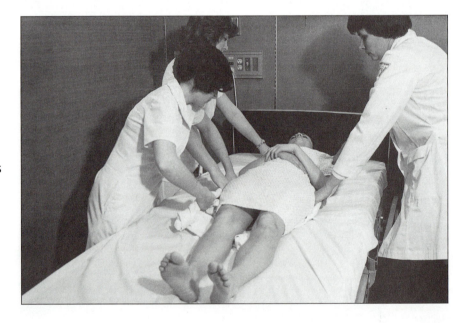

DANGLING THE CLIENT'S EXTREMITIES ON THE SIDE OF THE BED

ASSISTING THE MOBILE CLIENT

1 Clients who are on prolonged bed rest, those who are experiencing postural hypotension, and most individuals on the day of surgery are required to sit on the side of the bed and dangle their legs before getting out of bed to reestablish equilibrium. If your client has mobility, encourage her to do most of the moving and lifting with your assistance. Explain the procedure to her and raise the height of the bed to a comfortable working level. The procedure described next will be performed in stages to protect the client's back, minimize the strain to an abdominal or perineal incision, and exercise her upper extremities. With the client flat on her back, place a hand on her far hip to guide her (top). Explain that she should then roll toward you (bottom).

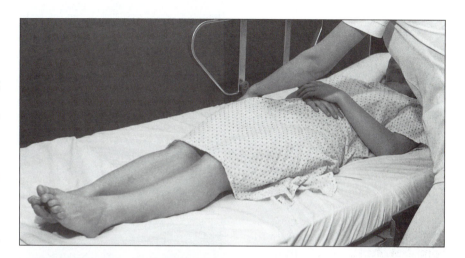

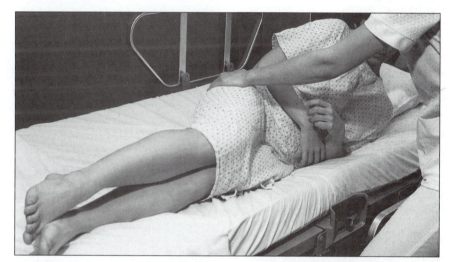

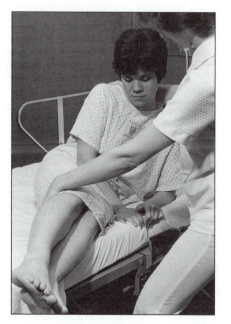

2 Once she is on her side, instruct her to flex her knees slightly and slide her legs off the side of the bed as she pushes up with her arms. You may assist her by guiding her legs and supporting her shoulders.

3 Support her at the edge of the bed until she feels comfortable and stable. Once she is secure, lower the bed so that her feet can dangle on the floor, or put a footstool under her feet.

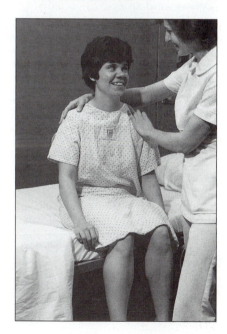

MOVING THE IMMOBILE CLIENT

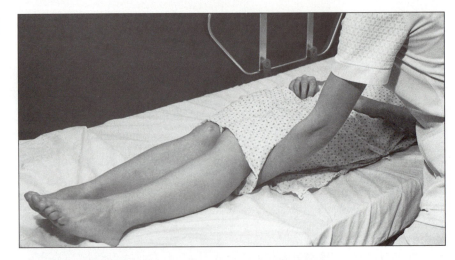

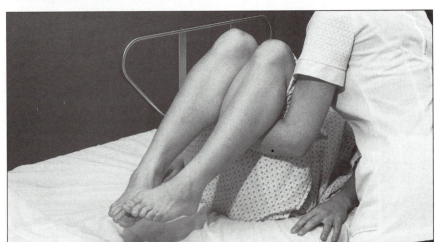

1 To dangle the extremities of the immobile client, you will need to do most of the lifting and moving yourself. Explain the procedure to the client and ask her to assist you as much as possible. Raise the bed to a comfortable working level, and place your hand under her knees (top) so that you can flex them and lift her feet off the bed (bottom).

2 Place your right arm around her shoulders and pivot her upper body up and around as you lower her legs over the side of the bed. For your own stability and safety, place your feet apart and pivot your weight from your right foot to your left foot as you lower her legs over the side. *Note: As an alternative, you can raise the head of the bed 90 degrees and pivot the client to the side of the bed, using the same hand positioning depicted in this photo.* Because she may experience dizziness for a while, continue to support her until she is stable enough for you to rest her feet on a footstool or to lower the bed for her feet to rest on the floor.

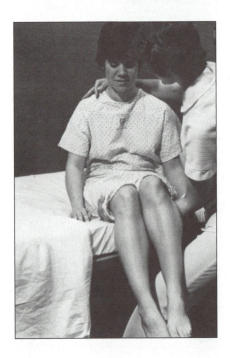

MOVING THE CLIENT FROM THE STRETCHER TO THE BED

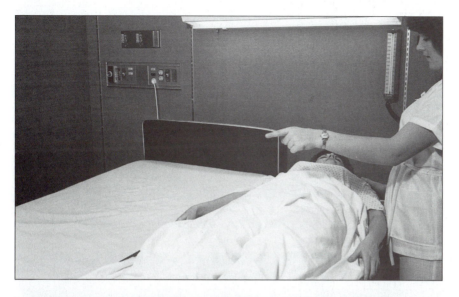

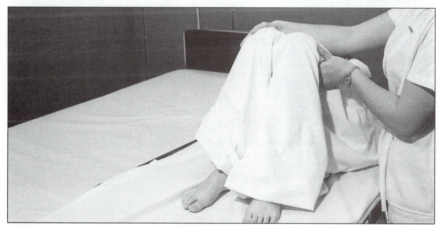

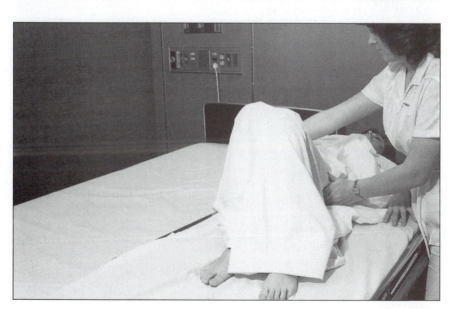

TEACHING THE SEGMENTAL TRANSFER TECHNIQUE

1 If your client can assist in the transfer, you can instruct her to move onto the bed from the stretcher by employing the segmental transfer technique. Before she begins the move, ensure that both the bed and the stretcher are locked in place to prevent them from separating during the move; adjust the bed to a height as close to that of the stretcher as possible. If the rails of the bed or stretcher do not lower completely, consider folding a sheet or blanket for light padding over the obstruction. Explain to the client that she will move her head, trunk, and feet in stages.

2 Ask her to flex her hips and knees so that her feet are flat on the stretcher.

3 She should press down on her feet and slide her trunk, her buttocks, and then her head over to the side of the stretcher.

➡

4 Instruct her to lift her feet and move them to the edge of the stretcher.

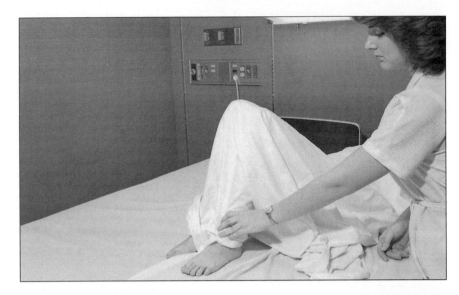

5 She should move her trunk and then her head as close to the edge of the stretcher as possible.

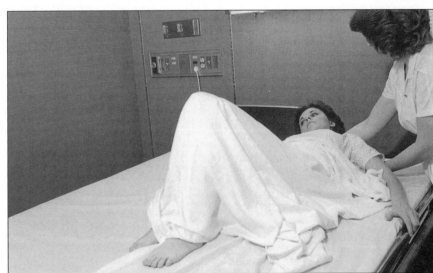

6 Tell her to place her feet on the side of the bed.

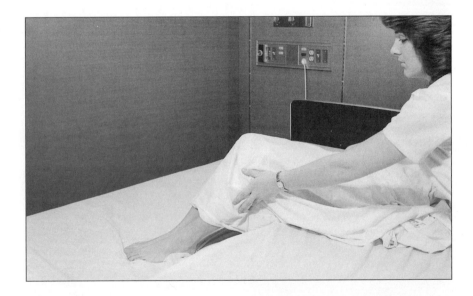

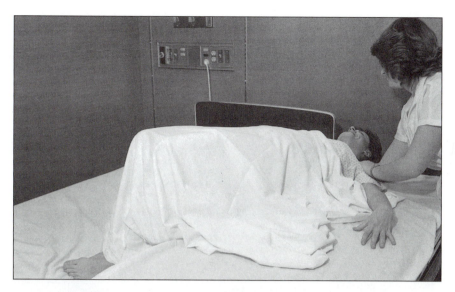

7 Instruct her to make a bridge with her trunk by lifting her pelvis off the stretcher.

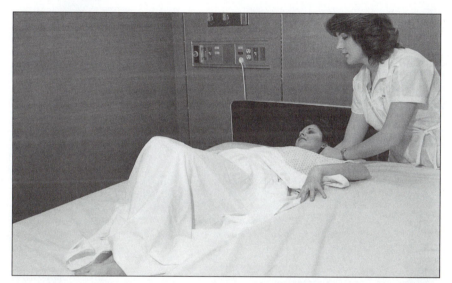

8 She will then move her pelvis and trunk onto the bed.

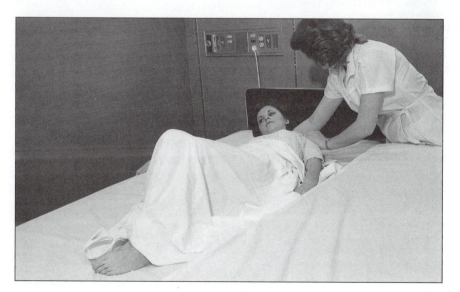

9 While her knees are still flexed, instruct her to press down on her feet to move her trunk and then her head to the center of the bed.

TRANSFERRING THE IMMOBILE CLIENT

1 If your client is immobile, seek the assistance of one or more helpers to transfer her from the stretcher to the bed. When three persons perform the move, two of the three movers should be on the side to which the client will be transferred (as shown). Explain the procedure to the client and then raise the bed to a height as close to that of the stretcher as possible and position her on a draw sheet that extends from the head to the mid-thighs. Lock the bed and stretcher in place to prevent their separation during the move. It is important to be close to the client during the lift, so the nurses who will do the initial lifting should get up onto the bed. (Nurses with slip-on shoes can remove them prior to getting up onto the bed. A towel or bed-saver pad can be placed under oxford-type shoes.) Roll the draw sheet close to the client's body, and cross her arms over her chest to prevent them from dragging on the bed during the transfer.

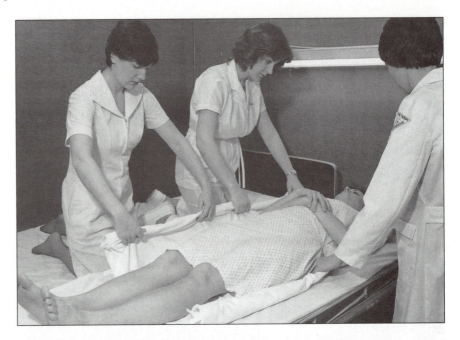

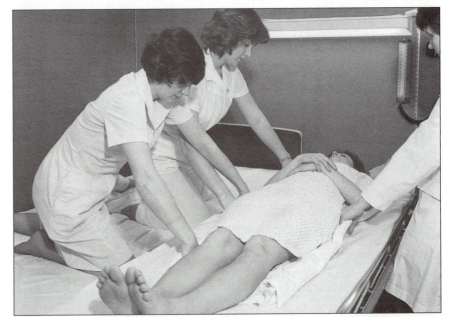

2 In preparation for lifting the client to the edge of the stretcher, the nurses on the bed will each place one knee behind the other to establish a wide base of support. They then cross their adjacent arms to distribute the client's weight evenly between them. The helper adjacent to the stretcher gasps the draw sheet, placing one hand at the level of the client's pelvis and the other hand at the level of the shoulder girdle.

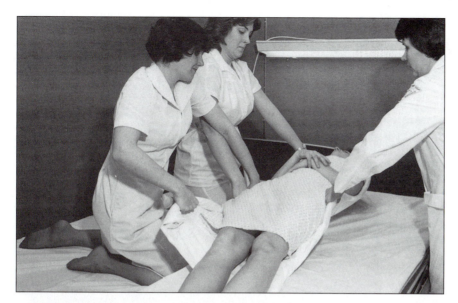

3 On a preestablished signal, the nurses on the bed will elevate and move the client by pulling back on the sheet. At the same time, the helper adjacent to the stretcher maintains tension on the sheet and follows the movement of the client by shifting her weight onto her forward leg. Note that as the client is moved to the edge of the stretcher, she is lifted only high enough to clear it.

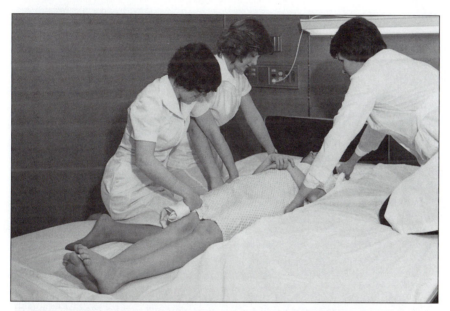

4 As the client is moved from the edge of the stretcher to the bed, the helper adjacent to the stretcher gets up onto its surface so that she can be as close to the client as possible, and the nurses on the bed move back toward the bed's edge. The client is then moved onto the bed using the same procedure that was employed to transfer her to the edge of the stretcher.

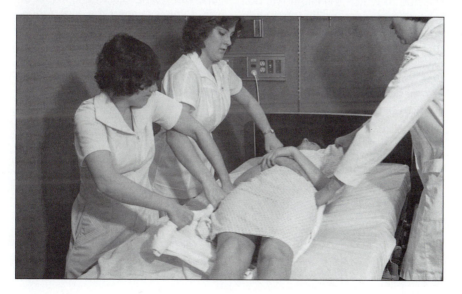

5 Remove the stretcher and move the client from the edge of the bed to the center of the bed following the same technique.

LOGROLLING THE IMMOBILE CLIENT

1 If your client has a neck injury or a spinal disorder, it will be necessary for you to logroll her when you change her position so that you maintain the alignment of her vertebral column during the turn. Logrolling is also indicated for clients with hip pinnings or hip prostheses to keep the hips in extension. Seek the assistance of a helper (find a third person if the client's head and neck require support), and explain the procedure to your client. Raise the bed to an optimal working level, and using a draw sheet, move the client to the edge of the bed opposite the side toward which she will be turned. (Review the steps in the preceding procedure.)

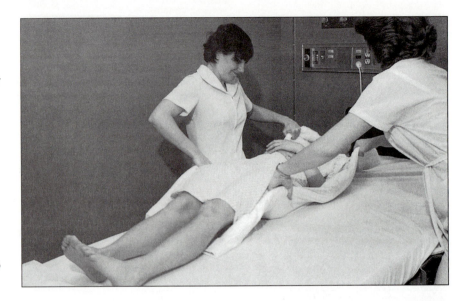

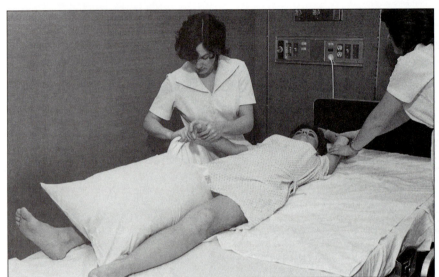

2 Straighten the draw sheet on the side to which the client will be turned, and place a pillow between her legs to maintain the position of the lower extremities. To roll the client toward the left side of the bed, you should first place her right arm beside her body; then flex her left arm over her head so that she will not roll over it during the turn. However, if your client has limited shoulder movement, keep the arm in extension next to the body.

Caution: If your client has a neck injury, you will need a second helper at this point to support the neck during the turn.

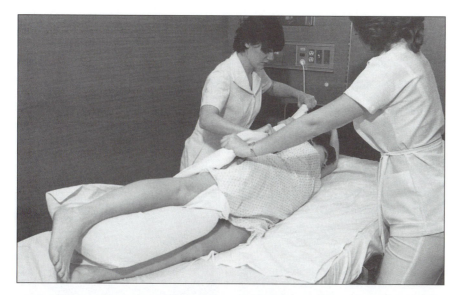

3 The nurse on the left side of the bed will flex her knees, maintain a wide base of support with her feet, and then grasp and lift up on the rolled draw sheet to guide the client toward herself. The nurse on the right side of the bed will maintain tension on the sheet to ensure the client's proper alignment. Note that the nurses' hands are alternated on the sheet to distribute the client's weight evenly. Either support the client in a side-lying position (see page 57) or continue to the prone position (as shown in step 4).

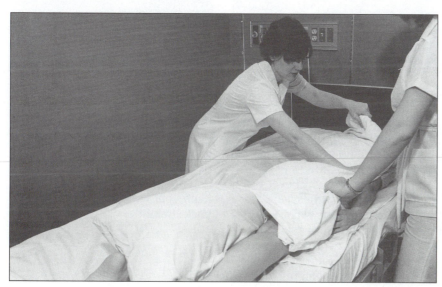

4 Continue the turn with the nurse on the right side of the bed guiding the client onto her abdomen. Place the client in a proper prone position (see page 58).

ASSISTING THE CLIENT FROM THE WHEELCHAIR (OR CHAIR) TO THE BED

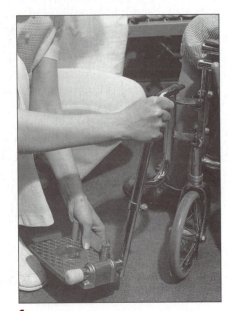 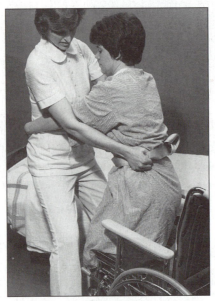 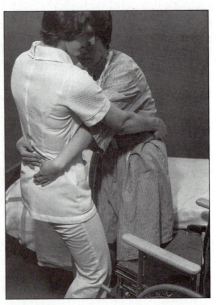

1 Clients who have enough mobility to help support themselves during the transfer may be assisted from the wheelchair or chair to the bed with the standing-pivot technique. Before starting, however, you must ensure that the client's transfer belt is fastened securely around her waist. The belt must be tight enough that it does not slide up the rib cage when an upward force is applied. Position the wheelchair at a 45-degree angle to the bed and lock both the wheelchair and the bed to ensure their stability. If the client will be transferred from a chair, make sure it is stable and will not slide on the floor. It is important either to remove the wheelchair's leg rests or to swing them out of the way so that they will not obstruct the move. Explain the procedure to the client and ensure that she understands each step and her role during the transfer. Encourage her to assume as much of the lifting and weight bearing as she can comfortably handle, using her stronger leg, if this is appropriate.

2 Flex your knees and position your feet into a wide base of support with one foot slightly in front of the other. Grasp the client's transfer belt, and instruct her to position her arms around your waist or shoulders, whichever is more stabilizing for the client. On the cue to stand, the client will prepare to stand on her stronger leg as you assist her into the standing position by pulling her trunk forward and up. As you pull her forward, transfer your weight from your forward leg to your back leg.

3 To ensure the stability of the your client's stronger leg, position the side of your knee against the side of her knee to maintain it in extension. Pivot the client and guide her until the backs of her legs are positioned against the bed. Keep your knees flexed and your back straight.

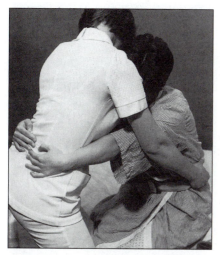

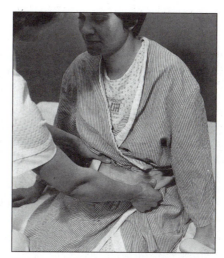

4 Shift your weight from your back leg to your front leg. Then, assist the client in lowering herself to the sitting position by using a slow bending of your knees to control the rate of descent.

5 Support her until she is stable and comfortable. Then remove the transfer belt and robe and assist her into bed. Reverse the procedure to move her from the bed to the chair.

USING A MECHANICAL LIFTING DEVICE

Mechanical lifts, such as the Hoyer, are excellent devices for lifting and transferring the immobile client. They are, however, contraindicated for clients with certain types of spinal disorders that require the vertebral column to be maintained in static alignment.

1 Be sure to read the operating instructions for the mechanical lifting device your agency employs. Be certain that the client's weight does not exceed the device's weight limit. Although it is possible to use the lift alone, a helper will both facilitate the process and ensure the client's safety by guarding him during the lifting procedure. First, explain the procedure to the client and assure him that he will be safe and comfortable during the transfer. Then, adjust the bed to a comfortable working height and roll the client into a side-lying position. Place the canvas sling along the client's body, extending it from his head to no farther than the popliteal fossa of his knees. While your helper supports the client's position, fanfold (accordion-pleat) the sling.

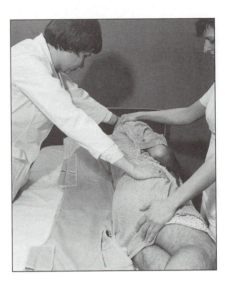

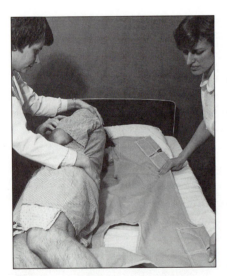

2 Roll the client to his opposite side and straighten the sling.

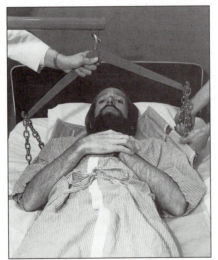

3 Return the client to his back, and cross his arms across his chest. Ask the client to keep his arms crossed. Move the lift to the side of the bed. Center the boom over the sling so that the chains can be attached to its upper section.

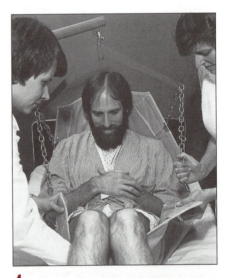

4 Elevate the boom slightly so that the chains can be attached to the lower section of the sling. The shorter chain is attached to the back support, and the longer chain is connected to the seat portion. While one nurse attaches the chains, the other should support and flex the client's knees. Ensure that the client's weight is evenly distributed in the sling.

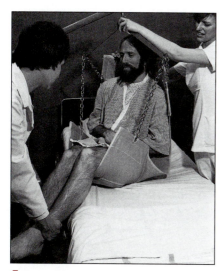

5 Either elevate the lift slightly, or lower the bed just enough so that you can clear the client of the bed and guide his legs over the side. The client's arms must remain crossed at the chest or folded in his lap.

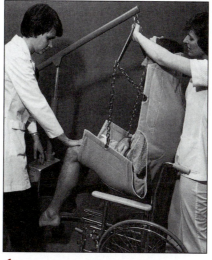

6 Move the client and the lift away from the bed and push a wheelchair or other transfer device under the client. Lock the wheelchair and then lower the lift so that the client is seated securely in the wheelchair. Protect his head as the boom is being lowered. Instruct the client to keep his arms folded during the transfer. This keeps the device balanced and prevents the client's arms from striking against the chair.

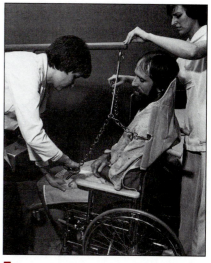

7 Unhook the chains, and either remove the sling if the client will be in the chair for an extended period of time or adjust it to remove the wrinkles. Place a security belt around the client's pelvis to ensure his stability in the chair.

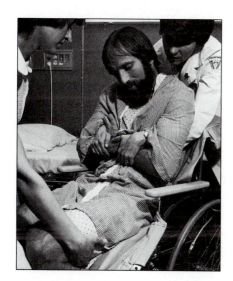

8 If your client slides down in his chair and is sitting on his sacrum, it will be necessary for you to lift him up so that he is positioned correctly. To do this, first cross his arms across his chest. Then, while one nurse stabilizes his legs and feet and prepares to push his pelvis back into the chair, the other stands behind the chair and positions her arms under the client's axillae and grasps his forearms. By grasping the crossed forearms rather than under the axillae, you will avoid the application of a force that could potentially separate the humerus from the glenoid fossa.

←

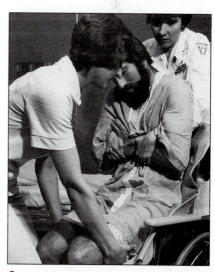

9 On a predetermined signal, the person behind the wheelchair will pull the client back and up in the chair while the nurse in front pushes his legs toward the back of the wheelchair to slide his pelvis into the correct position.

REFERENCES

Adler SS, Beckers D, Buck M: *PNF in Practice: An Illustrated Guide.* New York: Springer-Verlag, 1993.

Donatelli RA, Wooden MJ: *Orthopaedic Physical Therapy,* ed 2. New York: Churchill Livingstone, 1994.

Hertling D, Kessler RM: *Management of Common Musculoskeletal Disorders: Physical Therapy Principles and Methods,* ed 2. Philadelphia: Lippincott, 1990.

Indiana University Hospitals: *Nursing Procedures and Policies.* Indianapolis: 1994.

Kisner C, Colby LA: *Therapeutic Exercise: Foundations and Techniques,* ed 2. Philadelphia: FA Davis, 1990.

Meyers RS: *Saunders' Manual of Physical Therapy Practice.* Philadelphia: Saunders, 1995.

Palmer LM, Epler ME: *Clinical Assessment Procedures in Physical Therapy.* Philadelphia: Lippincott, 1990.

Pierson FM: *Principles and Techniques of Patient Care.* Philadelphia: Saunders, 1994.

Rantz MJ, Courtial D: *Lifting, Moving, and Transferring Patients,* ed 2. St Louis: Mosby, 1981.

Rice R: *Handbook of Home Health Nursing Procedures.* St Louis: Mosby-Year Book, 1995.

Sullivan PE, Markos PD: *Clinical Decision Making in Therapeutic Exercise.* Norwalk, CT and Los Altos, CA: Appleton-Lange, 1995.

CHAPTER 3

Administering Medications and Monitoring Fluids

CHAPTER OUTLINE

ADMINISTERING TOPICAL MEDICATIONS

Giving Ophthalmic Medications

Instilling Ointment
Instilling Drops
Instilling Ear Drops
Instilling Nose Drops

Giving Inhalant Medications

Using a Metered-Dose Inhaler
Using a Nebulizer

Giving Nitroglycerin

Applying Nitroglycerin Ointment
Applying a Nitroglycerin Disk
Administering Medications Through a Nasogastric Tube
Performing a Vaginal Irrigation (Douche)

Giving Rectal Medications

Inserting a Suppository
Instilling Ointment

ADMINISTERING INJECTABLE MEDICATIONS

Giving Intradermal Injections

Locating the Site
Injecting the Medication

Giving Subcutaneous Injections

Locating the Site
Injecting the Medication
Administering Heparin

Giving Intramuscular (IM) Injections

Mapping Muscle Sites for IM Injections
Providing an Air Lock
Injecting the Medication
Performing the Z-Track Technique

Disposing of Needles and Sharp Instruments

Nursing Guidelines: Managing Insulin Pumps

ADMINISTERING INTRAVENOUS FLUIDS AND MEDICATIONS

Preparing the Solution and Infusion Set

Inspecting the Container
Assembling the Infusion Set
Spiking the Container
Priming the Infusion Set
Labeling the Tubing and Container

Inserting a Peripheral Vascular Access Device

Assembling the Materials
Choosing a Venipuncture Site
Dilating the Vein
Preparing the Site
Inserting a Wing-Tipped Needle
Taping the Wing-Tipped Needle
Inserting an Over-the-Needle Catheter
Taping the Over-the-Needle Catheter
Applying Antimicrobial Ointment and a Gauze Dressing

Immobilizing the Extremity

Using an Armboard or Splint
Applying a Commercial Wrist Restraint
Applying a Gauze Restraint

Administering Intravenous (IV) Medications

Injecting Medications into Hanging IV Containers
Giving Medications by IV Bolus
Inserting a Saline/Heparin Lock for Intermittent Infusion Therapy
Giving Medications via a Partial-Fill (Piggyback) Container
Assembling a Volume-Control IV Set

COLLECTING, MONITORING, AND ADMINISTERING BLOOD

Collecting a Blood Sample with a Vacuum Collection System

Teaching the Diabetic Client Self-Monitoring of Blood Glucose

Initiating and Monitoring Blood Transfusions

Nursing Guidelines: Safe Administration of Blood

Administering Blood or Blood Components

INITIATING PATIENT-CONTROLLED ANALGESIA

MANAGING VENOUS ACCESS DEVICES (VADs)

Nursing Guidelines: Managing Chronic (Long-Term) Central Venous Catheters

Nursing Guidelines: Managing Acute (Short-Term) and Intermediate (Medium-Term) Multilumen Central Venous Catheters

Nursing Guidelines: Managing Peripherally Inserted Central Venous Catheters (PICCs)

Nursing Guidelines: Managing Midline Catheters (MLCs)

Nursing Guidelines: Managing Implantable Subcutaneous Ports

Changing the Exit Site Dressing for a Chronic Central Venous Catheter

Drawing Blood from a Chronic (Hickman®-Type) Central Venous Catheter and Flushing the Catheter Following Blood Withdrawal

Performing a Routine Irrigation of a Chronic Central Venous Catheter

Changing the IV Solution and Tubing for a Chronic (Hickman®-Type) Central Venous Catheter

Repairing a Multilumen Central Venous Catheter

Accessing the Implantable Subcutaneous Port

Withdrawing Blood from an Implantable Subcutaneous Port

Establishing a Heparin Lock in an Implantable Subcutaneous Port

Assessing and Intervening for an Air Embolism

Administering Topical Medications

GIVING OPHTHALMIC MEDICATIONS

INSTILLING OINTMENT

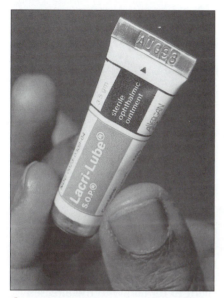

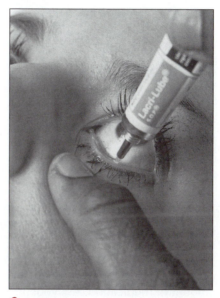

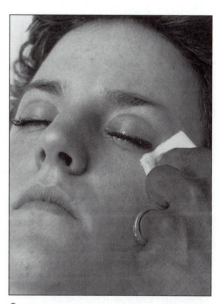

1 Before instilling anything into the eye, ensure that the medication is a sterile ophthalmic solution and that the date for usage has not expired. Because sight is so valuable and the tissues are delicate, wash your hands thoroughly and use aseptic technique when you instill anything into the eye, even though the eye itself is not sterile.

2 With the client either sitting or lying flat, the head should be tilted back slightly. If secretions adhere to the lashes or corners of the eye, remove them with a sterile 2 X 2 gauze pad or a sterile cotton ball, wiping from the inner to the outer canthus. Instruct the client to look upward as you instill the medication. This will minimize the chance of stimulating the corneal reflex, which could potentially cause the client to jerk and injure the eye. Expose the lower conjunctival sac by exerting gentle traction on the area that is just distal to the center of the lower lashes. This will form a pocket into which you will instill the ointment. With your dominant hand, gently squeeze a strip of medication along the conjunctival border. Start at the inner canthus and extend the medication outward toward the outer canthus. Generally, a 1–2 cm (⅓–¾ in) strip is adequate. If a small dose of medication has been prescribed, squeeze a small strip of ointment into the center of the sac.

3 Release the lower lid and ask the client to close her eyelids and move her eye around gently to distribute the ointment. Remove excess ointment by wiping gently across the lashes from the inner to the outer canthus with a sterile cotton ball or soft gauze pad.

INSTILLING DROPS

INSTILLING EAR DROPS

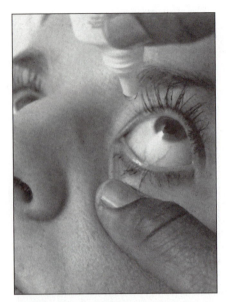

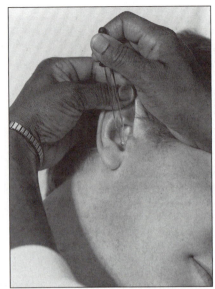

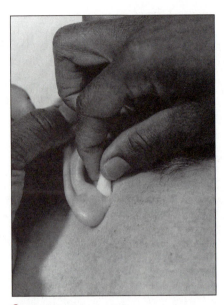

Review the preceding technique for instilling ointment. Follow the same guidelines, but dropper the medication into the center of the conjunctival sac (as shown). After administering the medication, instruct the client to close her eyelid and move her eye around to distribute the medication. At the same time, apply gentle pressure to the inner canthus for 30 seconds to 1 minute to minimize the potential for systemic absorption through the tear ducts.

1 Wash your hands. For your client's comfort, make sure the medication has been warmed to body temperature; then fill the dropper with the prescribed amount of medication. Ask your client to turn his head to the side so that the affected ear is uppermost. With your nondominant hand, pull up and back on the auricle to straighten the auditory canal. For an infant, pull down and back on the earlobe instead. Rest the wrist of your dominant hand on the client's head. This will allow your hand to move with the client rather than potentially injure the ear with the dropper, should he jerk during the instillation. Administer the medication, aiming it toward the wall of the canal rather than directly onto the eardrum. This will make the instillation less startling and hence more comfortable and safe for the client.

2 Unless the physician requests that the solution drain freely from the ear, you may insert a small piece of cotton loosely into the external auditory canal. Instruct the client to remain with the affected ear uppermost for 10–15 minutes to retain the solution.

INSTILLING NOSE DROPS

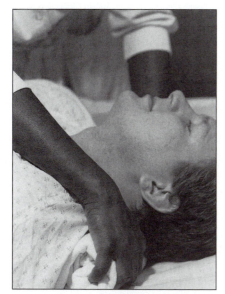

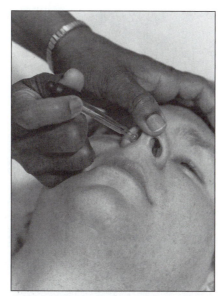

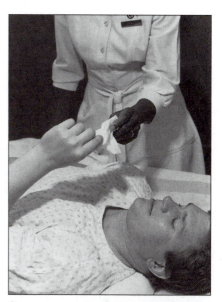

1 Wash your hands. Instruct your client to blow his nose gently. Assist him into a supine position with his head tilted back. It may be helpful to place a small pillow or a rolled towel under his shoulders to help maintain this position.

2 With your nondominant hand, press back gently on the tip of the nose to open the nares. Rest your dominant hand lightly on the face so that your hand will move along with the client should he move suddenly. This will prevent the dropper from accidentally injuring the nasal mucosa. Insert the dropper just inside the naris and instill the prescribed medication.

3 To ensure that the medication has time to drain through the nasal passages, encourage the client to maintain this position for a few minutes. Provide him with tissues in which to expectorate the solution that drains into the throat and mouth.

GIVING INHALANT MEDICATIONS

USING A METERED-DOSE INHALER

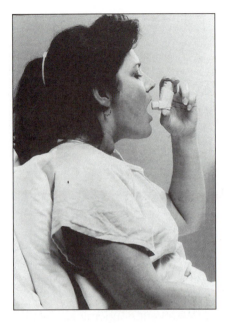

Clients who require bronchodilator aerosol (eg, for relief of broncho-spasm in reversible obstructive air-way disease or prevention of exercise-induced bronchospasm) may use metered-dose inhalants. Teach the client to follow these steps:

- Shake the inhaler immediately before use. Remove the protective cap, making sure the metal cannister is firmly inserted in the plastic case.

- Sit upright and exhale fully through the mouth.

- Position the mouthpiece 2.5–5.0 cm (1–2 in) from the mouth, holding it in an upright position. Holding the mouthpiece away from the mouth rather than in it will reduce the amount of aerosol hitting the oropharynx. A 4-cm (1.6 in) spacer to ensure appropriate distance of the mouthpiece to the mouth may be used by children or clients with coordination problems.

- While inhaling deeply and slowly through you mouth, depress the top of the metal cannister with your fingers, as shown.

- Hold your breath as long as you can. Before exhaling, release your fingers from the cannister.

- Wait 1 minute. Repeat the steps above, as prescribed.

Instruct the client to cleanse the inhaler at least once a day. Demonstrate by removing the metal cannister from the plastic case and rinsing it thoroughly in warm running water. Dry thoroughly and replace the cannister in the plastic case. Finally, recap the case.

USING A NEBULIZER

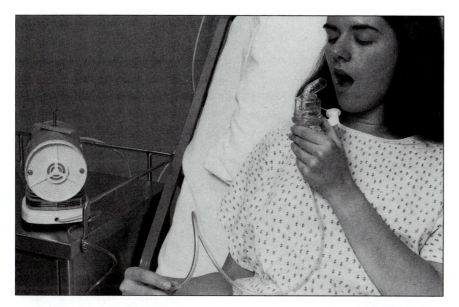

If your client has a pulmonary disorder, it may be necessary for you to use a nebulizer to administer an inhalant solution. The prescribed amount of solution is poured or droppered into the nebulizer (in the client's left hand, as shown). The compressor (on the bedside table) is then plugged in. With the client sitting upright to enhance chest expansion, instruct her to hold the nebulizer 2.5–5 cm (1–2 in) from her mouth. She should first exhale and then inhale as she closes off the finger valve (adjacent to her right index finger) to deliver the fine mist into the alveoli or other areas of the lungs. Explain that she should hold her breath for 3 seconds and then repeat the process until all the medication has been delivered from the nebulizer. ***Caution:*** *Some bronchodilators, such as metaproterenol, significantly alter the heart rate. Monitor the client's pulse rate frequently throughout the therapy and record the pretreatment and posttreatment measurements. Be sure to stay with the client throughout the treatment.* Ensure that the nebulizer and tubing are thoroughly cleaned and dried daily, according to your agency's guidelines. This practice reduces the likelihood that the nebulizer will become a reservoir for bacteria.

GIVING NITROGLYCERIN

APPLYING NITROGLYCERIN OINTMENT

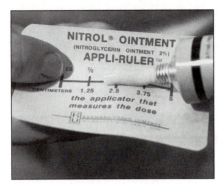

1 Nitroglycerin ointment is applied directly to the skin of clients with angina pectoris and cardiac ischemia to produce systemic vasodilation. This results in a decreased cardiac workload and improved myocardial tissue perfusion for a period of 4–6 hours. Before administering the medication, check your client's blood pressure and apical pulse to establish a baseline for subsequent comparison. Squeeze the prescribed dose directly onto the manufacturer's applicator paper. To ensure an accurate dosage, use an even pressure to produce a continuous column of medication. *Caution: Be sure to avoid direct contact with the nitroglycerin because it could give you a headache if it is absorbed through your skin. Wash your skin immediately with soap and water if this occurs.* Remove any residual ointment from previous applications prior to applying this dose.

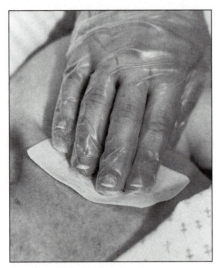

2 If desired, put on a clean glove to protect yourself from potential contact with the medication. Apply the ointment via the applicator paper directly to your client's skin. For optimal absorption, apply the ointment to skin that is hairless and dry. Application sites commonly used are the shoulder, anterior and posterior chest, abdomen, and legs. Rotate application sites to prevent sensitization and dermal inflammation. Be sure that you have initialed the patch and written the time and date of application.

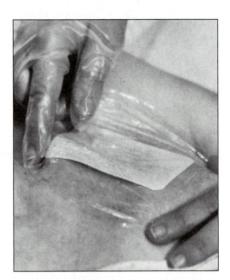

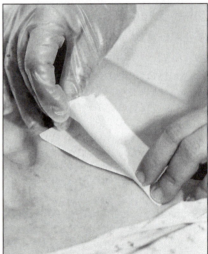

3 If the client is not receiving the desired effect from the medication, the physician may request that you cover the applicator paper with an occlusive plastic wrap (top) or with a wide strip of air-occlusive tape (bottom). Either will enhance absorption. However, if your client is achieving the desired effect without an air-occlusive dressing, avoid applying one because the increased absorption from the dressing could result in headache and dizziness.

4 Check your client's blood pressure a few minutes after applying the ointment. There should be a moderate decline in the systolic pressure. Continue to monitor your client for headaches, fainting, or dizziness. If these symptoms occur, alert the physician, who will probably decrease the dosage until the client develops a tolerance to the side effects of the drug.

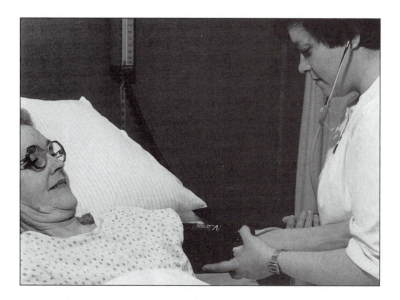

APPLYING A NITROGLYCERIN DISK

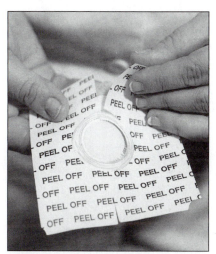

1 Review the previous steps for applying the nitroglycerin ointment because the principles for application and usage are similar to the disk's. The advantages in using the disk are its neatness, its dose accuracy, and its known duration of action. In addition, it poses less of a hazard for the person administering the drug. Disks produce a continuous release of medication over approximately a 24-hour period, starting approximately 30 minutes after application. First, remove the disk from the previous application. Then, to apply the new disk, peel off the strip of protective paper backing from one side of the disk.

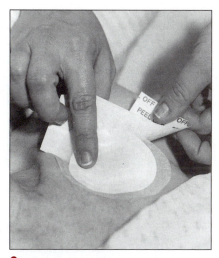

2 Adhere that side of the disk to a dry, hairless area of your client's skin. Then remove the remaining protective paper strip.

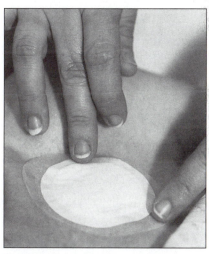

3 Securely adhere the disk's sticky surface to the client's skin. Write the date and time and initial the disk.

ADMINISTERING MEDICATIONS THROUGH A NASOGASTRIC TUBE

Have medications been prescribed that must be administered through your client's nasogastric tube? Administration can be easily performed using a large bulb or piston syringe, an emesis basin and bed-saver pad (to protect the linen when confirming proper tube positioning), and approximately 30 mL tap water.

1 First, attach a Luer-type adapter to the syringe you will use.

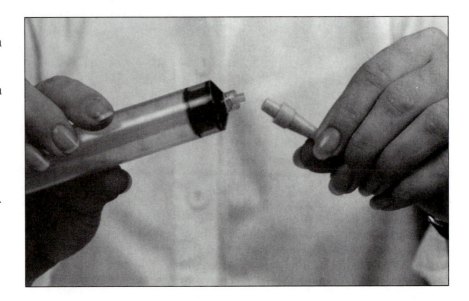

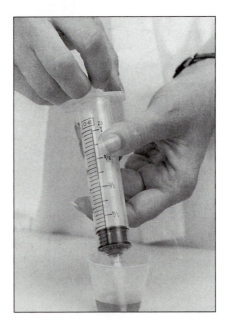

2 *For a small-bore feeding tube:* Pour the prescribed amount of medication into a measured dosage cup, and aspirate the medication into a piston syringe that is at least 30 mL in volume. Syringes of smaller volume could generate too much pressure and damage the tube. *For a large-bore feeding tube:* Leave the medication in the dosage cup. **Note:** *Use liquid dosage forms when administering medications through a nasogastric tube. Consult with a pharmacist before crushing tablets or opening capsules because this changes the product form and may alter therapeutic effects.*

HOME HEALTH CARE CONSIDERATIONS

Clients may reuse syringes, syringe adapters, and plastic cups. These supplies should be washed in warm, soapy water and allowed to dry thoroughly. Once they are dry, these supplies may be stored in a clean plastic bag.

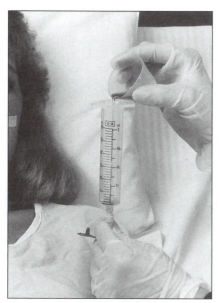

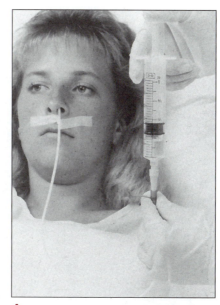

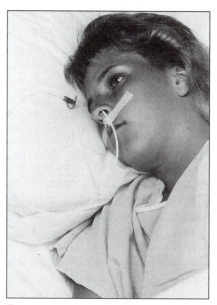

3 *For a large-bore tube:* Put on clean gloves, and confirm that the distal end of the tube is properly positioned in the stomach by aspirating for the presence of gastric contents (see page 256). Applying gentle pressure to the piston, reinstall the aspirate to prevent loss of electrolytes and gastric fluid. Remove the syringe and cap the nasogastric tube to prevent air ingestion and backflow of gastric contents. Remove the piston from the syringe barrel, uncap the nasogastric tube, and reattach the barrel to the nasogastric tube. Pour the medication into the barrel as shown and allow it to drain by gravity. After the medication has been instilled, flush the tube by adding 20–30 mL tap water into the barrel to ensure that none of the medication adheres to the tube's lumen. Hold the syringe 30–45 cm (12–18 in) above the client's abdomen and allow it to drain via gravity.

4 *For a small-bore tube:* Put on clean gloves. Ensure that recent radiology has confirmed the tube's proper gastric position. Signs of a tube's retrograde migration include choking and patient complaints of something in the esophagus. Indirect measurements of proper tube position used with large-bore tubes are unreliable with small-bore tubes. Attach the medication syringe, and then infuse the medication by applying gentle pressure on the piston. Remove the syringe and cap the nasogastric tube. Aspirate approximately 10 mL tap water. Uncap the tube, reattach the syringe, and instill the tap water (as shown) using gentle pressure. Instilling water will ensure that none of the medication adheres to the tube's lumen.

5 When you have completed the instillation, close the tube by inserting the tube plug. Place the client in high-Fowler's or a slightly elevated right side-lying position, as shown, to facilitate absorption of the medication. Clean and return the syringe to the client's bedside. Finally, chart the medication and record the amount of instillation on the client's intake and output (I&O) record, if appropriate.

PERFORMING A VAGINAL IRRIGATION (DOUCHE)

Vaginal irrigations are prescribed for preoperative cleansing (for example, with a povidone-iodine solution), for soothing inflamed vaginal mucosa, and for applying heat or medications to the vaginal mucosa and cervix. They are contraindicated in late pregnancy and during postpartum and menstruation. Use clean technique, and wear clean gloves for your own protection unless the client has an open wound. In that case, use sterile technique to protect the client from the potential spread of infection.

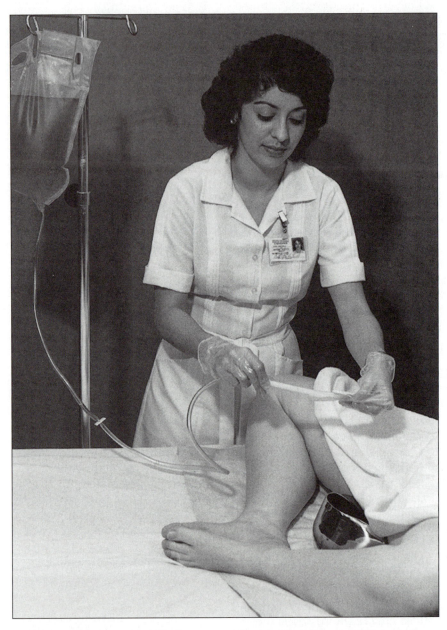

1 Prepare the prescribed solution, and check the solution's temperature with a thermometer to ensure that it is not too hot. Usually, 40.5 C (105 F) is the recommended temperature. Bring the solution and equipment to your client's room, and hang the container on an IV pole 30–45 cm (12–18 in) above the level of the client's vagina. This height will provide adequate gravity flow yet prevent the solution from entering the vagina with too great a force. Explain the procedure to the client and ask her to void if she hasn't recently done so. An empty bladder will make the procedure more comfortable and allow greater expansion of the vaginal canal. Provide privacy, and drape the client with a bath blanket or bedsheet. Assist her into a dorsal recumbent position, and place a bed-saver pad and bedpan under her buttocks. Her knees should be flexed and separated (as shown). Apply clean gloves. Remove the protective cap from the nozzle, and inspect the nozzle for cracks or other irregularities that could harm the vaginal mucosa.

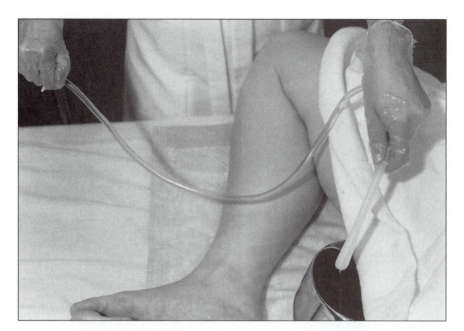

2 Direct the nozzle over the bedpan, and then open the tubing clamp to run the solution to the end of the nozzle. This will flush the tubing of air and lubricate the nozzle to facilitate its insertion into the vagina.

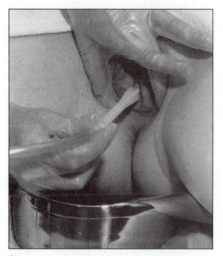

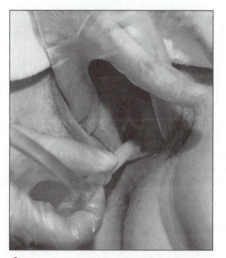

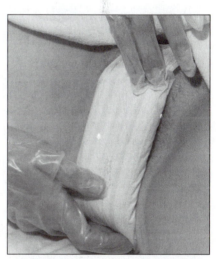

3 Separate the labia and allow the solution to flow over the external genitalia and vulva to prevent the introduction of contaminants into the vagina and uterus. Then close the clamp. *Note: If the client has copious discharge, cleanse the area with cotton balls soaked in a soapy solution. Use a fresh cotton ball for each single downward stroke.* Gently insert the nozzle into the vagina.

4 Direct the nozzle approximately 5.0–7.5 cm (2–3 in) into the vagina, angling it toward the sacrum to follow the anatomic structure of the vagina. Open the clamp again and allow the solution to flow. Unless the client has had cervical or vaginal surgery, gently rotate the nozzle to irrigate all the vaginal surfaces. When the solution has drained from the container, clamp the tubing and remove the nozzle. Then raise the head of the bed to permit the solution to drain out into the bedpan.

5 Dry the perineum with tissues, wiping from the front toward the anus. Then apply a sterile peripad to the perineum to absorb the residual solution and protect the clothing or bed linen from the irrigant. Remove the equipment from the bedside, and either dispose of it or clean it according to agency procedure.

GIVING RECTAL MEDICATIONS

INSERTING A SUPPOSITORY

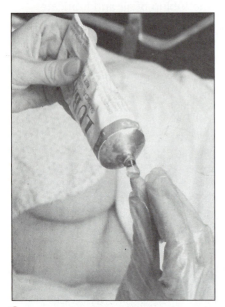 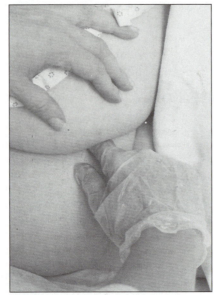 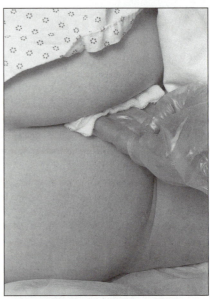

1 To insert a suppository, provide privacy and assist the client into a position in which the rectum is easily accessible, for example, a side-lying position with the upper leg flexed (Sims') as shown. Put on a clean glove, and generously lubricate the suppository with a water-soluble lubricant.

2 With your free hand, gently lift the uppermost buttock. With your index finger, guide the suppository into the anus, directing it along the rectal wall and away from fecal masses. To prevent immediate expulsion, be sure to insert the suppository beyond the internal sphincter.

3 With a tissue or gauze pad, press gently on the anus for a few moments to help the client retain the medication; then clean the rectal area with the tissue or pad. Encourage the client to retain the suppository for at least 20 minutes before using the bedpan or going to the bathroom, if it is appropriate for the suppository to be expelled.

INSTILLING OINTMENT

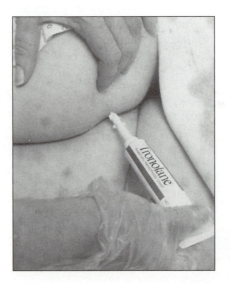

Review the preceding technique for inserting a rectal suppository. To lubricate the applicator, remove its protective cover and squeeze the tube (as shown). This will push the ointment through the small openings on the applicator and facilitate its insertion into the rectum. Insert the applicator gently to avoid injury to the rectal canal or to hemorrhoids. Squeeze the prescribed amount of ointment. Clean the rectal area with tissues, and assist your client to a comfortable position.

Administering Injectable Medications

GIVING INTRADERMAL INJECTIONS

LOCATING THE SITE

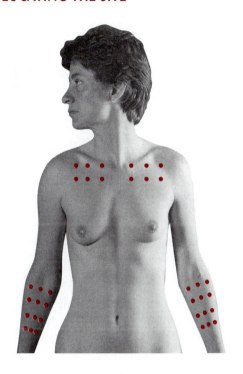

Anterior

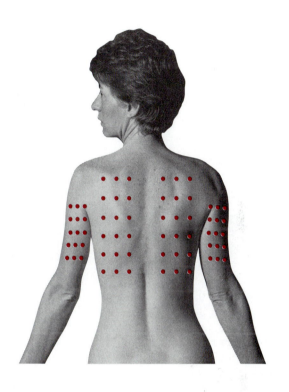

Posterior

Review these anatomic overlays to assist you in locating the proper sites for intradermal injections. The most common uses for intradermal injections are tuberculin skin testing (Mantoux test) and allergy testing.

The most frequently injected site is the ventral aspect of the forearm. To locate an appropriate injection site for this area, measure a hand's breadth from the antecubital space and a hand's breadth from the wrist. You can safely inject into the ventral area bordered by your two hands, provided the site is not scarred, covered with hair follicles, or inflamed, because these conditions would interfere with the reading.

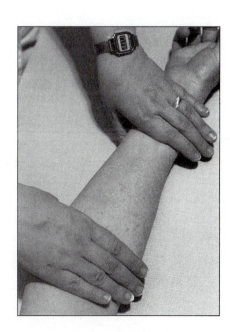

INJECTING THE MEDICATION

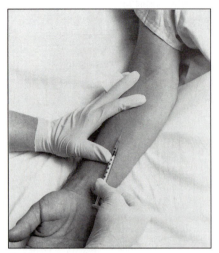 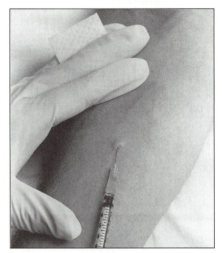

1 Wash your hands, prepare the medication, and draw it up into a tuberculin syringe that has a ⅜-inch to ⅝-inch, 26-gauge, short-beveled needle. Ask your client to sit facing you, flex the elbow, and rest the forearm on a flat surface. Prepare the skin with an alcohol sponge, starting at the injection site and working your way outward in a circular fashion to cover an area 5 cm (2 in) in diameter. Allow it to dry. With one hand, stretch the skin at the injection site between your thumb and index finger to facilitate the needle's penetration into the area just underneath the skin's surface. Hold the syringe between your thumb and index finger with the needle positioned at a 10- to 15-degree angle to the skin with the bevel up. *Note: Wear gloves if it is your agency's policy to do so.*

2 Insert the needle just under the surface of the skin, and slowly inject the medication. *Note: If the needle is inserted correctly, you should feel some resistance as you inject the medication. You might have inserted the needle too deeply if the medication can be injected too easily.* While injecting the medication, observe for the development of a wheal approximately 0.5 cm in diameter. Withdraw the needle. Do not massage the site because this could distort the eventual reading. If appropriate, closely observe the client for signs of an anaphylactic reaction to the substance that was injected. Discard the syringe and needle unit uncapped into a puncture-resistant container (see page 110). Be sure to document the type and amount of medication, the date, the exact time you administered it, and the injection site. In addition, document any reactions to the solution that was injected. Explain to the client that the reading of the test will be done in 2–3 days.

GIVING SUBCUTANEOUS INJECTIONS

LOCATING THE SITE

Review these diagrams to help you select a site for subcutaneous injection. Rotate sites for medications that are administered repeatedly, for example, insulin or heparin.

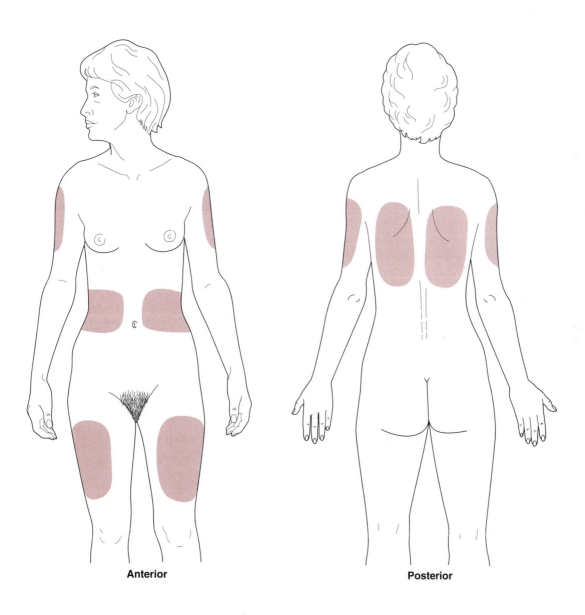

Anterior

Posterior

INJECTING THE MEDICATION

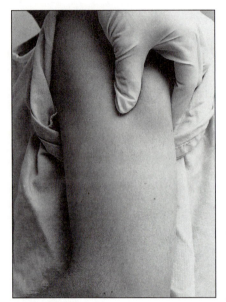 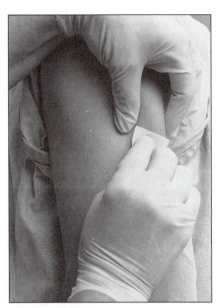 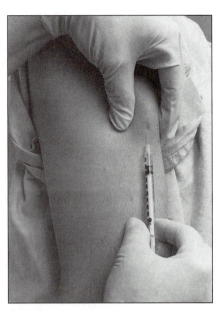

1 A subcutaneous injection is properly given into the layer of tissue that is above the muscle and below the skin and fat. To reach this layer effectively, you will need to assess each client to help determine the correct angle of insertion and, occasionally, the need for a longer or shorter needle. With a ⅝-inch needle you can usually vary the angle of insertion to penetrate the subcutaneous layer correctly. However, for very obese clients, a ⅝-inch needle may not be long enough to penetrate past the fatty layer. The same needle may be too long for children or very thin clients. Form a skin fold (as shown) to assess the amount of fat at the selected injection site and to determine the correct angle of insertion for reaching the subcutaneous tissue. If your client has an average build, a 45-degree angle is usually effective. An obese client may require a 90-degree angle, and a thin client may require an angle ranging from 15 to 45 degrees.

2 Draw up the prescribed medication into a 1- to 3-mL syringe with a 25-gauge, ⅝-inch (or the correct length) needle. The use of an air bubble (see page 106) should be determined by your agency's policy to ensure consistency in the amount of medication routinely delivered to each client. For example, if you use an air bubble and your coworker does not, the amount of medication you deliver will be slightly more than that delivered by your coworker because the air will clear the needle of medication. Consistency is especially crucial for diabetic clients receiving insulin. Prepare the site with an alcohol sponge. Start at the insertion site and work your way outward from the center in a circular fashion to cover an area 5 cm (2 in) in diameter. Allow the alcohol to dry.

3 Bunch the skin between your thumb and index finger. This will minimize your client's discomfort as the needle is inserted. Insert the needle with the bevel up, at the angle appropriate for your client.

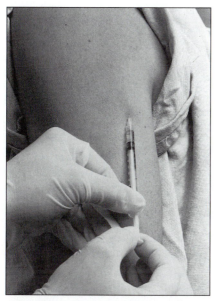
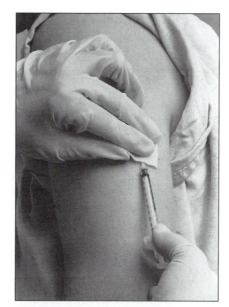

4 Release the skin and pull back on the plunger (as shown) to aspirate for blood. If you do aspirate blood, withdraw the needle because injecting a medication into a vascular area could result in a systemic reaction to the medication. Obtain a new syringe and needle, as well as new medication, and try again. When you are certain you are in a nonvascular layer of subcutaneous tissue, slowly inject the medication. ***Caution:*** *Do not aspirate if you are injecting heparin because it could cause a hematoma to form at the injection site (see next procedure).*

5 When the medication has been injected, withdraw the needle at the same angle in which it was inserted to minimize trauma to the tissues. Apply pressure with an alcohol sponge at the insertion site to avert bleeding. If massage has not been contraindicated, as it would be with heparin, it can be employed to facilitate absorption of the medication. Discard the syringe and needle unit uncapped into a puncture-resistant container (see page 110). ***Note:*** *Apply clean gloves to give injections if it is your agency's policy to do so.*

HOME HEALTH CARE CONSIDERATIONS

- Some clients may reuse syringes with the attached needles for the length of time determined by the home health agency or health care provider.

- Some health care providers do not mandate use of antiseptic wipes as long as client's skin is clean.

- Puncture-resistant containers (eg, coffee cans and detergent bottles) should be used in the home for disposing of syringes and needles. These containers can be returned to the health care agency for disposal when they are full or the client no longer requires them.

ADMINISTERING HEPARIN

Heparin is administered subcutaneously because intramuscular injection can cause hemorrhage and hematoma formation. Heparin's effects are also longer lasting when administered subcutaneously rather than via the intramuscular route.

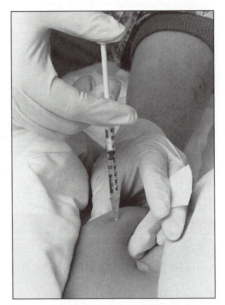

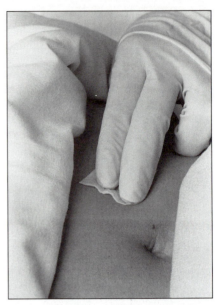

1 Use a 1-mL tuberculin syringe with a ⅝-inch, 25-gauge needle. After drawing up the prescribed amount of medication, change needles to prevent bruising or tracking through the subcutaneous tissues. Form a fat roll on the iliac or abdominal tissue by grasping the tissue gently. Avoid any areas that are bruised, and avoid needle insertion within 5 cm (2 in) of the umbilicus or any scar. Cleanse the site gently with an alcohol swab. Then insert the needle at a 90-degree angle, as shown, into the elevated fatty tissue. Reduce finger pressure on the tissue slightly and slowly inject the heparin. *Note: Apply clean gloves if it is your agency's policy to do so.*

2 When the medication has been injected, withdraw the needle at the angle at which it entered the tissue, releasing the skin roll as you do to minimize tissue damage. Press an alcohol swab over the injection site for 2–3 minutes to prevent oozing or bruising. ***Caution:*** *Do not massage the injection site, as this could damage the tissue.* To prevent hematoma formation, rotate injection sites with each administration of heparin. Document the medication and the site used.

GIVING INTRAMUSCULAR (IM) INJECTIONS

MAPPING MUSCLE SITES FOR IM INJECTIONS

Dorsal Gluteal

1 Review this anatomic overlay of the posterior gluteal (dorsal gluteal) area to assist you in locating the correct site for IM injections. Although this site is commonly used, extreme caution must be employed to avoid the sciatic nerve and gluteal artery. Notice that the nerve and trunk of the artery are distal to the diagonal line that extends from the posterior superior iliac spine to the greater trochanter of the femur. *Caution: Do not use this site for children under the age of 2 who have not been walking long enough to have developed adequate musculature. This site also may be contraindicated for the older adult or immobile client whose gluteal muscle could be deteriorated.*

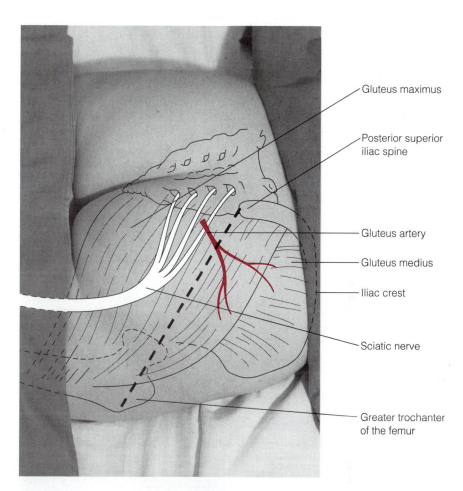

Gluteus maximus

Posterior superior iliac spine

Gluteus artery

Gluteus medius

Iliac crest

Sciatic nerve

Greater trochanter of the femur

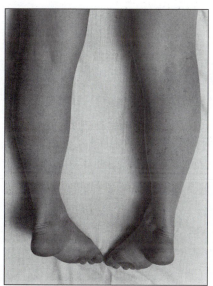

2 Ask the client to assume a prone, toe-in position. Internal rotation of the hips will relax the muscle and make the injection less painful.

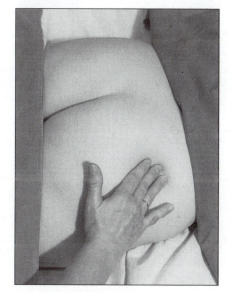

3 Although it is essential that you provide the client with as much privacy as possible, you must fully expose the buttocks to ensure complete visualization of the anatomic landmarks. Also, inspect and palpate the skin and tissue to assess for edema, fibrous areas, nodules, lesions, or draining wounds, which could either prevent adequate absorption or promote the spread of infection. *Note: Explain to the client what you are doing so that you do not cause unnecessary alarm.*

➤

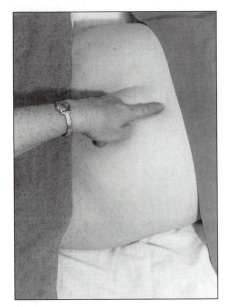

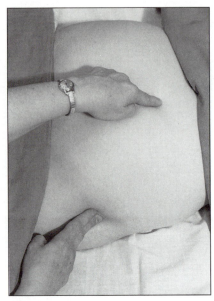

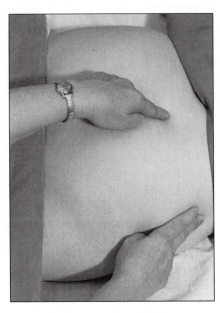

4 If the tissue is healthy, inspect and palpate the anatomic landmarks. Locate the posterior superior iliac spine. On many clients, this landmark can be identified as a dimpled area in the skin. It also can be palpated as a bony ridge approximately 2.5–5.0 cm (1–2 in) lateral and slightly superior to the separation between the buttocks.

5 Locate the greater trochanter of the femur. You can locate this site visually on most clients by following the lower curve of the buttock outward toward the lateral hip. You can also palpate the indentation at the hip where the hip and thigh join. The greater trochanter is just distal to the indentation.

Note: *If you are still unable to locate the landmark, press and slide your fingers from the waistline (as shown) downward until you feel the indentation.*

6 The diagonal line that extends from the posterior superior iliac spine toward the greater trochanter of the femur, and the horizontal line extending from the posterior superior iliac spine to the lateral hip two fingers' breadth below the iliac crest, form the boundary for the area that is safe for IM injections.

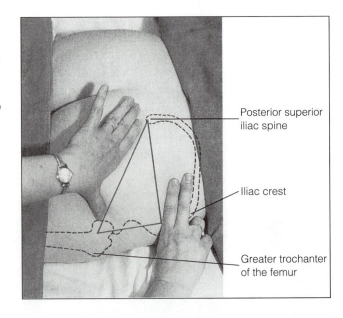

Posterior superior iliac spine

Iliac crest

Greater trochanter of the femur

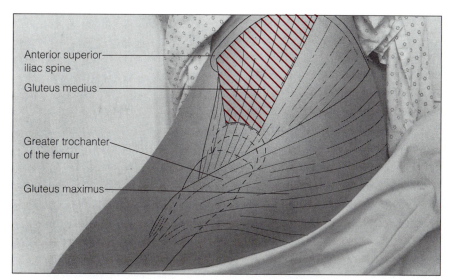

Anterior superior iliac spine

Gluteus medius

Greater trochanter of the femur

Gluteus maximus

Ventrogluteal

1 Review this anatomic overlay of the ventrogluteal area of the hip to assist you in locating the correct site for IM injections. Note that compared to the dorsal gluteal area, it is free of major nerves and blood vessels, and it is farther from the rectum, minimizing the risk of contamination. In addition, it has a dense muscle and minimal fat.

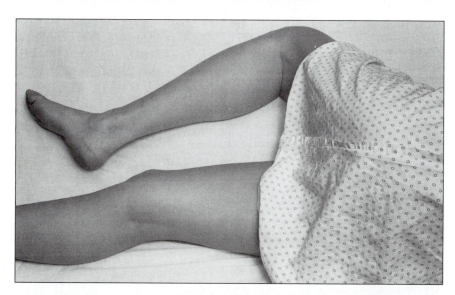

2 Although the client can be supine or prone for injections into this site, a side-lying position with the upper leg flexed and in front of the lower leg (as shown) will better expose the anatomic landmarks and relax the gluteal muscle.

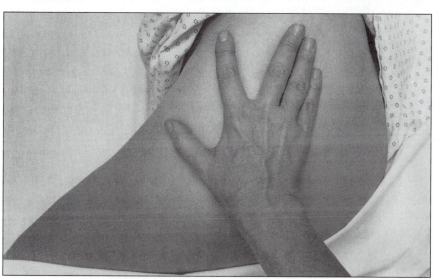

3 To inject the medication into the client's left hip (as shown), place your right palm over the greater trochanter (or use your left hand on the client's right hip). Position your index finger on the anterior superior iliac spine and form a "V" by placing your middle finger along the iliac crest. You may safely inject the medication into the center of the "V." Spread the tissue and angle the needle slightly, toward the client's head.

Vastus Lateralis

1 Review this anatomic overlay of the anterior lateral aspect of the thigh to locate the vastus lateralis muscle. This site is also free of major nerves and blood vessels, and it is usually well developed in both adults and children.

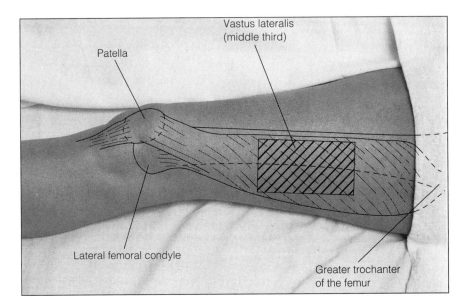

Patella

Vastus lateralis (middle third)

Lateral femoral condyle

Greater trochanter of the femur

2 The preferred position for your client is supine with the hip internally rotated (toes pointing toward the midline) to better expose the lateral aspect of the thigh. The site then may be divided into thirds, beginning at the greater trochanter of the femur to the lateral femoral condyles at the knee. The middle third is the correct area. You may also measure a hand's breadth above the knee (as shown) and select the site central to this boundary.

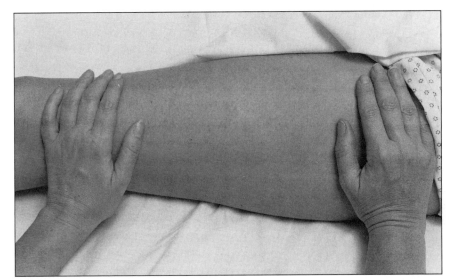

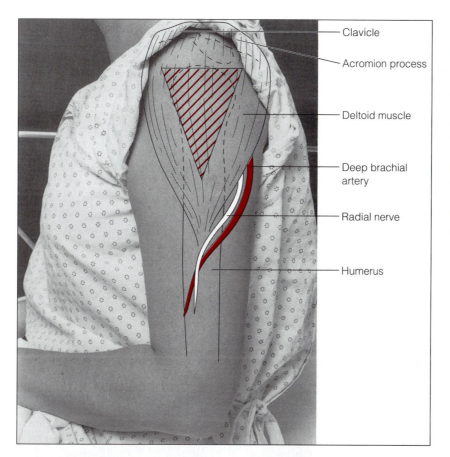

Clavicle

Acromion process

Deltoid muscle

Deep brachial artery

Radial nerve

Humerus

Mid-Deltoid

1 Review this anatomic overlay of the lateral aspect of the upper arm to help you locate the mid-deltoid area. Although an advantage of this site is its easy access, the deltoid muscle covers a relatively small area, and it is close to major bones, nerves, and arteries. In addition, this muscle cannot tolerate frequent injections or large doses of medication (not more than 1 mL in the average-sized adult). Thus, you should limit your injections into this muscle to adults and teenagers with well-developed muscle mass.

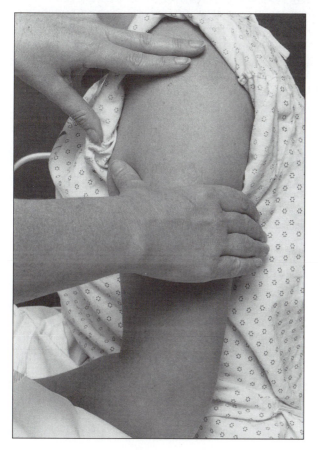

2 The client may sit, stand, or lie down to receive an injection in the mid-deltoid area, but it is important for the elbow to be flexed and supported so that the deltoid muscle can be relaxed. To map the muscle, locate the lower edge of the acromion process with one hand and then identify the area on the lateral aspect of the upper arm that is in a line with the axilla (as shown). Be certain that the gown or clothing does not interfere with your visualization of the site. The mid-deltoid muscle is bounded by an imaginary triangle that can be envisioned between the two hands (review top photo).

PROVIDING AN AIR LOCK

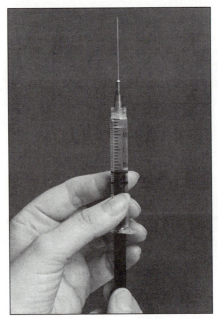

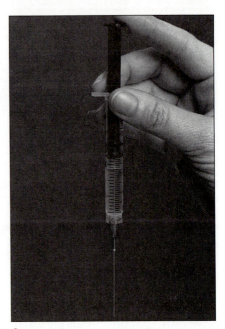

1 An air lock is used with an IM injection when the medication may be potentially harmful to the subcutaneous tissue. A bolus of air follows the administration of the medication to ensure that all the solution is ejected from the needle, thereby preventing tracking of the medication into the subcutaneous tissue after the needle has been withdrawn. After drawing up the prescribed amount of medication (and changing the needle, if appropriate), pull back on the plunger to aspirate approximately 0.5–1.0 mL of air into the syringe. Point the needle toward the ceiling (as shown) and expel all except 0.2–0.5 mL of air. The required amount of air will depend on the length and gauge of the needle. A 21-gauge, 1½-inch needle, for example, will require 0.2–0.3 mL of air to provide an effective air lock.

2 Note that the air rises to the top of the barrel when the syringe is held perpendicular to the floor. If the syringe were positioned parallel to the floor, for example, to inject the mid-deltoid area with the client sitting, the air bubble would move to the side of the syringe and become ineffectual. So if you wish to use an air lock for ventrogluteal or deltoid sites, the client must be side-lying. Similarly, a prone position is necessary for dorsal gluteal injections, and supine or sitting positions are required for injections into the vastus lateralis muscle. *Note: Air locks are usually contraindicated for the pediatric population.*

INJECTING THE MEDICATION

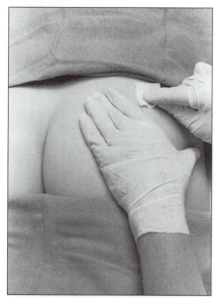

1 After you have prepared the medication, identified the client, and selected the appropriate injection site, prepare the skin with an alcohol sponge. Start at the proposed injection site and work your way outward from the center in a circular motion. Be sure to cover an area at least 5 cm (2 in) in diameter. Allow the alcohol to dry.
***Note:** Wear clean gloves, if it is your agency's policy to do so.*

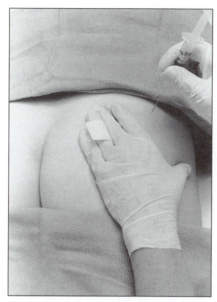

2 Spread the tissue between your thumb and index finger to make the skin taut, and then insert the needle in a quick dartlike motion. It is helpful to hold an alcohol swab between your middle fingers so that it is readily available after the needle has been withdrawn.
***Note:** For children and thin adults it may be necessary to bunch the tissue when injecting into the mid-deltoid area or vastus lateralis muscle.*

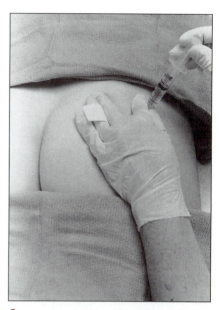

3 Support the barrel with your nondominant hand and pull back on the plunger with your dominant hand to aspirate for blood. If blood is aspirated, withdraw the needle and replace the syringe, needle, and medication.

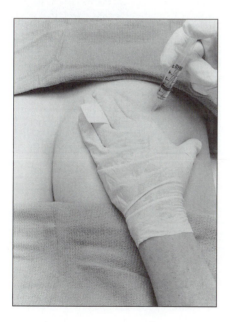

4 Inject the medication slowly to minimize your client's discomfort and distribute the solution evenly. Then, withdraw the needle, place the alcohol swab at the injection site, and apply pressure. This will minimize the chance for the medication to seep into the subcutaneous tissues. If rapid absorption is desired, massage the site for 1–2 minutes with the swab.
***Note:** To minimize trauma to the tissues, withdraw the needle at the same angle at which it was inserted.* Discard the syringe and needle unit into a puncture-resistant container (see page 110). Remove and discard your gloves and wash your hands. Finally, document the procedure and the site that you used.

PERFORMING THE Z-TRACK TECHNIQUE

Z-track injections are indicated when complete absorption of the medication is crucial or when medications such as iron preparations may seep into the injection track and stain the skin or surrounding tissues. Some agencies require the Z-track method for all injections into the gluteal muscle. The tissue is displaced downward and toward the median before, during, and after the injection so that when the tissue is released, the needle track that normally would have formed becomes instead a broken, non-continuous line. This method keeps the medication deep in the muscle by preventing its seepage up through the tissues.

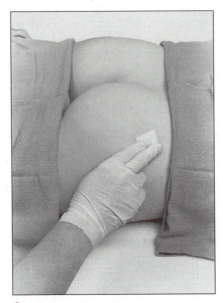

1 Draw up the medication, and then change the needle to one that is at least 5 cm (2 in) long (for the average adult). Because you will need to inject deeply to reach the muscle, the size of the needle will depend on the size of the client. Draw up a 0.5-mL air bubble (or larger, depending of the length and gauge of the needle). This will enable you to clear all the medication from the needle as well as eject the residual medication from the needle's end to prevent tracking the solution as the needle is withdrawn. Now you are ready to prepare the site with an alcohol sponge (as shown). Prepare the skin before displacing the tissue because it is difficult to maintain the required traction on the tissue for the length of time it takes for the alcohol to dry. Cleanse an area that is at least 10 cm (4 in) in diameter to ensure that you will have covered the injection site. *Note: Wear clean gloves if it is your agency's policy to do so.*

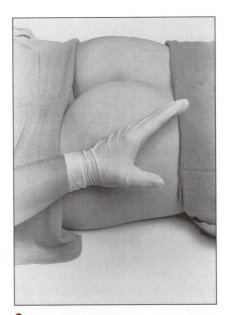

2 After preparing the skin, place the ulnar side of your nondominant hand along the diagonal that extends from the posterior superior iliac spine to the greater trochanter of the femur.

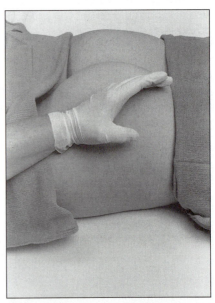

3 Displace the tissue downward and toward the median as far as you can and yet comfortably maintain the traction on the tissue.

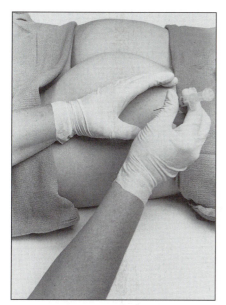

4 Continue to displace the tissue as you insert the needle.

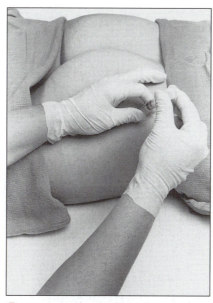

5 Carefully extend the thumb and forefinger of the hand that is displacing the issue to support the base of the syringe. Aspirate with your other hand. ***Note:*** *Do not release the traction on the tissue.*

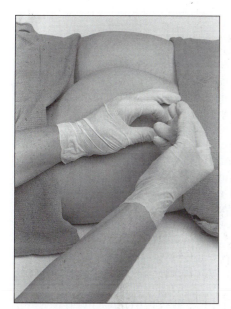

6 Continue to maintain the traction on the tissue as you slowly inject the medication. When you have competed the injection, wait 10 seconds to provide the necessary time for the medication to disperse into the muscle and to give the muscle time to relax after having been stimulated by the needle and medication.

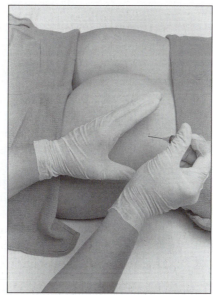

7 After waiting 10 seconds, remove the needle and immediately lift your other hand to release the tissue. Do not massage the injection site, and advise your client not to exercise or wear tight clothing following the injection. This will minimize the chance for the medication to spread into other layers of tissue. Discard the syringe and needle unit uncapped into a puncture-resistant container (see page 110). Then, remove and discard your gloves, wash your hands, and document the procedure.

DISPOSING OF NEEDLES AND SHARP INSTRUMENTS

As often as possible, place puncture-resistant containers in all work areas for the disposal of nonreusable needle-syringe units, scalpel blades, and other sharp items. These containers are intended for the disposal of needle-syringe units that are uncapped and unbroken (as shown).

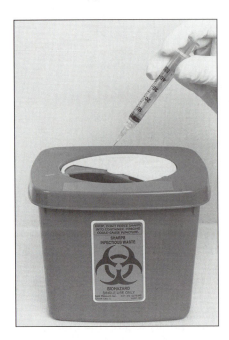

NURSING GUIDELINES: MANAGING INSULIN PUMPS

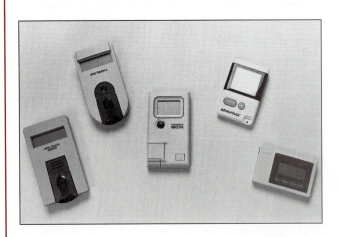

1 An insulin pump is a computerized device that delivers a constant insulin infusion throughout the day and night (called the basal delivery), with the capability of administering boluses manually at specified times, for example just prior to meals.

Thus, unlike conventional insulin therapy, which relies on single or multiple daily injections, the insulin pump acts more like the client's own pancreas. However, unlike the pancreas, an insulin pump can respond to the client's programming, based on frequent self-monitoring of blood glucose. There are several pumps available to the diabetic client, and each varies in method of operation and programming. Each pump has batteries, a syringe, a programmable computer, and a motor and drive mechanism. Buffered or Humulin R (short-acting) insulin is used, and it is contained by the syringe that inserts directly into the pump. A 60 or 105 cm (24 or 42 in) length of plastic tubing attaches on one end to the syringe, and at the other end to a 27-gauge needle or softset catheter that is inserted into the subcutaneous tissue. The client may attach the pump to a leather belt, fabric belt, or shoulder strap or carry it in a purse or pocket.

NURSING GUIDELINES: MANAGING INSULIN PUMPS

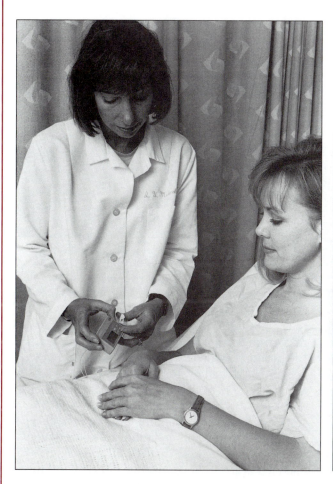

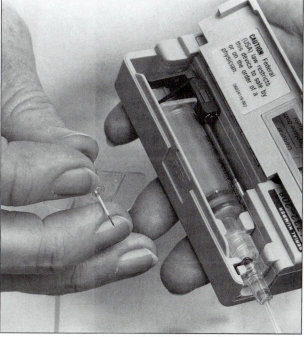

2 If the physician decides that your client is a good candidate for insulin-pump therapy, it may be your responsibility to explain the operational principles of the pump (each pump has a detailed manufacturer's manual, and sales representatives are also available to assist you). You might also need to reinforce the client's knowledge about dietary management and review self-monitoring of blood glucose (see pages 142–143). Initially, the basal rate and the meal boluses will be regulated by the physician, based on blood glucose measurements. Frequent testing of the blood glucose must be performed, and it should become a part of the daily regimen of every client with an insulin pump. It is the client's best assessment tool for measuring the effectiveness of diabetes management.

3 To ensure a proper flow rate, instruct the client to use only the syringe and tubing supplied by the manufacturer. It is also important to check the tubing periodically for kinks. With some pumps, the tubing may be primed manually; with others, the tubing is primed automatically by programming the pump. In either case, the syringe is routinely changed every 48 hours. Most pumps have alarms that alert the user to a low battery, kinked tubing, or an empty syringe.

➤

NURSING GUIDELINES: MANAGING INSULIN PUMPS (continued)

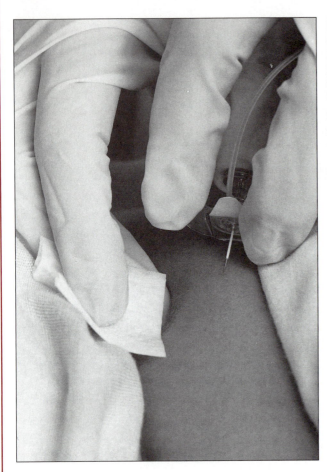

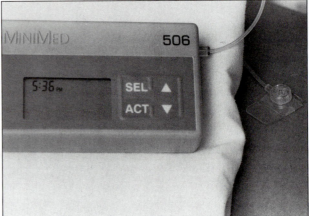

4 Rotate the sites for needle insertion as you would for conventional insulin therapy. However, because the needle or catheter will be indwelling, the choice for a potential site is limited by the length of the plastic tubing, the style and fit of the clothing, and the client's personal preference. Most clients choose the abdomen as an insertion site, but others occasionally use the upper thigh, hips, and arms. Apply clean gloves. Prepare the skin with an alcohol sponge, and insert the straight or bent needle at a 45-degree angle. Or, insert the softset catheter (shown) at a 90-degree angle. After inserting the softset catheter, withdraw the needle, leaving the catheter in place. If desired, povidone-iodine ointment may be applied to the insertion site.

5 Secure the catheter's self-adhering wings to your client's abdomen as shown. The needle or catheter can be reinforced with strips of hypoallergenic tape. A 10-cm (4-in) loop of tubing just proximal to the needle is also taped to minimize the traction on the catheter. Encourage the client to check the needle periodically to ensure that it has not become dislodged or disconnected from the tubing. With proper care, the same needle or catheter may be left indwelling for as long as 72 hours for some adult clients, depending on infusion set type and physician recommendation. However, it generally is recommended that the infusion set be changed every 48 hours to reduce the risk of infection, skin irritation, changes in the absorption of insulin, and infusion set obstruction. At the first sign of inflammation, the client should change both the site and the needle or catheter. With the physician, establish the protocol for intervention during insulin shock (hypoglycemia) and acute hyperglycemia. In most cases, you will treat the hypoglycemia—for example, by giving orange juice, dextrose, or sugar—rather than altering or discontinuing the pump.

Administering Intravenous Fluids and Medications

PREPARING THE SOLUTION AND INFUSION SET

INSPECTING THE CONTAINER

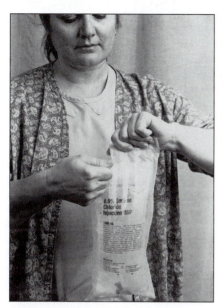 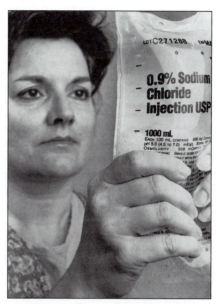

1 Wash your hands. Inspect the label on the container to ensure that the solution and amount match the physician's prescription and that the date for usage has not expired. Remove the plastic container from its overwrap by tearing along the perforated edge.

2 Hold the container against a light source and observe for discoloration, cloudiness, particulate matter, and tears in the plastic. Then, gently squeeze the bag and observe for leakage. Any irregularities, including leakage, necessitate replacement. *Note: If using a glass container, inspect in the same manner, but also be alert to cracks in the glass.*

ASSEMBLING THE INFUSION SET

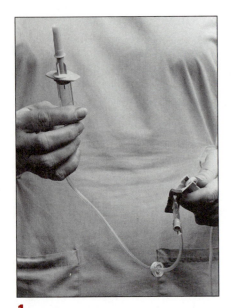

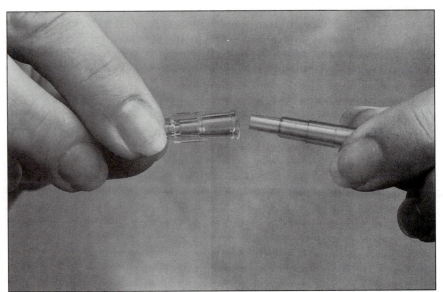

1 Inspect the package that contains the infusion set to ensure that it is intact, and then remove the tubing. If possible, slide the roller clamp directly under the drip chamber. If the tubing has a backcheck valve for the administration of piggyback fluids (as shown), slide the roller clamp up under the backcheck valve. By sliding the clamp up as high as possible, you will have quick access to the clamp for controlling the drip rate, and it will enable you to adjust the rate while closely monitoring the drip chamber. Then close the roller clamp.

2 If you want to allow the client more mobility or to provide extra ports for the administration of medication, you can attach extension tubing to the distal end of the IV tubing. Then close its clamp. Ensure that all connections are securely attached.

SPIKING THE CONTAINER

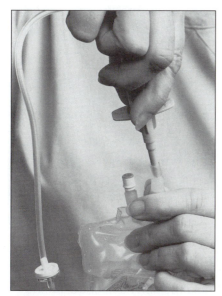

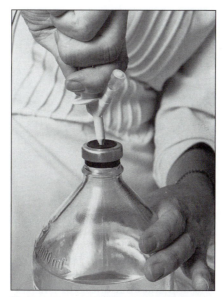

1 To spike a plastic container, hold the neck securely and remove the protective cap from the spiking port. Then slide the spike through the port. With plastic containers, nonvented tubing is used.

2 To spike a bottle, place the container on a flat, secure surface. Remove the protective cap from the spike on the infusion set, squeeze the drip chamber, and insert the spike into the rubber port of the glass container. Vented tubing, such as shown above, is more often used with glass containers unless the container itself has a vent.

PRIMING THE INFUSION SET

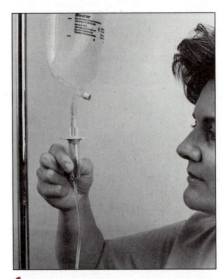

1 Hang the solution on an IV pole and, prior to opening the clamps and priming the tubing, squeeze the drip chamber and prime it with solution to the half-full line. This will minimize the formation of air bubbles in the tubing when you prime the tubing.

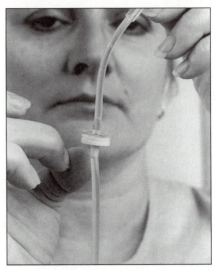

2 Open the clamps and let the solution flow to the end of the tubing to clear it of air. As you do this, hold the distal end of the tubing over a waste container or emesis basin. If the tubing has a back-check valve (as shown), invert the valve as you prime the tubing and snap it lightly to disintegrate the bubbles. Reclamp the tubing and perform a venipuncture, or attach the primed tubing to the indwelling needle or catheter.

LABELING THE TUBING AND CONTAINER

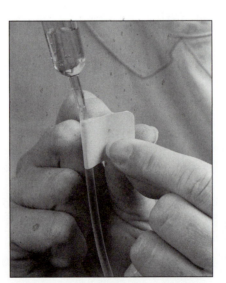

1 Attach a tape tab to the proximal end of the IV tubing, documenting the time and date the solution was hung. Change the tubing according to agency policy.

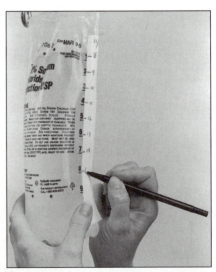

2 Label the bag with the time and date it was hung. The container should be replaced with a fresh one according to agency policy. Attach a timing label to enable you to gauge carefully the number of milliliters that must be infused hourly.

INSERTING A PERIPHERAL VASCULAR ACCESS DEVICE

ASSEMBLING THE MATERIALS

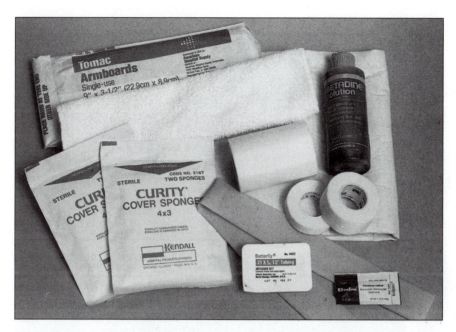

Before selecting the puncture site and assembling the materials, determine whether the client will receive short-term or long-term therapy, and note the viscosity of the prescribed solution. Clients with faster running infusions, viscous solutions, and presurgical and obstetric clients who may require blood transfusions all will require the use of larger needles, and hence, larger veins. Smaller wing-tipped needles are more often used for short-term therapy, children, older clients, or for clients with small, fragile veins. To insert a peripheral vascular access device, assemble the following materials (or variations thereof), depending on agency routine:

- ☐ sterile gauze pads
- ☐ tourniquet
- ☐ air-occlusive 7.5-cm (3-in) tape
- ☐ 1.25-cm (½-in) tape
- ☐ 2.5-cm (1-in) tape
- ☐ bed-saver pad
- ☐ antimicrobial ointment (depending on agency policy) such as povidone-iodine
- ☐ antimicrobial skin preparation such as povidone-iodine
- ☐ the appropriate needle (we have chosen a wing-tipped needle for this procedure)
- ☐ clean gloves
- ☐ arm board (optional)

CHOOSING A VENIPUNCTURE SITE

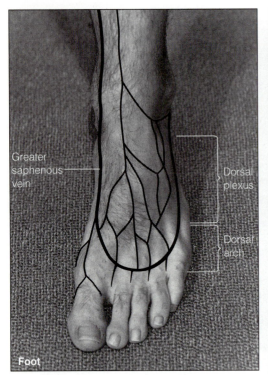

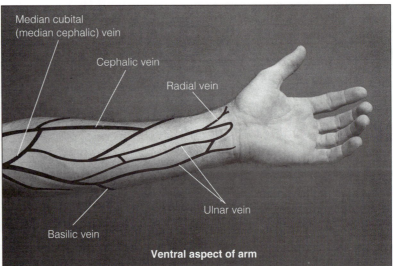

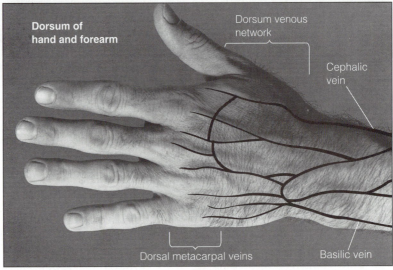

1 Review these anatomic overlays to assist you in locating the proper sites for a venipuncture.

2 Wash your hands and explain the procedure to the client. Plan to use the nondominant arm if your client will have short-term therapy. Never use an arm with an arterio-venous fistula or the involved arm for a client who has had a radical mastectomy. Begin by inspecting the median, distal basilic, and cephalic veins in your client's hand and forearm. Observe for large, superficial, full veins in a site that is neither inflamed nor irritated. Palpate the site to ensure that the vein is soft, unscarred, and rela-tively straight. Always begin at the distal end of the vein, if possible, to preserve the proximal vein for future IV sites. If you can, stay away from joints such as the wrist and elbow because needles are easily dislodged in these areas.

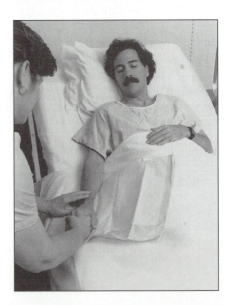

DILATING THE VEIN

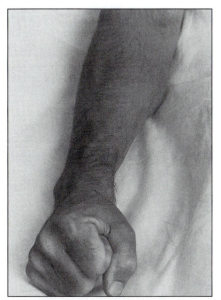

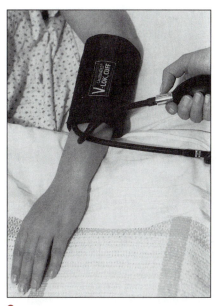

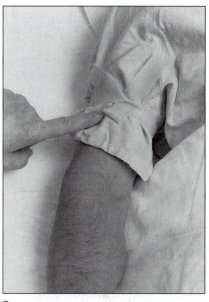

1 If the veins are not readily prominent, ask the client to open and close his fist. You may also apply manual pressure by wrapping your hands around the area just proximal to the potential insertion site and squeezing moderately to help dilate the vein. Applying hot, moist towels around the insertion site is also effective for many clients.

2 *Note: If you still have difficulty palpating the veins, wrap a blood pressure cuff below the antecubital fossa and inflate it to just below your client's systolic pressure (usually around 100 mm Hg). Deflate the cuff after palpating the veins. If you plan to use the cuff instead of a tourniquet to dilate the veins, deflate it to 40 mm Hg after having dilated the veins.*

3 When you have selected a viable site, wrap a tourniquet a few inches above it. To prevent pinching the skin, position the tourniquet over an article of clothing such as the sleeve of the hospital gown. The tourniquet should be tight enough to impede venous flow, but not so tight that it occludes the arteries. You should still be able to palpate an arterial pulse distal to the tourniquet.

PREPARING THE SITE

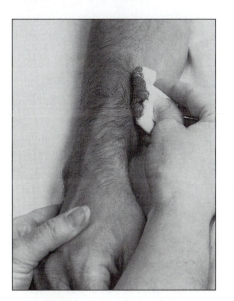

Prepare the insertion site by swabbing the skin with an antimicrobial solution such as povidone-iodine or 70% isopropyl alcohol. Apply the solution directly to the center of the site with a sterile applicator such as a gauze pad. Prepare the surrounding skin using a circular motion and working outward to cover an area at least 5 cm (2 in) in diameter. Allow the solution to dry thoroughly (at least 30 seconds) before inserting the needle.

INSERTING A WING-TIPPED NEEDLE

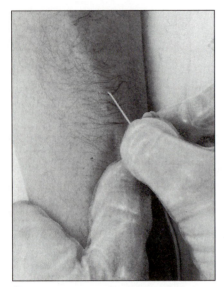

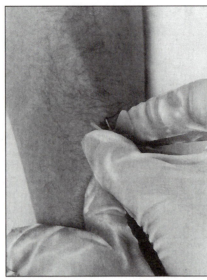

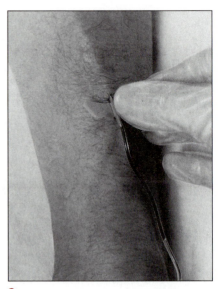

1 Wash your hands and apply gloves. With your free thumb, stabilize and anchor the vein distal to the insertion site. Ask the client to sustain a fist if his vein is not prominent. With the needle's bevel up, squeeze the wings together and position the needle at a 30- to 40-degree angle over the vein.

2 As you pierce the skin and enter the vein, decrease the angle to around 15 degrees. Advance the needle into the vein and continue to decrease the angle of the needle until it is parallel to your client's skin. You will feel a release or gentle pop as the needle enters the vein. Then ask your client to open his fist. Release the tourniquet.

3 In most instances if you have inserted the needle properly, you will see a backflow of blood in the tubing. To prime the needle's tubing, allow the blood to fill its entire length. If the venipuncture has been unsuccessful, withdraw the needle; insert a new, sterile needle; and attempt the venipuncture again proximal to the initial site or in another vein.

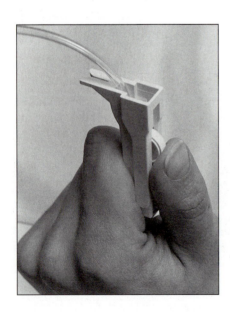

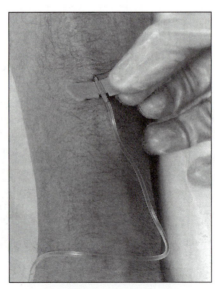

4 If the needle is to be used for the infusion of IV fluids, carefully attach the adapter of the primed infusion tubing to the needle's connector; slowly open the roller clamp (left) to start the infusion. Observe the drip chamber for an easy flow and inspect the insertion site for the presence of swelling, which would occur if the needle were positioned improperly. When you are certain that the venipuncture has been successful, decrease the flow and prepare to tape the needle and tubing.

TAPING THE WING-TIPPED NEEDLE

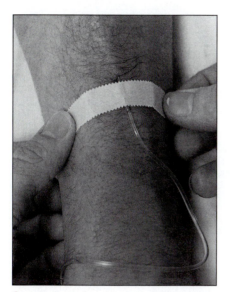

1 We recommend the following method for taping the wing-tipped needle. Cut three 7.5-cm (3-in) strips of 1.25-cm (½-in) tape. Place the first strip directly over the wings of the needle.

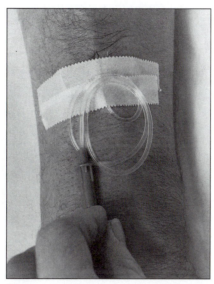

2 Attach the second strip of tape over the distal edge of the first strip. Then loop the tubing.

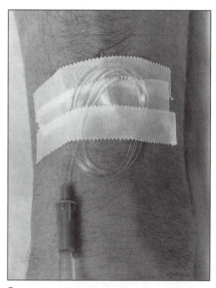

3 Place the third strip of tape over the looped tubing. Remember to keep the connector hub exposed so that you will have access to it for changing the tubing, for example, or for attaching an adapter plug.

INSERTING AN OVER-THE-NEEDLE CATHETER

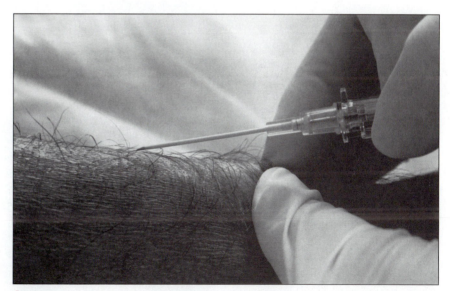

1 Review the preceding steps for preparing the skin and inserting a wing-tipped needle. Position the tip of the over-the-needle catheter over the selected vein at a 30- to 40-degree angle to the skin. With your free thumb, firmly anchor the vein distal to the insertion site.

2 As you pierce the skin, reduce the angle of the needle to around 15 degrees. Advance the catheter into the vein, reducing the angle as you do until the needle is parallel to the skin. Continue to insert the needle until you see a flash of blood in the chamber distal to the needle (as shown).

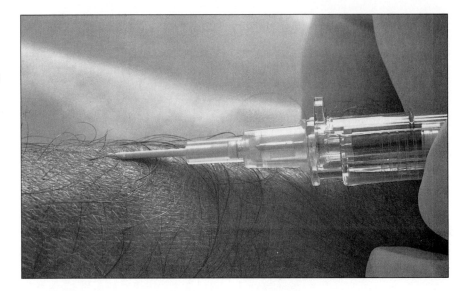

3 Slide the needle guard forward (left hand in photo) until the catheter hub is flush with the skin. Simultaneously hold the ribbed needle housing unit (shown in right hand in photo).

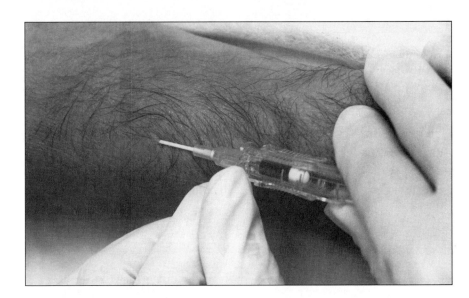

4 When the catheter hub is flush with the skin, gently pull back on the needle housing unit until the needle is enclosed completely (signified by a "click" with the product shown here). This is a safety feature to reduce the risk of puncture injury to the nurse.

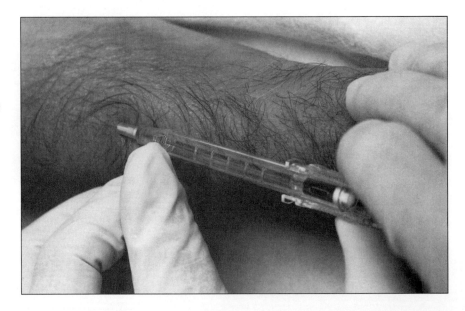

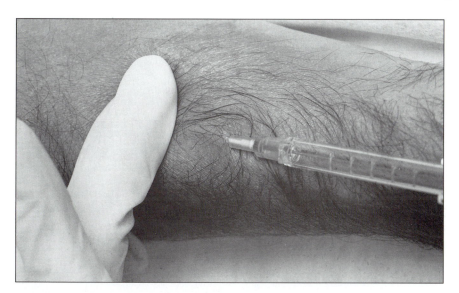

5 Occlude the vein proximal to the insertion site by pressing lightly with your finger. This will prevent backflow of blood once the needle is removed.

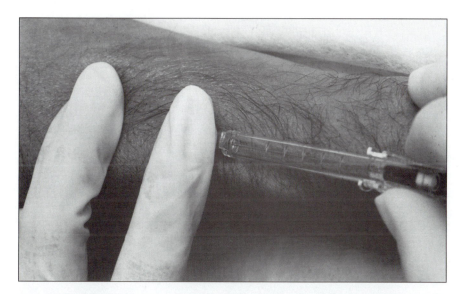

6 Hold gentle pressure on the hub of the catheter (left) as you gently twist and withdraw the sheathed needle (bottom).

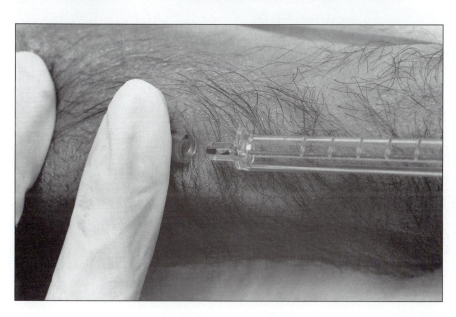

➜

7 After removing the sheathed needle, attach the distal end of the primed infusing tubing (as shown). Open the roller clamp and observe for an easy flow of solution into the drip chamber. To double-check, you also can apply pressure to the vein just proximal to the insertion site. If the dripping stops in the drip chamber at this time, you can be quite certain that the vein is patent and the needle has been positioned properly.

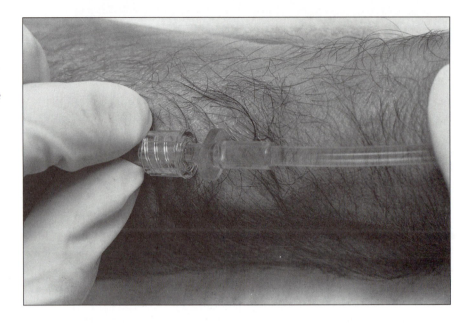

TAPING THE OVER-THE-NEEDLE CATHETER

1 An effective way to tape the over-the-needle catheter is to employ the "U" method. To do this, you will need three 7.5-cm (3-in) strips of 1.25-cm (½-in) tape. Place the first strip sticky side up under the needle's hub. Fold the end over (as shown) so that the sticky side adheres to the skin.

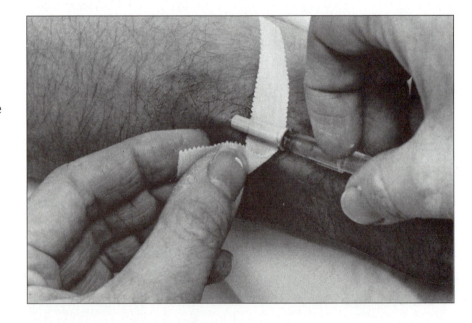

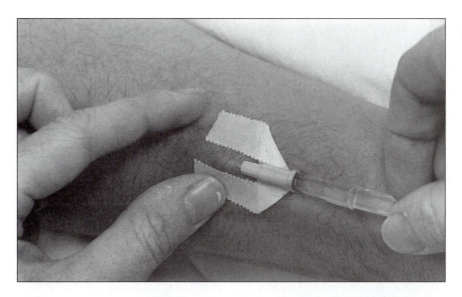

2 Fold the opposite end over and up in the same manner.

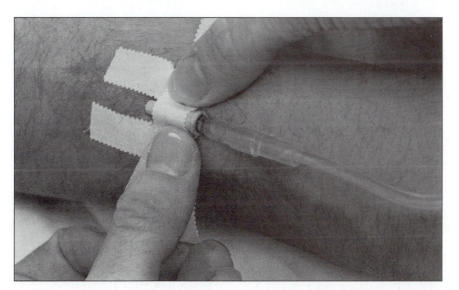

3 Place a second strip of tape sticky side down over the needle's hub.

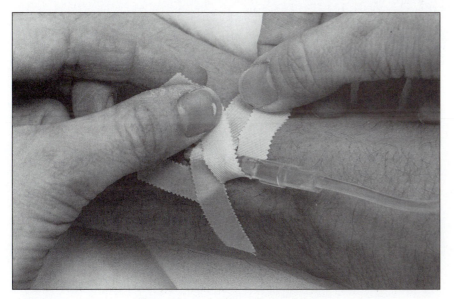

4 Place the third strip of tape sticky side up under the catheter hub and distal to the second strip. Then fold it diagonally across the hub sticky side down (as shown). Do the same for the opposite side of the tape.

APPLYING ANTIMICROBIAL OINTMENT AND A GAUZE DRESSING

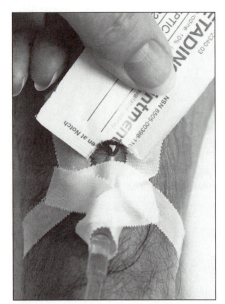 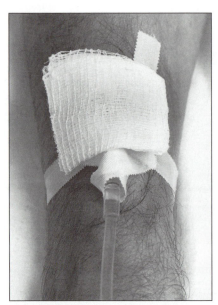 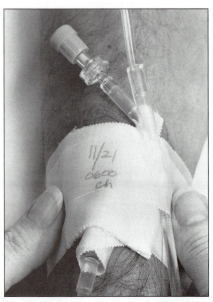

1 If antimicrobial ointment is used by your agency, apply a small amount directly to the taped insertion site.

2 Cover the area with a sterile gauze pad and tape securely. *Note: Dressings are often avoided in the neonate to ensure better site observation. Transparent sterile dressings, such as Op-Site, are also used. These dressings allow close observation of the insertion site without the removal of the dressing.*

3 Loop the tubing over the tape. Secure it with a 2.5-cm (1-in) strip of tape on which you have written the time and date and your initials. At least daily, gently palpate the insertion site through the dressing to assess for tenderness. If the client has tenderness at the insertion site or an unexplained fever, you must visually inspect the site for redness or discharge. The needle or catheter should be changed at least every 72 hours unless another peripheral insertion site cannot be found at that time.

IMMOBILIZING THE EXTREMITY

USING AN ARMBOARD OR SPLINT

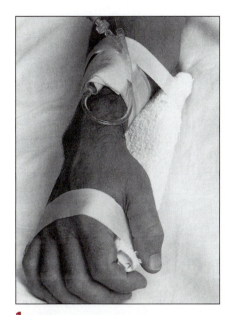

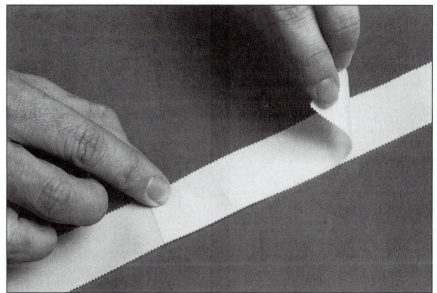

1 When a client is disoriented or combative, or when the venipuncture site is at or near a joint such as the wrist or elbow, you will need to splint the extremity to prevent the needle or catheter from dislodging. For your client's comfort, be sure to pad the armboard or splint with a small towel or washcloth. A short splint usually will be adequate if the venipuncture site is in the lower arm or hand, but use a long splint if the site is near the antecubital fossa. The hand should be prone (as shown) and well supported by the splint if the needle is in the hand or wrist. However, the fingers should be free to both extend and flex around the armboard.

2 Secure the splint to the arm with two or three tape strips. To make a tape strip, you will need two pieces of tape of equal widths. Tear one piece long enough to encircle the arm and splint. The shorter piece should be just long enough to face the longer piece over the area that would otherwise cover the skin. Place the shorter piece of tape in the center of the longer piece with the sticky surfaces together (as shown). Then wrap the tape strip snugly around the arm and the splint. Be certain, however, that you do not impede circulation. Monitor the client frequently to ensure that color, sensation, and pulses are normal in the hand and arm.

APPLYING A COMMERCIAL WRIST RESTRAINT

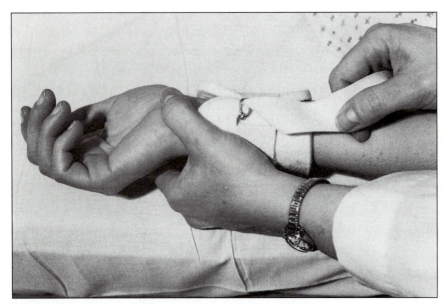 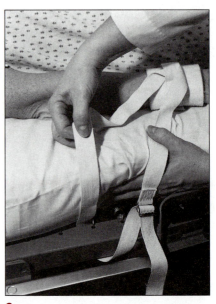

1 If you have a physician's prescription (a prescription may not be necessary for the pediatric population), you can restrain the wrist of a disoriented or combative client who might dislodge the needle or catheter in the opposite arm. Wrap a commercial restraint snugly (but not tightly) around the wrist to prevent the client from pulling the hand through the opening.

2 Attach the restraint to the bed frame. ***Caution:*** *Never attach the restraint to the side rails because this could result in injury to the arm when the side rails are lowered.* Allow enough slack in the restraint to provide the client adequate range of motion yet prevent contact with the opposite arm. Because the restraint will prevent normal movement, it is essential that you remove the restraint and change your client's position every 2 hours. Provide range of motion (ROM) exercises if the client must be restrained on a long-term basis. Also, ensure that color, sensation, and pulses are normal distal to the restraint, and provide skin care, such as massages with a moisturizer, if the skin under the restraint shows any sign of irritation.

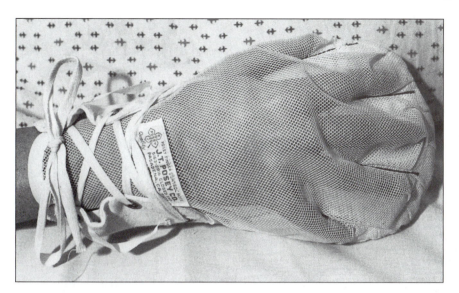

3 As an alternative, a mitt restraint may be applied to prevent the client from removing the needle or catheter in the opposite arm. Ensure that it is tied snugly but not tightly around the wrist and that it is removed at least once per shift (or according to agency protocol) to provide skin care and perform ROM exercises on the wrist and fingers.

APPLYING A GAUZE RESTRAINT

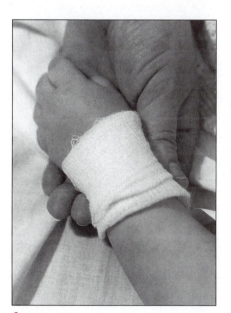

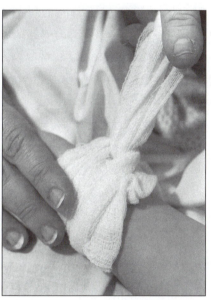

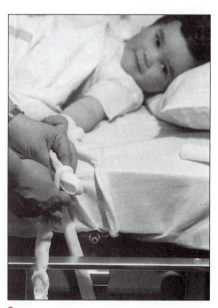

1 If commercially made restraints are unavailable, you can improvise with gauze pads and a strip of gauze roll at least 125 cm (50 in) in length. First pad around the wrist with a double thickness of gauze padding.

2 Tie the gauze roll around the gauze pad using a knot, such as a slip knot (as shown), that can be readily released in the event of an emergency.

3 Wrap the gauze roll around the bed frame (not the side rails), and tie it in a bow so that you can easily release it in an emergency. When using gauze rather than a commercial restraint, it is especially important that you monitor the client frequently for signs of neuro-vascular impairment because of the difficulty in controlling the degree of tension on the wrist. Remove the restraint every 2 hours, and ensure that color, sensation, and pulse are normal. Provide skin care as necessary.

ADMINISTERING INTRAVENOUS (IV) MEDICATIONS

INJECTING MEDICATIONS INTO HANGING IV CONTAINERS

Plastic Container

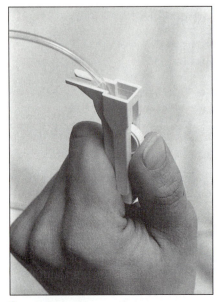

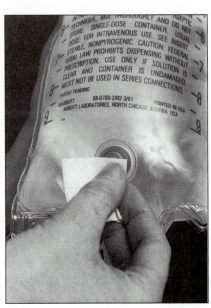

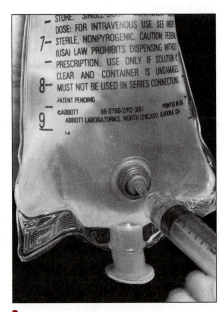

1 Prepare the prescribed medication, and close the roller clamp to stop the flow of solution. This will prevent the delivery of a medication bolus to your client.

2 Clean the injection port with an alcohol sponge (as shown).

3 Insert the needle into the injection port and inject the medication. Gently rotate the bag between your hands to mix the medication; open the roller clamp to achieve the desired rate of flow. Make a medication label, noting the type and amount of medication, the time and date you added it, and your initials. Attach the label to the IV container and document the medication.

Glass Container

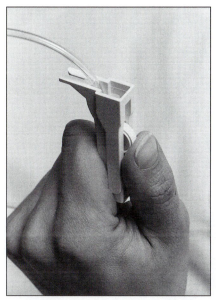

1 Prepare the prescribed medication. Then close the roller clamp to stop the infusion and prevent the delivery of a medication bolus to the client.

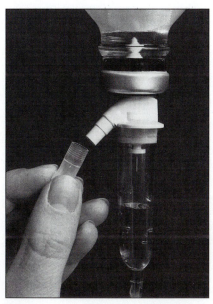

2 Aseptically remove the air vent cap (as shown).

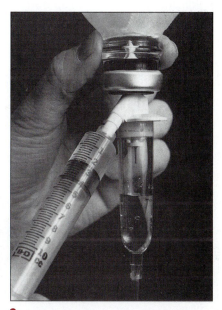

3 Remove the needle from the medication syringe and insert the syringe directly into the air vent. Inject the medication, and then gently rotate the bottle between your hands to mix the medication. Vigorous shaking would produce air bubbles. Replace the air vent cap and open the roller clamp. Adjust the rate of flow to the prescribed amount. Label the bottle with the type and amount of medication, the time and date it was added, and your initials. Document that medication was added to the IV infusion.

GIVING MEDICATIONS BY IV BOLUS

Through a Primary Line

1 After drawing up the prescribed medication, remove the cap from the injection port and set it aside in a manner that ensures asepsis. Pinch the tubing or close off the roller clamp close to the injection port to ensure that medication will be delivered directly into the client's vein.

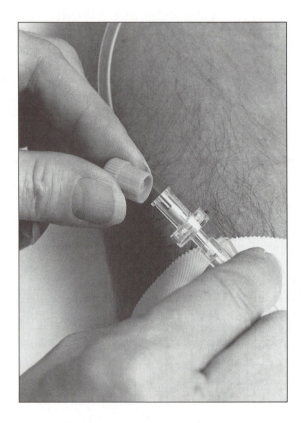

2 If the hanging solution is compatible with the medication, insert the medication syringe into the injection port. To avoid contamination, stabilize the port between the thumb and index finger of your free hand; then aspirate for a blood return to ensure that the catheter is safely in the vein. *Caution: Aspiration is usually contraindicated in infants and small children. Be especially alert to the signs of infiltration in this population.*

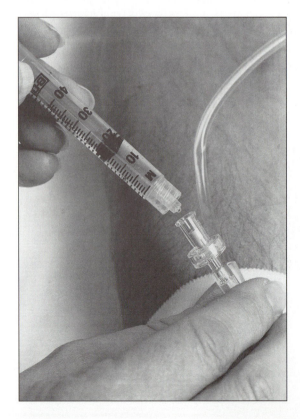

3 Inject the medication at the prescribed rate. Stop the infusion immediately if your client exhibits a reaction to the drug. *Note: If the medication is incompatible with the IV solution, flush the tubing before and after the bolus with 5 mL normal saline or other compatible solution.* Open the clamp and allow the hanging solution to flow again at the prescribed rate. Replace the cap on the injection port. Discard the syringe according to agency policy. Document the medication.

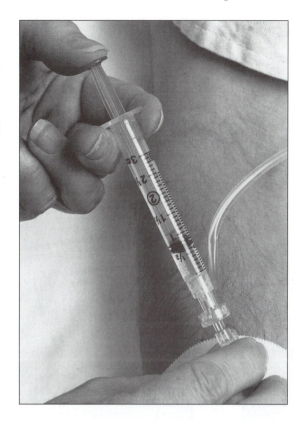

Through a Wing-Tipped Needle

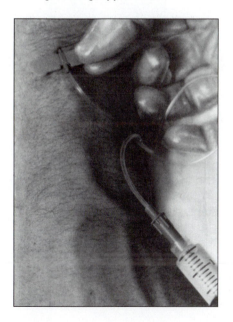

If an intravenous medication has been prescribed for a client who does not have an indwelling catheter or needle, first prepare the medication and then insert a wing-tipped needle (see steps page 120). A wing-tipped needle with an extension set will be more stable than a needle that is attached to a syringe, and it will be less likely to become dislodged and traumatize the client's vein. After inserting the needle, attach the medication syringe to the administration port of the extension tubing. Anchor the wings of the needle with your free thumb and index finger as you aspirate for a backflow of blood. This will not only ensure that the needle is in the vein, it will also fill the extension tubing with blood so that you can inject the medication without forcing air into your client's vein. Then slowly inject the medication at the prescribed rate. This may take anywhere from a minute to several minutes. Stop the infusion immediately if your client shows any signs of an allergic reaction. When the medication has been infused, remove the needle and apply pressure at the insertion site with a sterile gauze pad. Maintain the pressure for a minute or until the client stops bleeding. Dispose of the needle and syringe in the appropriate sharps container (see page 110).

INSERTING A SALINE/HEPARIN LOCK FOR INTERMITTENT INFUSION THERAPY

An intermittent infusion set (saline or heparin lock) is an indwelling reservoir in the vein for intermittent infusion therapy when continuous infusion therapy is not indicated. Periodic injections of saline and/or heparin into the device keep the needle or catheter patent. Be sure to follow your agency's protocol for injections of normal saline and heparin both before and after infusions into the lock. Indications for either solution vary from agency to agency.

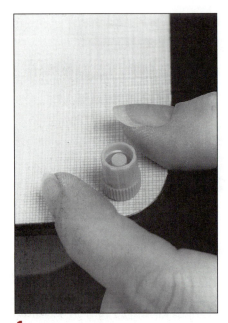

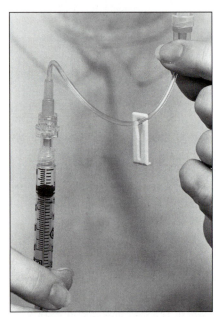

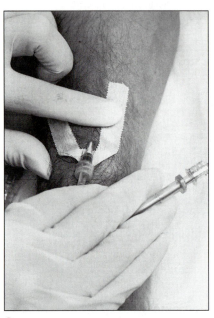

1 When continuous infusion therapy has been discontinued for your client who has an indwelling over-the-needle catheter, you can insert a saline/heparin lock into the catheter to enable intermittent infusion therapy. Before inserting the lock device, remove the cap from the infusion port (if the needleless system you are using has a cap) and place it aseptically on a tabletop (as shown). *Note: This lock, for safety, does not require a needle for access.*

2 Prime the intermittent infusion set with the prescribed amount of normal saline to keep it patent and to remove air from the tubing and port. Leave enough solution in the syringe (1 mL) for flushing the set once it is attached to the hub of the over-the-needle catheter. *Note: Heparin may be used to prime the set in some agencies.*

3 Close the roller clamp on the infusion set to stop the infusion. Apply clean gloves because there is a risk of contact with blood as you remove the tubing from the catheter hub. Detach the IV tubing and insert the intermittent infusion set into the catheter hub as shown. Apply a dressing to the insertion site as pictured on page 126. Then flush the remaining solution as described in step 2.

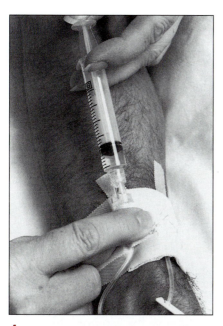

4 To inject medications into the lock, follow this general procedure. Remember to modify it according to your agency's protocol.

a. Into one syringe draw up the prescribed medication and into two syringes draw up 2–3 mL normal saline for each. If you will be using heparin to flush the lock, draw up the prescribed amount into a fourth syringe.

b. Remove the cap from the injection port, and place the cap aseptically on a nearby table.

c. Insert one syringe containing the normal saline into the insertion port and aspirate for blood return to ensure that the catheter is in the vein.

d. Inject the normal saline to flush the blood back into the vein.

Remove the syringe, which you will discard in a biohazardous waste container.

e. Attach the medication syringe. Inject the medication slowly at the prescribed rate of infusion. Observe for adverse reactions to the medication. Remove the medication syringe.

f. Attach the second syringe containing the normal saline to flush the medication, and prepare the lock for capping. Remove the saline syringe. *Note: If your agency uses heparin, you would instill the heparin at this time, after the second saline flush.*

g. Recap the infusion set.

h. Every 8–12 hours, ensure patency by aspirating and flushing with 2–3 mL of normal saline. Unless another peripheral insertion site cannot be found, the lock should be changed at least every 72 hours.

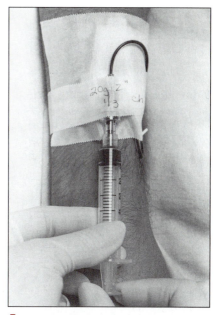

5 To administer intermittent infusions of a hanging solution, remove the cap from the intermittent infusion set and attach a syringe. Validate that there is a blood return, as shown, by pulling back on the plunger. See step 4d for discarding this syringe.

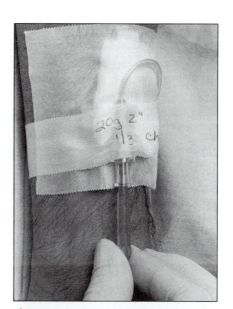

6 Remove the cap from the male (plug) end of the infusion tubing for the hanging solution that contains the medication, and insert the infusion tubing into the infusion port of the lock device. Adjust the roller clamp to achieve the desired rate of flow.

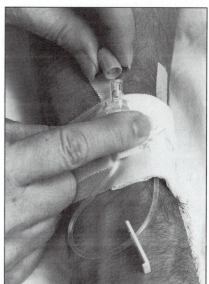

7 After the medication has completely infused, remove the infusion tubing and flush the intermittent infusion set as described in steps 4f and 4g. Replace the cap on the infusion port as shown.

GIVING MEDICATIONS VIA A PARTIAL-FILL (PIGGYBACK) CONTAINER

Piggyback medications are administered through an established IV line via a secondary (piggyback) set, which attaches to the upper injection port on the primary line. The primary line must have a backcheck valve to prevent the tubing from running dry after the piggyback bottle empties. The backcheck valve allows the primary solution to run after the piggyback solution reaches the level of the drip chamber on the primary infusion tubing.

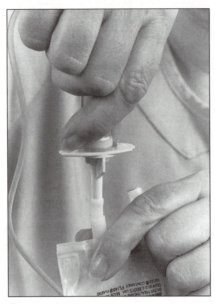

1 The piggyback infusion set may be primed by following the same general steps for priming a primary set (see pages 114–116). However, the following steps for priming piggyback tubing will ensure that none of the medication is wasted during the priming. This is especially important when minute quantities of medication are to be infused. Close the clamp on the piggyback infusion set. Spike the piggyback bag containing the medication (as shown).

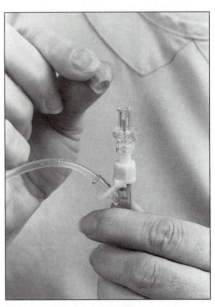

2 Remove the cap from the injection port on the primary line (if the product you are using has a cap).

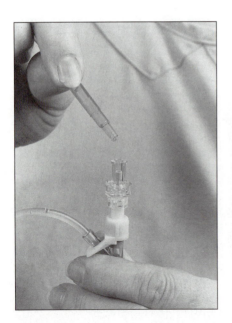

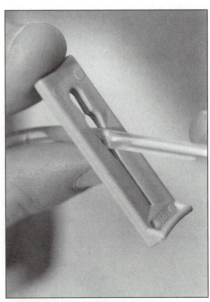

3 Close the roller clamp on the primary line to stop the infusion. Attach the piggyback tubing hub to the end of the infusion injection port (left). Open the clamp on the piggyback infusion set (right). Solution from the primary container will run into the piggyback tubing, clearing out all the air. When the solution reaches the drip chamber on the piggyback tubing, close the clamp.

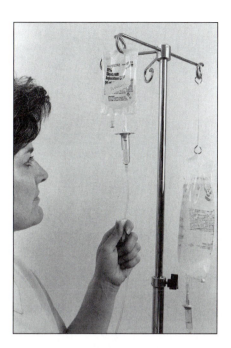

4 Hang the piggyback bag on the IV pole. You will need an extension hook to rehang the primary set, making it lower than the piggyback container. This will activate the backcheck valve. Squeeze the drip chamber on the piggyback tubing and fill the drip chamber to the half-full mark. Adjust the roller clamp on the primary tubing to regulate the rate of flow. Finally, label the piggyback's infusion tubing with the time and date. Document the medication. Once the infusion is complete, close the roller clamp on the piggyback set (as shown), and adjust the primary infusion to the prescribed rate.

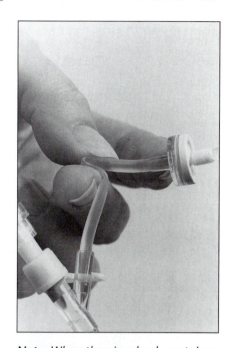

Note: *When the piggyback container empties, you can administer the residual medication in the tubing by pinching the primary tubing just above the upper injection port until the fluid level reaches the hub at the upper injection port. When you release the pressure on the tubing, solution from the primary container may move into the piggyback tubing, but the backcheck valve will prevent it from entering the piggyback bottle.*

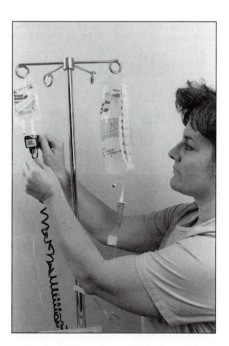

5 If you are going to deliver the piggyback infusion via an infusion pump, plug the piggyback tubing into the infusion pump (procedure will vary by manufacturer). Place the pump's drip counter on the piggyback drip chamber, and set the rate on the pump to deliver the medication in the prescribed amount of time (usually a period of 15–60 minutes).

6 When the infusion is complete, clamp off the piggyback infusion set, return the drip counter to the regular infusion drip chamber, and reset the rate as prescribed.

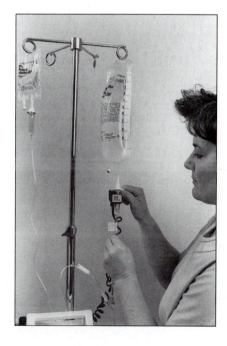

ASSEMBLING A VOLUME-CONTROL IV SET

When it is necessary for you to administer precise doses of dilute medications to a child (or to an adult) over an extended period of time, a volume-control set will make this a safe and effective procedure for your client. Hang it as a primary line for a child. For an adult, it is most often used on a secondary line.

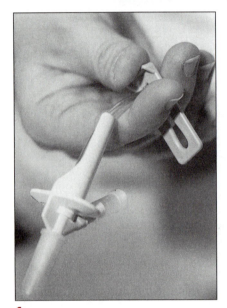

1 Prepare the IV container. Then slide the roller clamp up under the drip chamber and close it off. Close the main slide clamp under the spike (as shown). Remove the spike's protective cover, spike the container, and suspend it on an IV pole.

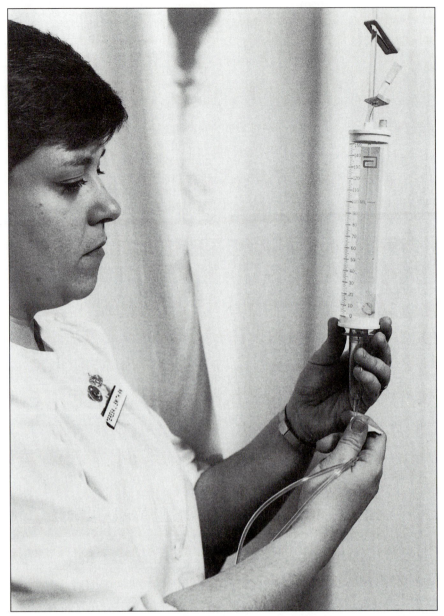

2 Open the main slide clamp and allow 25 mL of the solution to enter the burette (the fluid chamber). Close the main slide clamp.

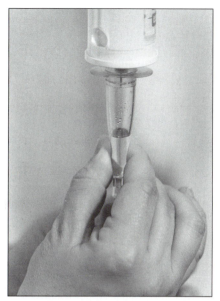

3 Squeeze the drip chamber to fill it to the half-full line. This also should float the diaphragm at the base of the burette. Then open the roller clamp and allow the solution to flush the air from the tubing. Close the roller clamp. *Note: If the drip chamber becomes overfilled, close all the clamps and invert the burette. Squeeze the drip chamber to expel the excess fluid into the burette.*

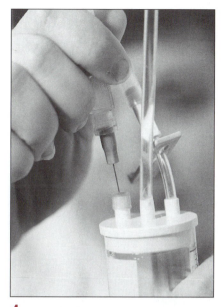

4 To add medication to the burette, first ensure that the air filter (on the right in photo) is open. Then clean the medication port with an alcohol sponge, and inject the prescribed medication (as shown).

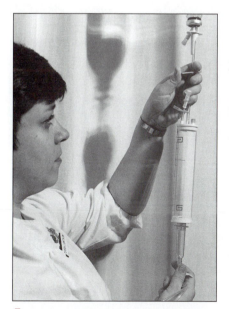

5 If the medication requires diluting, open the main slide clamp to add the desired amount of solution to the burette. Then close the slide clamp.

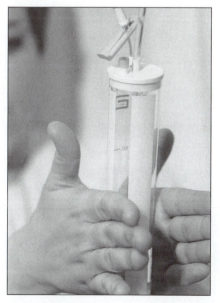

6 Gently roll the burette between your hands to mix the medication with the solution. Attach the distal end of the tubing either to your client's indwelling needle or catheter or to the injection port on the primary tubing. Open the roller clamp and administer the medication at the prescribed rate. The flow will automatically shut off when the burette empties. To refill the burette, repeat steps 2 and 3 above. Be sure to label the burette with the name and dose of the medication and your initials. Document the medication.

Collecting, Monitoring, and Administering Blood

COLLECTING A BLOOD SAMPLE WITH A VACUUM COLLECTION SYSTEM

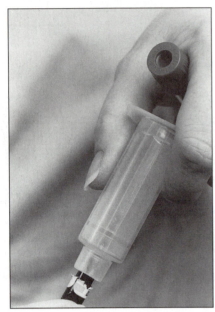

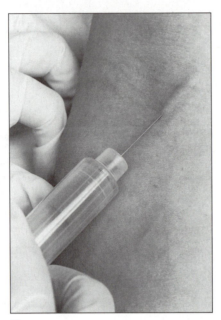

1 Aseptically screw the double-ended needle into the plastic outer container, with the shorter needle positioned inside the outer container (as shown). Then insert the vacuum tube into the outer container with the rubber stopper of the tube resting against the shorter needle. *Note: The vacuum collection system depicted has a sheathed needle protector that reduces the risk of puncture injury to the nurse.*

2 Review the procedures earlier in this chapter for preparing the skin, dilating the vein, and performing a venipuncture. Apply clean gloves and proceed with the venipuncture at the antecubital space.

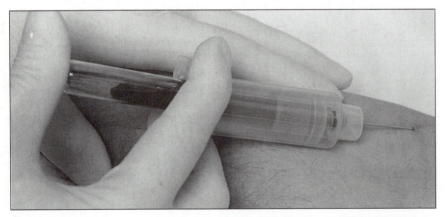

3 After puncturing the vein, stabilize the plastic outer container, and gently but firmly advance the vacuum tube to pierce the rubber stopper with the short needle.

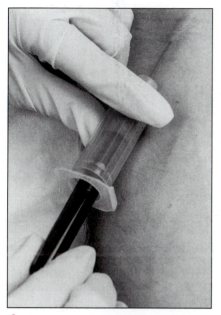

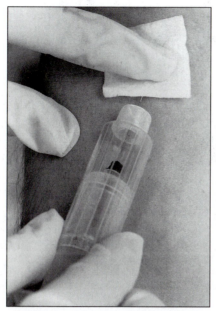

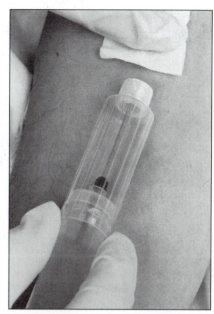

4 Because of the vacuum, blood immediately should begin filling the vacuum tube. As soon as it does, release the tourniquet to prevent the blood from seeping into the surrounding tissues. Remove the vacuum tube when it becomes full and set it aside. If required, insert another vacuum tube.

5 For your client's comfort be sure to remove the vacuum tube, thus preventing vacuum, before you remove the needle from the vein. To remove the device shown, which is a sheathed needle protector, place a 2 X 2 gauze pad just proximal to the insertion site and depress the vein with a finger of your free hand. Hold the outer barrel steady as you withdraw the inner barrel to which the needle is attached.

6 The needle will be covered by the outer barrel, thus reducing your risk of a needlestick. Apply a sterile sponge to the site, and ask your client to press on the sponge for 1–3 minutes to stop the bleeding. Once the bleeding has ceased, place a bandage over the puncture site. Arrange for the delivery of the blood to the laboratory, and document the procedure.

TEACHING THE DIABETIC CLIENT SELF-MONITORING OF BLOOD GLUCOSE

Until a few years ago, urine testing was the only method available to the diabetic client for testing of glucose levels at home. Now, however, there are several blood glucose testing products available that provide a much more accurate indicator of current glucose levels. In addition, they give greater control over the management of the disease and help in the prevention of such acute complications as hypoglycemia and hyperglycemia, as well as chronic complications such as blindness, renal failure, and neuropathies. Of course, the client must continue to test the urine for ketones if he or she is ill or if blood glucose levels are high. Blood glucose can be monitored both visually and with an electronic meter. Blood glucose levels for the client with diabetes will vary, depending on such conditions as food intake, exercise, or insulin dose. Capillary blood glucose values for the nonpregnant, nondiabetic adult are as follows: *fasting* <100 mg/dL (5.6 mmol/L); *2-hour glucose tolerance test* 140 mg/dL (7.8 mmol/L). Because electronic monitors vary greatly, we are showing only the procedure for visual monitoring.

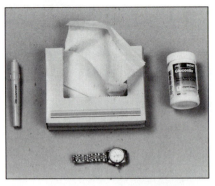

1 For visual monitoring of blood glucose, assemble facial tissue, reagent strips for showing glucose levels, and a watch with a second hand. In addition, you will also need a device for puncturing the skin (usually at the fingertip) to obtain the capillary blood. Either a manual device, such as a needle or lancet, or an automatic device (as shown) may be used. *Caution: If you are performing this procedure, rather than your client, be sure to apply clean gloves.*

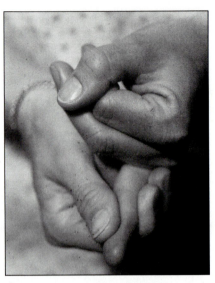

2 Have the client wash both hands with soap and warm water to remove surface bacteria and increase peripheral dilatation; the hands should then be dried thoroughly. Instruct the client to squeeze the fingertip while holding the arm below the level of the heart. This will well the blood at the puncture site.

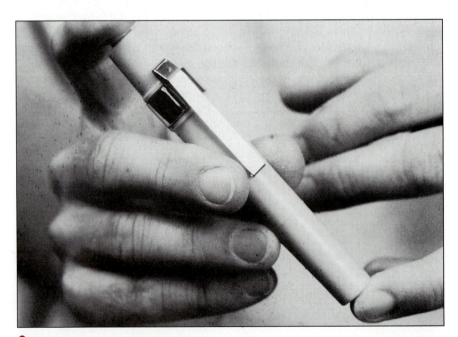

3 The platform of the automatic puncturing device should be placed directly over the puncture site. The periphery of the fingertip should be used because it is less sensitive to pain, and, in many clients, it has fewer calluses than other areas of the finger. To lower the lance and puncture the skin, instruct the client to depress the button (under the client's right index finger).

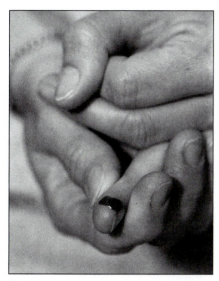

4 The client should then milk the finger by alternately squeezing and releasing the pressure until a drop of blood is produced that is large enough to cover the reagent pad on the test strip.

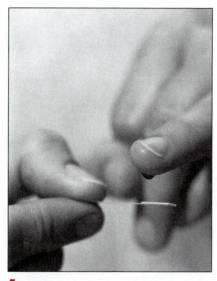

5 Have the client position the test strip just under the droplet of blood (as shown) and cover the entire surface area of the reagent pad with the blood. Smearing the blood onto the surface, however, could cause the blood to soak in unevenly and distort the reading.

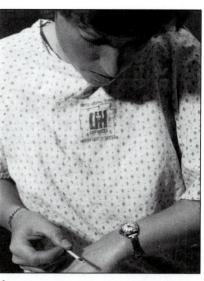

6 The moment the blood touches the strip, the client must begin timing the strip for a period of 30 seconds (or the specified time).

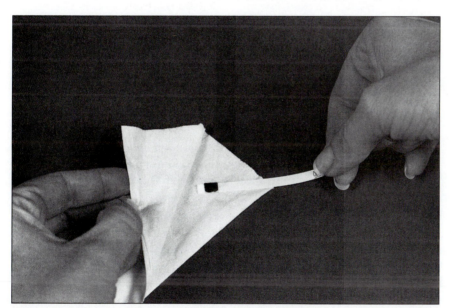

7 When 30 seconds have elapsed, instruct the client to blot the blood gently between the folds of the facial tissue. *Note: This step will vary depending on the manufacturer of the test strip. Follow the instructions for the reagent strips your agency uses.* After blotting the blood, wait 90 seconds (or the specified time).

➤

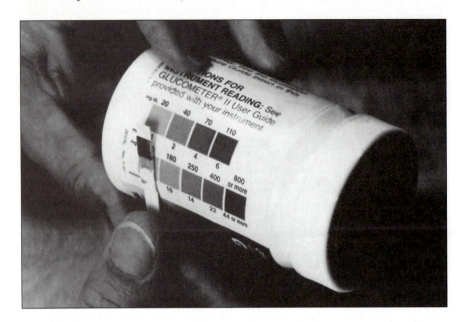

8 Compare the reagent pad to the colored blocks on the back of the container from which the strip was obtained. If the color of the reagent pad falls between two of the color blocks, instruct the client to take the average of the two values to estimate the glucose level. This is called interpolation. The client should then record the result in a log book, along with the time and date, the time and dose of the last insulin injection, and the amount of stress or activity currently being experienced.

INITIATING AND MONITORING BLOOD TRANSFUSIONS

NURSING GUIDELINES: SAFE ADMINISTRATION OF BLOOD

- To decrease the risk of bacterial growth, a blood infusion should be started within 30 minutes after it has been issued from the blood bank.

- For normal, healthy adults, use an 18- to 19-gauge needle or catheter to enhance the flow rate and to prevent injury to the red cells (hemolysis). Children and clients with small or thin-walled veins may require needles as small as 23 gauge. Monitor these clients carefully for adverse reactions and expect a much slower infusion rate.

- Use a special blood administration set with a filter specified by your agency for filtering out cellular debris.

- If indicated, hang only 0.9% normal saline with the blood. Dextrose, Ringer's solution, medications and other additives, and hyperalimentation solutions are incompatible and may result in hemolysis or clumping.

- To prevent incompatibilities with a primary solution, and for a more secure insertion site, avoid piggybacking the blood into the injection port of an existing primary line. Perform a venipuncture at a different site, or (with a physician's prescription) remove the infusion set from an existing

indwelling 18- to 19-gauge needle and attach the primed blood infusion set directly to the indwelling needle. Remember to flush an existing needle with 50 mL of 0.9% normal saline before infusing the blood.

- Hang the blood approximately 1 m (3–4 ft) above the client's heart for an optimal flow rate.

- Administer the blood at the rate of flow prescribed by the physician. Obtain a prescription for the administration rate if one has not been written.

- The maximum time for infusing a unit of blood is 4 hours. There is an increased potential for bacterial growth in blood that is allowed to hang for a longer period of time.

- To prevent circulatory overload for clients with cardiac disorders, administer the transfusion slowly.

- Blood should be warmed *only* when large amounts are infused rapidly and could otherwise cause hypothermia and dysrhythmias. Rapid infusions more typically occur in the operating room, in the emergency room, or in the critical care setting.

ADMINISTERING BLOOD OR BLOOD COMPONENTS

Assessing and Planning

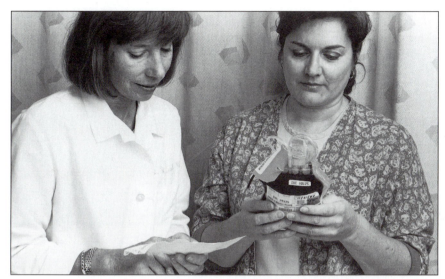

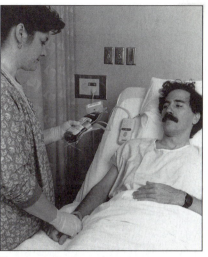

1 Prior to administering the blood, carefully compare the data on the crossmatch report and requisition form to the blood unit information. Check the following data with another health care professional: the client's name and hospital number, blood unit number, blood expiration date, blood group, and blood type. Inspect the blood for abnormalities, such as gas bubbles or black sediment, which are indicative of bacterial growth and necessitate returning the blood to the blood bank.

2 Explain the procedure to the client. Both you and a coworker should then compare the blood unit information to the data on the client's wristband. Ensure that the client's name and hospital number positively match the data on the blood unit; then sign the blood transfusion form according to agency policy. Reconfirm data from the client history regarding known allergies or previous adverse reactions to blood transfusions. Be sure to take and record the vital signs to provide a baseline for subsequent assessments during the transfusion.

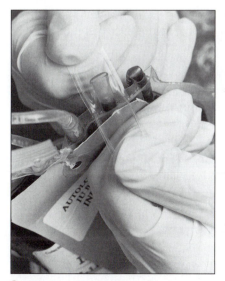

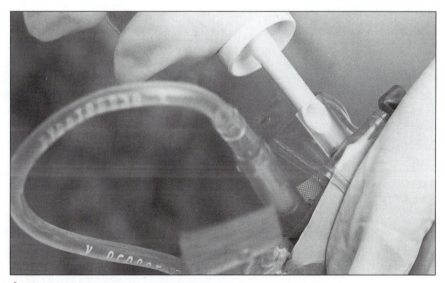

3 Wearing clean gloves, aseptically pull apart the plastic tabs on the blood container (as shown) to expose the blood port.

4 Insert the blood infusion set spike into the blood port, and hang the blood.

5 Perform a venipuncture with an 18- to 19-gauge needle or catheter, or, if the physician has prescribed its discontinuation, remove the infusion tubing from an indwelling 18- to 19-gauge catheter. Attach the primed infusion set to the catheter hub, tape it securely, and, if necessary, secure a splint or armboard to the client's arm to ensure stability. If appropriate, flush a preexisting needle of an incompatible solution with normal saline. Otherwise, open the clamp to the blood. Adjust the clamp to deliver approximately 5–10 mL/minute over the next 15 minutes.

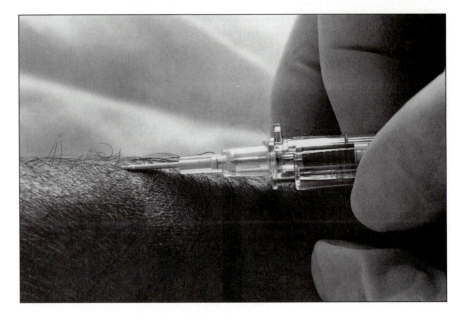

Evaluating

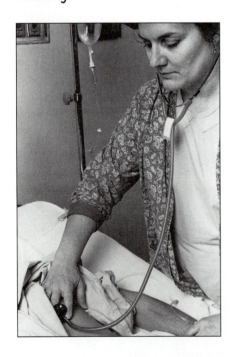

6 Assess the client frequently over the next 15–30 minutes, and monitor him for signs of an adverse reaction to the transfusion (Table 3.1). After the first 15 minutes of the transfusion, check the vital signs again and compare them to the baseline. Be especially alert to a sudden decrease in blood pressure or a rise in temperature. If the vital signs are stable, gradually increase the rate of flow to the prescribed rate. Continue to monitor the client and document the vital signs at least hourly, or more frequently, depending on agency guidelines. If your client has a cardiac disorder, or if large amounts of blood are being infused over a short period of time, auscultate the lung bases for adventitious breath sounds such as crackles (rales) that could indicate circulatory overload. When the blood has been infused, flush the tubing with 20–50 mL of normal saline to deliver the residual blood. Then either hang the prescribed solution (after changing the blood administration set) or change the IV to a saline/heparin lock (see pages 134–135) as indicated. Maintain the venipuncture site in case the client develops a delayed reaction to the blood. Dispose of the blood bag and tubing in the appropriate biohazardous container. Document the procedure.

Table 3.1 Acute Transfusion Reactions

Reaction	Cause	Clinical Manifestations	Management	Prevention
Acute hemolytic	Infusion of ABO-incompatible whole blood, red blood cells, or components containing 10 mL or more of red blood cells. Antibodies in the recipient's plasma attach to antigens on transfused red blood cells, causing red blood cell destruction.	Chills, fever, low back pain, flushing, tachycardia, tachypnea, hypotension, vascular collapse, hemoglobinuria, hemoglobinemia, bleeding, acute renal failure, shock, cardiac arrest, death.	Treat shock, if present. Draw blood samples for serologic testing slowly to avoid hemolysis from the procedure. Send urine specimen to the laboratory. Maintain blood pressure with IV colloid solutions. Give diuretics as prescribed to maintain urine flow. Insert indwelling catheter or measure voided amounts to monitor hourly urine output. Dialysis may be required if renal failure occurs. Do not transfuse additional RBC-containing components until transfusion service has provided newly cross-matched units.	Meticulously verify and document client identification from sample collection to component infusion.
Febrile, nonhemolytic (most common)	Sensitization to donor white blood cells, platelets, or plasma proteins.	Sudden chills and fever (rise in temperature of greater than 1 C), headache, flushing, anxiety, muscle pain.	Give antipyretics as prescribed—avoid aspirin in thrombocytopenic clients. Do not restart transfusion.	Consider leukocyte-poor blood products (filtered, washed, or frozen).
Mild allergic	Sensitivity to foreign plasma proteins.	Flushing, itching, urticaria (hives).	Give antihistamine as directed. If symptoms are mild and transient, transfusion may be restarted slowly. Do not restart transfusion if fever or pulmonary symptoms develop.	Treat prophylactically with antihistamines.

➡

Table 3.1   Acute Transfusion Reactions (*continued*)

Reaction	Cause	Clinical Manifestations	Management	Prevention
Anaphylactic	Infusion of IgA proteins to IgA-deficient recipient who has developed IgA antibody.	Anxiety, urticaria, wheezing, progressing to cyanosis, shock, and possible cardiac arrest.	Initiate CPR if indicated. Have epinephrine ready for injection (0.4 mL of a 1:1,000 solution subcutaneously or 0.1 mL of 1:1,000 solution diluted to 10 mL with saline for IV use). Do not restart transfusion.	Transfuse extensively washed RNC products, from which all plasma has been removed. Alternatively, use blood from IgA-deficient donor.
Circulatory overload	Fluid administered faster than the circulation can accommodate.	Cough, dyspnea, pulmonary congestion (rales), headache, hypertension, tachycardia, distended neck veins.	Place client upright, with feet in dependent position. Administer prescribed diuretics, oxygen, morphine. Phlebotomy may be indicated.	Adjust transfusion volume and flow rate based on client's size and clinical status. Have transfusion service divide unit into smaller aliquots for better spacing of fluid input.
Sepsis	Transfusion of contaminated blood components.	Rapid onset of chills, high fever, vomiting, diarrhea, and marked hypotension and shock.	Obtain culture of client's blood and send bag with remaining blood to transfusion service for further study. Treat septicemia as directed—antibiotics, IV fluids, vasopressors, steroids.	Collect, process, store, and transfuse blood products according to blood banking standards and infuse within 4 hours of starting time.

Source: National Blood Resource Education Programs, Transfusion therapy guidelines for nurses, September, 1990, NIH Publication No. 90-2668a.

INITIATING PATIENT-CONTROLLED ANALGESIA

Patient-controlled analgesia (PCA) involves the use of a programmed syringe pump that delivers pre-determined amounts of analgesia at preset intervals. PCA enables the client to titrate analgesia to maintain a consistent serum level of narcotic rather than experience the peaks and troughs that occur with prn injections. Client populations for whom this device is indicated include those in need of parenteral analgesia, those willing to operate the device, and those mentally alert and able to follow instructions. Populations for whom the device is usually contraindicated include those with chronic pulmonary diseases, those with a history of allergies to morphine or meperidine, those with a history of drug abuse, and those with major psychiatric disorders.

The nursing staff programs the pump as prescribed by the physician for the following: dose increment to be delivered, minimum time interval between delivered doses ("lockout" interval), and total doses available over a 4-hour period. Clients initiate infusions by pressing a handheld control button that is connected to the pump. The client has an IV infusion running to keep the vein open between analgesia infusions.

Client instruction is a critical part of this therapy. The client must verbalize understanding of how the PCA device works before the therapy is initiated. Provide the client with verbal instructions, and reinforce this information with reading materials such as booklets about PCA therapy. In addition, instruct the client to notify staff for the following: inadequate pain relief, change in the severity or location of pain, machine appearing to malfunction, alarms sounding, or any questions arising regarding the machine or pain relief. ***Note:*** *The following procedure applies to the Abbott pump. These guidelines will vary depending on the manufacturer of the PCA equipment.*

Assessing and Planning

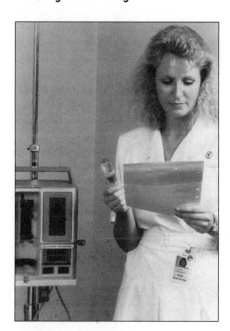

1 Verify physician prescription for the PCA, comparing it to the vial of analgesia that was obtained from the pharmacy and noting prescribed settings. ***Note:*** *If the pump is for a pediatric client, it is recommended that two nurses verify pump settings.* Morphine is supplied in 30-mL vial injectors with a concentration of 1 mg/mL, and meperidine (Demerol) is supplied in 30-mL vial injectors with a concentration of 10 mg/mL.

Be aware that administration of blood or any other medication incompatible with morphine or meperidine requires a second IV site. If a triple-lumen catheter is to be used for the infusion, the narcotic infusion is usually administered through the proximal port.

Perform a baseline assessment of your client's respiratory system (see Chapter 6) for ongoing comparison throughout the PCA therapy. Also verify that your client is not allergic to morphine or meperidine, whichever is prescribed. Reinforce client teaching information as described at left. Assemble the PCA pump and infusion tubing.

Implementing

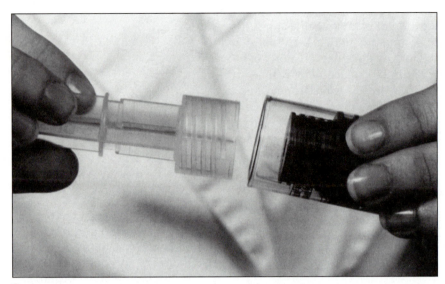

2 Snap off the caps from the injector (plunger) and prefilled vial, and connect the injector to the vial by screwing them together.

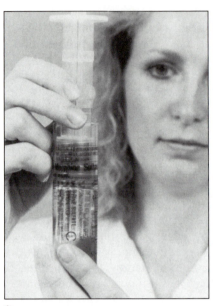

3 Prime the unit by pushing down on the injector to eject the air.

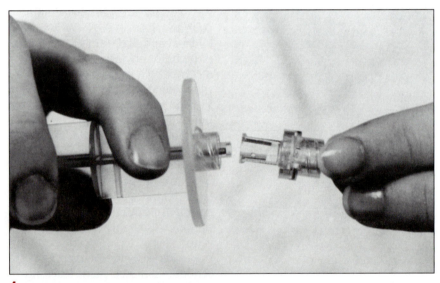

4 Next, attach the female (socket) connector on the long end of the PCA tubing to the male (plug) end of the injector in the vial.

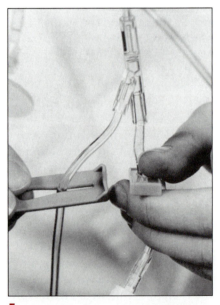

5 Flush the tubing *only* as far as the Y-branch (Y-injection site back-check valve port). ***Caution:*** *Flushing all the tubing would administer more than the prescribed dose of IV narcotic when it is attached to the client.* Close the slide clamp on the PCA tubing, as shown.

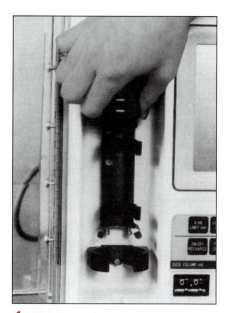

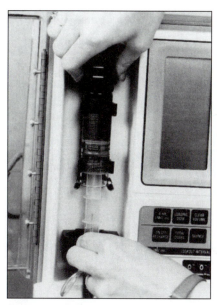

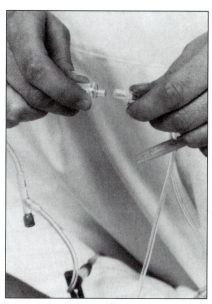

6 Open the machine door by turning the key. Activate the drive release mechanism on the pump by pinching the spring-loaded lever, as shown, and retracting the drive assembly (moving it all the way up).

7 Load the vial into the drive assembly and clamp it securely in place, with the graduations on the vial facing out. After the vial has been clamped in place, activate the drive release mechanism again by pinching the spring-loaded lever (as shown), and slide the drive assembly down until it securely locks the vial in place. The flange on the injector (behind the nurse's lower hand) must "click" into its locked position in the holder. Then close the door on the pump and take it to the client's room. Plug the pump into an appropriate outlet unless battery operation is desired.

8 Remove the protective cap from the Y-site on the PCA tubing, and attach it to the distal end of the client's maintenance IV fluid tubing.

If the client already has maintenance fluids running, stop the infusion by clamping off the fluids using the roller clamp on the tubing. Disconnect the maintenance fluid tubing from the client's connector tubing, being certain to maintain sterility. Remove the protective cap from the Y-site on the PCA tubing, and attach the distal male (plug) connector of the maintenance IV tubing to the female (socket) connector of the PCA tubing.

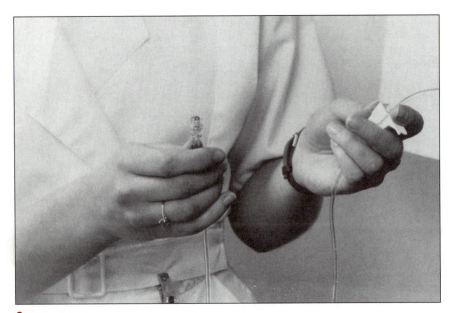

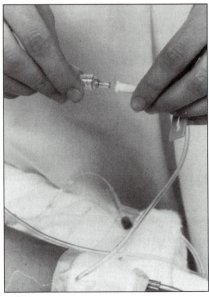

9 Prime the remainder of the PCA tubing by adjusting the roller clamp on the maintenance infusion tubing.

10 Attach the male (plug) end of the PCA tubing to the female (socket) end of the client's connector tubing. Open the slide clamps on the main IV infusion tubing, the PCA tubing, and the client's connector tubing. Or, as another option, remove the client's connector tubing and insert the PCA tubing directly into the hub of the intravenous catheter.

11 If appropriate at this time, press the ON/OFF button to turn on the machine. DOOR OPEN and VOLUME DELIVERED messages will appear once the machine is turned on. CHECK SYRINGE and ALARM messages also will appear if the injector is not positioned securely in the injector holder.

Adjust the pump dials according to the physician's prescribed limits. If a loading dose has been prescribed, establish this before setting the other limits. Set LOCKOUT LIMIT at 00 minutes, and then set the prescribed volume to be delivered, using the DOSE VOLUME control (set in tenths of a cc). Then press LOADING DOSE. The pump's screen will reflect the volume delivered.

If a loading dose has not been prescribed (or after a loading dose has been delivered), establish the limits as follows: DOSE VOLUME: as prescribed for client delivery and given in tenths of a cc; LOCKOUT INTERVAL: the interval between allowable doses given in minutes (9 minutes will appear as 09; 15 minutes will appear as 15).

Set the FOUR-HOUR LIMIT as prescribed by the physician. This represents the maximum amount of medication the patient can receive in a 4-hour period, and it is prescribed in increments of 50 (eg, 1 cc q10min with a 4-hour limit of 20 cc).

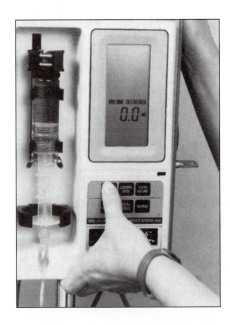

Evaluating

12 Close the pump's door, making sure it is locked securely. Remove the key and put it with the narcotics keys, or follow the agency-established protocol. On a piece of tape, write the time and date when the vial was inserted and attach it to the pump. Usually the container is discarded within 24–48 hours after it was placed in the pump, depending on agency policy. Any drug remaining in the pump after 24–48 hours or when PCA is discontinued is wasted according to pharmacy protocol for narcotic waste.

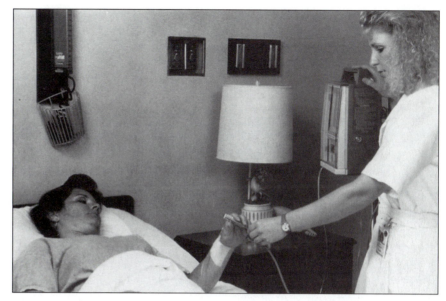

Give the handheld button to the client or tie it to the side rail for easy access. Review instructions for the use of the machine and button with the client.

The READY message that appears indicates that the PCA infuser is now in the patient control mode, and the first dose is available to the client. When the client presses the handheld button, a beep will acknowledge the request, the dose will be delivered, and READY will disappear.

VOLUME DELIVERED will display the increments of medication as the dose is delivered (as well as the loading dose that was given).

LOCKOUT INTERVAL message appears as the dose delivery is completed. When the allotted time has elapsed following the last delivered dose, the LOCKOUT INTERVAL message will disappear and READY will reappear. If the client desires, pressing the handheld button at this time will deliver another dose.

Adjust these dials accordingly if the physician changes the PCA prescription during the course of therapy.

Continue to assess the client throughout the therapy at frequent intervals (q2h during the first 24 hours; q4h thereafter). Compare each respiratory system assessment to the baseline for potential changes. Be alert to bradypnea (<12 breaths/minute) as well as to

hypotension, dizziness, nausea, and vomiting. Remember that the goal of PCA is relief of pain without sedation. Also check patency of the IV lines q2h. Change PCA and maintenance IV tubing according to agency protocol.

Note: To change an injector vial: First close the manual slide clamp that is most proximal to the Luer-lock connector on the plunger. This will maintain the primed tubing and prevent entry of air. Assemble the replacement plunger and vial and remove air according to instructions in steps 2 and 3 on page 150. Remove the empty vial from the clamping mechanism on the pump. Attach the male Luer-lock connector on the vial's plunger (injector) to the female end of the PCA tubing (see step 4). Load the vial and plunger device into the drive assembly, and lock it in place by following steps 6 and 7. Release the manual slide clamp when therapy is to be resumed. Affix a piece of tape to the pump, noting the date and time this and subsequent injector vials were placed in the pump.

To stop an infusion in progress: Close the slide clamp that is most proximal to the Luer-lock connector on the injector vial, unlock and open the security door, and press the ON/OFF button to turn the unit off. This will stop the infusion automatically. *Note: The history*

of the infusion will be lost if the machine is turned off for more than 1 hour; therefore, record the amount of medication administered before turning the machine off.

To discontinue the infusion: Close the slide clamp that is most proximal to the Luer-lock connector on the injector vial, unlock and open the security door, remove the injector from the infuser, and disconnect the set. Press the ON/OFF button to turn the unit off. Continue or discontinue the maintenance IV as prescribed.

Documentation: Document PCA infusion on proper chart forms, usually q8h or according to agency protocol. To determine the amount of morphine or meperidine given, press TOTAL DOSES and multiply by the number of "ccs" prescribed for the increment dose. For example, if the prescribed dose was 1 cc and the client administered 10 doses, multiply 10 X 1 = 10 cc. Pressing CLEAR VOLUME at the end of each 8-hour period will indicate the amount of analgesia used by the client. *Note: LOADING DOSES are usually charted separately on the medication record and are documented according to the exact time they were administered.* Finally, remember to document the level of pain relief obtained from the PCA medication.

Managing Venous Access Devices (VADs)

NURSING GUIDELINES: MANAGING CHRONIC (LONG-TERM) CENTRAL VENOUS CATHETERS

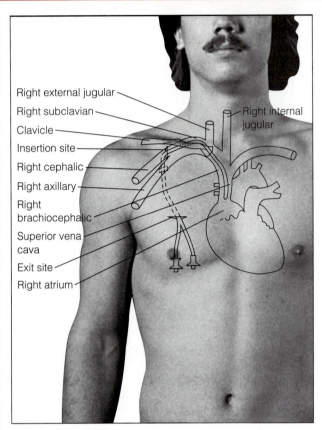

Right external jugular
Right subclavian
Clavicle
Insertion site
Right cephalic
Right axillary
Right brachiocephalic
Superior vena cava
Exit site
Right atrium
Right internal jugular

Description

Long-term catheters that have single, double, or triple lumens. They are inserted either percutaneously into the subclavian vein or by cut-down into the external jugular vein. The catheter is tunneled subcutaneously and externalized at a convenient site on the chest wall. The catheter tip is positioned at the junction of the superior vena cava and right atrium and subcutaneously anchored with a Dacron cuff.

Uses

Provide long-term (ie, 6 months to 2 years or more) venous access for blood drawing and administration of drugs, antibiotics, chemotherapy, total parenteral nutrition (TPN), blood, and blood products.

Nursing Considerations

- Lower infection rate than the acute multilumen central venous catheters because (1) the entrance and exit sites are separated and (2) the Dacron cuff forms a barrier against ingress of organisms.

- More invasive insertion and removal than with the acute multilumen central venous catheters.

- Catheter occlusion is usually the most common complication.

- Mechanical problems (eg, leakage in the external catheter) usually can be resolved with the line repair kits that are issued by the catheter manufacturer.

- To prevent blood loss or air embolus in the presence of a damaged external line (eg, cut, puncture, or leakage), clamp the catheter with a padded hemostat or smooth-edged clamp as close to the chest wall as possible (or proximal to the damaged lumen). If an air embolus is suspected, position the client in a left side-lying position with the head lower than the heart (see page 176). Set up equipment for catheter repair.

- The silicone material is biocompatible and makes the catheter more durable and comfortable than the polyurethane material used in most acute central venous catheters.

- When the catheter lumens are not being used for infusion of IVs or medications, keep them sealed with Luer-lock caps or rubber injection caps.

- Irrigation protocol varies according to manufacturer, client condition, and agency. Follow specific guidelines established for each client.

NURSING GUIDELINES: MANAGING ACUTE (SHORT-TERM) AND INTERMEDIATE (MEDIUM-TERM) MULTILUMEN CENTRAL VENOUS CATHETERS

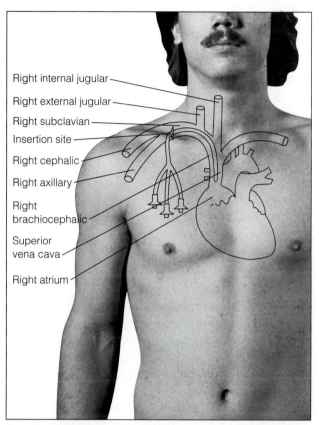

Right internal jugular

Right external jugular

Right subclavian

Insertion site

Right cephalic

Right axillary

Right brachiocephalic

Superior vena cava

Right atrium

Description

Temporary venous access devices that have two or three separate polyurethane or silicone lines encased in one catheter. They are usually inserted into the subclavian vein by percutaneous stick and sutured in place.

Uses

Acute Catheters: Provide short-term (5 to 7 days) delivery of multiple infusions through one venipuncture, including continuous TPN, chemotherapy, antibiotics, blood, and blood products; simultaneous delivery of physically incompatible drugs; and frequent blood drawing for clients who require therapy for approximately a week. They also enable monitoring of central venous pressure (CVP).

Intermediate Catheters: Provide medium-term (6 to 8 weeks) delivery of multiple infusions as discussed above. These catheters are indicated for conditions that necessitate 6- to 8-week courses of antibiotics (eg, with osteomyelitis) or nutrition (eg, before and after gastrointestinal surgery or with Crohn's disease).

Nursing Considerations

- Seen more frequently in critical care areas.

- Higher rate of infection and migration than with the chronic central venous catheters.

- Catheters made with silicone are more biocompatible than those made with polyurethane and can stay in place longer.

- These lumens are more likely to clog with fibrin sheaths than the lumens of the chronic central venous catheters because of the vessel injury that occurs with the percutaneous insertion. If clogging occurs, a dye study and x-ray usually reveal the location of the fibrin, which is then lysed with thrombolytic therapy. Urokinase is usually the drug of choice.

- Mechanical problems (ie, leakage) usually necessitate line replacement.

- To prevent blood loss or air embolus in the presence of a damaged line (eg, a cut, puncture, or leakage), clamp the catheter with a padded hemostat or smooth-edged clamp as close to the chest wall as possible (or proximal to the damaged lumen). If an air embolus is suspected, position the client in a left side-lying position with the head lower than the heart (see page 176). Set up equipment for line replacement.

NURSING GUIDELINES: MANAGING PERIPHERALLY INSERTED CENTRAL CATHETERS (PICCs)

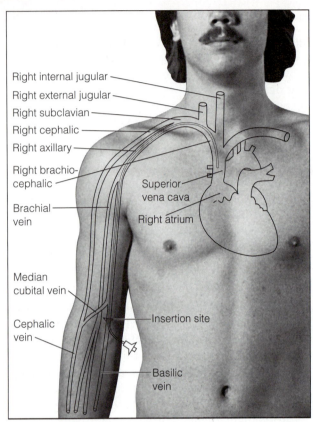

Right internal jugular
Right external jugular
Right subclavian
Right cephalic
Right axillary
Right brachio-cephalic
Brachial vein
Superior vena cava
Right atrium
Median cubital vein
Cephalic vein
Insertion site
Basilic vein

Description

A temporary or long-term venous access device that has a single or multiple lumen. The line, up to 60 cm (2 ft) in length, is inserted peripherally through the antecubital fossa into the basilic, median cubital, or cephalic vein and advanced through the subclavian vein and into the superior vena cava.

Uses

Provides short-term or long-term (up to 6 months) venous access for blood drawing and administration of drugs, antibiotics, chemotherapy, TPN, and blood and blood products. This catheter also can be used for CVP monitoring.

Nursing Considerations

- Chest x-ray indicated for verifying placement of the catheter tip.

- Frequently used in clients in acute care and home care settings who lack reliable access for short- and long-term therapy or who require frequent blood drawings.

- Contraindicated for clients who have antecubital veins that are bruised, sclerosed, or scarred from multiple venipunctures.

- Useful for infusions of hyperosmolar or vesicant solutions because of the catheter's placement in large blood vessels, which accesses high blood flow in the central circulation.

- Silicone polymer material, which is biocompatible, soft, and pliable.

- Catheter generally not sutured in place. Anchor it securely with sterile tape. Document the length of the catheter outside the client's insertion site. Consult physician promptly for any alteration in its position.

- Change dressing following the same procedure for central line catheter (see pages 159–162). If a gauze dressing is used, change it every 48–72 hours and once a week if a transparent film dressing is used (or per agency policy).

- Flush the line after any infusion. The volume of the flush will vary with the gauge and length of the catheter. Generally, flush with 2–5 mL normal saline followed by 2–2.5 mL of heparin, 100 u/mL. *Caution: Do not use smaller than a 5–10 mL syringe for flushing because the pressure generated by a smaller syringe may rupture the catheter.*

NURSING GUIDELINES: MANAGING MIDLINE CATHETERS (MLCs)

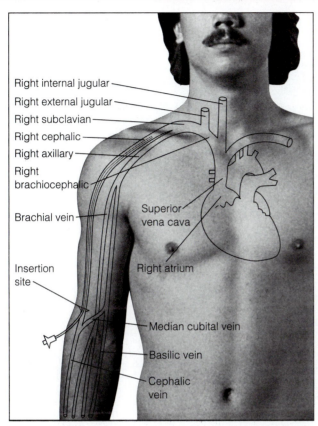

Right internal jugular

Right external jugular

Right subclavian

Right cephalic

Right axillary

Right brachiocephalic

Brachial vein

Superior vena cava

Insertion site

Right atrium

Median cubital vein

Basilic vein

Cephalic vein

Description

Peripherally inserted venous access device whose tip lies in a large vessel between the antecubital area and the head of the clavicle. This is a temporary device with a single or double lumen. The line is shorter than the PICC and is inserted through the antecubital space and advanced into the cephalic vein.

Uses

Provides short-term venous access (1–8 weeks) for blood drawing and administration of drugs, antibiotics, chemotherapy, and blood and blood products.

Nursing Considerations

- Chest x-ray indicated to verify placement of the catheter tip.

- Frequently used in clients in acute care settings who lack reliable access for short-term therapy or who require frequent blood drawings.

- Not indicated in clients whose antecubital veins are bruised, sclerosed, or scarred from multiple venipunctures.

- Elastomeric hydrogel material becomes 50 times softer within 2 hours after insertion, enabling the catheter to increase 2 gauge sizes and approximately 2.5 cm (1 in) in length.

- Anchor catheter securely with sterile tape or strips. Document the length of the catheter outside the client's insertion site. Consult the physician immediately for any alterations.

- Change dressing according to agency policy for central lines. Generally, this dressing is changed every 48–72 hours if a gauze dressing is used and once a week if a transparent dressing is used.

- Flush line after any infusion as for the PICC, adjusting for the smaller volume of the MLC.

NURSING GUIDELINES: MANAGING IMPLANTABLE SUBCUTANEOUS PORTS

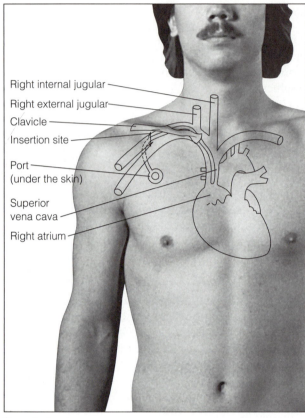

Right internal jugular
Right external jugular
Clavicle
Insertion site
Port (under the skin)
Superior vena cava
Right atrium

Description

Totally implanted devices that enable repeated access to the central venous system without multiple venipunctures. These devices consist of a silicone catheter and port with a self-sealing silicone-rubber septum that allows 1,000 to 2,000 punctures (depending on the manufacturer). Using local anesthesia, the physician creates a subcutaneous pocket for portal implantation. The catheter's distal end is threaded into the appropriate blood vessel, with the proximal end positioned at the port site. The port is sutured in place.

Uses

Enable repeated blood drawing and infusions of TPN, blood and blood products, continuous fluid replacement, antibiotics, chemotherapy, and bolus medications.

Nursing Considerations

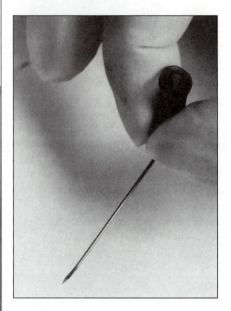

- Use only a special, noncoring (Huber) needle (above) to minimize trauma to the self-sealing septum.

- Advantages over the external central venous catheters include excellent client acceptance due to absence of external catheter, no dressing once the site has healed, minimal maintenance, and decreased risk of infection.

- Flush and fill the port with heparinized solution after every use.

- Observe the insertion site for wound hematoma, infection, and port rotation or extrusion.

- Before accessing the port, prepare the overlying skin using aseptic technique.

- Insert Huber needle firmly and perpendicular to the skin into the rubber septum until the needle tip reaches the bottom of the portal chamber.

- Generally, 90-degree Huber needles are used for long-term IV infusions, and the straight needles are used for blood samples or a single maintenance irrigation.

- Flush with normal saline or aspirate for blood to confirm catheter patency and proper needle placement prior to use.

CHANGING THE EXIT SITE DRESSING FOR A CHRONIC CENTRAL VENOUS CATHETER

Assessing and Planning

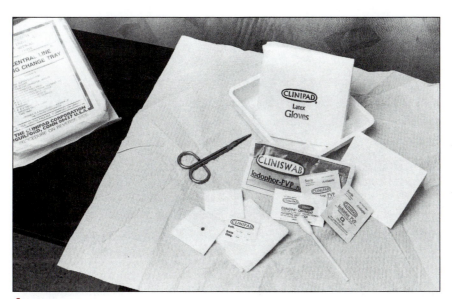

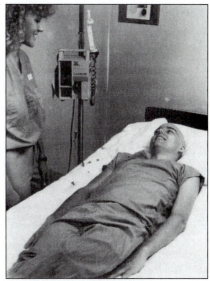

1 Assemble either a commercially prepared dressing change kit or a variation of the following sterile materials:

☐ either an antiseptic solution or swabsticks (eg, alcohol, povidone-iodine, or chlorhexidrine are commonly used). Check for client allergies before making your selection.

☐ overwrap for a sterile field

☐ sterile gloves

☐ cotton swabs

☐ gauze pads

☐ gauze or semipermeable dressing

☐ antiseptic ointment

☐ antiseptic wipes

☐ scissors

☐ basin in which to pour the antiseptic cleansing solution if swabsticks are not used

In addition, you will also need to assemble:

☐ tape

☐ clean gloves

☐ impervious bag for disposal of dressings and supplies

Generally, a sterile procedure is used for the first week following catheter placement, and the dressing is changed daily if the client has increased risk for localized infection (eg, with granulocytopenia or bleeding at the exit site). In addition, the dressing should be changed prn whenever it becomes contaminated (eg, with excess drainage, perspiration, or blood). A clean technique is usually followed the week after catheter placement, and the dressing is changed three times a week if a gauze dressing is used and one to two times a week if a transparent dressing is used (or more frequently if the client has drainage at the exit site). Bring the materials to the bedside.

2 Explain the dressing change procedure to your client. Adjust the height of the bed to facilitate the dressing application. If your client's catheter will be disconnected for an IV tubing change, flattening the head of the bed helps to increase intrathoracic pressure, thereby minimizing the risk of an air embolism. Then, either remove the pajama top or lower the gown at the exit site.

➤

Implementing

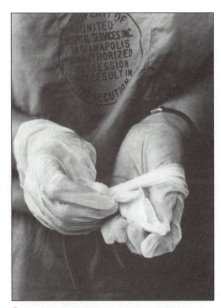

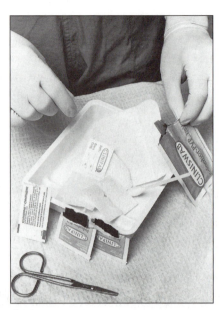

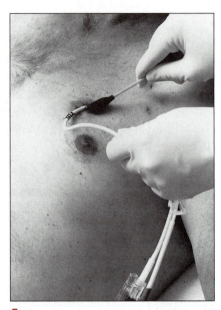

3 Wash your hands and put on the clean gloves. Instruct your client to turn his head away from the exit site, which will minimize the potential for contamination, and gently remove the old dressing. Assess for the presence of redness, drainage, swelling, tenderness, and odor—signs that the client may have a localized infection. For more information, see "Performing Wound Care," page 25, in Chapter 1. As appropriate, culture any drainage that appears to be purulent. Then encase the dressing in your gloves (as shown) and deposit them in the impervious plastic bag.

4 Wash your hands again. Establish your sterile field on a clean and dry surface, using either a sterile towel or the sterile wrap from the commercially prepared dressing change kit (see technique in Chapter 1, page 18). Then put on the sterile gloves. Open all the packets that are inside the sterile kit and set them in a convenient spot on the sterile field.

5 Using your clean hand (left hand in this photo), lift the catheter off your client's chest to facilitate cleaning around the insertion site. Using your sterile hand (right hand in this photo), cleanse the exit site with a sterile swab saturated with povidone-iodine. Cleanse in a circular motion, starting at the exit site, as shown. Never return to the exit site with a used swab.

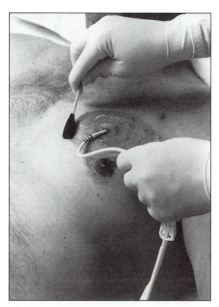

6 Continue to cleanse outward 5 cm (2 in) in diameter away from the exit site, using a circular motion. Discard the swab. As necessary, repeat this procedure using fresh swabs until the site is free of encrustations and particles and the entire area has been cleansed.

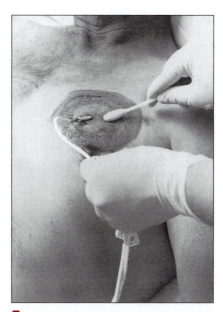

7 Dry the site with a sterile cotton swab, using a circular, outward motion.

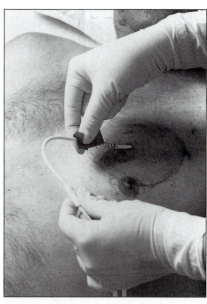

8 Use an antiseptic pledget to cleanse the proximal 7–8 cm (3 in) of the catheter.

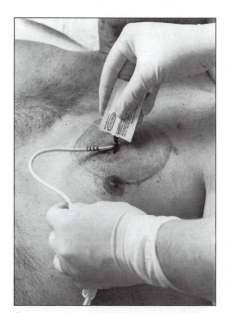

9 Apply a small amount of antiseptic ointment to the exit site.

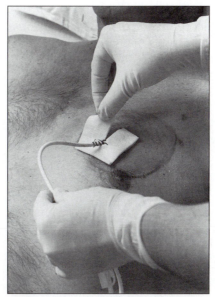

10 Place the split 2 X 2 gauze dressing around the exit site (as shown).

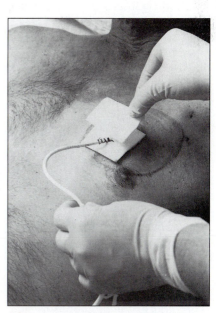

11 Place another 2 X 2 gauze dressing over the split dressing.

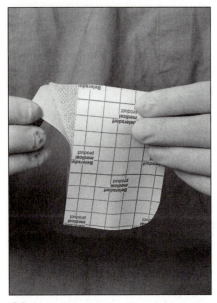

12 Peel the backing off half of the adhesive dressing.

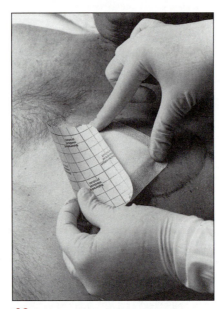

13 Place the dressing over the gauze and secure it with your fingers around the edges of the exposed section. Pull the remainder of the backing off the dressing as you apply it.

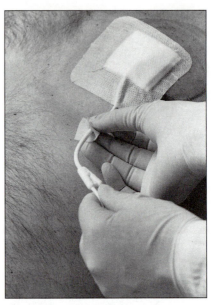

14 Cleanse the exposed catheter that is outside of the dressing with an alcohol wipe, wiping from its proximal to its distal end.

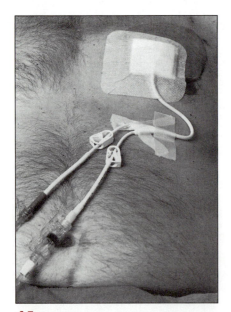

15 Loop the exposed catheter and adhere the loop to the client's skin. This reduces the drag on the catheter and insertion site.

Evaluating

Remove your gloves. Initial and write the dates of both the catheter insertion and dressing change on a label and adhere it to the dressing. Assist the client into a comfortable position. Remove the waste from the bedside and dispose of it according to agency policy. Wash your hands. Document the procedure in your nurses' notes, recording the date and time of dressing change, your assessment of the catheter exit site and adjacent skin, and the manner in which the client tolerated the procedure.

HOME HEALTH CARE CONSIDERATIONS

- After a catheter has been in place for 3 weeks, clean technique is usually followed for dressing changes for clients with catheters that will be indwelling long term.

- The dressing is changed 3 times a week if a gauze dressing is used and 1–2 times a week if a transparent dressing is used.

- The client should keep the dressing dry during bathing by taping plastic wrap securely over the entire dressing. The dressing should be changed if it gets wet. Taking showers is not recommended because the increased potential for splashing of water increases the risk of infection at the insertion site.

DRAWING BLOOD FROM A CHRONIC (HICKMAN®-TYPE) CENTRAL VENOUS CATHETER AND FLUSHING THE CATHETER FOLLOWING BLOOD WITHDRAWAL

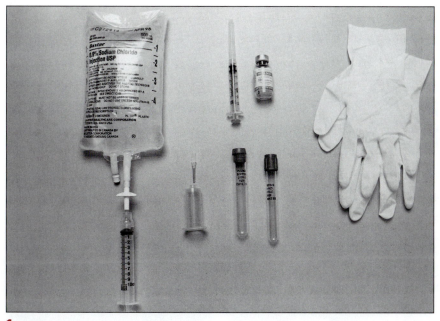

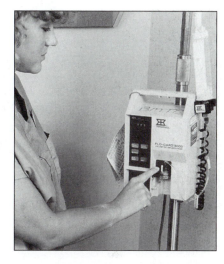

1 Wash your hands and assemble the following materials or as prescribed:

- ☐ vacuum collection system with multidraw adapter

- ☐ vacuum tubes for the blood sample

- ☐ normal saline with a syringe for flushing

- ☐ vial of heparinized solution if the line is to be capped and clamped following blood withdrawal

- ☐ syringe into which you will aspirate heparin (if heparin is to be used)

- ☐ capped needle (shown here on one of the syringes) to protect the end of the infusion tubing if the infusion will be restarted

- ☐ clean gloves (because of the possibility of coming in contact with blood)

You will also need antiseptic wipe and a needleless injection port if the client does not already have one.

2 Describe the procedure to the client; explain that you will obtain venous blood for diagnostic laboratory work. If the client's catheter is attached to IV infusion(s), stop the infusion(s) at this time.

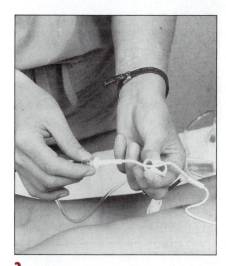

3 Clamp the catheter lumen (as shown). If the client has a double- or triple-lumen catheter, ensure that the other lumens are clamped as well.

➡

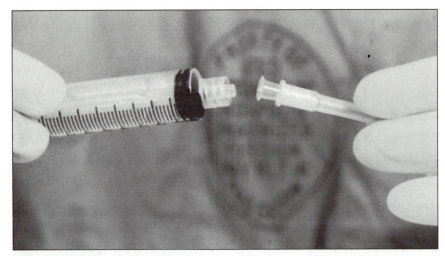

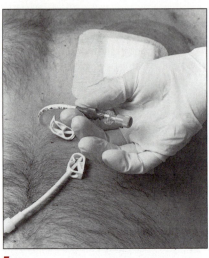

4 Apply clean gloves. If the client has a single-lumen catheter through which an IV infusion is running, remove the needle and cap from the syringe (as shown). Disconnect the infusion tubing from the catheter hub, attach the capped needle to the distal end of the infusion tubing to keep the tubing sterile, and set it aside.

5 Attach the needleless injection port to the end of the client's catheter.

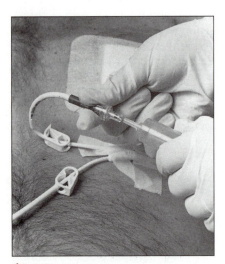

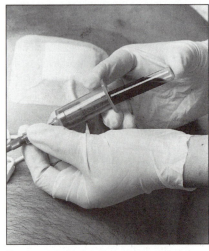

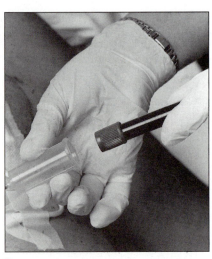

6 Remove the cap from the needleless injection port and set it aside in an aseptic manner (see step 1, page 134). Cleanse the catheter hub with an antiseptic wipe. Then attach the vacuum collection barrel with the multidraw adapter to the injection port as shown.

7 Unclamp the catheter, insert a vacuum tube, and aspirate approximately 5 mL of blood, or as prescribed, for discard. Laboratory values may be altered if the infusion solution or solution used to flush the catheter is not cleared adequately from the catheter; but because the external line holds, on average, no more than 1 mL, 5 mL usually is adequate for discard.

8 After drawing off the discard, remove that tube (as shown), and insert a new vacuum tube. Aspirate the amount of blood necessary to perform the prescribed tests.

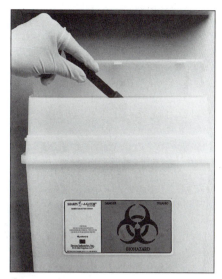

9 Dispose of the discard tube following agency policy for biohazardous waste.

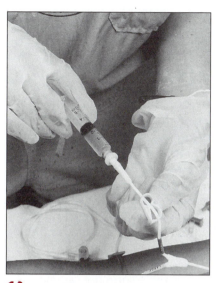

10 If the catheter lumen will be attached to an IV infusion following this procedure, attach the syringe containing the normal saline to the catheter, unclamp the catheter (as shown), and inject all but 0.5 mL of the solution to flush the tubing of residual blood.

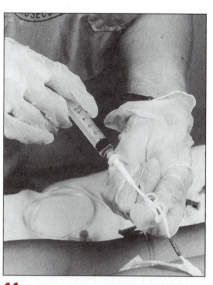

11 Then begin to clamp the catheter while simultaneously injecting the remaining 0.5 mL. Once the catheter has been clamped, however, stop injecting the solution. There may be a small amount of solution left in the syringe. *Caution: Do not inject solution against a clamped catheter because this could damage the catheter.* The simultaneous injection during the clamping procedure will provide enough positive pressure in the external line to prevent backflow of solution into the catheter tip.

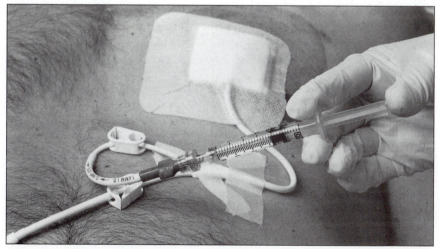

12 If the catheter will be capped and clamped following this procedure (rather than attached to an IV infusion), you will need to flush the catheter first with 3–5 mL normal saline, followed by a flush with 3–5 mL of 10 u/mL heparin, using steps 10 and 11.

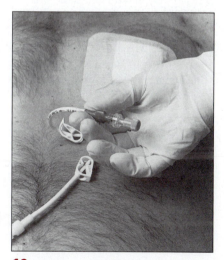

13 Replace the cap, and position the client for comfort.

PERFORMING A ROUTINE IRRIGATION OF A CHRONIC CENTRAL VENOUS CATHETER

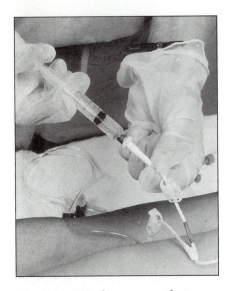

Chronic central venous catheters are flushed immediately following each infusion. Various concentrations of heparinized saline, from 10 to 1,000 USP units/mL, are commonly used for Hickman® and Broviac® catheters.* The Groshong™* catheter with the three-position Groshong valve eliminates the need for heparin and is flushed with normal saline only. For frequently (at least every 8 hours) accessed Hickman® and Broviac® catheters, flushing between infusions with 5 mL of normal saline without heparin has been shown to be effective. When the catheter has not been accessed in at least 8 hours, a periodic heparin flush is recommended to maintain patency. Flushing frequencies ranging from once a day to once a week have been found to be effective. Determination of the appropriate heparin concentration, volume, and flushing frequency is based on the client's medical condition, laboratory results, and prior clinical experience.

Prepare the prescribed amount of irrigant. Clamp the catheter and detach the infusion tubing. Cleanse the catheter hub with an antiseptic wipe and attach the syringe to the catheter hub. If the catheter has a needleless injection port, remove the injection port cap and insert the syringe directly into the injection port. Unclamp the catheter and inject the irrigant. For photo depiction of these steps, see the previous procedure. Wear gloves if this procedure follows either blood withdrawal or flushing that has been performed to prevent blood from backing up into the catheter.

---

*Hickman and Broviac are registered trademarks of C. R. Bard, Inc. Groshong is a trademark of C. R. Bard, Inc., or its subsidiaries.

CHANGING THE IV SOLUTION AND TUBING FOR A CHRONIC (HICKMAN®-TYPE) CENTRAL VENOUS CATHETER

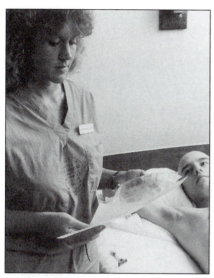

1 IV solution and tubing for a chronic central venous catheter are changed q48–72h, depending on agency protocol. Obtain the appropriate tubing and solution. Compare the prescribed infusion solution to the physician's prescription for your client.

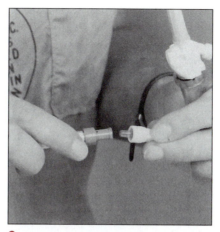

2 Attach extension tubing to the primary infusion set (as shown). Then spike the fresh solution container (see page 115), and prime the tubing (see page 116) to remove all the air. Turn off the infusion pump if the client has one, and clamp the client's central venous catheter.

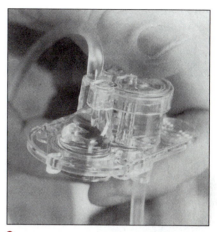

3 If your client has an infusion pump, follow manufacturer's instructions for priming the line, threading the tubing through the infusion pump, and purging the tubing as described by the infusion pump manufacturer. Invert the cassette (as shown) that is used by your agency's infusion pump, and depress the button on the cassette (or per manufacturer's instructions) to purge air from the cassette chamber.

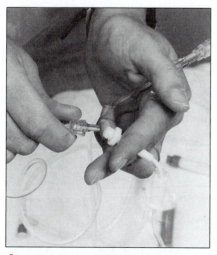

4 Clean the catheter/tubing junction with an antiseptic wipe, and detach the old infusion tubing from the catheter. Hold the hub of the catheter in such a way that you avoid contaminating it.

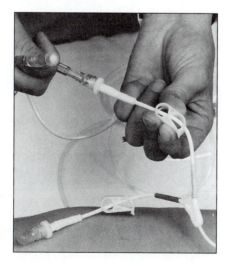

5 Remove the protective cap from the new infusion tubing, cleanse the catheter hub with an alcohol swab, and attach the new infusion tubing to the catheter hub. Unclamp the catheter. Then insert the new tubing into the infusion pump, following manufacturer's instructions. Clear the pump to determine the amount of fluids previously infused, and set the appropriate rate as needed. Unclamp the infusion tubing and turn the infusion pump on.

REPAIRING A MULTILUMEN CENTRAL VENOUS CATHETER

Many manufacturers of multilumen central venous catheters market repair kits that can be used if the central line breaks or tears somewhere external to the client. The lines are relatively easy to repair. Instructions vary. Be sure to follow specific steps outlined with each manufacturer's repair kits.

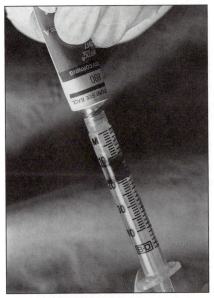

1 Wash your hands. Drape a sterile towel under the catheter to create a sterile field. Apply sterile gloves. Following manufacturer's instructions, aspirate into the sterile syringe the recommended amount of the adhesive that is included in the kit.

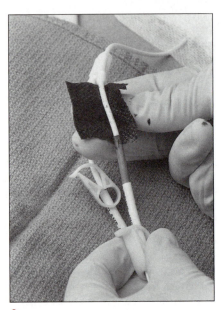

2 Using an antimicrobial wipe, thoroughly cleanse the area of the catheter that is to be repaired.

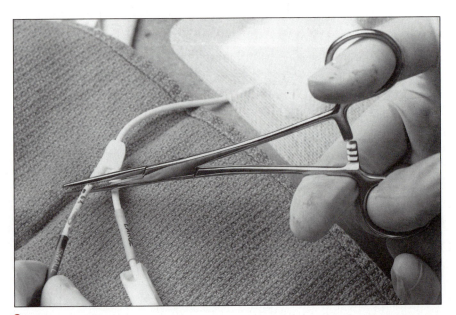

3 Firmly clamp the catheter proximal to the damaged area with forceps.

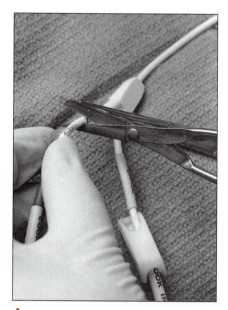

4 Cut off the damaged portion of the catheter using the sterile scissors included in the kit.

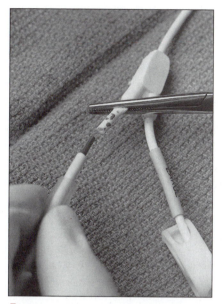

5 With a twisting motion, insert the replacement tubing into the cut end of the catheter until it is approximately 2–3 mm from being flush with the catheter. Apply a small amount of adhesive to the junction and slide the replacement tubing the rest of the way into the catheter.

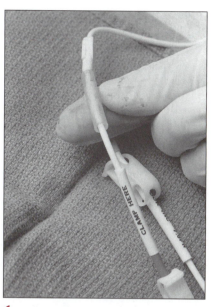

6 Slide the protective sleeve of the replacement tubing (shown in the photo between the nurse's thumb and index finger) over the junction.

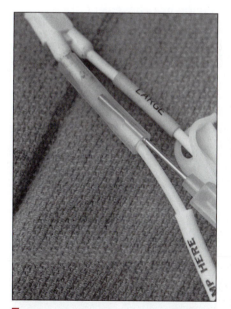

7 Using the blunt-ended needle supplied in the repair kit, inject adhesive into both ends of the sleeve. Wipe off any excess adhesive.

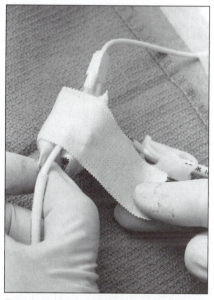

8 Splint the repaired junction with tongue blades that have been broken into 1-inch pieces and padded with gauze and tape.

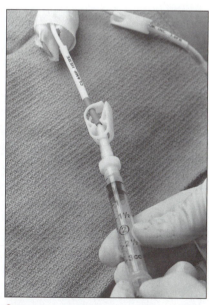

9 Once the repair has been completed, unclamp the line and aspirate for a blood return to ensure that the line is patent. See "Performing a Routine Irrigation of a Chronic Central Venous Catheter," page 166, for details.

ACCESSING THE IMPLANTABLE SUBCUTANEOUS PORT

1 Assemble the following materials:

☐ central line dressing kit or materials (see photo and description in "Changing the Exit Site Dressing for a Chronic Central Venous Catheter," page 159).

In addition, you will also need the following, as shown in this photo:

☐ normal saline for flushing the line. This bag of normal saline has a multidraw needleless adapter port (also known as a dispensing pin) to which a sterile syringe can be attached. In addition to the clean syringe that is attached to keep the dispensing pin sterile, you also will need another 5- or 10-mL sterile syringe.

☐ a noncoring bent Huber needle in 19, 20, or 21 gauge, 0.5–1.5 inch in length, with attached extension tubing (if the needle does not have attached extension tubing, obtain a 7-inch Luer Lok extension set)

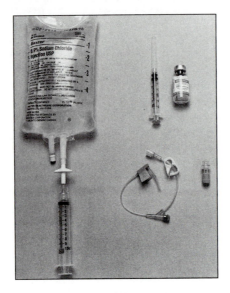

☐ needleless injection port

☐ heparin (usually 100 U/mL) and syringe if a heparin lock will be established after accessing the port (see page 175).

You will also need an impervious bag for disposal of dressings and supplies, a bag of prescribed fluids with primed infusion tubing (if fluids will be delivered), and an IV infusion pump (optional).

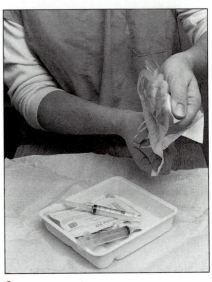

2 Wash your hands and open the sterile overwrap of the central line dressing kit for use as a sterile field. Drop the additional supplies onto this sterile field, including the 5- or 10-mL sterile syringe that you will use for drawing up the saline flush. Then, place the normal saline flush bag with the attached clean syringe in a convenient place on the bedside table or other table away from the sterile field. Remove the attached clean syringe, keeping the dispensing pin sterile by preventing its contact with the table's surface (eg, by letting it overlap the table).

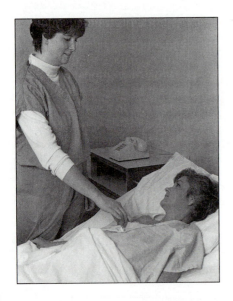

3 Explain the procedure to your client. Lower her gown to expose the skin over the implanted port. Palpate the position of the implanted port under the client's skin and locate the rubber septum.

4 Apply sterile gloves. Remove the sterile 5- or 10-mL syringe from the sterile field and attach it to the dispensing pin of the normal saline flush bag without touching the bag. Draw up 5 mL of the solution and place the filled syringe on the sterile field.

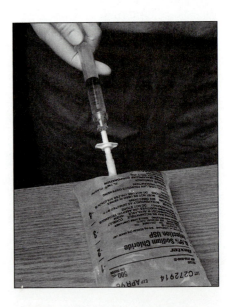

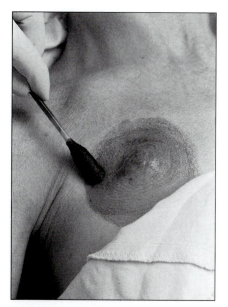

5 Open the package of antimicrobial swabsticks that are on your sterile field and place the opened package in a convenient place on your field. Remove one of the swabsticks and cleanse the area to be punctured, starting over the center of the port and circling outward to cover an area 10 cm (4 in) in diameter. Repeat with the two remaining swabs. Allow the area to dry at least 30 seconds while preparing the remaining supplies (step 6).

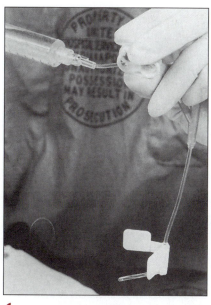

6 On the sterile field, connect the Huber needle, extension tubing, and injection port. Flush the needle-tubing-port assembly with the normal saline, leaving the syringe attached.

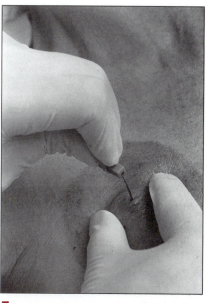

7 Stabilize the port between the thumb and finger of your non-dominant hand (this nurse is left-handed). With your dominant hand, insert the Huber noncoring needle perpendicular to the center of the port septum. Push firmly through the skin and septum until the needle touches the bottom of the port.

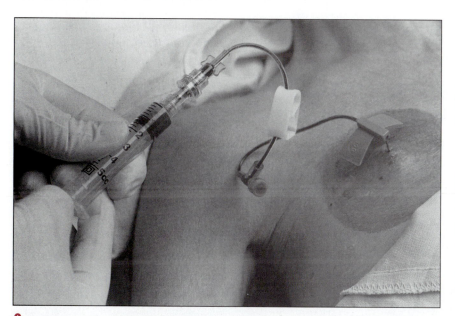

8 Aspirate gently until you note a blood return.

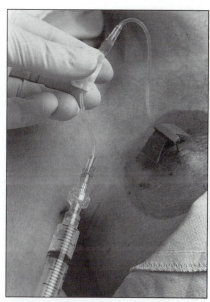

9 Flush with the normal saline to clear the line.

➤

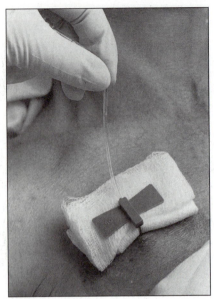

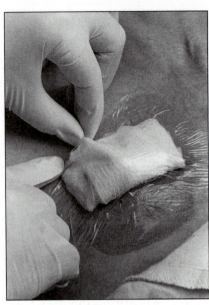

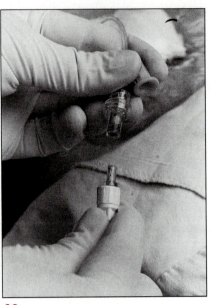

10 Place a folded 2 X 2 gauze pad under the hub of the needle (as shown) and another over the top.

11 Cover the entire site with adhesive, transparent dressing such as Tegaderm. You may secure the dressing further by taping down the edges.

12 To withdraw blood or establish a heparin lock, see pages 173–174 or page 175. To deliver fluids, remove the syringe and connect the primed IV tubing. Open the roller clamp and adjust it to the prescribed rate. Observe for free flow of the infusion and absence of any subcutaneous infiltration. Document the client's response to the procedure, the needle size used, and the date to ensure appropriate dressing and needle change. Dispose of the syringe into which you aspirated blood in a container for biohazardous waste and your used supplies in the impervious plastic bag. Or dispose of both per agency policy.

Note: For Home Health Care Considerations, see page 162, "Changing the Exit Site Dressing for a Chronic Central Venous Catheter."

WITHDRAWING BLOOD FROM AN IMPLANTABLE SUBCUTANEOUS PORT

1 Assemble the following materials:

☐ clean gloves (because of the possibility of coming into contact with blood)

☐ normal saline solution with a syringe for flushing

☐ vacuum container with multi-draw adapter

☐ vacuum tubes

☐ heparinized solution (usually 100 U/mL) if the heparin lock is to be capped and clamped after blood withdrawal

☐ capped needle (shown here on one of the syringes) to protect the end of the infusion tubing if an infusion is currently running.

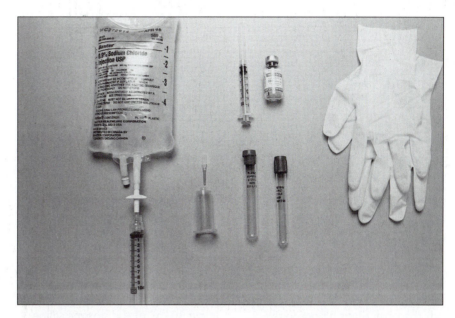

Explain the procedure to your client. Position her for comfort and to ensure that you have easy access to her implanted port. If your client's port is not already accessed, follow steps 1–8 in the previous section. After completing steps 1–8, go to step 2, below.

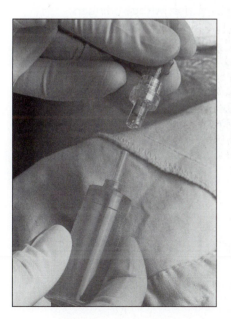

2 If your client's port has been accessed already (see previous procedure), wash your hands and apply clean gloves. If the port has a heparin/saline lock, remove the cap from the injection port and place it aseptically on the table (see step 1, page 134). If the client has an IV infusion running instead, stop the infusion, clamp the extension line, and detach the infusion tubing from the port's connector hub. Attach a sterile cap (eg, a needle cap) to the infusion tubing to keep it clean. Then, as shown, attach a vacuum container with a multidraw adapter to the port's extension set. *Note: This client's extension set has an attached injection port that is designed for safety inasmuch as it does not require a needle for access.*

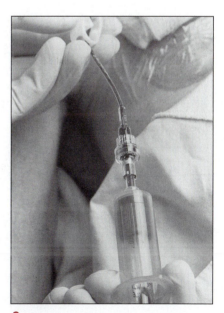

3 Unclamp the line, insert the vacuum tube fully into the vacuum container, and aspirate 10 mL of blood for discard.

➡

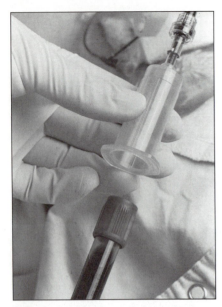

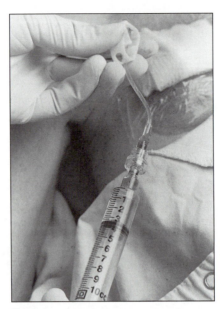

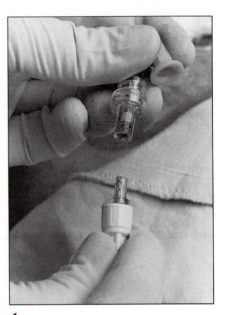

4 Remove the vacuum tube. Continue filling the vacuum tubes in this manner until the appropriate amount of blood has been drawn for the prescribed blood work.

5 Remove the vacuum container from the injection port. Attach the syringe containing the normal saline to the injection port or hub. Inject 10 mL of the normal saline. Because of the small diameter of the tubing, it is important that you inject the saline vigorously to prevent clotting of the tubing. Clamp the extension line and remove the syringe.

6 Either reattach the infusion tubing (as shown) and unclamp; flush with a heparinized solution (see page 175) and cap; or discontinue the needle access if appropriate. To prevent backflow of blood when discontinuing the needle access, maintain positive injection pressure while simultaneously withdrawing the needle and pressing down on the port with two fingers.

Remove your gloves and wash your hands; document the procedure. Dispose of the blood obtained for discard following agency protocol for disposal of body fluids. Arrange for delivery of the blood sample to the laboratory.

ESTABLISHING A HEPARIN LOCK IN AN IMPLANTABLE SUBCUTANEOUS PORT

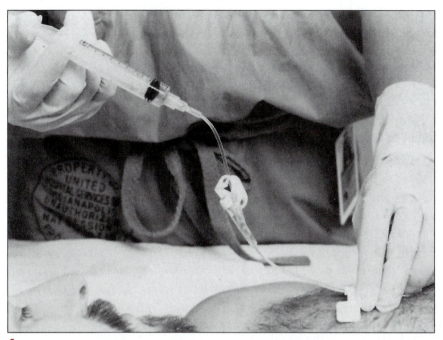

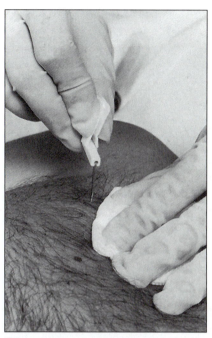

1 After each use, it is necessary to fill the port with sterile heparinized solution to prevent clot formation and subsequent catheter blockage. If the port is not used for prolonged periods of time, it should be flushed at least once every 4 weeks. Assemble the following materials:

- ☐ clean gloves (to prevent contact with blood)
- ☐ injectable normal saline solution
- ☐ heparin (100 U/mL)
- ☐ gauze pad
- ☐ antiseptic wipes
- ☐ 2 10-mL syringes with needles

Fill one syringe with 10 mL normal saline and the other with 5 mL heparin (100 U/mL), or as prescribed. Clamp the extension tubing and cleanse the connector hub with an antiseptic wipe. Attach the syringe containing the normal saline to the connector. Unclamp the line and inject the normal saline into the port. Reclamp.

Remove the empty syringe and attach the syringe containing the heparin. Unclamp and inject the solution.

2 When you have injected the solution and if you will be discontinuing the needle and extension tubing, squeeze the needle wings together and withdraw the needle straight up, pressing down on the port with two fingers. Blot the needle's exit site with a sterile gauze pad. Bleeding should be absent or minimal. Dispose of the needle in the nearest sharps container. Remove your gloves and wash your hands.

ASSESSING AND INTERVENING FOR AN AIR EMBOLISM

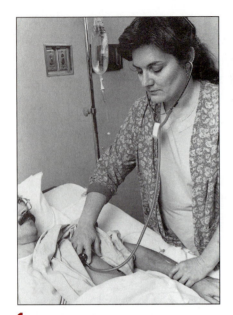

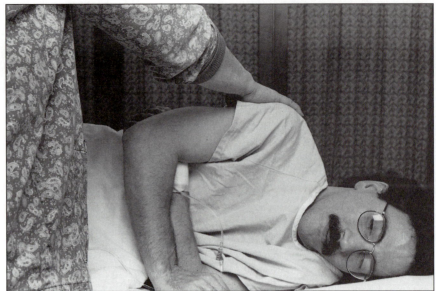

1 All clients with IV lines are at risk for an air embolism. Rapid infusion rates compound the risk by producing high vascular pressure—for example, the administration of a unit of blood over a 10–15 minute period. Because an air embolism can be fatal, it is essential that you monitor and observe the client for the presence of chest pain, coughing, hypotension, cyanosis, and hypoxia. In addition, if the client does have an air embolism, auscultation over the right ventricle may reveal a churning "windmill" sound.

2 Any indication of an air embolism necessitates an immediate intervention. Turn the client to his left side to displace the air into the apex of the heart and to help prevent its rapid movement into the pulmonary artery. Then remove the pillow and lower the head of the bed into Trendelenburg's position. Lowering the head of the bed will increase intrathoracic pressure, decreasing the flow of air into the vein during inhalation.

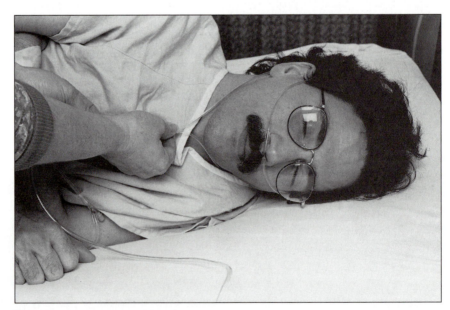

3 Administer oxygen, if it is at the bedside, and notify the physician immediately. If the air has not slowly and safely dissipated into the pulmonary system, the physician may aspirate the air from the apical area. Stay with the client and continue to reassure him.

REFERENCES

Christianson D: Caring for a patient who has an implanted port. *Am J Nurs* 94(11):40–44, 1994.

Dickerson R: Ten tips for easing the pain of intramuscular injections. *Nursing 92* 22(8):55, 1992.

Drass J: What you need to know about insulin injections. *Nursing 92* 22(11):40–43, 1992.

Dutcher JP. ed: *Modern transfusion therapy,* volume 1. Boca Raton, Florida: CRC Press: 1990.

Freedman S: Basserman G: Tunneled catheters: Technologic advances and nursing care issues. *Nurs Clins North Am* 28(4):851–858, 1993.

Gullo S: Implanted ports: Technologic advances and nursing care issues. *Nurs Clins North Am* 28(4):859–871, 1993.

Holder C. Alexander J: A new and improved guide to IV therapy. *Am J Nurs* 90(2):43–47, 1990.

Kelly C et al: A change in flushing protocol. *Oncology Nurse Forum* 19(4):599–605, 1992.

Lehmann S, Barber J: Giving medications by feeding tube: How to avoid problems. *Nursing 91* 21(11):58–61, 1991.

McGovern K: 10 golden rules for administering drugs safely. *Nursing 92* 22(3):49–56, 1992.

Meares C: PICC and MLC lines: Options worth exploring. *Nursing 92* 22(10):52–55, 1992.

Millam D: Starting IV: How to develop your venipuncture expertise. *Nursing 92* 22(9):33–48, 1992.

National Blood Resource Education Programs: *Transfusion guidelines for nurses.* NIH Publication No. 90-2668a, September 1990.

Newton M, Newton D, Fudin J: Reviewing the "big three" injection routes. *Nursing 92* 22(2):34–41, 1992.

Querin J, Stahl L: Twelve simple, sensible steps for successful blood transfusions. *Nursing 90* 20(10):68–81, 1990.

Rice R: *Handbook of Home Health Nursing Procedures.* St. Louis: Mosby, 1995.

Rountree D: The PIC catheter: A different approach. *Am J Nurs* 91(8):22–26, 1991.

Sheldon P, Bender M: High-technology in home care: An overview of intravenous therapy. *Nurs Clins North Am* 29(3):507–519, 1994.

Standards Committee, American Association of Blood Banks: *Standards for blood banks and transfusion services,* ed 16. Bethesda, Maryland, 1994.

Teplitz L: Responding to an air embolism. *Nursing 92* 22(7):33, 1992.

Viall C: Your complete guide to central venous catheters. *Nursing 90* 20(2):34–41, 1990.

Whitney R: Comparing long-term central venous catheters. *Nursing* 21(4):70–71, 1991.

Wickham R: Advances in venous access devices and nursing management strategies. *Nurs Clins North Am* 24(2):345–364, 1990.

PERFORMING SPECIALIZED NURSING PROCEDURES

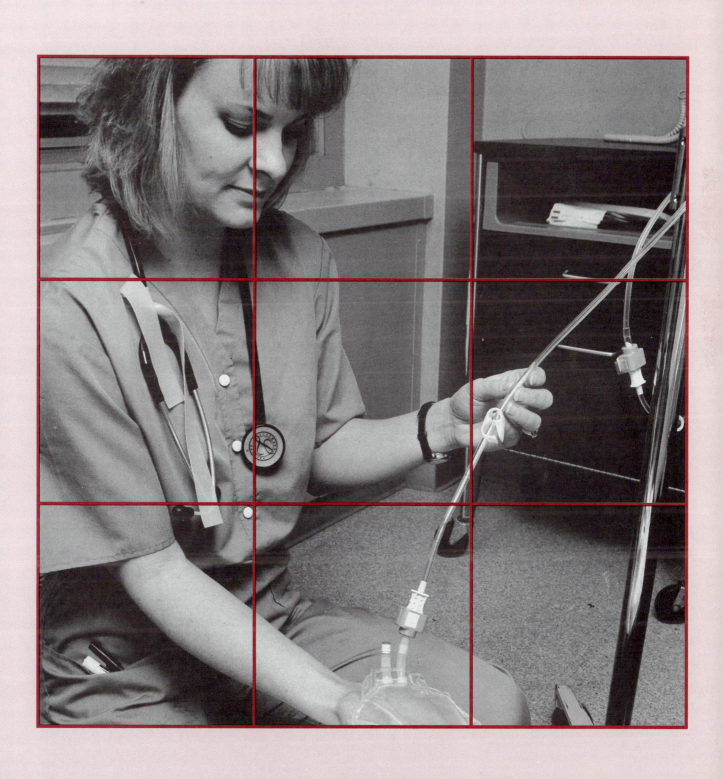

CHAPTER 4

Managing Female Reproductive Procedures and Immediate Care of the Newborn

CHAPTER OUTLINE

PERFORMING ROUTINE GYNECOLOGIC TECHNIQUES

The Female Reproductive System

Nursing Assessment Guidelines

Teaching Breast Self-Examination

Assisting the Client with Postsurgical Mastectomy Exercises

Providing Perineal Care

Using a Squeeze Bottle

Preparing a Sitz Bath

Using a Surgi-Gator

Providing Care for Clients with Cervical-Uterine Radiation Implants

PERFORMING PRENATAL TECHNIQUES

Assessing the Prenatal Abdomen

Measuring Fundal Height

Inspecting and Palpating Fetal Parts

Auscultating Fetal Heart Tones

Using Ultrasonic (Doppler) Auscultation

Performing External Electronic Fetal Monitoring

Assessing for Amniotic Fluid

Providing Comfort Measures

Applying Counterpressure to Relieve Leg Cramps

Applying Pressure to Relieve Back Pain

PERFORMING POSTPARTUM TECHNIQUES

Assessing the Mother

Inspecting and Palpating the Breasts

Palpating the Fundus and Bladder

Evaluating the Lochia

Inspecting the Perineum

Assisting with Infant Feeding

Positioning the Infant

Burping the Infant

Massaging the Breasts for Manual Expression of Breast Milk

Using Breast Pumps

Managing Hand Pumps

Assisting with Electric Breast Pumps

CARING FOR THE NEWBORN

Admitting the Neonate to the Hospital

Obtaining Footprints

Instilling Ophthalmic Erythromycin

Administering a Vitamin K Injection

Obtaining a Blood Sample

Obtaining a Urine Specimen

Assessing the Neonate

Performing a General Inspection

Auscultating

Taking an Axillary Temperature

Palpating

Measuring and Weighing the Infant

Taking an Arterial Blood Pressure

Providing Neonatal Care

Giving Umbilical Cord Care

Suctioning

Using Phototherapy

Performing Routine Gynecologic Techniques

THE FEMALE REPRODUCTIVE SYSTEM

Assessing and Planning

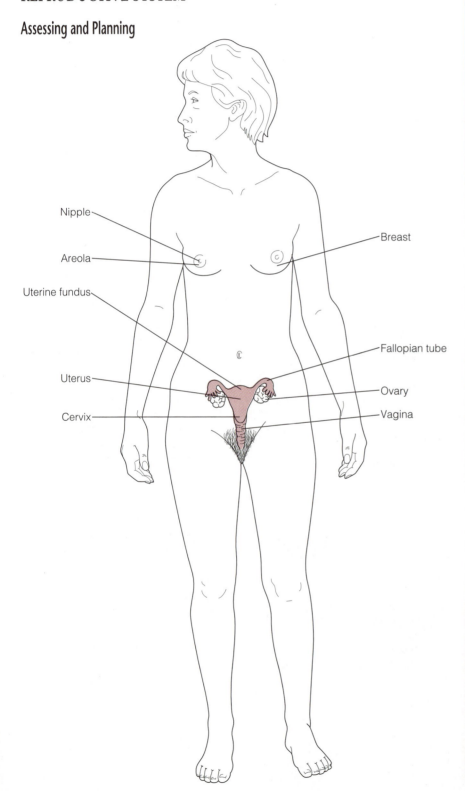

Nipple

Areola

Uterine fundus

Uterus

Cervix

Breast

Fallopian tube

Ovary

Vagina

Before teaching breast self-examination (BSE), gather subjective data from the client. A comprehensive history should include a complete evaluation for the following:

Risk Factors for Breast Cancer: client history of breast surgery, cancer, or fibrocystic disease; family history of cancer, fibroids, mother's taking of diethylstilbestrol (DES); history of smoking or exposure to carcinogens; history of obesity, diabetes mellitus, or hypertension; history of chronic psychological stress; use of estrogens; dietary intake high in animal fats.

Personal Factors: client's age—risk for breast cancer increases steadily after age 35, with the greatest risk occurring in clients over age 85; ages at which menstruation and menopause began—clients with early menstruation (11 years or younger) or late menopause (after 52 years) are at greater risk; age at first full-term pregnancy—clients over 30 years and nulliparous clients are at higher risk, and clients having their first child at age 20 or younger have decreased risk; discharge or secretions in nipples—color, amount, frequency; changes in breasts since adulthood—size, shape, color; mammography history and results; knowledge of BSE, frequency of performance, and time of month it is performed.

TEACHING BREAST SELF-EXAMINATION

Assessing and Planning

The most common site for cancer in the adult woman is the breast, and the single most effective means for improving survival rates in breast cancer is early detection of breast tumors using breast self-examination. This important procedure should be incorporated into the discharge planning for *all* your adult female clients.

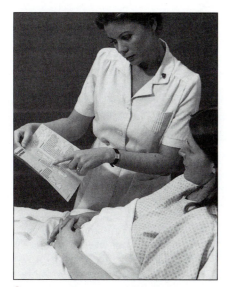

1 Provide a warm and private environment for your client, and arrange for her to sit facing away from the door. Explain that she should routinely perform breast self-examination (BSE) about a week after her menstrual period has begun because at that time her breasts will be the least swollen and a lump will be more readily detected. To ensure consistency, menopausal clients or those who have had hysterectomies or oophorectomies should perform the examination at the same time every month, for example on the first day of the month. Women who are breastfeeding should perform BSE when their breasts are empty.

Take your time, encourage questions, and give the client literature on breast self-examination, such as the free pamphlets provided by the American Cancer Society. The goal of this procedure is to familiarize your client with the way her breasts normally look and feel. Optimally, the examination will give her confidence in her knowledge base and skill in assessing abnormalities so that should cancer be detected, she will have found it at its earliest, most treatable stage. In addition, teaching your client breast self-examination will enable you to assess for abnormalities at the same time.

Implementing

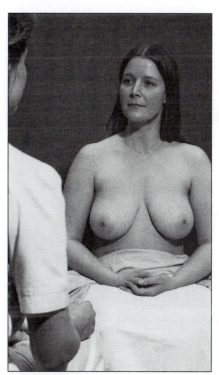

2 The assessment consists of both inspection and palpation. To begin the inspection segment of the examination, instruct the client to sit on the side of the bed and to lower her gown to the waist.

Explain that she should relax her arms in her lap and inspect her breasts in a large mirror. If a mirror is unavailable, she should pretend that you are a mirror so that she can follow each step without losing the continuity of the examination. As she looks in the mirror, explain that each breast may normally deviate slightly from the other in size and symmetry, but she should be alert to any monthly *changes* in contour and appearance. Instruct her to look for swelling, puckering, dimpling of the skin, changes in texture and color, as well as a change in a mole. Striae (stretch marks) are normal, and symmetrical venous patterns are fairly common in fair-complexioned women. Explain, however, that diffuse, blue casts, suggestive of an increased blood supply to an area, should be followed up with a physician's examination. The areolae also may vary slightly in size and shape from one another, but differences in color, rashes, scaling, or ulcerations should be noted. Discharge from the nipple is usually abnormal in the mature, nonlactating woman; an inverted nipple also can signal a problem, especially if it was recently everted. Explain also that an inverted nipple that becomes everted during movement can occur with an underlying pathology. *Note: At this time, you also should be alert to peau d'orange, skin that is large-pored and edematous caused by a tumor obstructing the lymph glands. This is an advanced sign of breast cancer and generally is not necessary to include for client education.*

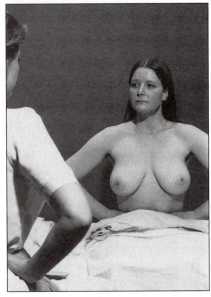

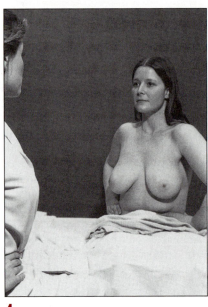

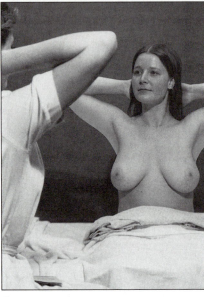

3 Instruct the client to tense her pectoral muscles by squeezing her waist. She should look again for asymmetry in size and contour, dimpling, puckering, or retractions of the skin.

4 While continuing to squeeze her waist, she should turn from side to side so that she can view all of the breast tissue.

5 Demonstrate raising the arms by placing them behind or high over the head. This will enable the client to look for unilateral changes in the symmetry and contour of each breast.

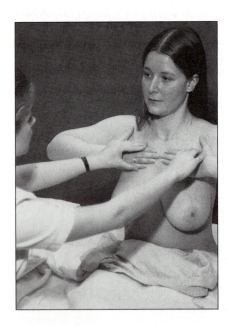

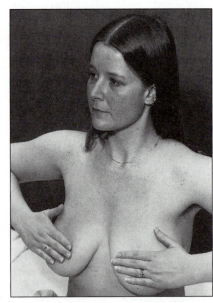

6 To being the palpation segment of the examination, wash your hands and then show your client how to sweep her breasts bilaterally. Explain that this is done to assess for lumps in the upper breast tissue, which begins just under the clavicles. Show her how to position her hands at the clavicles (left) and to sweep them downward onto the nipples (right). Occasionally, a hardened area will be palpated and most often it is a rib. To ensure that it is, the client should be shown how to palpate across the area to feel for the underlying rib. If the hardened area is not contiguous, she should see a physician. This segment of the examination can be facilitated if it is performed in the shower. The wet skin will enhance the sensitivity of the flats of the fingers.

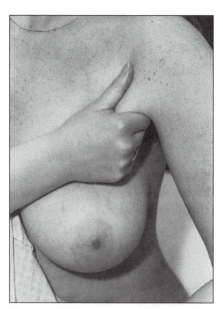

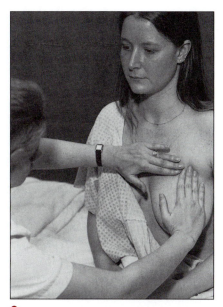

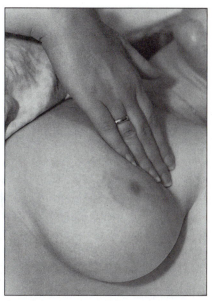

7 Show the client how to assess the muscle and lymph tissue at the axillae. To relax the muscle, she should rest an arm in her lap with the elbow slightly flexed. She should then grasp the tissue between the thumb and fingers of her opposite hand and palpate for lumps or swollen lymph glands using the flats of her fingers.

8 While she is sitting, teach her the procedure for palpating each breast in concentric circles. This is the portion of the examination that the woman will regularly perform in a supine position. Show her how to find the 12 o'clock position at the periphery of the breast tissue, the uppermost and outermost section (shown here). Explain that she should palpate around the breast in a circular fashion, using the pads of her middle three fingers, until she returns to 12 o'clock. In this photo, the nurse is showing her client how to palpate with the right hand and guide the movement with the left hand. Explain that a ridge of firm tissue at the curve of the lower breast is normal. However, she should see a physician if she detects lumps, knots, or thickened tissue. Typically, a malignancy is painless, is attached to underlying tissue, and occurs most often in the upper outer quadrant.

9 For self-examination, the client should lie down and, while supine, apply the above technique. To examine the left breast (as shown), the client should place a towel or a small pillow under the left side and shoulder and position her left hand behind her head. This position will distribute the breast tissue over the chest wall more evenly. A larger breasted woman should lie down on her left side to assess the right side of her left breast and on her right side to assess the left side of her left breast. Explain that she can facilitate the gliding motion and increase the sensitivity of her fingertips by generously applying lotion to her fingertips. After palpating in a complete circle around the outer breast tissue, she should advance an inch toward the nipple and repeat the process until the entire breast has been examined in this manner.

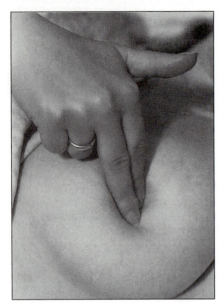

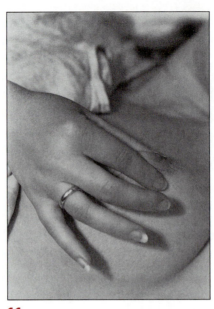

10 After the client has examined the breast, she should next examine the nipple. She should depress the nipple with her index and middle fingers to palpate the area underneath, which is referred to as the *well.* This is a common location for tumors, and it too often is missed during a cursory examination.

11 Instruct her to squeeze and milk the nipple gently to assess for discharge. Any new discharge in an adult nonlactating female is significant, and it should be referred to a physician.

Evaluating

12 After completing the assessment of the left breast, the client should repeat the examination with the right breast while you observe and answer any questions she may have.

When the assessment has been completed, compare your observations with those of the client. Arrange for a physician referral if you have detected any abnormalities. Reassure her that most lumps and abnormalities (eight out of ten) are benign, but that only a physician can make a diagnosis and arrange for the appropriate treatment. Suggest that women with fibrocystic breasts make a graph noting areas of lumps and thickened tissue. This will provide a comparison so they can quickly determine whether the lumps are preexisting or indicative of change.

ASSISTING THE CLIENT WITH POSTSURGICAL MASTECTOMY EXERCISES

Postsurgical arm and shoulder exercises are crucial to the full recovery of your clients who have had mastectomies because they help to maintain circulation in the involved arm, reduce edema, and promote maximum function. If your client is scheduled for a mastectomy, consult with her physician prior to the surgery to determine the type of mastectomy anticipated so that you can develop an individualized exercise plan that can be implemented as soon as the client arrives in the recovery room. In addition, with physician approval, you can arrange for a visit by a member of the American Cancer Society's "Reach to Recovery" support group or other similar groups in your community for the postsurgical period. To ensure that your client's progress warrants increased range of movement, check with her physician before initiating each new exercise. The movements depicted in the following photographs range from the simple to the advanced. As appropriate, teach the following exercises to the client *before* surgery. Review them with her during her hospitalization and again just prior to hospital discharge. ***Note:*** *The photos that follow demonstrate client teaching* ***before*** *surgery.*

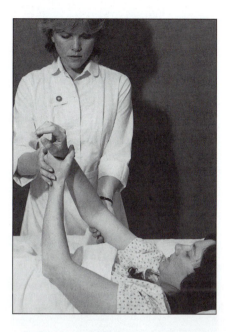

1 Passive range of motion (ROM) exercises can be initiated as soon as the client arrives in the recovery room; once she has returned to her room you can begin assisted ROM exercises on her involved shoulder (as shown). Review the procedures in Chapter 2 to assist you with the movements involved. Because the client may have both discomfort with and apprehension about stretching the incisional site, be sure to explain the reason for the exercises and reassure her that the movements will be adapted to her level of tolerance. For maximal joint mobility, these exercises should be performed in sets of 10, three times a day.

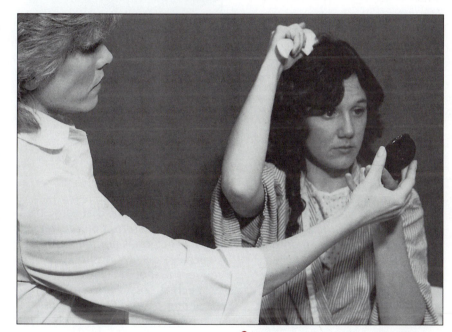

2 By the second postoperative day, activities of daily living using the involved arm should be encouraged as much as possible. For example, combing the hair, putting on makeup, or washing the face are all activities that will exercise the involved arm.

➡

3 When your client is able to lift her involved arm actively without assistance, instruct her to clasp her hands behind her head (as shown).

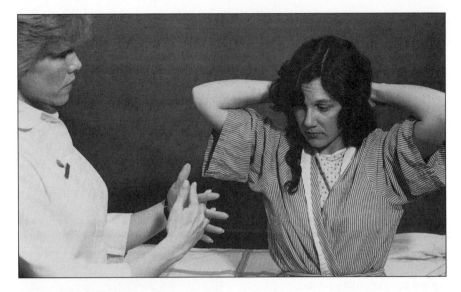

4 She should then attempt to touch her elbows together, or to bring them as close together as possible. This movement will flex, externally rotate, and adduct the involved shoulder.

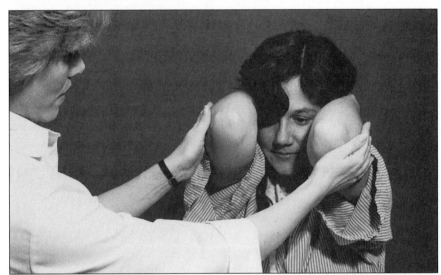

5 You also can use assistive devices to achieve shoulder flexion. With physician approval, assemble a rope and pulley system onto an overhead trapeze bar. The client should grasp the hand grips and begin the exercise with the involved arm in the lower position. Instruct her to pull down gently with the hand of the uninvolved arm, allowing the involved arm to be raised gradually (as shown). Explain to the client that some discomfort and a sensation of stretching the incision is normal, but that to achieve maximum shoulder range, she should flex the shoulder as much as possible. *Note: The client may adapt this exercise at home by placing a rope over a stable shower curtain rod or over a wall hook.*

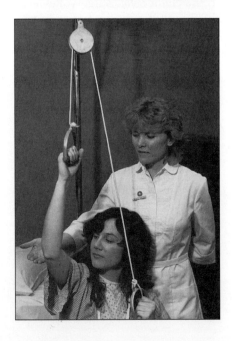

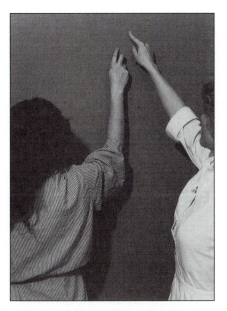

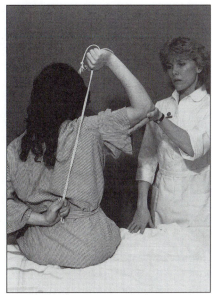

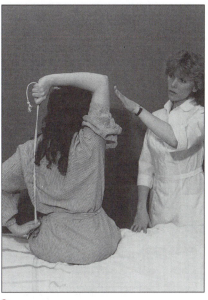

6 You can also teach the client how to "climb a wall," which will promote shoulder flexion without the use of an assistive device. The client should face the wall and position her involved arm at shoulder level. Gradually she will scale the wall by "walking" her fingertips upward (as shown). Encourage her to achieve maximum shoulder ROM. *Note: Place a tape marker on the wall to indicate her progress after each exercise. This will give her a goal to strive for with each new attempt.*

7 Around the second postoperative week, usually after the sutures have been removed, the client can begin exercises that will maximize external rotation and abduction of the shoulder. A 75-cm (30-in) rope can be used to assist the client in achieving maximum range. Instruct her to grasp the rope, holding the lower end in her uninvolved hand in the back at the level of her waistline. The top of the rope should be held in the hand of her involved arm at about the level of her head.

8 She should very gently pull down on the rope with the hand of her uninvolved arm, guiding the involved arm through abduction and external rotation. This exercise should be performed at least three times daily in sets of 10 each.

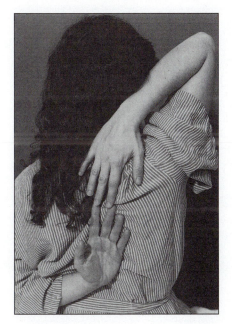

9 For implementation after the incision and underlying tissue have healed, teach the client how she can achieve maximum shoulder flexion by touching her fingertips behind her back with the involved arm uppermost. This exercise simulates the range required for zipping back zippers and fastening brassieres.

PROVIDING PERINEAL CARE

USING A SQUEEZE BOTTLE

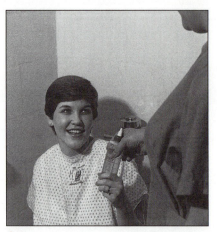 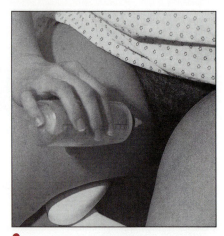

1 A very simple method for providing perineal care is the use of a squeeze bottle filled with tap water warmed to approximately 37.8 C (100 F). A postpartum client can use this method after every voiding to cleanse her perineum.

2 Instruct the client to insert the nozzle of the bottle between her legs and to squirt the bottle so that it sprays onto the perineum. Explain to the client that it will take several squirts to thoroughly cleanse the area. She should then blot her perineum from front to back when she has finished with the squeeze bottle, using either toilet paper or clean wipes provided by your agency.

PREPARING A SITZ BATH

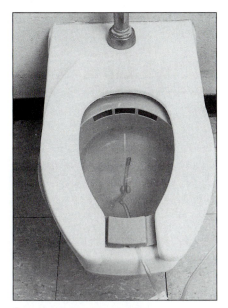

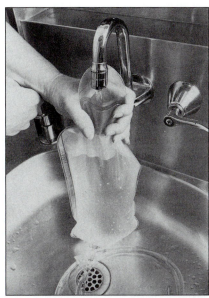

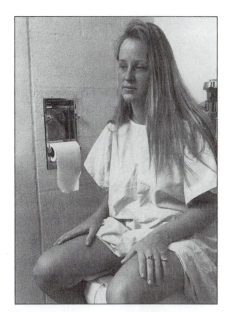

1 A sitz bath is prepared for clients who have vulvar pain and swelling and who require warmth to heal the perineal area, for example after vaginal hysterectomies, vulvec-tomies, childbirth, or hemorrhoid-ectomies. The disposable plastic basin shown here can be sent home with the client. The system functions as a warm water bath. Warm water flows from the plastic bag reservoir through the tubing into the basin and overflows into the commode. It takes 20–30 minutes for the reservoir to finish draining.

2 Fill the plastic basin with warm water and place it in the commode. Fill the plastic reservoir with warm water (as shown), being sure to clamp the tubing. Hang the reser-voir on an IV pole or wall hook, or place the reservoir on the sink beside the commode. Attach the tubing to the bottom of the plastic basin (shown in step 1), and ensure that the tubing is patent. When it is in use, the system will drain continuously to provide a source of fresh warm water to the client.

3 Test the temperature of the sitz bath to ensure that it is in the range of 37.8–40.5 C (100–105 F), using a bath thermometer to verify the temperature. Assist the client into the sitting position. After she is situated, unclamp the tubing. If you cannot stay with the client during the prescribed treatment time, make sure the emergency call light is within her reach. Because of the warmth of the water, the client must be monitored periodically for potential fainting. Sitz baths are usually recommended for periods of 20–30 minutes.

USING A SURGI-GATOR

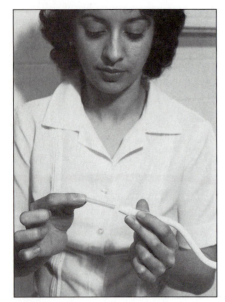

1 If your agency has a Surgi-gator perineal care system for cleansing and providing warmth to the perineum, you can teach your client how to use the system on her own for the times in which it is prescribed, as well as during the times she experiences perineal discomfort.

Every client is issued her own applicator. Explain to the client that she must first insert the soap cartridge into the proximal end of the applicator.

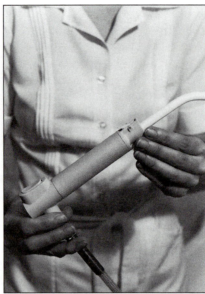

2 The proximal end is then inserted and snapped into the dispensing handle that connects to the wall-mounted unit. Explain that depressing the control button on the dispensing handle delivers both the cleansing cycle and the rinse cycle. Make sure the temperature is set at approximately 37.8 C (100 F).

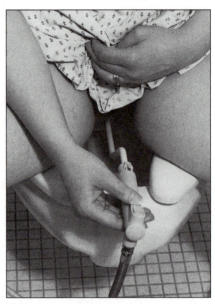

3 Instruct the client to sit on the toilet, spread her legs apart, and insert the Surgi-gator applicator between her legs so that it is just distal to her perineum.

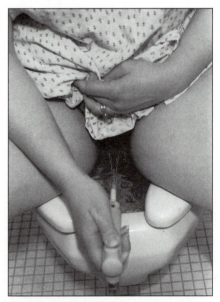

4 After depressing the control button, she can adjust the distance of the applicator to her perineum to achieve the desired force of spray. Remind her to return the applicator to the bedside for subsequent use.

PROVIDING CARE FOR CLIENTS WITH CERVICAL-UTERINE RADIATION IMPLANTS

If your client has gynecologic carcinoma, such as endometrial cancer, she may be treated with external radiation or sealed radioactive implants that are placed within her body. Because the implant is sealed within a metal capsule or supplied as a solid substance, the potential for contamination is negligible. The external radiation level associated with these implants is substantial, however, and necessitates that exposure to staff, other clients, and visitors be minimal. Therefore, clients undergoing internal radiation usually have private rooms. Women who are pregnant or who may be pregnant should not enter the room. Visitation is restricted to individuals older than age 18 and often to the client's spouse or significant other only.

Visitors under the age of 45, with the exception of the client's spouse, often are asked to limit their visits to 30 minutes a day. Clients with radiation implants must have warning signs posted on their closed doors and charts to alert staff and visitors that radiation therapy is in progress.

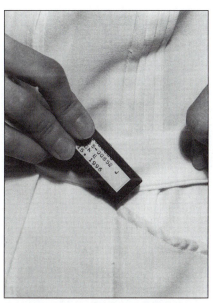

1 Before entering the client's room, attach a radiation badge to your clothing at about the level of the client's uterus. Monthly radiation levels, according to federal regulations, never should exceed 400 mrem. Nurses who care for these clients rarely receive monthly amounts this high.

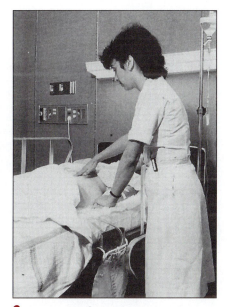

2 Plan client care carefully so that you can accomplish as much as possible in the shortest amount of time. If the client is allowed to move from a supine position for brief periods of time, plan care around the scheduled position changes. Comfort measures, such as upper back care, the use of sheepskin pads, and on-time administration of pain medications, are essential for helping to minimize the client's discomfort. Because the client will have an indwelling urinary catheter to decompress the bladder, inspect the catheter and drainage system and assess the bladder to ensure that the system is draining effectively. An obstructed catheter, causing bladder distension, could result in radiation burns to the bladder. Whenever possible, stand at the head of the bed to maximize the distance between yourself and the client's uterus. Be sure to inspect the vaginal introitus to ensure that the gauze packing and implants are intact. If you do find metal in the bed, *do not touch it.* Notify the radiation department so that they can remove the implant with forceps. However, be assured that the client's excretions and secretions are *not* radioactive. *Caution: Avoid use of oil-based lotions or creams on the client's back, abdomen, or buttocks. When used in conjunction with radiation, these products may cause burning of the skin. Use water-soluble lubricants instead.*

Performing Prenatal Techniques

ASSESSING THE PRENATAL ABDOMEN

MEASURING FUNDAL HEIGHT

Assessing uterine size by measuring fundal height is often initiated in the client's second trimester. It is continued into the third trimester as a routine assessment tool for monitoring fetal growth. Although it is not a precise indicator of fetal development, it will alert you to sudden growth spurts found, for example, in multiple gestations, or to a lag in progression indicating intrauterine growth retardation. To measure the fundal height, obtain a nonstretchable tape measure; position one end at the fundus and measure the distance to the symphysis pubis in centimeters. Up until the third trimester, the measurement, will, on average, correlate with the gestational age.

For example, at 24 weeks' gestation, the fundus measures around 24 cm for the average woman, and it is usually at the level of the umbilicus.

Using McDonald's Rule

When the client is in her third trimester, apply McDonald's rule to estimate gestational age. For example, if your client measures 28 cm from the fundus to the symphysis pubis, you can estimate gestational age in lunar months by calculating in the following manner:

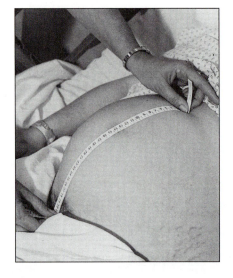

$$\frac{\text{Fundal height in cm}}{3.5} = \frac{\text{Gestational age}}{\text{in lunar months}}$$

$$\frac{28\ \text{cm}}{3.5} = 8\ \text{lunar months}$$

INSPECTING AND PALPATING FETAL PARTS

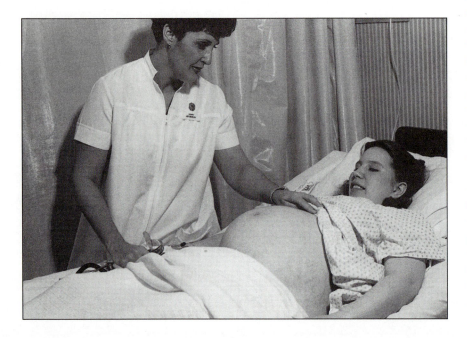

Palpate and locate fetal parts prior to auscultating for fetal heart tones (FHTs). Once you have identified the fetal back, you can readily elicit heart sounds because there is less bone and tissue through which to auscultate. Provide warmth and privacy for your client; for her comfort and to relax the abdominal wall, make sure she has recently voided. After explaining the procedure, elevate her head slightly and ask her to flex her knees, which will further relax the abdomen. Expose the abdomen from the xiphoid process to the symphysis pubis, and then inspect it to help you assess the position of the fetus. Does it appear to lie up and down in a longitudinal position or left and right in a transverse position?

Performing Leopold's Maneuvers

Leopold's maneuvers are performed to determine fetal position. Make sure your hands are warm, and perform the assessment between contractions, whether Braxton Hicks or labor contractions.

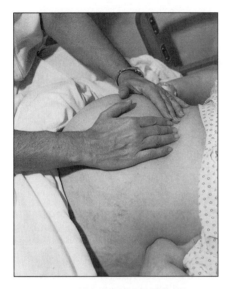

First Maneuver: Face the client and bilaterally palpate the upper abdomen. This will help you determine which of the fetal parts is in the uterine fundus. The breech is large, soft, and asymmetrical; the head is round, hard, and it moves more freely.

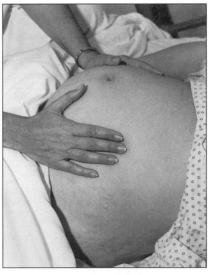

Second Maneuver: Continue facing the client, and place each hand along the sides of the abdomen. Gently but firmly palpate with your palms and fingers. Assess one side and then the other to determine the side on which the fetal back lies. One side should feel smooth and quite firm—the fetal back; the other side should be indentable and less resistant—the extremities on the opposite uterine wall.

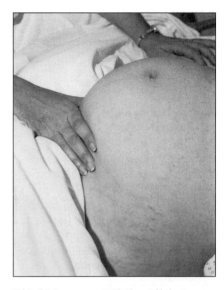

Third Maneuver: While still facing the client, position your dominant hand over the lower abdomen just proximal to the symphysis pubis, and firmly palpate with your thumb and index finger. Explain to the client that this maneuver may be uncomfortable. This maneuver helps to confirm the data gathered in the first maneuver. Again, the head will be round, hard, and ballotable (movable) if it has not already engaged. The breech will feel soft and asymmetrical. (This assessment will be much more difficult if the presenting part has already engaged.)

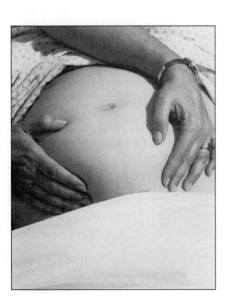

Fourth Maneuver: Face the client's feet and position your hands on both sides of the abdomen with your fingers curving downward toward, and immediately proximal to, the pubis. This maneuver will help you locate the cephalic prominence, which is the most prominent portion of the fetal head. Press deeply with your fingertips because you will need to palpate through several layers of tissue,

muscle, and fluid. The cephalic prominence is located on the side in which your fingers meet the greatest resistance. If it is located on the side opposite the back, the head is flexed and a normal delivery will probably ensue. If it is located on the same side as the back, the head is extended and the face or brow will probably present. Again, the greater the engagement, the more difficult the assessment.

AUSCULTATING FETAL HEART TONES

Once you have located the fetal back using Leopold's maneuvers, you can readily auscultate FHTs. This assessment will also reconfirm your assessment of the location of the fetal parts. However, in an emergency, auscultate in the midline between the umbilicus and symphysis pubis, the site in which FHTs are the loudest in the more typical cephalic presentation. With a fetoscope, the FHTs will be inaudible until weeks 18–20 of gestation, and at that time the point of maximum intensity is just above the pubis. Thereafter, the point of maximum intensity varies depending on the fetal position and presentation. Most often it can be heard best over the fetal back.

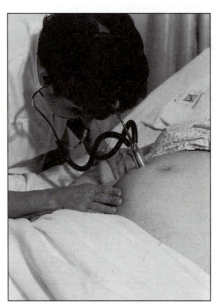

1 Position the warmed fetoscope over the palpated fetal back. Move the fetoscope around until you locate the point of maximum intensity. Generally, with cephalic presentations, the FHTs can be heard in the lower quadrant, toward the mother's flank. In breech presentations they can be heard closer to the midline around the level of the umbilicus. Apply slight pressure with the fetoscope bell to elicit the sounds.

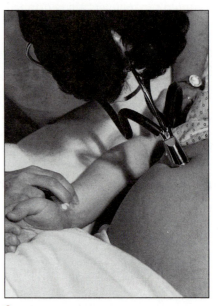

2 When the heart tones are at their loudest, palpate the mother's radial pulse as you count the FHTs. This will ensure that you have not confused the mother's *souffle* with the fetal heart tones. This souffle is a soft, rushing sound produced by blood moving through the uterine arteries and it is synchronous with the maternal heart rate. Count the FHTs for one full minute. They should range from 120 to 160 beats/minute.

USING ULTRASONIC (DOPPLER) AUSCULTATION

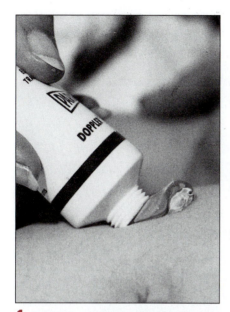 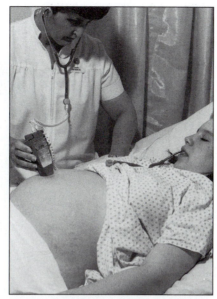

1 Preview Chapter 7 for a description of the Doppler. An ultrasonic transducer has the advantage of detecting FHTs by the 12th week, and occasionally as early as the 9th or 10th week. Lubricate an area over the fetal back using a thin layer of conducting jelly.

2 Position the transducer over the lubricated area. If the Doppler has an extra headset, allow the mother to listen simultaneously. Count the beats for a minute. You may also elicit a *bruit,* a hissing sound produced by blood moving through the umbilical arteries and other fetal vessels, as well as a souffle.

PERFORMING EXTERNAL ELECTRONIC FETAL MONITORING

Electronic fetal monitoring is used in the clinical setting to monitor both fetal heart rate and uterine activity. This is accomplished by means of an ultrasonic transducer, which uses the sonar principle to detect continuous sound waves from the fetal heart, and a toco-dynamometer, which is a pressure device that simultaneously transmits a signal that reveals frequency of uterine contractions. Both signals are recorded on the screen and graph paper.

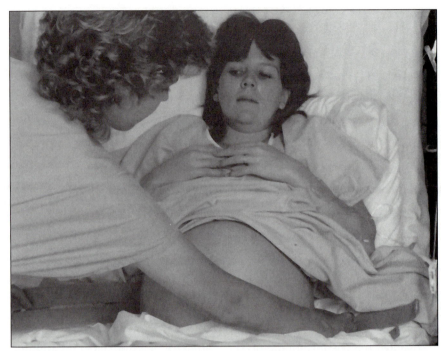

1 Wash your hands. Identify the client and explain the procedure to her. Tell the client that the top belt will be secured snugly to ensure an accurate reading. Place the client in a position of comfort, usually semi-Fowler's position. Slide the transducer belts under the client's abdomen, as shown.

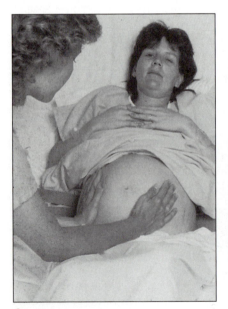

2 Identify fetal parts using Leopold's maneuvers (see page 195) to determine the position of the fetal back.

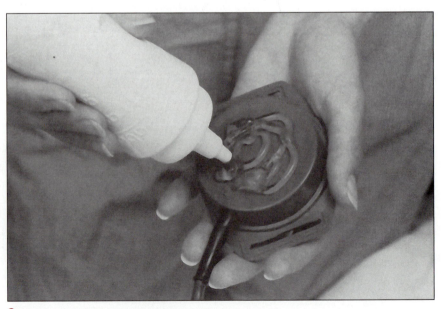

3 Apply conducting gel to the underside of the ultrasound transducer (as shown).

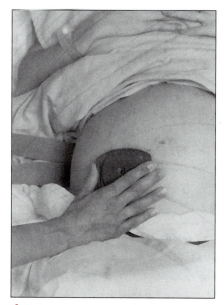

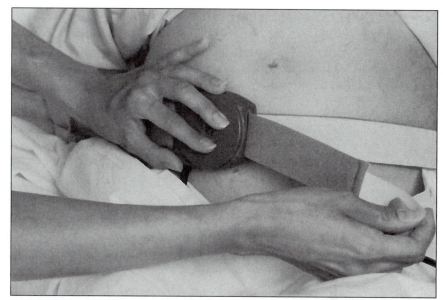

4 Caution the client that the transducer will be cold from the gel. Apply the transducer to the area over the fetal back proximal to the fetal head (as shown for this client). Start the tracing on the monitor and wait 3–5 seconds for the tracing to begin. If FHTs are not audible, reassess fetal position and repeat step 2.

5 If FHTs are audible, secure the transducer with the belt (as shown). Identify the graph tracing with client information, including client's name, medical record number, vital signs, date, time, and type of fetal monitor used.

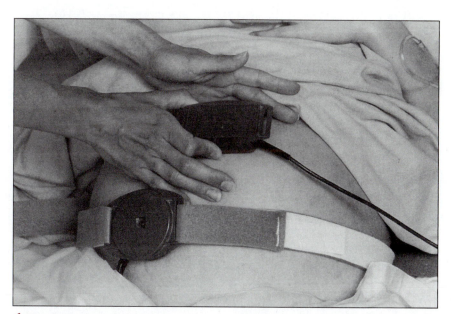

6 Next, position the tocotransducer over the fundus, where uterine contractions are most accurately assessed. Adjust the uterine activity on the monitor to the zero point. Secure the tocotransducer with the remaining abdominal belt, applying the belt snugly against the client's abdomen to ensure that uterine pressure against the tocotransducer is enough to record the contractions on the monitor.

➤

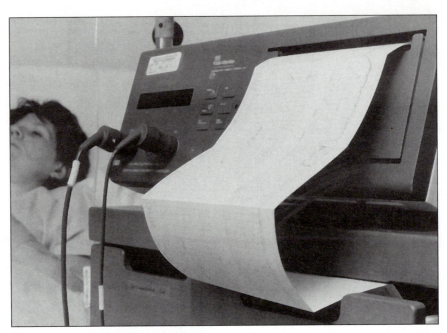

7 Let the monitor run for 20–30 minutes if checking fetal status. If the mother is in labor, let the monitor continue running as prescribed.

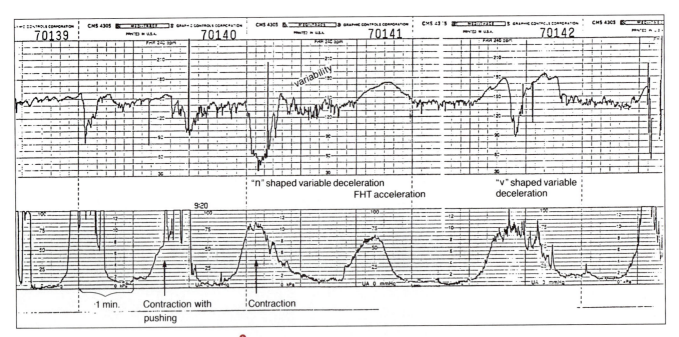

8 Inspect the strips to assess FHTs and uterine activity. Although it is not our purpose in this text to teach strip interpretation, the variable "n"-shaped segments in the FHT strip denote FHT acceleration. The variable "v"-shaped segments show FHT deceleration. The strip with uterine activity shows contractions with pushing and contractions without pushing. Note that the contractions are 1 minute apart.

ASSESSING FOR AMNIOTIC FLUID

If you or your client notes the presence of clear fluid on her peripad or garment and you suspect that her membranes have ruptured, the first priority is to inspect the perineum and introitus to determine the presence or absence of a prolapsed cord. Next, monitor FHTs. If severe bradycardia (≤100 beats per minute) is present, notify the physician at once. Then apply gloves and perform a vaginal examination to determine if the cord is being compressed by the presenting part. If you note cord compression, place the client immediately into Trendelenburg's position while pushing the presenting part upward to relieve the cord compression. Maintain this position while the physician evaluates the client further.

To determine if the fluid is amniotic, place a nitrazine test strip directly into the fluid and shake off any excess. ***Note:*** *Avoid placing the test strip on the peripad or garment itself, as this may result in a false reading due to the presence of blood, mucus, or diluted urine.*

Immediately compare the results to the color chart on the nitrazine container (as shown). Amniotic fluid is alkaline with a 7.2 pH, and the darker the test strip, the more likely it is that the membranes have ruptured. ***Note:*** *A false positive may result if the client has had a recent vaginal examination with a water-soluble lubricant or if the fluid contains blood.*

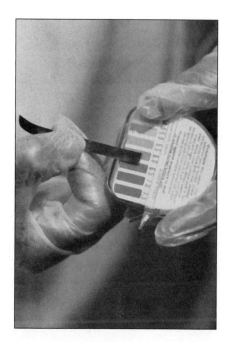

PROVIDING COMFORT MEASURES

APPLYING COUNTERPRESSURE TO RELIEVE LEG CRAMPS

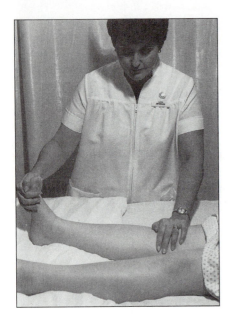

Your pregnant client may experience painful muscle spasms in her legs, especially during the third trimester when circulation is impaired in the lower extremities and the weighty uterus presses on the nerves in her legs. These cramps are often precipitated when the client is recumbent and extends her feet. They can be relieved by straightening the leg with one hand as you dorsiflex the foot with the other hand. Be sure to teach this technique to your client's partner.

APPLYING PRESSURE TO RELIEVE BACK PAIN

If your client experiences back pain, which may be caused from increasing curvature of the back or a relaxation of the pelvic joints, assist her onto her side and apply firm pressure with the heel of your hand into the sacrococcygeal area. Continue to exert pressure until the discomfort is diminished or relieved.

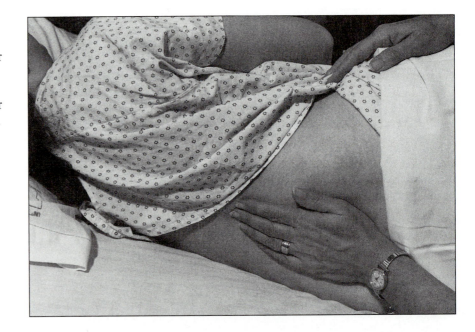

Performing Postpartum Techniques

ASSESSING THE MOTHER

Wash your hands and explain the procedure to your client. Be sure to provide privacy. To make the process as comfortable as possible, ensure that the client has recently voided. Begin the assessment by taking vital signs to ensure that they are within normal limits when compared to the baseline. Frequent assessment is essential, especially during the first 24 hours when the client is at the greatest risk for postpartum hemorrhage. Perform vital sign assessment before your hands-on assessment of the client because the discomfort of a fundal check could be reflected in an elevated blood pressure and pulse rate.

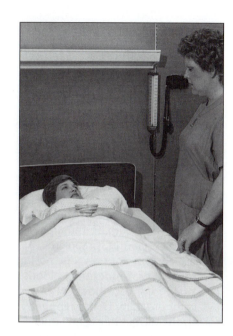

INSPECTING AND PALPATING THE BREASTS

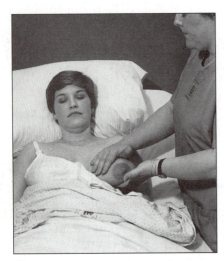

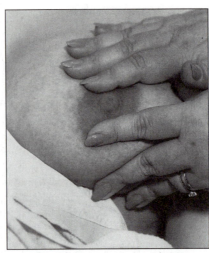

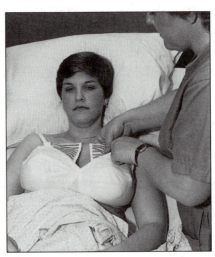

1 Raise the head of the bed, and ask your client to lower her gown so that you can examine her breasts. Inspect each breast, noting reddened areas or any irregularities such as asymmetry; and if present, assess the degree of engorgement. Palpate each breast, assessing for heat or nodules caused by occluded milk ducts. These occur most frequently in the upper outer quadrants.

2 Inspect and palpate the areolae and nipples. Gently spread the areola between your fingers, noting cracks, fissures, tenderness, blood, or a buildup of secretions. Also assess for erectility of the nipple by rolling the nipple between your thumb and index finger. If cracks or fissures are noted, encourage the client to keep the flaps of her bra unhooked and down to enhance air drying. Creams and ointments should be used only in instances of severe irritation because most require removal prior to breast-feeding, resulting in increased irritation to the area. It is acceptable to use pure hydrous lanolin, however, because it is more readily absorbed into the skin and does not require removal prior to breastfeeding.

3 Breast engorgement is usually indicative of inadequate feeding or expression frequency. In most cases, beginning breastfeeding immediately after birth and ensuring the infant's unlimited access to the breast as desired (usually every 1 1/2 to 3 hours) will prevent engorgement. If engorgement occurs, the mother should nurse her baby more frequently or express the milk by pump (see page 212) if the baby is unavailable. Using hot packs and massaging the breasts before feeding help promote milk ejection. In the non-nursing mother, ice packs, such as the chemical packs shown in the photo, and a supportive bra are recommended.

PALPATING THE FUNDUS AND BLADDER

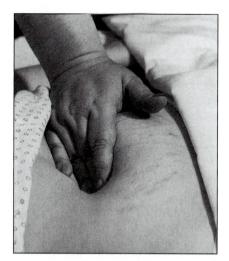

The fundus should be assessed for location and tone at frequent intervals, according to agency protocol, until around the 10th day postpartum when it is usually no longer palpable. Because most clients are discharged much earlier than this, instruct the client in self-examination so that she can be alert to changes in her uterus. To assess the fundus and bladder, lower the head of the bed so that the abdomen will be relaxed. Ensure that the client has recently voided because a full bladder will displace the

fundus. Fundal height is measured in relationship to its distance in finger breadths from the umbilicus. To measure the distance, position your ring finger directly over the umbilicus so that your small finger is closest to the client's head. Using your ring finger as a fulcrum, roll your hand back and forth gently. If the fundus is more than a finger's breadth (FB) above the umbilicus (U) or more than two below, reposition your fingers in the appropriate direction. Document the measurement accordingly, for example:

1 FB ↑ U; or 1 FB ↓ U; or @U.

At the same time, note the fundal relationship to the midline. Displacement to either side of the midline is usually caused by a distended bladder. Normally the fundus will be at the midline. If it is displaced, palpate the bladder gently, following guidelines in "Assessing the Bladder" in Chapter 8. Also, describe the uterine tone. Optimally, it will feel firm and well contracted; it should not be excessively tender to the touch.

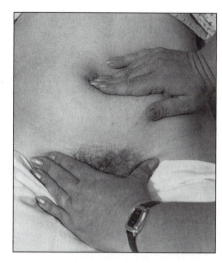

Performing Fundal Massage: If the uterus feels soft and boggy, perform a light massage in an attempt to contract and harden it. Ask the client to flex her knees to relax her abdomen and to release the peripad so that you can clearly assess the amount, color, and consistency of the lochia expelled during the massage. Place the flattened fingertips of your dominant hand at the client's fundus. To prevent uterine prolapse, provide support with your other hand (as shown). Lightly massage the fundus in a circular motion. If the uterus does not respond to a light massage, repeat with more vigorous movements. If the client's uterus is nonresponsive and remains soft and boggy, and if this is accompanied by copious bleeding, contact the physician for immediate intervention. ***Caution:*** *Never massage a well-contracted uterus. Overstimulation can result in muscle fatigue and uterine relaxation.*

EVALUATING THE LOCHIA

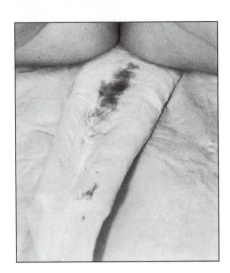

To assess the lochia, detach the peripad from the client's sanitary belt. Be sure to remove it from the front to the back to minimize the risk of contaminating the vagina with rectal discharge. Note the amount, character, and odor of the discharge. During the first few days, the lochia should resemble menstrual blood in that it should be dark and red (lochia rubra). After the third day it should appear more serous and brown in color (lochia serosa). Clots are usually abnormal and could mean that the client has retained placental tissue or has inadequate uterine contraction. If clots are found, further investigation is indicated, and a referral may be necessary. Be sure to ask the client about her evaluation of the bleeding and the number of pads she has saturated. Four to eight saturated pads may be considered normal over a 24-hour period. However, if your client has had a cesarean delivery, that amount would be excessive. Also, foul-smelling lochia on a fresh pad could be indicative of an infection. Document the amount and character of the lochia, for example: lochia rubra, moderate amount with a few small clots; or lochia serosa, scant.

INSPECTING THE PERINEUM

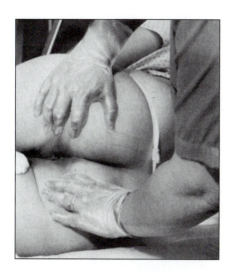

To inspect the perineum, instruct the client to assume a side-lying (Sims') position. It is important that she flex the top leg to minimize the strain on the episiotomy. Apply gloves and gently separate the buttocks, which will enable you to fully inspect the perineum. Assess the area for stage of healing, presence of edema, bruising, dehiscence, and signs of infection, as well as for hemorrhoids. Document your observations. If indicated, apply ice packs to the perineum for the first 12 hours to minimize edema. After the first 12 hours, apply heat, such as chemical heat packs or perilights, or encourage the use of a sitz bath. If your client has had a cesarean delivery, it is still important to assess the perineal area for the presence of hemorrhoids.

ASSISTING WITH INFANT FEEDING

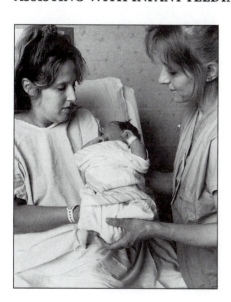

The infant should be nursed as often as she desires (approximately every 1½ to 3 hours) with unlimited feeding time. Provide time for the mother to prepare for infant feeding. For example, she may wish to void, and she should wash her hands and get into a comfortable position. To provide her with privacy, draw the curtain around her bed and shut her door. If the infant and mother are not rooming together, be sure to verify that the infant's name and identification numbers match those of the mother.

POSITIONING THE INFANT

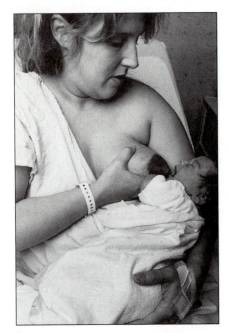 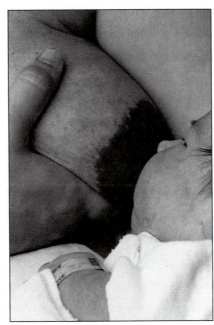 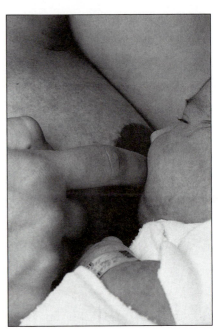

1 *The Cradle Hold:* A commonly used position for a breastfeeding is the cradle hold, in which the mother is sitting upright with the infant's head held in the crook of her arm, the spine supported by her forearm, and the buttocks cradled in her hand. Teach the mother to draw the infant close to her body to minimize traction on her nipple. Ensure that the infant's abdomen is against the mother's abdomen. Support her arm with pillows, as needed, to prevent maternal fatigue.

2 Note that the mother positions her hand in a "C" shape around the side and base of her breast, squeezing gently. This encourages the infant to place her mouth around as much of the areola as possible, which in turn stimulates the milk ducts underneath the areola. This hand position also prevents the breast from obstructing the infant's nose. Teach the mother to elicit the rooting response (see page 223) so that the infant will suck when placed at the breast.

3 When the mother desires to remove the infant from her breast, teach her to break the suction by inserting her finger into the corner of the infant's mouth (as shown).

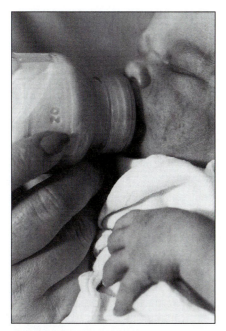

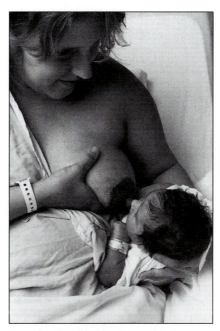

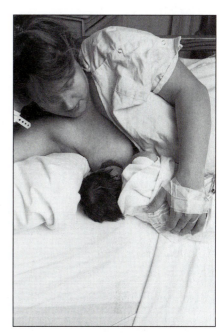

4 Bottle-fed infants are positioned in the cradle hold position because it enhances the warmth and physical closeness that occur with breast-feeding. The bottle *always* should be held rather than propped up, and the nipple must be full of milk to avoid introducing air into the infant's stomach.

5 *Football Hold:* This position is recommended for mothers who have had a cesarean delivery, because it enables them to support the infant's weight off their abdomens. The infant is held supine along the forearm with the head supported by the mother's hand. The infant's weight can be supported by a pillow. It is important for the mother to bring the infant to her breast rather than take her breast to the infant. This will help minimize traction on her nipple.

6 *Side-Lying:* When the mother wishes to rest, a side-lying position will enable her to lie down with the infant at her side rather than in her arms. Place a pillow between the mother's knees for comfort and proper body positioning. The infant can be supported in the side-lying position either with a rolled blanket or the towel placed behind her back or by being held in that position by her mother. This position is also excellent after cesarean deliveries. Ensure that the infant's abdomen is positioned against her mother's abdomen.

BURPING THE INFANT

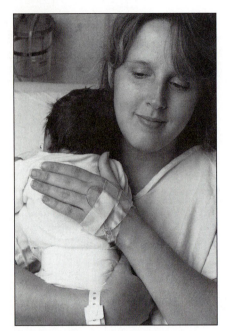 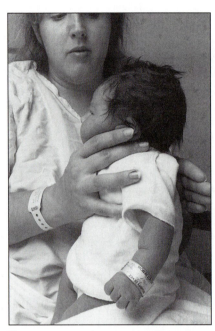 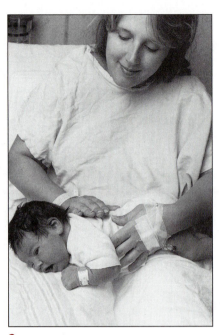

1 After feeding the infant at each breast, the mother should burp her gently by patting or rubbing her back to expel the air bubbles. She can hold the infant over her shoulder (as shown) with a diaper or towel placed under the infant's mouth to absorb any fluid that may be expelled.

2 In another burping position, the infant sits upright. The mother holds the infant across the jaw with one hand to support the head and neck and pats or rubs her back with the other.

3 The infant also can be burped in a prone position over the mother's thighs. *Note: Never place the infant on a pillow because the surface is too soft and the infant could suffocate.* Positions 2 and 3 are recommended for newborns because either position allows the mother to see the infant's face, which will alert her to choking and aspiration.

MASSAGING THE BREASTS FOR MANUAL EXPRESSION OF BREAST MILK

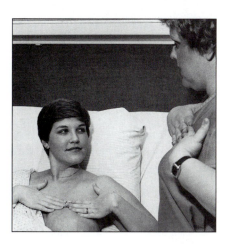

1 Teach your breastfeeding client how to massage her breasts to facilitate the manual expression of breast milk. This will enable her to produce a small amount of milk or colostrum, which will help entice a disinterested infant to eat. It also will allow her to relieve breast engorgement and to store milk for future feedings in her absence.

The mother should first wash her hands. Explain that breast massage will enhance the flow of milk through all the milk ducts. Show her how to sweep her fingers from the chest wall onto the upper surface of the breast.

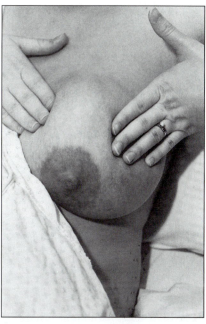

2 Next, she should slide her fingers down both sides of the breast.

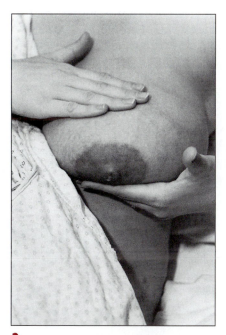

3 Her hands should then be positioned on the top side and underside of the breast, sweeping toward the areola.

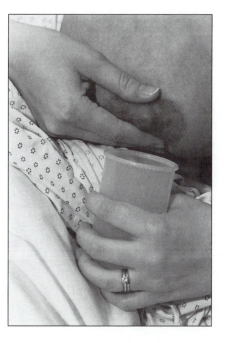

4 She can express the milk manually by grasping the areola between her thumb and index finger. As she presses the thumb and index finger together, the breast should be held along the chest wall to express the milk. She should then repeat the nipple compression as she repositions her thumb and index finger in a circular fashion around the breast. Instruct her to alternate massage with manual expression to facilitate complete emptying of each breast. Ensure that the expressed milk does not run over her fingers but rather runs directly into the sterile container.

USING BREAST PUMPS

Breast pumps are used to express milk for the relief of breast engorgement in the nursing mother, as a means of maintaining lactation, or as a method for milk storage when the mother must be absent from feedings. In the hospital, aseptic technique is used; after she is discharged, the mother can use clean technique.

MANAGING HAND PUMPS

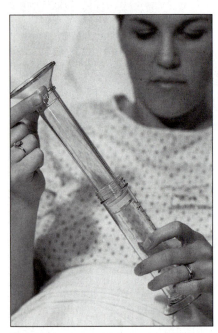

1 The manual breast pump is best used for the occasional expression of milk. The Marshall Kaneson breast pump is a popular brand of pump used for this purpose. After your client has washed her hands, teach her how to insert the inner cylinder into the outer cylinder (as shown), using aseptic technique.

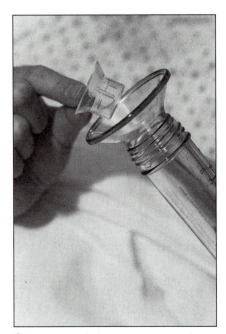

2 She then can select and attach the flange that most closely accommodates her nipple and breast size. The flange screws into the inner cylinder. The flange is important because it provides tactile stimulation to the areolar skin, which is necessary for the milk ejection reflex (letdown).

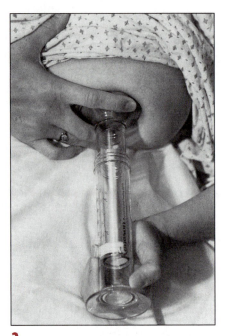

3 Instruct the client to place the flange over the nipple or slightly off center if the nipple is too small to contact the flange. Teach the client to slide the outer cylinder in and out gently, using small movements until letdown has occurred and the milk is flowing. At that point the client can increase the in-and-out movements to fill the inner cylinder with the milk. When the cylinder is nearly full of milk, she should pour the milk into a sterile plastic bottle or plastic liner from a commercial nurser if she wishes to store the milk for later use. Glass containers should be avoided because leukocytes in breast milk have a tendency to adhere to the sides of these containers.

After each use the breast pump should be cleaned thoroughly according to agency protocol, dried, and stored in a closed container at the bedside.

ASSISTING WITH ELECTRIC BREAST PUMPS

Electric breast pumps, such as the Medela, are an efficient and time-saving method of initiating lactation without the suckling baby for obtaining breast milk on a long-term basis.

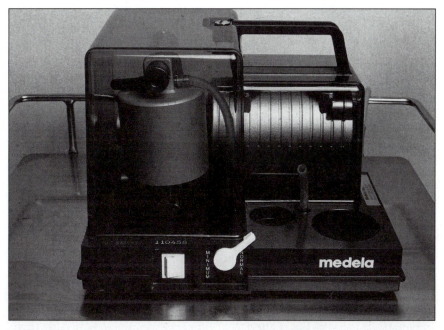

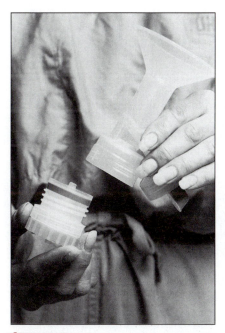

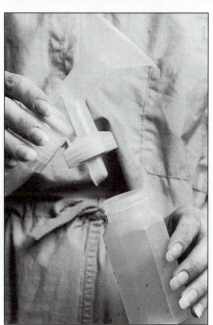

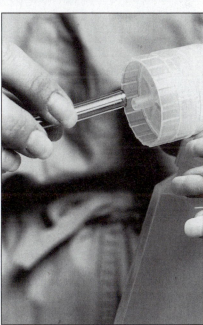

1 Wash your hands. Connect the pump adapter to the breast pump shield, being certain that the seal is tight.

2 Screw the breast shield onto the plastic container that will hold the expressed milk.

3 Attach the suction hose to the breast shield as shown.

➤

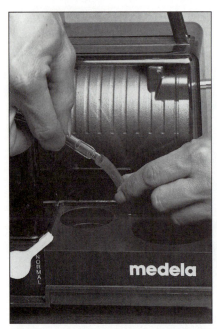

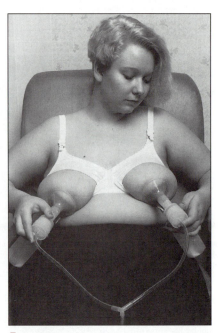

4 Attach the distal end of the hose to the pump. Set the suction to minimal and increase the suction as tolerated.

5 Instruct the mother to position the breast shield so that it is slightly off center on the areolar skin. This will maximize contact for milk ejection.

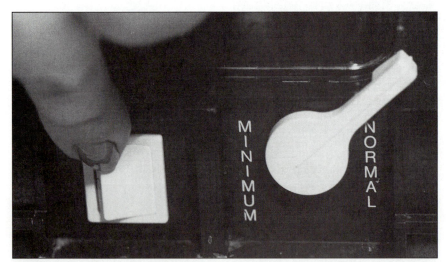

6 Turn the pump on. She can then adjust the control lever on the pump to the desired amount of suction. She can start expressing with the pressure level set at "minimum" and increase it if she desires by turning to "normal" to maximize maternal prolactin levels and milk supply. It is best to express the breasts simultaneously using a double-pump kit for 10–15 minutes at both breasts. If a single-pump kit is used, she should express for 5 minutes on the first side, turn off the power and gently remove the bell, and express for 5 minutes on the other breast. This should be repeated for 4 minutes on each side, followed by 3 minutes on each side, then 2 minutes, and then 1 minute. This alternating pattern will improve milk supply and hormone stimulation. *Note: To heal tender nipples, mother's milk is an excellent ointment to apply to them following milk expression.* Label and store the milk and cleanse the equipment according to the procedure for using hand pumps.

Caring for the Newborn

ADMITTING THE NEONATE TO THE HOSPITAL

OBTAINING FOOTPRINTS

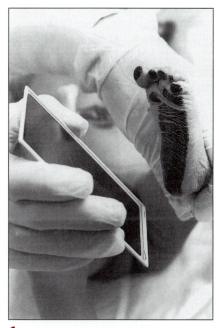 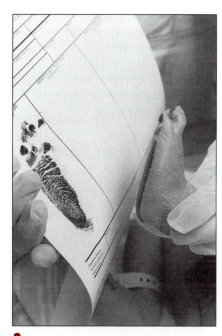

1 If your agency requires footprints and/or palm prints as a part of the permanent birth record, recording them may be the responsibility of the nurse who admits the newborn to the nursery. To obtain the footprints, apply clean gloves, wipe any vernix off the sole of the foot, and position the carbon plate over the entire length of the newborn's foot. Use moderate pressure as you ink the sole because too much ink can obscure the lines and creases.

2 After inking the foot, press the footprint sheet onto the inked sole. To stimulate the newborn to spread his toes, press the footprint sheet from the heel to the toes. Repeat the process on the other foot, and then file the prints in the infant's chart. Making an extra set of prints for the parents is usually appreciated. After obtaining the footprints, rub the soles of the feet with a towel or cloth diaper to remove the ink. Your agency may also file the mother's fingerprint along with her newborn's footprints.

INSTILLING OPHTHALMIC ERYTHROMYCIN

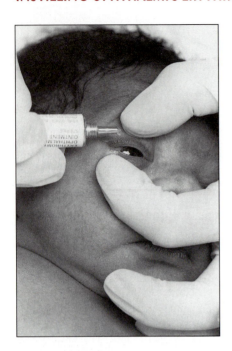

The instillation of an antibiotic ophthalmic solution, such as erythromycin, is a procedure mandated by most states as a prophylaxis for gonococcal ophthalmia neonatorum. Although many agencies require the immediate instillation in the delivery room, others delay the process until the neonate's admission into the nursery to facilitate the newborn's bonding with the parents.

Wash your hands and apply clean gloves. Lightly touch the upper lid, which will cause the neonate to open the eye, and then apply gentle pressure on the lower lid to expose the lower conjunctival sac. Instill the ointment into the conjunctival sac from the inner to outer canthus (see page 83). Avoid instilling the medication directly onto the cornea because this could cause corneal irritation. Allow the eye to close so that the medication can be spread over the surface of the eye. Repeat the procedure in the other eye. Because this medication could result in a mild conjunctivitis, be sure to explain to the parents that this is a temporary condition.

ADMINISTERING A VITAMIN K INJECTION

A vitamin K injection is administered as a prophylaxis for transient coagulation deficiency in the neonate. It usually is given on the day of birth because the coagulation disorder potentially would appear between the second and fifth day after birth.

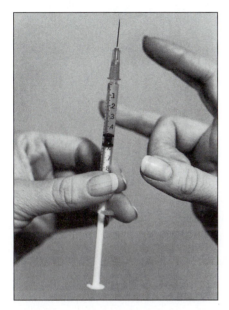

1 Wash your hands and draw up the prescribed dose of the medication into a tuberculin syringe that has a 25-gauge needle. Usually, 0.5–1.0 mg is administered.

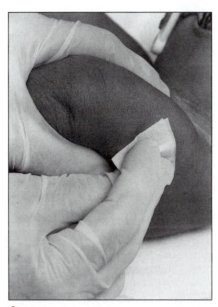

2 Swab the anterolateral segment of the upper thigh (the vastus lateralis muscle) with an alcohol sponge. Allow the alcohol to dry. *Note: Apply clean gloves if it is your agency's policy to do so.*

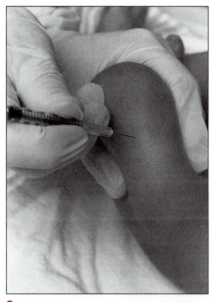

3 Bunch the tissue between your thumb and index finger, and quickly insert the needle at a 90-degree angle to the thigh. Aspirate to check for a blood return. When you are certain you are in a nonvascular area, slowly inject the solution so that you will evenly distribute the medication and minimize the newborn's discomfort. Remove the needle and massage the site with an alcohol sponge. Document the administration of the medication.

OBTAINING A BLOOD SAMPLE

Blood samples are obtained during the first few hours of birth as an assessment for hypoglycemia. Those at especially high risk include the following: infants of diabetic mothers, premature infants, infants small or large for gestational age, infants who are ill, and infants of prolonged or very stressful labor.

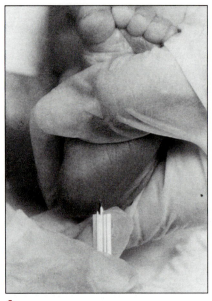

1 Apply gloves. To obtain the blood sample, dorsiflex the foot and prepare the lateral aspect of the heel with an alcohol sponge. When the alcohol has dried, firmly pierce the skin with the lancet, just deeply enough to elicit a large droplet of blood.

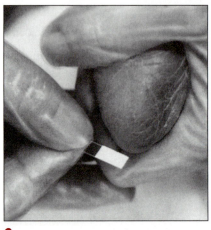

2 Position the pad of a reagent strip directly under the puncture site and collect a large droplet of blood onto the pad without smearing the blood. Review the steps on pages 142–143, for visually monitoring blood glucose.

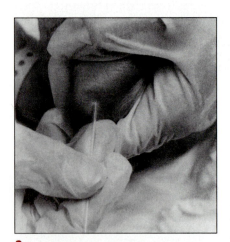

3 When a hematocrit has been prescribed for evaluation of blood volume, prepare the heel and pierce the skin, according to step 1. Warming the heel prior to making the puncture will improve both the blood flow and the accuracy of the test. Place the capillary tube at the puncture site and allow it to become at least half full of blood.

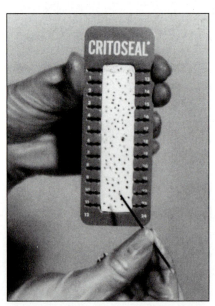

4 After obtaining the blood, place one end of the capillary tube into Critoseal (above) or cap the tube (right) to prevent specimen loss. Follow agency guidelines for spinning the tube in a centrifuge and reading the value.

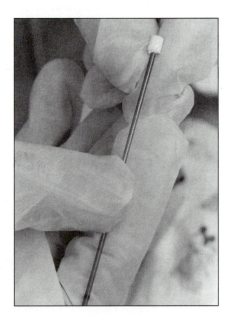

OBTAINING A URINE SPECIMEN

Applying an External Urine Collection Device

If a urine specimen is required for routine urinalysis or assessment of latex agglutination for beta *Strepto-coccus,* a specimen can be obtained using an external urine collection device. If the infant is quiet, this procedure can be performed easily by one person. A crying or restless infant may require two people.

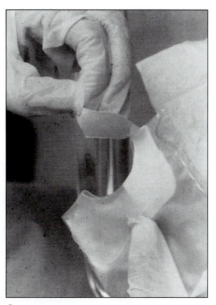

1 Apply clean gloves, remove the neonate's diaper, and cleanse the genitalia. Then detach the backing from the adhesive surface of the urine collection device (as shown).

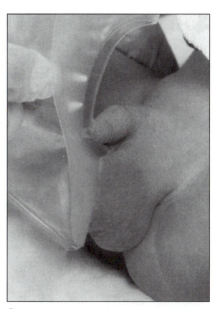

2 Abduct the neonate's legs and position the opening of the collection device over the perineum and along the labia for a female or under and around the penis for a male (as shown).

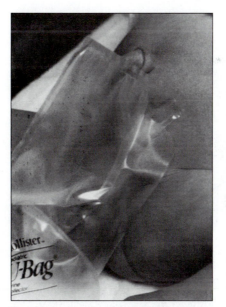

3 Gently smooth the adhesive sides around the groin to seal the contact with the baby's skin.

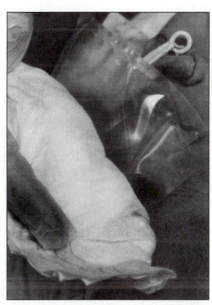

4 Cover with a diaper and recheck in 30–60 minutes.

Removing an External Urine Collection Device

After the infant has voided, apply gloves and gently peel the adhesive surface of the collection device from the top downward, exerting gently pressure with your opposite hand (as shown) to break the seal of the adhesive surface to the infant's skin.

Once you have removed the collection device, transfer the urine to a rigid specimen container. Label the container and send it to the laboratory, following agency protocol for transporting specimens.

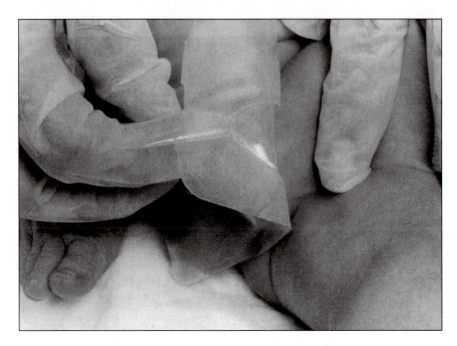

ASSESSING THE NEONATE

PERFORMING A GENERAL INSPECTION

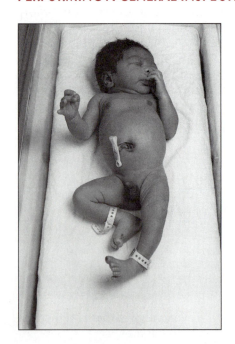

Wash your hands, and prepare to assess the infant in a warm environment such as the radiant warmer or at the mother's bedside. Wear gloves if the neonate has not had his first bath or if it is your agency's policy to do so. Remove the diaper and shirt.

Observe the resting posture. A normal-term infant's posture is flexed even when he is asleep. Also, note the color. In white infants, the color is normally ruddy or pink-tinged. Darker-skinned infants can be assessed by inspecting the lips and mucous membranes, which are normally pink. A yellow cast may indicate jaundice; a blue tint at the feet, hands, and mouth is often indicative of sluggish peripheral circulation. This is usually transient and clears in several hours. However, cyanosis, along with restlessness and choking, necessitates

immediate suctioning to remove esophageal mucus. Count the respirations for a full minute and note their quality. Normally, they range between 40 and 60 breaths per minute. Because neonates are diaphragmatic breathers, observe the abdomen rather than the chest for respirations. Respirations greater than 60 after the first 4 hours of birth or less than 30 per minute at any time, as well as substernal and subcostal retractions, are abnormal. With cyanosis, they could be indicative of aspiration or of disorders such as respiratory distress, transient tachypnea, or congenital heart disease. Slow respirations may be indicative of narcotic depression from drugs given to the mother during labor, central nervous system disorders, or deep sleep. These infants should be referred to the attending physician immediately.

AUSCULTATING

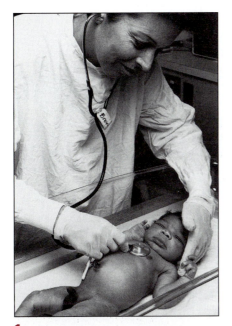

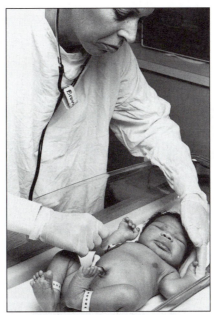

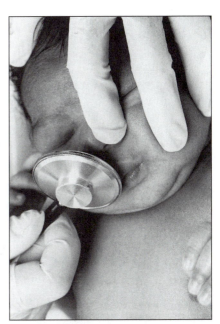

1 Auscultation, especially for heart sounds, should be performed when the infant is quiet. It is usually a good idea, therefore, to auscultate before initiating the hands-on assessment. Auscultate over the precordium for a full minute to assess apical pulse. Note the rate, rhythm, and intensity of the pulse. It should range from 130 to 160 beats/minute. However, the pulse may be as low as 90 at rest or as high as 200 when the infant cries. Be alert to irregularities, such as dysrhythmias, or to murmurs, which are heard as slurs or clicks between lub and dub.

2 Auscultate over the lung fields to assess breath sounds. Review Chapter 6 to assist you with auscultation sites and breath sounds. Be alert to diminished breath sounds when comparing one side to the other, especially if breath sounds were normal immediately following birth. Crackles may be heard immediately following birth because of unabsorbed amniotic fluid. Within the next few hours, the breath sounds should become clear as the fetal lung fluid is absorbed and the alveoli open throughout the lungs.

3 Assess the patency of the nares by alternately obstructing each naris with an index finger. Listen with the stethoscope over the open naris to assess airflow. If the airflow is abnormal, either suction with a bulb syringe or attempt to pass a sterile catheter gently down the naris. Notify the physician if one or both nares are obstructed.

TAKING AN AXILLARY TEMPERATURE

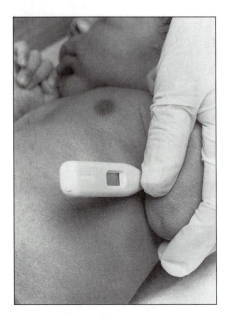

1 While the infant is quiet, insert a thermometer into the axillary area; hold it in place for 3–5 minutes. An axillary temperature is often preferable to a rectal temperature because the rectum maintains the core temperature longer than the skin. Therefore, the axillary temperature will alert you more readily to rapid temperature changes that frequently occur in the newborn. The axillary temperature should register around 36.5–37 C.

PALPATING

1 Begin your hands-on assessment of the neonate at the head by palpating the fontanelles (soft spots)—both the anterior fontanelle (as shown) and the posterior fontanelle at the occiput. It is a good idea to measure your own fingers in centimeters to give yourself a built-in tape measure. The anterior fontanelle is normally 2–3 cm (0.75–1.2 in) in width, 3–4 cm (1.2–1.6 in) in length, and diamondlike in shape. It can be described as soft, which is normal, or full or bulging, which could be indicative of increased intracranial pressure. Conversely, a depressed fontanelle could mean that the neonate is dehydrated. The posterior fontanelle is smaller and triangular in shape, and it closes within 6–12 weeks; or it may be closed at birth. The anterior fontanelle usually closes within 12–18 months.

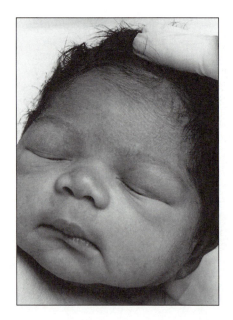

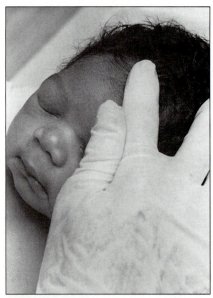

2 Palpate the sutures, which are the junctions of the cranial bones and are normally movable. Overriding sutures are normal in the first week of life secondary to the molding of the head during birth. Fixed sutures are abnormal and should be called to the physician's attention.

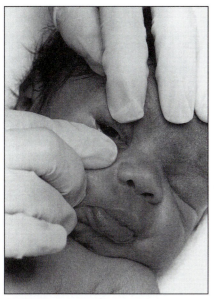

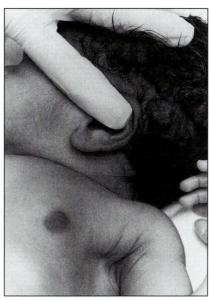

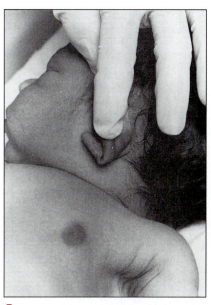

3 Inspect the eyes by gently separating the lids. Assess the pupillary reflex with an ophthalmoscope or penlight to ensure that the pupils react equally to light. Also observe for the equality of pupil size. Unequal pupils could suggest birth trauma. Note whether the corneas appear cloudy, which is indicative of a congenital infection, or hemorrhagic, which is usually transient and caused from pressure during delivery.

4 Assess the infant for low-set ears, which may be indicative of chromosomal abnormalities and are often associated with genitourinary disorders. Normally, the pinna of the ear is in a straight line with the outer canthus of the eye.

5 Next, assess the development of the ear cartilage. If the auricle stays in the position in which it is pressed, or returns to its original position slowly, it usually means that the gestational age is less than 38 weeks. Also, inspect for preauricular skin tags, which are usually normal and often are removed for cosmetic reasons.

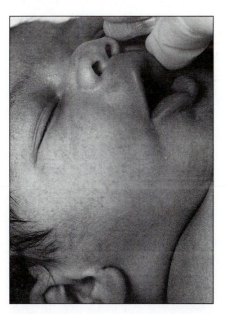

6 To assess the rooting reflex, lightly stimulate the cheek by stroking from the outer corner of the mouth toward the ear on the same side. The infant should turn toward the finger in an attempt to suck. Teach this technique to the breastfeeding mother.

➤

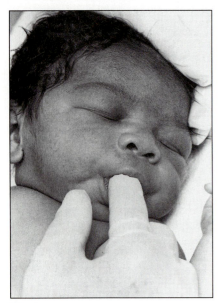

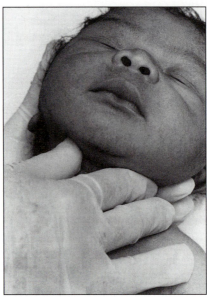

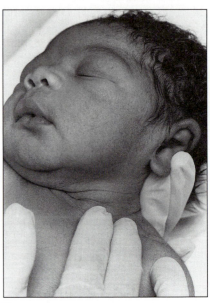

7 Assess the sucking reflex by donning a clean glove and inserting a finger in the neonate's mouth. In addition, inspect and palpate the hard and soft palates to assess for clefts as well as for Epstein's pearls, which are white specks occasionally found on the gums and hard palate and may be palpated as hardened areas. These are normal and usually disappear after several days. You also might palpate neonatal teeth on the gum line. Because there is a potential for aspiration, notify the physician that you have found them in the event that removal is indicated. Deciduous teeth, however, are not removed.

8 Bilaterally palpate the neck to assess for masses, trachial deviation, an enlarged thyroid, or swollen lymph glands. Although the trachea normally is slightly at the right of the midline, the other findings are abnormal and should be referred to the physician. Also, assess the sternocleidomastoid muscles for symmetry and the shoulder joints for full range of motion.

9 Palpate the clavicles to ensure that they are symmetric and contiguous. A lump along one of the clavicles could be a fracture site caused from a difficult delivery.

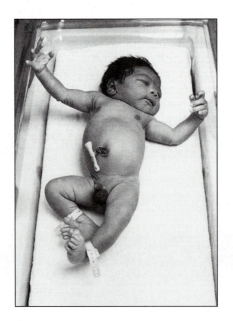

10 Elicit the startle reflex with a loud noise—for example, by clapping your hands together or by pulling up gently on his arms and releasing quickly. Normally, the newborn will abduct and extend his arms. The fingers will extend and then flex into a "C." An asymmetric response suggests a fractured clavicle or an injury to the brachial plexus. Lack of a response is indicative of a hearing loss or brain damage.

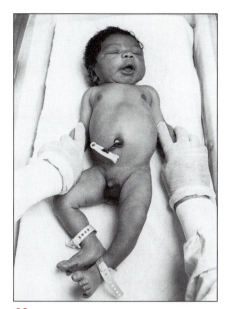

11 Continue your palpation of the upper extremities. Assess for adequate range of motion and bilateral symmetry of bones, muscles, and movement.

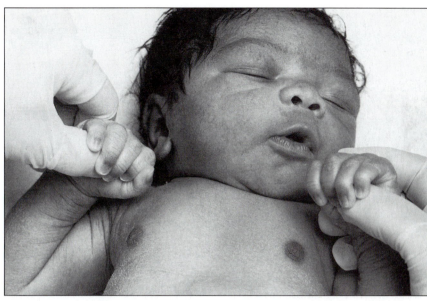

12 Assess the grasp reflex by stimulating the newborn's palms with your fingers. He should grasp your fingers tightly enough to be lifted off the surface on which he is lying. An asymmetric or weak grasp suggests possible central nervous system damage. Also, assess the hands for extra digits. If present, a physician likely will tie them off, and they will usually drop off after 2–3 days.

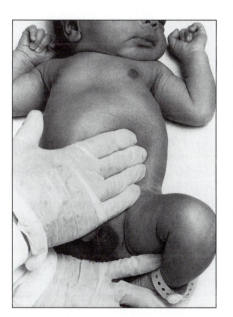

13 While the infant is relaxed, palpate all four quadrants of the abdomen, noting masses and/or tenderness. Normally it feels soft to the touch. To feel the tip of the spleen, press down and sweep upward when palpating the left upper quadrant (as shown). To palpate the liver's edge, follow the same sweeping motion on the right upper quadrant. Palpate the suprapubic area to assess the bladder.

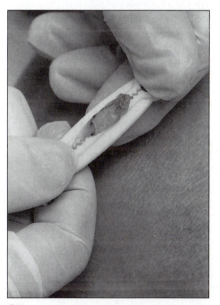

14 Inspect the umbilical cord for the presence of three vessels—a vein and two arteries. An absence of an artery may be associated with abnormalities of the genitourinary tract and should be noted on the chart.

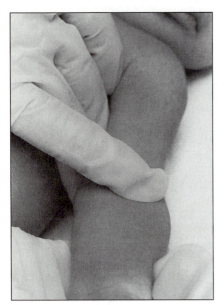

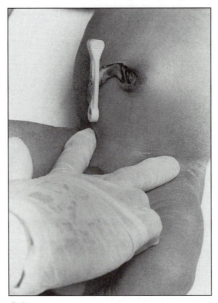

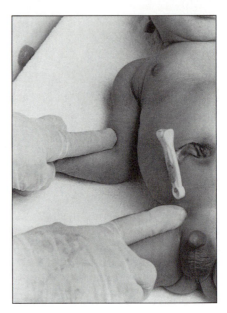

15 Assess the pulses, beginning with the brachial pulse. According to the American Heart Association's Standards and Guidelines for Cardiopulmonary Resuscitation (CPR) and Emergency Cardiac Care (ECC), the brachial pulse often is a more accurate indicator of true heart rate in the infant than the apical pulse because the precordium may transmit impulses rather than pulsations. Bilaterally assess the brachial pulses for equality in rate and intensity. Palpate for the brachial pulse above the antecubital fossa.

16 Bilaterally palpate the femoral arteries for rate and intensity of the pulses. Press each fingertip gently at the groin (above). Compare the femoral pulses to the brachial pulses by palpating the pulses

simultaneously (as shown) for a comparison of rate and intensity. If the pulsations are less intense in the femoral arteries, the newborn may have a coarctation of the aorta.

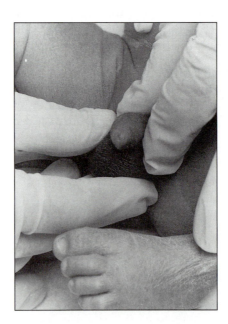

17 Assess the genitalia next. In the female, examine the labia for appropriate size and symmetry and the clitoris for appropriate size. Assess for both a vaginal and urinary os, and observe for a vaginal discharge, which may be blood-tinged. This is normal, and it is caused by the presence of the mother's hormones in the neonate. In the male, examine the penis and assess for hypospadias, a condition in which the urethral meatus appears on the underside of the penis. Palpate the scrotum to assess both testes if they are not readily visible. The testes may be undescended, or they may be drawn up into the abdomen if the infant is chilled.

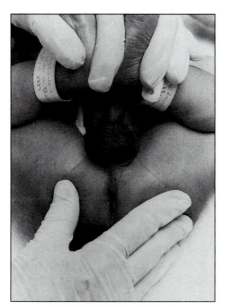

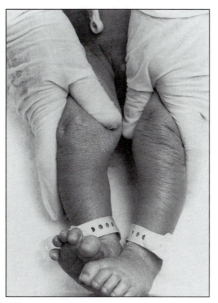

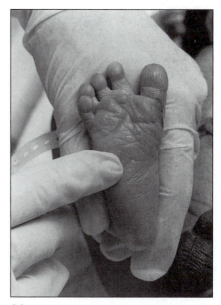

18 Spread the buttocks and assess the anus for patency and placement. If the anus appears to be either anteriorly or posteriorly positioned, the physician should be notified. In females, a rectal-vaginal fistula may be present, or this could represent a blind pouch with the true rectum correctly positioned but not patent. Patency is confirmed by the passage of the first meconium stool.

19 Continue to palpate the lower extremities for range of motion and bilateral symmetry of bones, muscles, and movement.

20 Inspect each foot to assess for clubfoot. Normally the foot is positioned at the midline of the tibia. A foot that is both inverted and plantarflexed and cannot be manipulated to midline necessitates a referral to the physician for further assessment. Also, inspect the soles of the feet for creases. If the creases do not cover the sole, the infant is probably less than 38 weeks' gestational age.

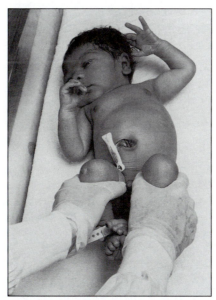

21 To assess for congenital hip dislocation, perform the test for Ortolani's click. Position your middle fingers over the greater trochanters and your thumbs along the medial thighs. Then flex the hips and knees.

➡

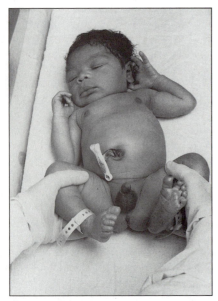

22 Gently abduct the hips and flex them to an even greater degree.

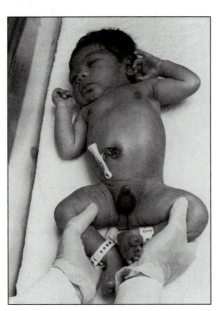

23 Externally rotate the hips. Unilateral or bilateral limitations in mobility, along with clicking, occur with hip dislocation or subluxation. Notify the physician for further evaluation.

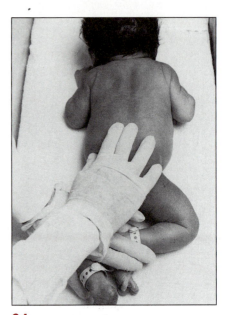

24 Place the neonate in a prone position and inspect and palpate the spine to assess for missing vertebrae and defects. Assess for dimples, sinuses, and tufts of hair, especially in the sacrococcygeal area, where a nevus pilosus (hairy nerve) is often indicative of spina bifida. Mongolian spots also may be present on the buttocks and in the dorsal lumbar area. These are bluish areas found usually in dark-skinned ethnic and racial groups. Be sure to explain to the parents that these spots are normal and that most fade within the first or second year.

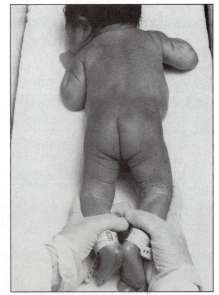

25 Straighten the legs; observe for symmetry in the creases of the buttocks and legs. Asymmetry could suggest a congenital hip dislocation.

MEASURING AND WEIGHING THE INFANT

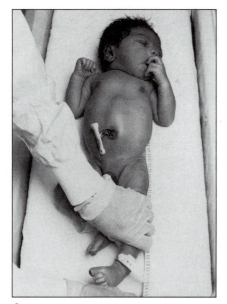

1 To measure the infant's length, place him in a supine position and extend one of his legs. The tape measure is then positioned from the top of the head to the heel.

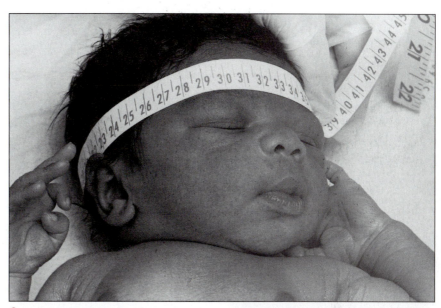

2 The head circumference is measured along the broadest part of the occiput with the tape positioned just slightly above the eyebrows. If the head is severely molded from the delivery, repeat the measurement daily.

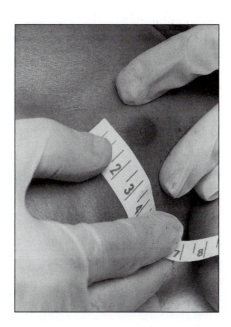

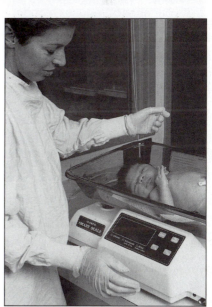

3 You also may measure the breast tissue to further evaluate gestational age. Compress the tissue between your thumb and index finger and measure the tissue in centimeters. At a normal gestational age, the tissue should measure between 0.5 cm (0.2 in) and 1 cm (0.4 in). An absence of or decreased breast tissue is often indicative of prematurity or a newborn who is small for gestational age. Also observe for supernumerary nipples, which are not harmful and may be removed at a later date. Both female and male infants may have breast engorgement with actual milk production caused by the presence of maternal hormones. Be sure to explain to the parents that this is normal.

4 The neonate may lose 5%–10% of his body weight over the first 3–5 days because of normal fluid loss and low intake. Therefore, you must weigh the infant daily to monitor weight loss or gain. The scale should be balanced, cleaned, and covered with a fresh paper or pad before weighing each infant to prevent cross-contamination and to minimize heat loss. Always place your hand above the infant to prevent him from falling off the scale.

TAKING AN ARTERIAL BLOOD PRESSURE

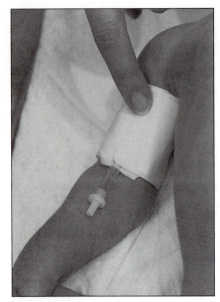

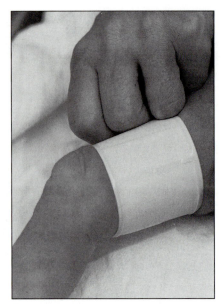

1 If your agency requires blood pressure monitoring for the neonate, you probably will use an ultrasonic device such as the Doppler. Wrap a blood pressure cuff of the appropriate size around the newborn's upper arm (see Chapter 7). Attach the cuff to the Doppler device and obtain the pressure reading according to the manufacturer's instructions. A diastolic pressure less than 40 and a systolic pressure greater than 100 require further investigation. If the newborn is crying, the reading may be falsely elevated.

2 If the femoral pulses are weak or absent, suggesting coarctation of the aorta, assess the blood pressure in the leg. Wrap the cuff around the upper thigh and obtain the pressure reading. The reading should be slightly higher in the leg than in the arm. A vast difference between the two, however, helps to confirm coarctation of the aorta, and you should obtain a pressure reading in all four extremities.

PROVIDING NEONATAL CARE

GIVING UMBILICAL CORD CARE

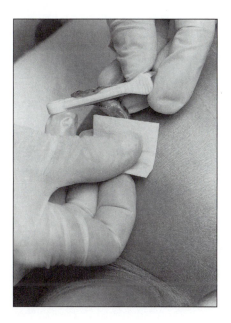

1 To help prevent infection and promote drying of the umbilical cord, cleanse the cord daily with alcohol or antibiotic ointment, according to agency guidelines. Be sure to swab around the entire surface of the cord base. The cord will usually fall off on its own after 7–10 days. Observe for redness or discharge, which are signs of infection, and be certain to keep the diaper below the cord. Instruct the parents in cord care.

SUCTIONING (BULB)

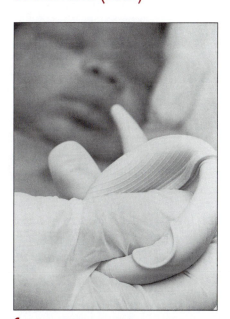

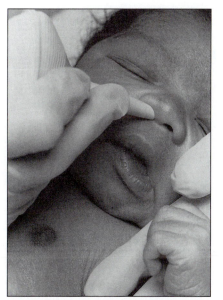

2 Insert the tip of the nozzle into each naris, and allow the bulb to expand slowly. Be sure to stabilize the infant's head with your free hand to minimize the risk of injuring the nasal mucosa. If indicated, suction the mouth as well. To remove the drainage from the bulb syringe, compress the bulb and point the nozzle over a tissue. Be sure to instruct the parents in the proper use of the bulb syringe. ***Caution:*** *Limit nasal suctioning to an "as-needed" basis. Frequent suctioning can irritate the mucous membrane and stimulate the vagal nerve.*

1 *Using a Bulb Syringe:* A bulb syringe is kept in the newborn's crib for removing secretions in the nose and mouth. To use the bulb syringe correctly, first depress the bulb with your thumb. ***Note:*** *Apply clean gloves before suctioning.*

SUCTIONING (MECHANICAL)

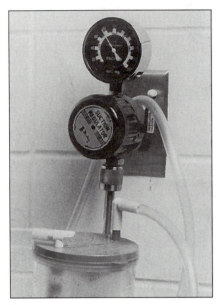

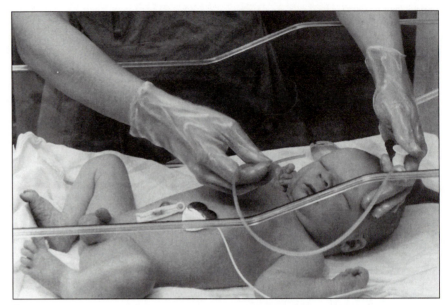

1 *Using Mechanical Suctioning:* Set the suction pressure gauge at or less than 80 cm H₂0.

2 Review the suctioning procedure on pages 330–334. Suction no deeper than the infant's pharynx.

USING PHOTOTHERAPY

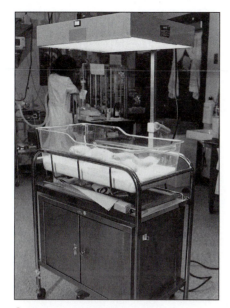

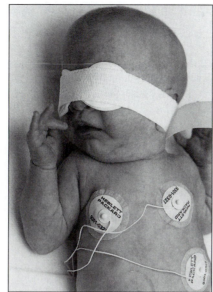

1 Premature infants commonly experience jaundice due to increased serum bilirubin levels. To help prevent the bilirubin from reaching dangerous levels or to help decrease the bilirubin count, phototherapy is used. The infant's entire skin is exposed to the light for prescribed time periods. Monitor serum bilirubin test results closely to assess the efficacy of the therapy. Be alert to potential side effects of the therapy: skin rash, loose green stools, increased water loss necessitating fluid replacement, and increased temperature. The infant's position should be changed every 2 hours to facilitate exposure of the light to all skin surfaces. ***Note:*** *The dose of phototherapy is determined by the irradiance levels of the light bulbs and the infant's distance from the lights. The standard distance is 45 cm (18 in).*

2 Always make sure the infant's eyes are well protected from the light. Eye patches or masks must be used with each treatment. To prevent corneal abrasion, make sure the infant's lids are closed before applying the patches. Some agencies suggest the use of protective covering over the genitalia as well. ***Note:*** *This infant's electrode patches are unrelated to his phototherapy.*

REFERENCES

Avery GB, Fletcher MA, MacDonald MG: *Neonatology: Pathophysiology and Management of the Newborn,* ed 4. Philadelphia: Lippincott, 1994.

Bobak IM, Jensen M, Lodermilk DL: *Maternity and Gynecologic Care: The Nurse and Family,* ed 5. St Louis: Mosby, 1993.

Bowers AC, Thompson JM: *Clinical Manual of Health Assessment,* ed 4. St Louis: Mosby, 1992.

Indiana University Hospitals: *Nursing Procedures and Policies,* Indianapolis, 1994.

Johnson J: Caring for the woman who's had a mastectomy. *Am J Nurs* 94(5):24–32, 1994.

Ladewig PW, London ML, Olds SB: *Essentials of Maternal-Newborn Nursing,* ed 3. Redwood City, CA: Addison-Wesley, 1994.

Lawrence RA: *Breastfeeding: A Guide for the Medical Professional,* ed 4. St Louis: Mosby, 1994.

May KA, Mahlmeister LR: *Maternal and Neonatal Nursing: A Family-Centered Care,* ed 3. Philadelphia: Lippincott, 1994.

Merenstein GB, Gardner SL: *Handbook of Neonatal Intensive Care,* ed 3. St Louis: Mosby, 1993.

Phillips CR: *Family-Centered Maternity/Newborn Care: A Basic Text,* ed 3. St Louis: Mosby, 1992.

Rice R: *Handbook of Home Health Nursing Procedures.* St Louis: Mosby, 1995.

Riordan J, Auerbach K: *Breastfeeding and Human Lactation.* Boston: Jones and Bartlett, 1993.

Sims LK et al: *Health Assessment in Nursing.* Redwood City, CA: Addison-Wesley, 1994.

Spence AP: *Basic Human Anatomy,* ed 3. Redwood City, CA: Addison-Wesley, 1991.

Thompson JM: *Mosby's Manual of Clinical Nursing,* ed 3. St Louis: Mosby, 1993.

Tucker SM: *Pocket Guide to Fetal Monitoring,* ed 2. St Louis: Mosby, 1992.

Wardell DW: Reproductive disorders. In Swearingen PL, ed: *Manual of Medical-Surgical Nursing Care,* ed 3. St Louis: Mosby, 1994.

CHAPTER 5

Managing Gastrointestinal Procedures

CHAPTER OUTLINE

ASSESSING THE GASTROINTESTINAL SYSTEM

The Gastrointestinal System

Nursing Assessment Guidelines

Examining the Oral Cavity

Inspecting the Mouth

Inspecting the Tongue and Pharynx

Examining the Abdomen

Inspecting the Abdomen

Auscultating the Abdomen

Percussing the Abdomen

Palpating the Abdomen

Measuring Abdominal Girth

Examining the Rectum

Inspecting the Rectum

Palpating the Rectum

MANAGING GASTRIC TUBES

Nursing Guidelines: Managing Gastric Tubes

Single-Lumen Tube

Double-Lumen Tube

Triple-Lumen Esophageal-Nasogastric (Blakemore) Tube

Four-Lumen (Minnesota Sump) Tube

Gastrostomy Tube

Percutaneous Endoscopic Gastrostomy (PEG) Tube

Gastrostomy Button

Inserting a Nasogastric Tube

Inserting a Small-Bore Feeding Tube

Inserting an Orogastric Tube

Removing a Nasogastric Tube

Irrigating a Nasogastric Tube

Administering Nasogastric Tube Feedings

Giving an Intermittent Tube Feeding

Giving a Continuous-Drip Tube Feeding

Giving Gastrostomy Tube Feedings

Administering Gastric Lavage

Aspirating Stomach Contents for Gastric Analysis

MANAGING INTESTINAL TUBES

Nursing Guidelines: Managing Intestinal Tubes

Single-Lumen Tube

Double-Lumen Tube

Jejunostomy Tube

MANAGING RECTAL ELIMINATION AND DISTENTION

Administering a Nonretention Enema

Administering a Retention Enema

Inserting a Rectal Tube

Testing Stool for Occult Blood

MANAGING STOMA CARE

Nursing Guidelines: Managing Ostomies

Ascending Colostomy

Transverse Colostomies

Descending or Sigmoid Colostomy

Ileostomy

Continent Ileostomy

Ileoanal Reservoir

Patch Testing the Client's Skin

Applying a Drainable Pouch

Dilating a Stoma

Irrigating a Colostomy

Draining a Continent Ileostomy

Assessing the Gastrointestinal System

THE GASTROINTESTINAL SYSTEM

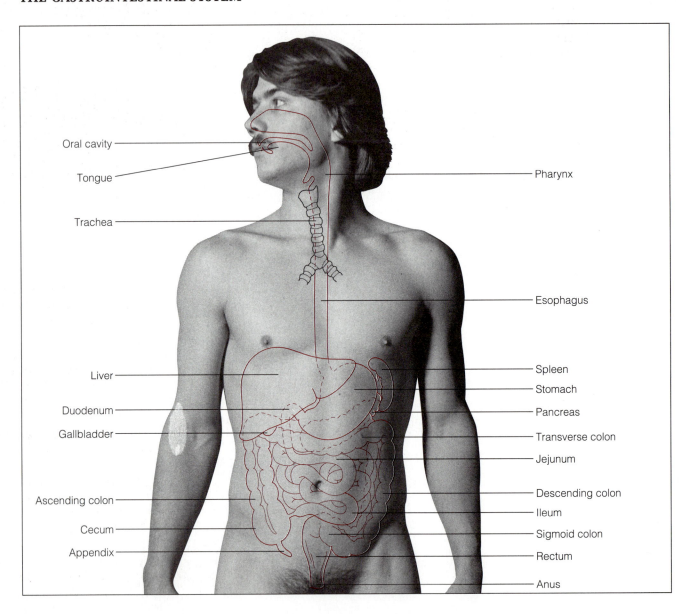

Oral cavity

Tongue

Trachea

Liver

Duodenum

Gallbladder

Ascending colon

Cecum

Appendix

Pharynx

Esophagus

Spleen

Stomach

Pancreas

Transverse colon

Jejunum

Descending colon

Ileum

Sigmoid colon

Rectum

Anus

Nursing Assessment Guidelines

To assess your client's gastrointestinal system, you will need to interview him or her for subjective data; take vital signs; and examine the oral cavity, abdomen, rectum, and sacrum. A comprehensive nursing care plan will include a complete evaluation for the following subjective data:

Personal factors: age, occupation, marital status, cultural/religious/economic lifestyle indicators (for example, those that would affect diet)

History of medically related problems of nutrition: alcoholism, hyperlipidemia, obesity, diabetes mellitus, peptic ulcer disease, ulcerative colitis, Crohn's disease, malignancy, paralysis

History of: previous oral, nasal, abdominal, or intestinal surgery

Risk factors: psychologic stressors, smoking, environmental pollutants

Presence of: dentures, loose (or missing) teeth, ostomy, hemorrhoids

Medications: type; use of laxatives, enemas, vitamins

Pain: onset; location; intensity; radiation; intensified or relieved by food (type), change in position, activity

Appetite impairment: early satiety; compulsive eating patterns; anorexia nervosa; precipitated by stress, depression, activity

Alterations in abdominal status: distention, rigidity, tenderness

Food intolerances/allergies: special diet

Recent weight gain/loss

Description of daily dietary intake: amount and type of food and fluid

Alterations in oral intake: anorexia, dysphagia, nausea, reflux, vomiting, eructation

Emesis: frequency, character, amount, hematemesis

Alterations in bowel elimination: diarrhea, constipation, incomplete evacuation, flatulence, anal discomfort

Stool: frequency, character, color, amount, presence of mucus or blood

EXAMINING THE ORAL CAVITY

A complete evaluation of your client's gastrointestinal system will include an assessment of the oral cavity. For adequate visualization, you will need a penlight and a tongue depressor.

INSPECTING THE MOUTH

Wash your hands and explain the procedure to your client. Observe for drooping of the mouth and the presence of drooling. These are indications of paralysis, which can interfere with dietary intake. If your client wears dentures, check for optimal fit, and then remove them before initiating examination of the oral cavity. Assess the lips for color and moistness. Note any bleeding, cracks, or lesions. Inspect the teeth for looseness, cracks, and gross caries and the gums for inflammation and bleeding, which occur with gingivitis or periodontitis. To visualize the buccal surface, retract

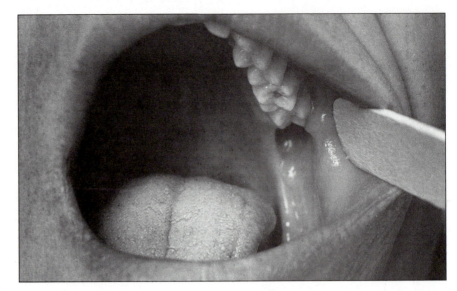

the cheeks with a tongue depressor and use your penlight to examine the membranes. They should be reddish-pink, smooth, and moist. Abnormalities may include canker sores or inflammation, generally referred to as stomatitis. Bluish patches are considered normal in

the black client. Also, be aware that halitosis can occur with such disorders as an infection, abscess, dehydration, or esophageal problems. *Note: Be sure to examine both sides of the mouth, because diseases can be manifested on one side only.*

INSPECTING THE TONGUE AND PHARYNX

Depress the tongue. Note the color and observe for the presence of edema or an abnormal, thick coating, which is an indicator of thrush. A thin, white coating is usually considered to be normal. Assess the tonsils for inflammation or exudate. Normally, they are small and pink. The uvula should rise with the soft palate when the client says "aah." The hard palate should be pale and moist, but a yellow hue is often

indicative of jaundice. Stimulate the gag reflex by pressing the tongue depressor on the back of the tongue. You should be able to see the involuntary contraction at the oropharynx. Finally, ask your client to move his tongue from side to side. An inability to do so suggests a pathology of the 12th cranial nerve. Palpate the tongue with a gloved finger, noting any lumps or sores.

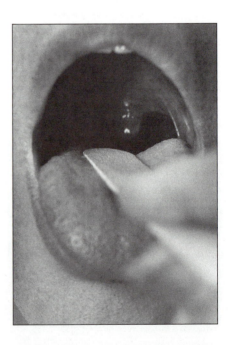

EXAMINING THE ABDOMEN

To examine the client's abdomen, provide a quiet, warm, and private environment. Explain the assessment procedure, and ensure that the client has recently voided. Assist the client into a supine position, and place pillows under his head and knees and ask him to position his arms at his side or across his chest to help relax the abdominal muscles. As you are preparing the client, observe his body alignment and facial expression for objective indicators of discomfort, such as grimacing or flexing the legs, which often occurs with acute appendicitis or peritonitis. Remember that your examination should begin with a visual inspection of the abdomen, followed by auscultation, and finally percussion and palpation. Because touching and temperature variations stimulate both peristalsis and muscle guarding, these reactions would alter the frequency and character of bowel sounds.

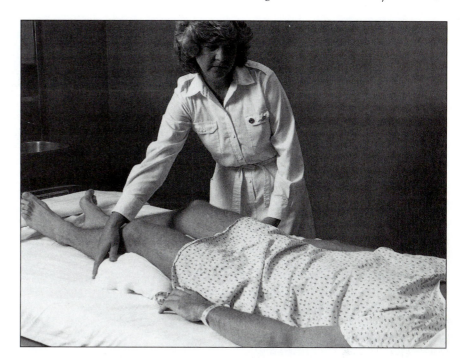

INSPECTING THE ABDOMEN

Expose the abdomen from the sternum to the pubis. Note the contour of the abdomen, which can be described as protruberant (eg, with pregnancy or obesity), rounded, flat, or scaphoid (concave). Observe for distention; asymmetry, which could indicate the presence of a mass; or peristaltic waves, which although not often seen, are indicative of intestinal obstruction in the adult or pyloric stenosis in the infant. Also observe for unusual pigmentation; striae, which occur after a pregnancy or weight gain; and loose skin folds, which can occur with weight loss. Assess the umbilicus for infection in the neonate, for inversion, or for eversion in clients with umbilical hernias or extreme ascites, and make a note of any abdominal scars. Also, observe the epigastrium for the presence of pulsations. Mild pulsations normally may be seen in very thin clients; however, vigorous pulsations occur in clients with right ventricular hypertrophy or with masses anterior to the aorta. Be alert to a pronounced venous network in the abdominal area. This is seen in adults with hepatic obstruction, portal hypertension, or ascites. However, it may be normal in infants and children. Note the presence of any ostomies, the color and character of the stoma, the appearance of the peristomal skin, and the amount and character of the effluent (fecal drainage) in the pouch. Question the client about the presence of scars, which may be indicative of previous surgery. Also be alert to abdominal breathing, which can signal

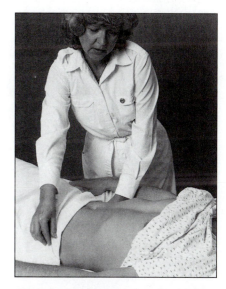

thoracic problems in the client older than 6 or 7. Children younger than 6 or 7 normally breathe using their abdominal muscles.

AUSCULTATING THE ABDOMEN

Review this anatomic overlay to assist you in dividing your client's abdomen into quadrants. The epigastric, umbilical, and hypogastric areas are further delineated. For auscultation, palpation, and percussion, you should develop your own pattern of assessment—for example, a clockwise examination of each of the four quadrants—and follow the same pattern consistently. Always auscultate before palpating and percussing, since the latter two assessments can interfere with normal bowel sounds.

To auscultate the abdomen, warm the diaphragm of the stethoscope and then place it in the center of each of the four quadrants, counting the frequency and character of the bowel sounds for a full minute. Move the stethoscope to various areas within the quadrant if you are unable to elicit sounds in the center. Generally, you will be able to hear 5–34 bowel sounds per minute. With hyperperistalsis you will hear more frequent, high-pitched gurgling. These sounds will occur with diarrhea, gastroenteritis, or intestinal hemorrhage. In a late obstructive process, paralytic ileus, or peritonitis, bowel sounds are typically absent. However, with a developing obstruction, bowel sounds may be absent in the quadrant in which the obstruction

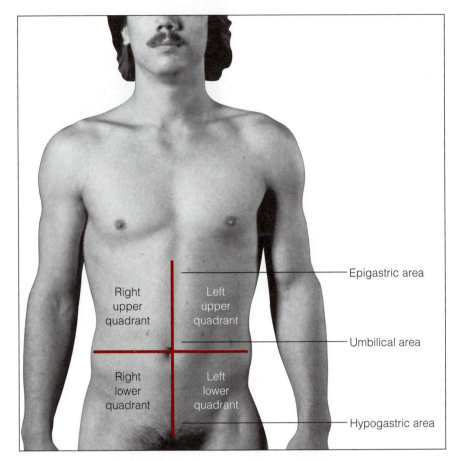

Right upper quadrant

Left upper quadrant

Right lower quadrant

Left lower quadrant

Epigastric area

Umbilical area

Hypogastric area

occurs, yet increase in frequency proximal to the point of obstruction. Hypoactive bowel sounds may be heard in the postoperative client.

During auscultation you should be alert to circulatory sounds such as *bruits*. These are swishing sounds, which may be heard in the midepigastric area in clients with diseased aortas or over the renal or femoral arteries. *Venous hums* are softer and more continuous than bruits and may be heard in the upper epigastric area and over the liver in clients with advanced cirrhosis. *Friction rubs* sound like sandpaper rubbing together, and they are heard best with the client taking deep respirations. They may be heard over diseased livers, spleens, and gallbladders. Auscultation should be performed at least daily.

PERCUSSING THE ABDOMEN

To percuss the abdomen, place your middle or index finger on the client's skin, and then strike that finger with the same finger on your opposite hand to elicit sounds. This assessment technique will reveal the density of the underlying structures. Hollow cavities, such as the empty intestine, will elicit high, tympanic sounds. Dull, flat sounds are heard over a distended bladder or over an organ, such as the liver in the right upper quadrant or the spleen in the left upper quadrant. You may also hear dullness while percussing the left lower quadrant over the sigmoid colon prior to the client's defecation. Dull sounds in other locations may be indicative of an abnormality, such as a mass.

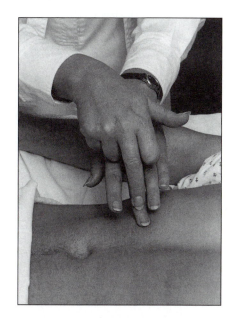

PALPATING THE ABDOMEN

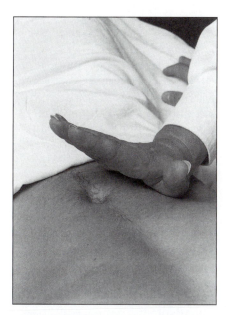
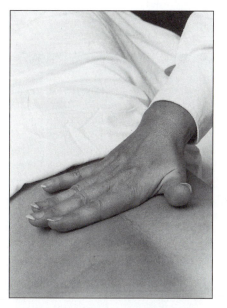
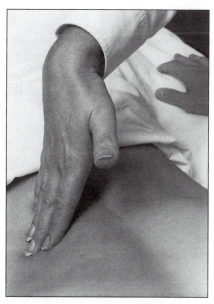

Lightly palpate the abdomen to determine muscle tone, tenderness, distention, organ size, pulsations, or the presence of a mass. You might use your entire hand not only because it is more comfortable for the client and the process will produce less muscle guarding, but also because you will have a larger surface area from which to assess abnormalities. Roll the hand over an abdominal area starting with the heel of the hand, (left photo), progressing to the palm (middle photo), and finishing at the fingertips. If you prefer, palpate with flattened fingertips (right photo). A healthy abdomen should feel soft and supple, but you will feel resistance with a distended abdomen and it will be less pliant. *Caution: Clients with peritonitis, who have boardlike abdomens, will find even light palpation extremely uncomfortable. Do not palpate the abdomen for an individual in whom Wilms' tumor is suspected.*

Deep palpation: Deep palpation is employed after light palpation to assess for enlarged organs or for the presence of masses. In addition, if your client feels discomfort over a particular area during light palpation, you can use this technique to assess for rebound tenderness. This is found in client's with peritoneal inflammation or appendicitis. Gently and slowly press your flattened fingertips approximately 6–8 cm ($2\frac{1}{3}$–$3\frac{1}{8}$ in) in the adult; 2–3 cm ($\frac{3}{4}$–$1\frac{1}{5}$ in) in the neonate; and 3–6 cm ($1\frac{1}{5}$–$2\frac{1}{3}$ in) in the child into the quadrant *opposite* that in which you elicited pain; then quickly release the pressure. Your client will feel a sudden, sharp pain over the original area of discomfort if rebound tenderness is present. ***Caution:*** *Never deeply palpate the right lower quadrant if*

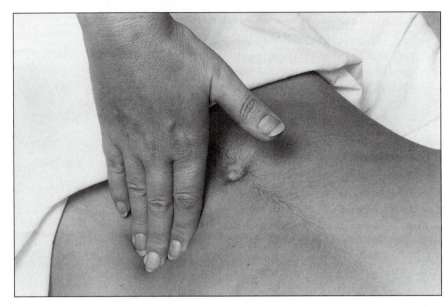

appendicitis is suspected. Deep palpation is also contraindicated in clients with rigid abdomens or in those who may have pancreatitis or *ectopic pregnancy because the procedure can be very painful and it could cause serious injury to the client.*

MEASURING ABDOMINAL GIRTH

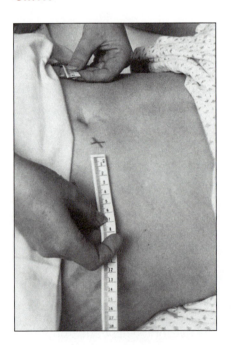

To assess for increasing degrees of distention, including ascites, you will need to measure the abdominal girth daily and at the same time of day—for example, before breakfast. Place the client in a supine position. Mark a spot on the abdomen with indelible ink to ensure that you measure around the same circumferential site with each measurement. Measure the girth of the abdomen, using a nonstretchable tape measure, and record the result. Daily increases in girth are significant and should be reported to the attending physician. (Note the presence of striae on this client.)

EXAMINING THE RECTUM

INSPECTING THE RECTUM

Before inspecting the rectum, provide your client with privacy, explain the procedure, and assist her into Sims' position. Expose the buttocks and inspect the rectal and sacral areas for the presence of external hemorrhoids, alterations in the integrity of the skin, pilonidal cysts, and fissures.

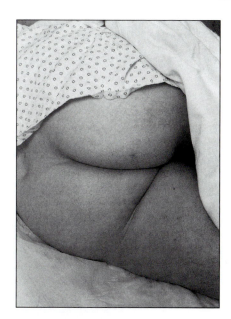

PALPATING THE RECTUM

Put on a disposable examination glove, and lubricate your index finger with water-soluble lubricant. Ask the client to breathe deeply and to bear down. Gently and slowly insert your index finger 5–10 cm (2–4 in) into the rectum, past the external and internal sphincters. Palpate along the circumference of the rectal wall to assess for the presence of masses, fistulae, or stool. Use special care if the client has external or internal hemorrhoids. Assess sphincter tone by asking the client to tighten the sphincter around your finger. After removing your finger, inspect the glove for the presence of stool, blood, or mucus. *Caution: If this procedure is performed for infants or small children, use the small finger rather than the index finger. Because of the risk of vagal stimulation with a rectal examination, this procedure may require a physician's prescription.*

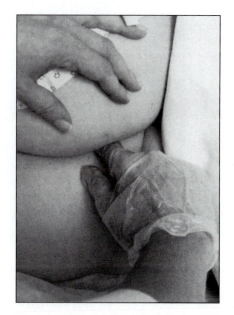

Managing Gastric Tubes

NURSING GUIDELINES: MANAGING GASTRIC TUBES

Single-Lumen Tube

Description

76–125 cm (30–50 in) in length, rubber or plastic material, may have radio-paque tips for x-ray film detection; smaller-lumen tubes may have insertion guides.

Sizes

Levin-type tubes:	12–18 French (F) for adults
	8–12F for children
	5–8F for infants
Pediatric feeders:	5–8F
Oral tubes:	30–40F

Uses

Gavage, administration of medications, lavage, diagnostic evaluation, decompression

Nursing Considerations

- Chill rubber tubes in icy water prior to insertion, if desired.
- Warm plastic tubes in hot water prior to insertion, if desired.
- Most tubes are inserted through the nose unless the nasal route is contraindicated.
- Larger-lumen tubes cause more irritation to the stomach, esophagus, and nose.
- For decompression, the tube should be connected to intermittent suction or placed to gravity drainage.

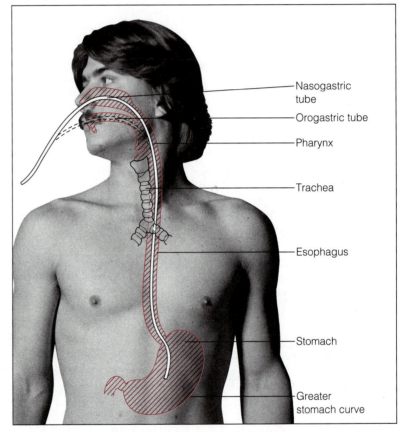

- Smaller tubes (8F) may require insertion guides (contraindicated for the neonate) for easier intubation.
- Check tube placement in stomach before any instillation.
- Provide oral and nasal hygiene at least three to four times a day.

NURSING GUIDELINES: MANAGING GASTRIC TUBES (continued)

Double-Lumen Tube

Description

85–125 cm (35–50 in) in length, plastic or rubber material, may have radiopaque tip for x-ray film detection and mercury-weighted tip to facilitate movement to the stomach.

Sizes

12–18F for adults

8–12F for children

5–10F for infants

Oral tubes: 30–40F

Uses

Decompression, lavage, gavage

Nursing Considerations

- Irrigate sump tubes through large port only.

- Inject only air into pigtail port of sump tubes, after reconnecting the large port to suction.

- For decompression, sump tubes work best when connected to continuous suction at 30 mm Hg.

- Check for correct stomach placement before any instillation.

- Provide oral and nasal hygiene at least three to four times daily.

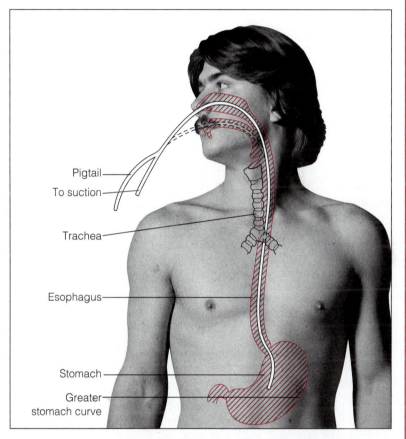

Pigtail

To suction

Trachea

Esophagus

Stomach

Greater stomach curve

- Remove tube only after an assessment that reveals active bowel sounds, the passing of flatus, and an undistended or minimally distended abdomen.

NURSING GUIDELINES: MANAGING GASTRIC TUBES (continued)

Triple-Lumen Esophageal-Nasogastric (Blakemore) Tube

Description

86–98 cm (36–39 in) in length; x-ray film opaque; latex rubber; has ports for gastric balloon, esophageal balloon, and gastric aspiration.

Sizes

16–20F for adults
12F for children

Uses

Compression; as a tamponade for control of esophageal bleeding; decompression; lavage

Nursing Considerations

- The tube is usually inserted by a physician.

- The client requires constant observation while the balloons are inflated.

- A Levin or sump tube is sometimes inserted into the opposite naris for aspiration of the esophagus.

- Provide comfort measures while the tube is in place: blankets during lavage, backrubs and skin care, oral and nasal hygiene.

- A football helmet may be positioned on client's head so that exterior traction on the tube can be achieved by taping the tube to the face guard.

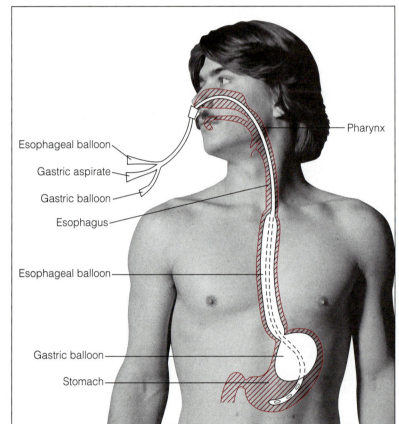

- The esophageal balloon is deflated for 5 minutes every 8–12 hours to prevent erosion to the esophagus.

- Tape scissors to the head of the client's bed for emergency tube cutting (deflating both balloons) in the event of acute respiratory distress.

NURSING GUIDELINES: MANAGING GASTRIC TUBES (continued)

Four-Lumen (Minnesota Sump) Tube

Description

Has a fourth port for esophageal aspiration; thus, the need for a Levin or sump tube is eliminated.

Uses

See Blakemore tube, page 246.

Nursing Considerations

See Blakemore tube, page 246.

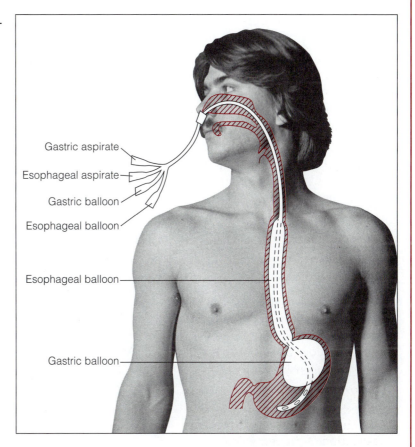

Gastric aspirate

Esophageal aspirate

Gastric balloon

Esophageal balloon

Esophageal balloon

Gastric balloon

NURSING GUIDELINES: MANAGING GASTRIC TUBES (continued)

Gastrostomy Tube

Description

35 cm (14 in) in length; 20–28F; rubber or latex material, often with an inflatable balloon (as shown).

Uses

Gavage; or it may be inserted during intestinal surgery for decompression

Nursing Considerations

- The tube is surgically inserted into the stomach.

- Unless the client has nausea, discomfort, or distention, keep the tube plug attached to the tube when the tube is not being used for feedings.

- The skin at the abdominal exit site requires careful observation because leaking gastric contents can cause skin irritation. Use skin barriers or pouches as needed.

- Follow aseptic technique for dressing changes.

- Two weeks after surgery, the tube usually can be removed and inserted as needed for tube feedings.

- Clean the inside and outside of the feeding port with a cotton-tipped applicator.

- Clean around the stoma with a cotton-tipped applicator or a moist cloth. For the healthy stoma, soap and water are usually adequate cleansing agents.

- Irrigate the tube with 30–50 mL water (10–25 mL for the infant or child), or as recommended by the tube's manufacturer.

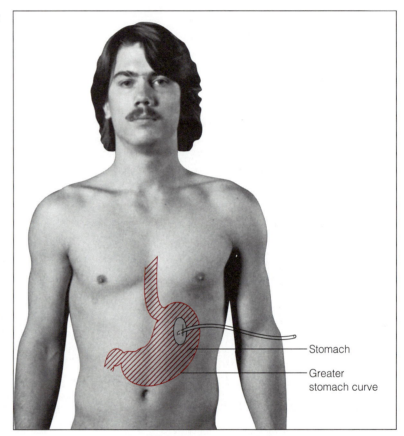

Stomach

Greater stomach curve

HOME HEALTH CARE CONSIDERATIONS

- For the first 2–3 weeks after tube insertion, antiseptic soap or hydrogen peroxide solution may be used to clean around the exit site, followed by a thorough rinsing. After 2–3 weeks, the caregiver or client may clean around the exit site with warm, soapy water.

- Dressings usually are not required, but the client may cover the exit site with gauze if the clothing irritates the site.

NURSING GUIDELINES: MANAGING GASTRIC TUBES (continued)

Percutaneous Endoscopic Gastrostomy (PEG) Tube

Description

Flexible silicone tube that is inserted endoscopically into the stomach and held in place internally with a radio-paque bumper and externally with a retention disk.

Uses

To provide long-term enteral nutrition in clients who have difficulty swallowing or who cannot tolerate indwelling nasogastric tubes. These tubes also are inserted into clients for whom surgical placement of a gastrostomy tube is contraindicated. Generally they are not used in individuals who are morbidly obese or who have ascites.

Nursing Considerations

- Client must have an intact, patent gut from the pharynx through the esophagus and into the stomach.

- A detachable adapter is used for attaching the feeding tube. The adapter may be capped off when feedings are discontinued.

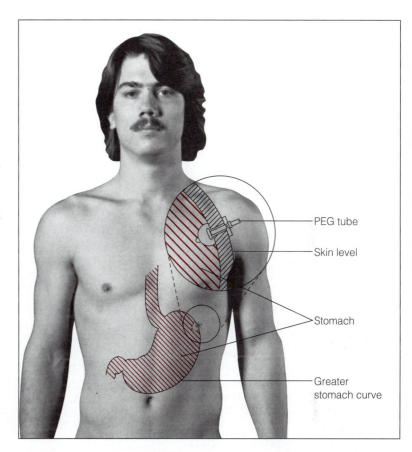

PEG tube

Skin level

Stomach

Greater stomach curve

- Gently clean the abdominal exit site with cotton-tipped applicators moistened with water. Apply a topical antibiotic ointment to the site as prescribed. After the exit site is well-healed (usually after 2–3 weeks), clean with soap and water as prescribed.

- The exit site will have a dressing for the first 7–10 days. Change this dressing according to agency protocol.

- Monitor the skin around the exit site for evidence of irritation caused by leaking of gastric contents. Apply skin barriers as needed.

- Mark the PEG tube with indelible ink at the point where it exits the abdomen. If the tube moves, withhold the feedings and notify physician accordingly.

- The PEG tube can be changed 10–14 days after insertion, when the tract has been well-established. This may be indicated for a clogged tube or for client comfort or aesthetics.

- See "Gastrostomy Tubes," page 248, for Home Health Care Considerations.

Gastrostomy Button

Description

Flexible silicone device with a radio-paque dome on the distal end that secures the button in the stomach, two small wings at the proximal end that are flush with the abdominal skin, and an outer plug that is attached to the wings. Sizes include small (18F), medium (24F), and large (28F); and lengths range from 1.7 cm (²⁄₃ in) to 4.3 cm (1²⁄₃ in). An antireflux valve at the distal end helps prevent backflow and leakage of gastric contents. Each button comes with a kit that includes an obturator for ease of insertion, a stoma-measuring device, and a special feeding apparatus.

Use

Long-term gavage of 6–8 months to 1 year

Nursing Considerations

- Insertion requires a well-established gastrostomy site. Usually the site is dilated over a 3–4 week period with increasingly larger Foley catheters prior to the initial button insertion. Once positioned, the button can stay in place until malfunction occurs.

- Stoma depth is measured with a stoma-measuring device (left photo, page 251) to facilitate button size selection.

- Because the button is flush with the skin, it has a more cosmetically pleasing appearance than a gastrostomy tube.

- Most clients experience greater mobility and independence with the button than with a tube.

- Be alert to gastric contents leakage, which can signal malfunction of the antireflux valve.

- If gastric contents leak, insert the obturator gently into the button shaft (middle photo, page 251) to return the antireflux valve to its closed position. If this fails, it may be necessary to replace the button with a new one.

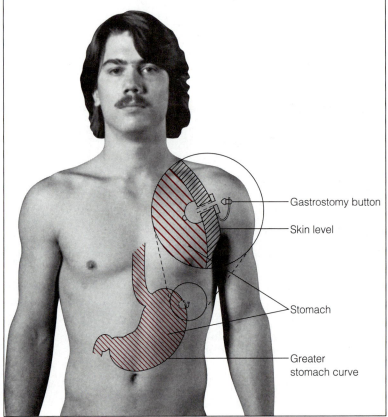

Gastrostomy button

Skin level

Stomach

Greater stomach curve

- See "Gastrostomy Tube," page 248, for Home Health Care Considerations.

- Rotate the button in a full circle during site care to facilitate thorough cleaning.

- Use mild soap and water to clean around the stoma one to two times each day. This can be accomplished during the daily bath, since the button can be immersed safely in water. To ensure thorough drying, allow the stoma site to be exposed to air for 20 minutes before covering with clothing.

- If the peristomal skin becomes reddened and irritated when cleansing with soap and water, try cleaning the site with water alone, followed by povidone-iodine swabs or liquid. Another option for impaired skin integrity is the use of stoma-hesive powder or a pectin wafer skin barrier on the peristomal skin.

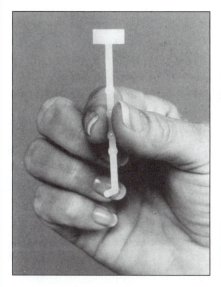 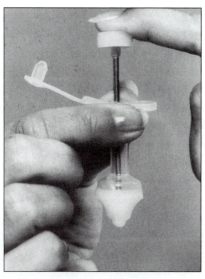 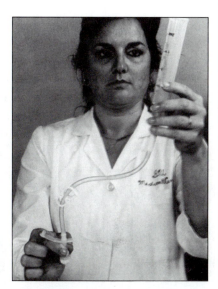

- For bolus feedings, attach special feeding catheter and syringe (right photo) to the proximal end of the button. This equipment comes as part of a special kit with each button. Check for residual from previous feedings (see page 264) before administering new feeding.

- Continuous feedings also can be administered via gravity or infusion pump over a 16–24 hour period. Check residual from previous feedings q8h.

- To prevent clogging of the button with formula, rinse with water (10 mL for pediatric client, 30–50 mL for the adult) after every feeding or insertion of medication.

- Crush medication tablets and contents of capsules, and mix with water prior to instillation.

- Maintain client in Fowler's or slightly elevated right side-lying position for at least 30 minutes during and after feedings or medication instillation to reduce the risk of aspiration of stomach contents.

- Rinse feeding apparatus with water after every feeding. Once a day, wash the feeding apparatus in warm, soapy water, and rinse well. Soak in mild vinegar solution weekly and rinse well.

- Weight gain and growth, especially in the pediatric population, will necessitate a larger and longer button.

- Avoid using oily substances around the stoma, which would deteriorate the silicone button and make it difficult to keep the outer plug in place.

- Insertion steps are as follows:

  —Measure depth of the stoma with stoma-measuring device (left photo) to ensure proper size selection of the button.

  —Lubricate the tip of the obturator with a water-soluble lubricant. Insert obturator into the button's lumen (middle photo), and distend the button several times to ensure patency of the antireflux valve.

  —Lubricate the button's dome and the client's stoma with water-soluble lubricant, and insert the button into the stoma to the stomach.

  —Rotate the obturator slightly on removal to prevent its adherence to the antireflux valve.

  —After removing the obturator, look through the button's lumen to ensure that the antireflux valve is in the closed position.

  —Insert the outer plug into the button's lumen, keeping the plug in place between feedings.

INSERTING A NASOGASTRIC TUBE

Caution: Nurses should not insert, withdraw, or irrigate nasogastric tubes for postoperative clients with gastric or esophageal resections. Hemorrhage could result from an injury to the suture line.

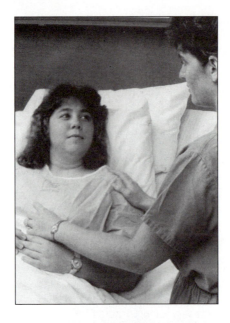

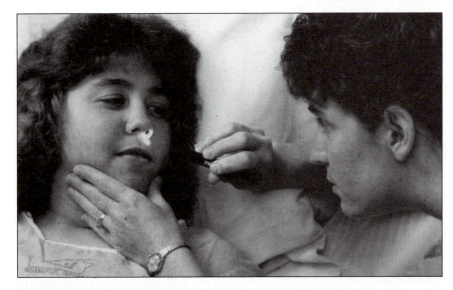

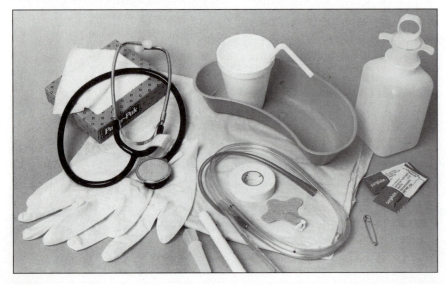

Assessing and Planning

1 Wash your hands and assess the client to obtain her baseline gastrointestinal status (see pages 237–242). Assess her knowledge of the procedure, and explain why the tube has been prescribed and how her assistance can facilitate the procedure. Evaluate the need for premedication, and obtain a prescription if appropriate. Together, agree on a signal she can use, such as tapping your arm, that will alert you to stop momentarily if the procedure becomes too uncomfortable. A thorough explanation, combined with a relaxed and empathetic manner, will help to ensure a successful and quick insertion.

2 With your penlight, inspect both nares to determine which is more patent. Alternately close each naris to check airflow. Ask the client which nostril breathes more easily, and whether she has ever had a fractured nose, which could affect passage of the tube. If both nares are obstructed, you may need to intubate through her mouth (see page 260).

3 Gather the following materials:

- [ ] the prescribed nasogastric tube
- [ ] irrigation set with a 50-mL syringe
- [ ] tissues
- [ ] glass and a straw
- [ ] penlight
- [ ] stethoscope
- [ ] 1.25 cm wide hypoallergenic tape (or a commercially available tube-securing device)
- [ ] bed-saver pad
- [ ] emesis basin
- [ ] water-soluble lubricant
- [ ] clean gloves
- [ ] safety pin for securing tube to the client's gown
- [ ] tube plug (if indicated)

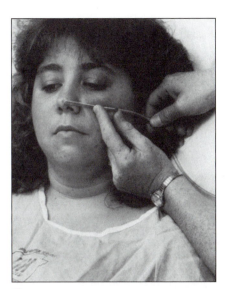

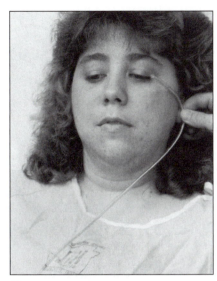

4 Measure the tube against the client to help ensure its proper placement into the stomach. Measure the distance from the tip of the nose to the ear.

5 Measure the distance from the ear to the xiphoid process. The total measurement, referred to as NEX (nose-ear-xiphoid), should be either marked on the tube with tape or indelible ink or compared against the markings on the tube and remembered. Many tubes are marked at 45 cm and 55 cm, the average length to an adult's stomach. Compare these marks to your measurement. They should be within a comparable range.

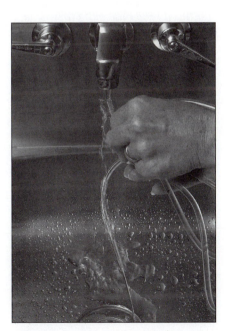

6 Ensure patency of the tube by flushing it with water. Also, check for rough edges that could harm delicate mucosa. If you are inserting a rubber tube, you may need to chill it in icy water to firm it up. A stiff plastic tube can be made more pliant by immersing it in warm water.

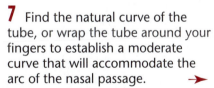

7 Find the natural curve of the tube, or wrap the tube around your fingers to establish a moderate curve that will accommodate the arc of the nasal passage. →

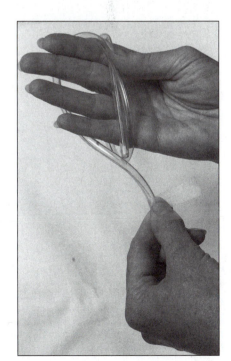

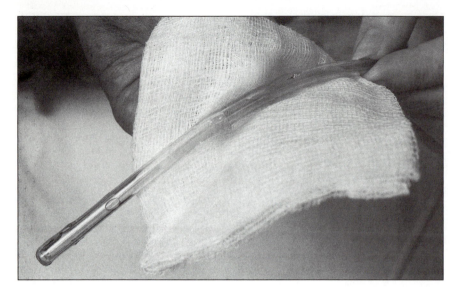

8 Lubricate the first 15–20 cm (6–8 in) of the tube with water-soluble lubricant to facilitate insertion. *Caution: Never use an oil-based lubricant because it will not dissolve, and respiratory complications could result if the tube is mistakenly inserted into the trachea.*

Implementing

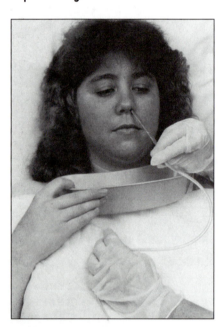

9 Drape the client with a bed-saver pad, and ask her to remove her glasses and dentures, if she has them. Give her an emesis basin and explain that the tube could activate her gag reflex as it enters her throat. Provide her with tissues for excessive tearing, which can occur as the tube passes the nasopharynx. Fowler's position is advised because it will lessen the potential for aspiration, making swallowing easier, and promote the tube's movement into the stomach via gravity. If this position is contraindicated, a right side-lying position is also acceptable. Because there is the risk of activating the gag reflex and causing vomiting, apply clean gloves at this time. Insert the tube into the naris and gently advance it along the floor of the nasal passage. Slight pressure is sometimes necessary to pass the nasopharynx. *Caution: Never force the tube. If you meet resistance, remove the tube, relubricate it, and intubate the other naris if it is patent.*

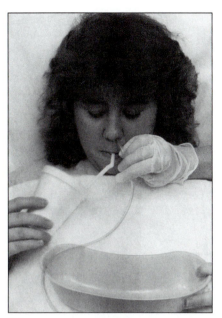

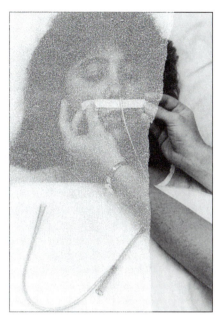

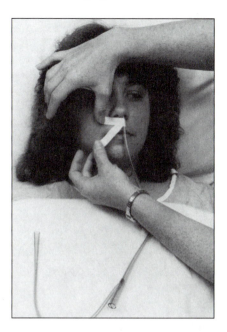

10 When the tube enters the oro-pharynx, pause briefly to minimize the potential for emesis. Ask the client to flex her head forward and sip water (or dry swallow if fluids are contraindicated). This will ease the tube's insertion into the esophagus. *Caution: Never have the client hyperextend her neck at this point. Doing so opens the airway and could permit the tube to enter the trachea.* Advance the tube 5–10 cm (2–4 in) with each swallow. If the client starts to cough or gasp for air, remove the tube immediately because you may have inserted the tube into the airway.

11 When the predesignated mark on the tube is at the level of the client's nostril, secure the tube to the client's nose, following agency protocol. If you plan to use tape, cut a strip 10 cm (4 in) in length. Slide it sticky-side up under the tube between the client's nose and mouth. As an alternative, you may use a commercially available tube securing device (shown on page 264).

12 Next, grasp one end of the tape and transfer it around and to the opposite side of the tube, adhering the sticky side to the tube and the client's face.

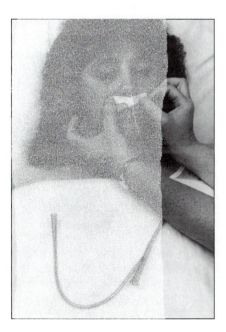

13 Finally, do the same with the remaining tape end and adhere it to the tube and the client's face.

Evaluating

14 Check the back of your client's mouth with a penlight to ensure that the tube is not curled at the oropharynx.

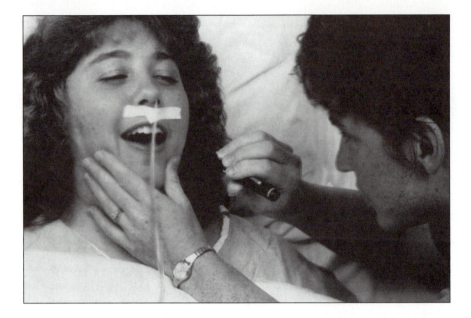

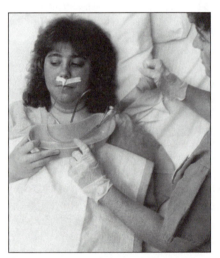

15 To ensure that the tube is correctly positioned in the stomach, aspirate for stomach contents by attaching a 50-mL syringe to the open end of the tube. If the tube is positioned correctly, gastric contents will return after you have squeezed the bulb or pulled back on the piston. Unless the stomach contents appear to contain blood, reinstill the aspirate to maintain the electrolyte balance. Hold the syringe barrel 30–45 cm (12–18 in) above the client's abdomen and allow the aspirate to return via gravity flow. *Caution: X-ray confirmation is the only valid test for stomach position in small-bore tubes (6–12F). See pages 258–259.*

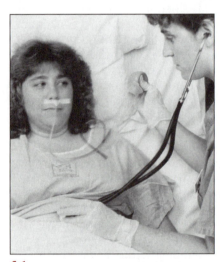

16 To perform another test for correct stomach placement, inject approximately 5–10 mL of air into the open end of the tube ($\frac{1}{2}$–1 mL for premature and small neonates and up to 5 mL for the larger child) as you auscultate the epigastric area with your stethoscope. With a properly positioned tube, you will hear a "whoosh" as air enters the stomach. If the client eructates instead, the tube may be in the esophagus. You also can ask the client to hum or speak. If the tube is in the trachea, she will be unable to do so. *Caution: Always perform these tests to confirm correct stomach placement of larger-bore tubes before instilling anything into the tube. Follow agency policy accordingly.*

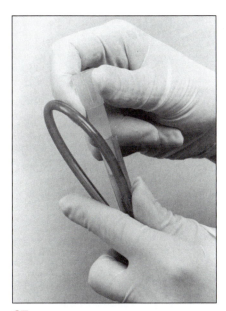

17 Either connect the tube to suction or insert a tube plug (as shown).

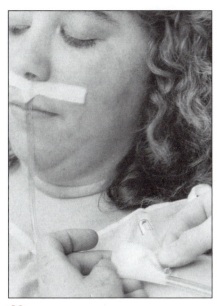

18 Attach the tube to the client's gown by inserting a safety pin through a tape tab. Document the procedure.

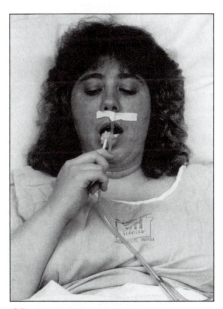

19 *Providing Oral and Nasal Hygiene:* Clean and refresh the client's mouth after inserting the nasogastric tube. A Toothette is being used here. Lip balm also can be applied to the lips for moisture and comfort.

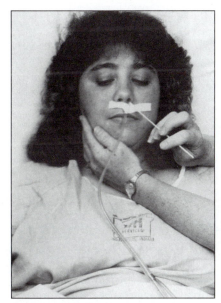

20 The cotton-tipped swab has been moistened with a water-soluble lubricant to clean and help protect the naris from potential skin irritation. Frequently assess the client for the need for oral and nasal hygiene. If possible, keep lip balm and Toothettes at the bedside.

INSERTING A SMALL-BORE FEEDING TUBE

Note: *Follow the guidelines for inserting a nasogastric tube, with the following variations.*

Assessing and Planning

1 If inserting the small-bore feeding tube into the stomach, measure the distance as described on page 253, and mark. If the tube will be inserted into the intestine, add approximately another 23 cm (9 in) for the adult (as shown), and mark accordingly.

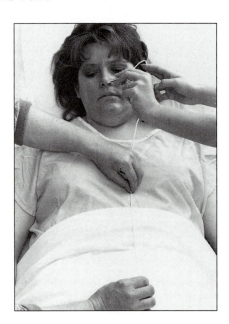

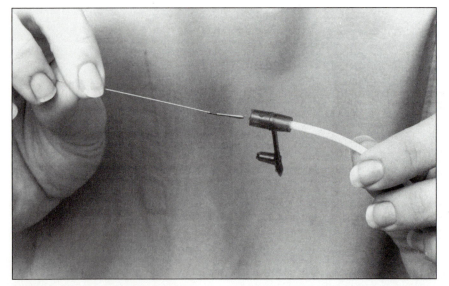

2 To facilitate ease of insertion through the nasal passageway and into the stomach, the stylet that is packaged with the feeding tube can be introduced into the proximal end of the tube and threaded through the length of the tube. First, irrigate the tube with 10 mL of water by attaching a 30-mL syringe to the proximal end of the tube. This will activate the internal Hydromer lubricant and facilitate insertion of the stylet. Insert the stylet until it reaches the weighted tip and its Luer connector firmly attaches to the feeding tube's Luer connector at the proximal tip.

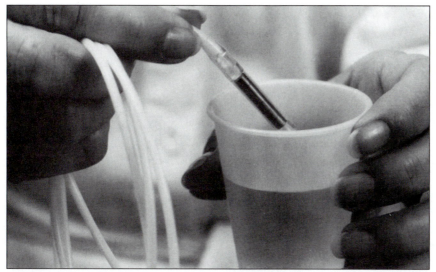

3 For most small-bore feeding tubes, external lubrication at the tip's distal end is not necessary. Instead, insert the distal (weighted) end of the tube into a small amount of water, as shown, to activate the Hydromer lubricant.

Implementing

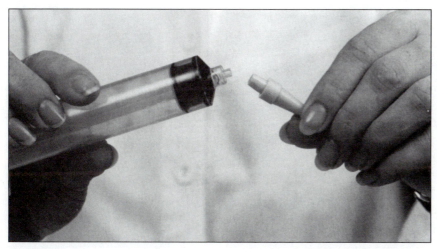

4 Always use syringes ≥30 mL when aspirating or instilling anything into the small-bore feeding tube. Syringes smaller in size could generate too much pressure in the small-bore tube, damaging the tube. Use 5–10 mL water to flush this tube. *Caution: Before instilling anything into the tube, ensure that proper stomach position has been confirmed by radiography. Small-bore tubes become displaced relatively easily, and there is risk of instilling fluid into the client's respiratory tract.* After confirming proper position of the feeding tube, remove the stylet, if it was used, by applying gentle traction. Never reinsert the stylet into the tube once the tube has been inserted into the client.

INSERTING AN OROGASTRIC TUBE

Note: Follow the guidelines for inserting nasogastric tubes, with the following variations for assessing and implementing.

Assessing

1 If nasal intubation is contraindicated, you may be required to insert the tube through your client's mouth. Measure the distance from the tragus of the ear to the mouth to the tip of the xiphoid process to determine the approximate distance to the stomach. Mark the site with indelible ink.

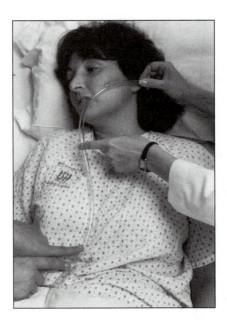

Implementing

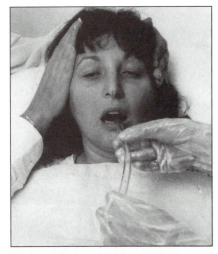

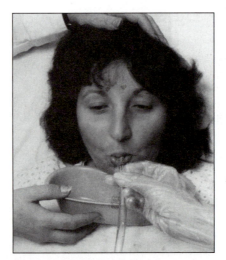

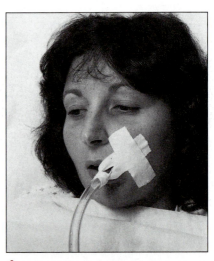

2 Ask the client to open her mouth, and then glide the tube toward the back of her throat. If necessary, depress the tongue with a tongue depressor.

3 At the oropharynx, pause briefly to minimize the potential for emesis. Then instruct the client to flex her head forward and begin swallowing. She may, at this point, guide the tube with her lips and teeth, as if it were a spaghetti noodle. *Note: Alert clients who require frequent oral intubations should be taught to insert their own tubes.*

4 When you have determined correct stomach placement, tape the tube to the client's cheek.

REMOVING A NASOGASTRIC TUBE

Caution: Nurses never insert or remove nasogastric tubes for postoperative clients with gastric or esophageal resections. Hemorrhage could result from an injury to the suture line.

Assessing and Planning

1 Before removing the nasogastric tube, assess the client's abdomen by auscultating for bowel sounds and inspecting and palpating for distention. If you do not hear bowel sounds, or if the abdomen is quite distended, check with the physician to make sure the tube should be removed. Assess the client's knowledge of the procedure, and explain why the tube will be removed. If the tube is connected to suction, disconnect it at this time. Because there is the risk of stimulating the gag reflex and causing vomiting, apply gloves.

2 Cover the client's gown with a bed-saver pad to protect her from drainage of gastric contents. Place her in Fowler's position to prevent aspiration of the gastric contents as the tube is removed. Remove the tape from the client's nose and rotate the tubing back and forth to ensure that it is mobile.

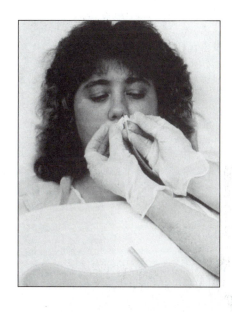

Implementing

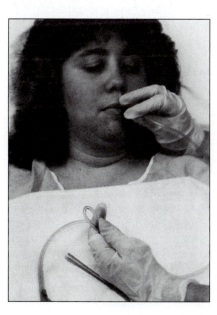

3 Clamp the tube or squeeze it firmly between your fingers. Ask the client to take a deep breath and to exhale slowly as you withdraw the tube. This will relax the pharynx and prevent aspiration as well. Then remove the tube in one continuous movement.

4 Cover the tube with the bed-saver pad and remove it from the bedside; remove your gloves. Wash your hands. Provide the client with materials for oral and nasal hygiene, and document the procedure.

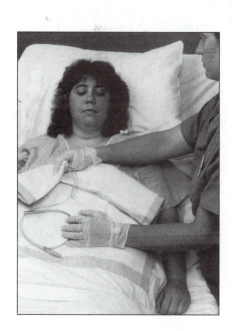

Evaluating

5 Continue to monitor the client for distention, alterations in nutrition, nausea, or any of the symptoms that necessitated the tube's insertion.

IRRIGATING A NASOGASTRIC TUBE

Caution: Irrigation is contraindicated for clients with gastric resections without a specific physician's prescription to do so.

Assessing and Planning

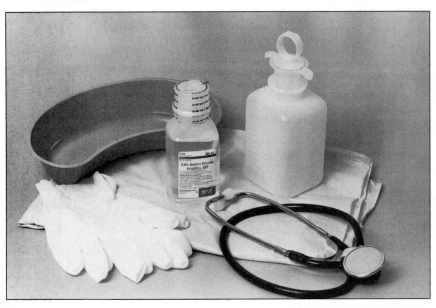

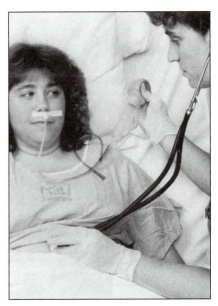

1 If you have determined that the nasogastric tube is no longer patent, obtain a physician's prescription for an irrigation. Wash your hands and assemble the following materials:

- ☐ normal saline (or the prescribed irrigant)—usually 60–90 mL
- ☐ irrigation set with a 50 or 60 mL syringe (3–15 mL for the pediatric population)
- ☐ bed-saver pad
- ☐ stethoscope for confirming stomach placement
- ☐ emesis basin for return of the irrigant
- ☐ clean gloves

2 Assess your client's knowledge of the procedure, and explain why it has been prescribed. Place her in semi-Fowler's or Fowler's position, put on clean gloves, and disconnect the tube from suction or unclamp it, and confirm the tube's correct stomach placement. If the client can speak and if you are able to hear the "whoosh" of air over the epigastric area as you inject 5–10 mL of air into the tube as shown ($\frac{1}{2}$ to 1 mL for premature and small neonates and up to 5 mL for larger children), you can assume that the tube is correctly positioned in the stomach. Be sure to drape the client's gown for the procedure.

Implementing

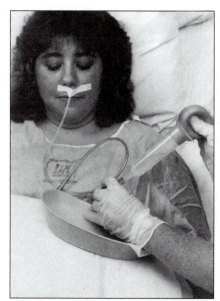

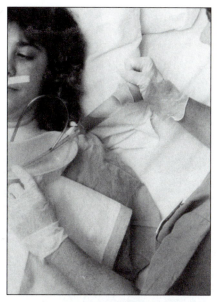

3 Draw up 20–30 mL of the irrigant into the syringe (see physician's prescription for the amount of irrigant for the pediatric population), attach it to the open end of the tube, and apply gentle pressure as you inject it into the tube. To prevent injury to the tissues, do not force the irrigant through the tube.

If you cannot instill the irrigant, check the tubing for kinks, have the client turn from side to side, or pull back slightly on the tube to change its position at the distal end. Remember to recheck for stomach placement if you have altered the position of the tube.

4 After instilling the irrigant, gently pull back on the piston or decompress the bulb to get an equal return, and empty the return into the emesis basin. ***Note:*** *If you are unable to get a return, or if the return is less than the instilled amount, be sure to note this on the intake and output record.* Instill and withdraw the irrigant two more times or until the returns become clear. Then reclamp the tube or reconnect to suction, as indicated. Document the procedure and the results.

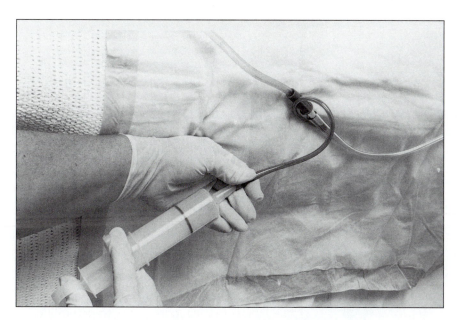

5 ***Note:*** *If the client has a double-lumen sump tube, you will need to instill 15–20 mL of air (1–5 mL for the pediatric population) into the pigtail port after you have reconnected the larger lumen to suction. Never instill liquid into this port because doing so could result in tube malfunction.*

Evaluating

6 Periodically assess the patency of the tube and irrigate if indicated, provided you have a physician's prescription.

ADMINISTERING NASOGASTRIC TUBE FEEDINGS

GIVING AN INTERMITTENT TUBE FEEDING

Assessing and Planning

1 If tube feedings have been prescribed for your client, determine the problems the client may have regarding food allergies or medically related problems of nutrition. If the client has had a previous feeding, determine if alterations in bowel elimination, nausea, and flatulence have occurred. These are indications that there may be an intolerance to the feeding solution. Inspect and palpate the client's abdomen for distention, which would suggest nonabsorption of the previous feeding.

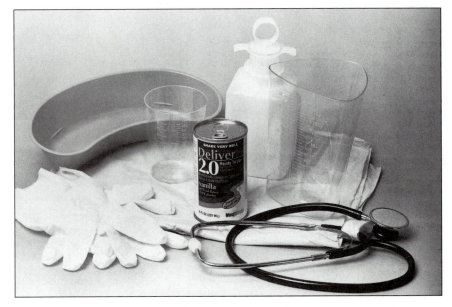

2 For an intermittent tube feeding, assemble the following equipment:

☐ irrigation set with a 50-mL syringe

☐ emesis basin

☐ clean measured container for the feeding solution (residual solution can be a medium for bacterial growth)

☐ clean measured container for instilling the water

☐ prescribed feeding solution warmed to room temperature to prevent vasoconstriction and cramping (check expiration date to ensure the solution is fresh)

☐ bed-saver pads

☐ stethoscope for confirming correct stomach placement

☐ 30–50 mL tap water

☐ clean gloves

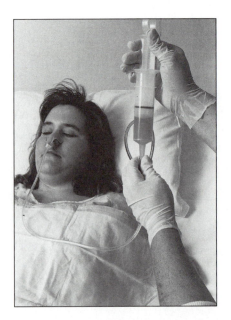

3 Explain the procedure to the client; place her in Fowler's position to enhance the solution's gravitational flow and to prevent aspiration. If a sitting position is contraindicated, a slightly elevated right side-lying position is acceptable. Apply clean gloves, remove the tube plug, and attach the syringe to the opened end of the tube. Aspirate all the stomach contents (as shown), and measure the absorption of the last feeding. If your client has residual volume, check your agency's aspiration precautions policy to determine whether or not to withhold this feeding. The standard protocol for withholding the feeding is a residual of ≥75–100 mL.

Implementing

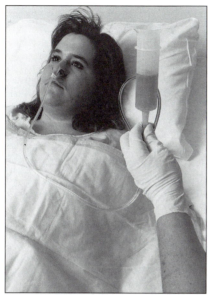

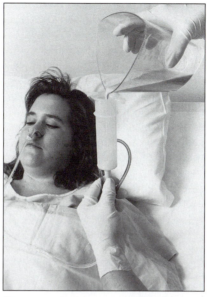

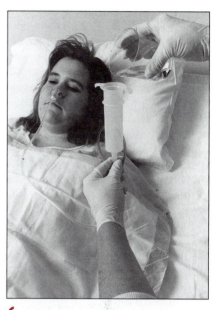

4 Remove the piston from the irrigation syringe, and reinstill the measured aspirate via the syringe barrel to prevent loss of electrolytes and gastric juices. For effective gravity flow, hold the syringe 30–45 cm (12–18 in) above the client's abdomen. To make this feeding as pleasant as possible, try to avoid instilling the gastric contents directly in front of the client.

5 Before the aspirate drains completely from the neck of the syringe, begin pouring the feeding solution into the syringe barrel. This will prevent the aspiration of air into the client's stomach. Raise or lower the syringe if you need to adjust the flow to ensure a slow instillation of the feeding.

6 When the desired amount of feeding has been instilled, flush the tubing with 30–50 mL of water, unless contraindicated. For the pediatric population, flush with 1–2 mL of water for small tubes and approximately 5 mL for larger tubes, or as prescribed. Be sure to add the water before the feeding solution has drained from the neck of the syringe. Clamp the tube before removing the syringe to prevent reflux of the feeding.

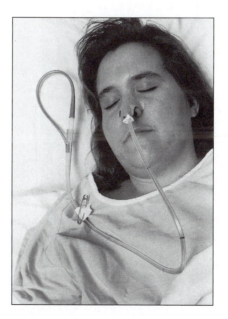

7 For better absorption, have your client remain in Fowler's position for 45–60 minutes after the solution has been instilled. If this is uncomfortable, she may be positioned in a slightly elevated right side-lying position so that the solution can flow by gravity from the greater stomach curve to the pylorus. Wash and dry the syringe and the other feeding containers, and return them to the bedside stand. Document the feeding in the chart and on the intake and output record.

Evaluating

8 Assess for alterations in fluid volume, nutrition, and bowel elimination. If alterations occur, the rate of infusion or the concentration of the feeding solution may need to be changed. Monitor the fluid and electrolyte status by checking laboratory values, and assess the client's vital signs, skin turgor, intake and output balance, and mucous membranes. Query the client about the presence of thirst, the primary indicator of dehydration. Tube feedings that are high in protein tend to increase the risk of osmotic diuresis, which can result in depletion of extracellular and cellular water. To help prevent this, periodically instill water into the nasogastric tube, basing the amount and frequency on your assessment and the tube-feeding guidelines. Perform urine glucose tests every 6–8 hours to assess for glycosuria, which can be caused by the high osmolarity of the feeding solution. Administer nasal and oral hygiene after each feeding, and weigh the client daily, if prescribed.

HOME HEALTH CARE CONSIDERATIONS

- Once the client has received enteral feedings for a long period of time, checking for residual feeding volume usually is not necessary unless there are indications of problems such as excessive gagging with the feeding.

- Equipment can be washed in warm, soapy water; rinsed well; and dried thoroughly.

- If the nasogastric tube is indwelling, it should be removed every 2 weeks; washed in warm, soapy water; rinsed; and reinserted into the opposite naris to prevent skin breakdown.

- The nasogastric tube can be washed and reused repeatedly until it loses its pliability.

GIVING A CONTINUOUS-DRIP TUBE FEEDING

Note: *Review the guidelines for giving an intermittent tube feeding, and make the following variations.*

There are several ways to administer a continuous-drip tube feeding.

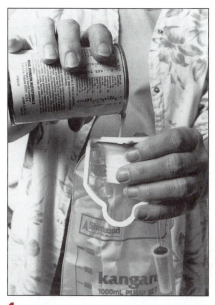

1 One method is to pour the prescribed feeding solution into a feeding container, as shown. Pour only enough of the solution for the prescribed amount and time of the feeding, usually 3–4 hours.

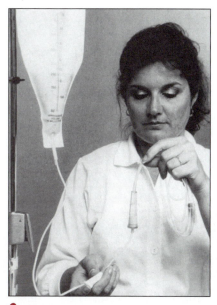

2 Hang the feeding container and prime the tubing to remove the air. Attach the primed tubing to the client's gastric tube. ***Note:*** *Feeding containers should be discarded after 24 hours or the timeframe recommended by the manufacturer.*

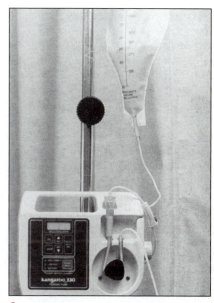

3 Feeding pumps are often used for clients who have either smaller-bore gastric tubes or intestinal tubes for which gravity flow or drip-regulated methods of infusion are inadequate. Pumps are also indicated for clients who require careful monitoring of their intake or who need a specific amount of formula infused over a specified period of time. Familiarize yourself with the types of feeding pumps your agency uses, and follow the operating instructions for those pumps.

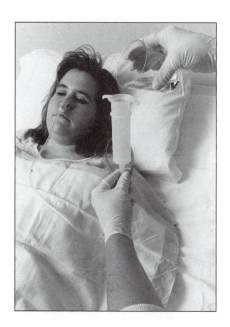

4 To ensure adequate absorption of any continuous-drip feeding and to verify correct stomach placement, discontinue the feedings every 6 hours, or as indicated, and aspirate and measure gastric contents. The protocol for most agencies is to withhold the feeding if more than 75–100 mL of gastric contents is measured. Then, flush the tubing with 30–50 mL of water to ensure patency as well as to increase fluid intake. ***Note:*** *To prevent spoilage, the same solution should not be hung for longer than 3–4 hours at a time (or the manufacturer's recommended time).*

GIVING GASTROSTOMY TUBE FEEDINGS

Assessing and Planning

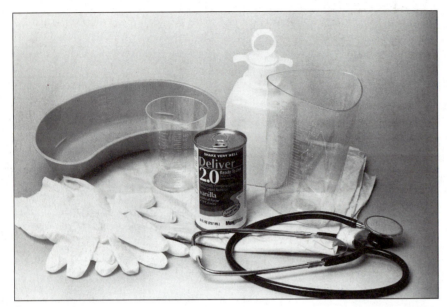

1 If tube feedings have been prescribed for your client who has a gastrostomy tube, determine whether the client has a history of food allergies or medically related alterations in nutrition. If the client has already received a tube feeding, inspect and palpate the abdomen to assess for gastric distention. If the abdomen is distended, the previous feeding may not have been adequately absorbed. Monitor the client for indications of intolerance to the previous feeding: alterations in bowel elimination, flatulence, and nausea. Assess the client's understanding of the procedure and intervene accordingly.

Assemble the following materials and equipment for an intermittent feeding:

- ☐ 50-mL syringe (10–20 mL for the pediatric population)
- ☐ stethoscope
- ☐ 30–50 mL water
- ☐ clean measured container for instilling the feeding solution
- ☐ clean measured container for instilling the water
- ☐ emesis basin
- ☐ bed-saver pad
- ☐ clean gloves
- ☐ prescribed solution for tube feeding warmed to room temperature to minimize the potential for cramping and vasoconstriction

Note: To administer feedings via continuous drip, follow procedure on page 267.

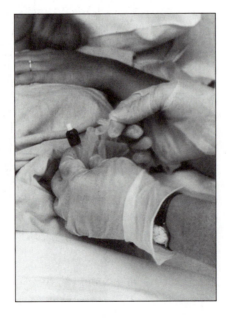

2 Place the client in semi-Fowler's or a right side-lying position. Protect the client's gown and bed linen with a bed-saver pad, apply clean gloves, and detach the feeding port plug from the tube's lumen.

Implementing

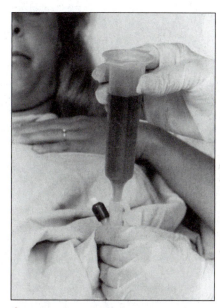

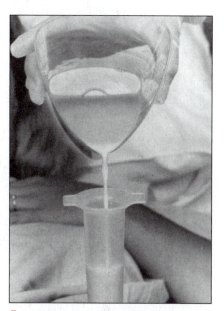

3 Insert the syringe into the open end of the tube and aspirate the residual stomach contents to evaluate the absorption of the previous feeding. Follow your agency's aspiration precaution rule to determine whether to give this feeding. The usual protocol for withholding a feeding is a residual amount of ≥75–100 mL of gastric contents. *Note: If this is the client's first tube feeding, ensure patency of the tube by instilling 10–20 mL of water first (1–2 mL for small children and 5 mL for larger children).*

4 Remove the bulb or piston and reinstill the measured aspirate via the syringe barrel, allowing it to flow into the stomach by gravity.

5 Pour in the premeasured formula, instilling it before the aspirate has drained from the neck of the syringe barrel to avoid introducing air into the client's stomach. If the client complains of discomfort or cramping during the feeding, lower the syringe barrel and pause for a few moments. If the solution oozes around the abdominal exit site, the balloon may not be flush with the gastric wall. Applying slight tension on the tube may correct this problem.

➤

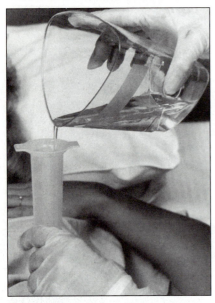

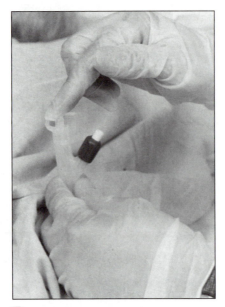

6 Flush the tubing with 30–50 mL of water, unless otherwise prescribed, to help maintain tubal patency, as well as increase the fluid intake and aid in the excretion of waste products. Pour the water into the syringe barrel before the formula has drained completely from the barrel neck.

7 When the feeding has been completed, reinsert the plug into the feeding port. If the client complains of abdominal discomfort, nausea, or distention, detach the feeding port plug, and place the tube's open end over an emesis basin to release the gastric contents. Document the procedure in the chart and on the intake and output record.

Evaluating

8 Assess the client for alterations in fluid volume, bowel elimination, and nutrition; observe for indicators of fluid and electrolyte imbalance: thirst, change in vital signs, and alterations in skin and mucous membrane moisture. Tube feedings that are high in protein content tend to increase the risk of osmotic diuresis, which can result in depletion of extracellular water. To help prevent this, periodically instill water into the tube, basing the amount and frequency on your assessment and the tube-feeding guidelines. Monitor laboratory values as well. Every 6–8 hours, test the urine for increased glucose levels, potentially caused by the high osmolarity of the feeding solution. Change the dressing as prescribed, and observe for leaking gastric contents that could cause skin excoriation. Cleanse the area thoroughly and use skin barriers if they are indicated (see pages 299–300). Evaluate the patency of the tube, and if you have a prescription for irrigation, do so when it becomes necessary.

ADMINISTERING GASTRIC LAVAGE

Assessing and Planning

1 Take the client's vital signs to establish a baseline for subsequent assessment, and inspect and palpate the abdomen to assess the degree of distention. Explain the procedure, tell the client why it is being done, and reassure her or him. Insert a nasogastric tube if one is not already in place (see pages 252–257).

2 Assemble the following:

☐ prescribed irrigant, either tap water or normal saline at room temperature (usually 1,000–1,500 mL for adults and 500 mL for the pediatric population)

☐ measured container for evaluating the amount of aspirate

☐ irrigation set with a 50-mL piston syringe (20-mL for the pediatric population)

☐ bed-saver pads

☐ emesis basin or larger container such as a bath basin if a large amount of lavage is anticipated

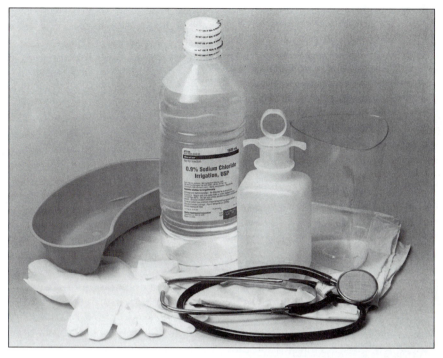

☐ stethoscope

☐ clean gloves

You also should have blood pressure monitoring equipment, a rectal or axillary thermometer, and blankets at the bedside. *Note: If*

iced lavage has been prescribed you may pour the irrigant into a metal container for faster chilling, but do not pour the solution directly over ice because you would dilute the irrigant and make it difficult to keep accurate intake and output records.

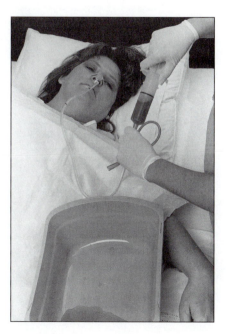

3 Place the client in a semi-Fowler's or Fowler's position. If this position is contraindicated because of hypovolemia or other conditions, lower the head of the bed and turn the client to her side to prevent aspiration. Drape the client with a bed-saver pad, apply clean gloves, and confirm correct stomach placement of the nasogastric tube by aspirating gastric contents with the syringe (see page 256). Rather than reinstill the aspirate, inject it into a container for later measurement and disposal.

→

Implementing

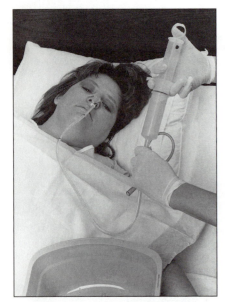

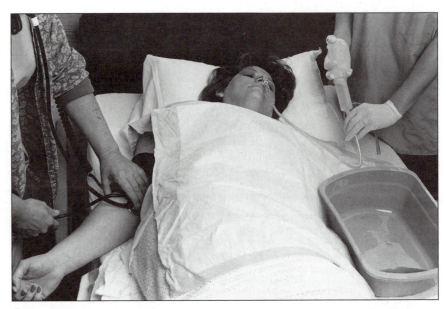

4 Draw up approximately 50 mL of the irrigation solution into the syringe and instill it into the tube using gentle pressure. Do not use force. Aspirate and inject the return into the collection container. Continue to instill and aspirate until the returns are clear or pink-tinged.

5 Have a coworker monitor vital signs as you perform the lavage. If a decrease in blood pressure occurs, lower the head of the bed. After 20–30 minutes (or the prescribed amount of time) if the aspirate has not become clear or pink-tinged, the physician should be notified for medical intervention.

Evaluating

6 Accurately record the amounts of both the irrigant and return to evaluate the quantity of blood loss. Continue to monitor the variations in blood pressure and pulse rates as an assessment for hypovolemia and potential shock. Provide materials for oral and nasal hygiene; document the procedure describing the type and amount of irrigant, the amount and character of the return, and your assessment of the client's condition and tolerance of the procedure.

ASPIRATING STOMACH CONTENTS FOR GASTRIC ANALYSIS

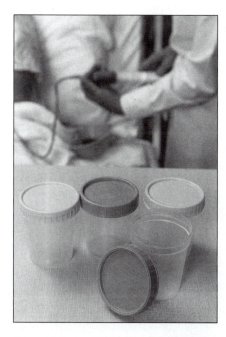

If possible, explain the procedure to the client at least a day ahead of time because he or she must fast for at least 8 hours before the test. A gastric analysis evaluates the amount of acid produced by the parietal cells when the stomach is in a state of rest. Therefore, fluids, smoking, and anticholinergics are also contraindicated because they will affect the gastric contents. At the prescribed time, insert a nasogastric tube (see pages 252–257) and aspirate the residual stomach contents with a 50-mL syringe. Usually, you will discard the first aspirate unless the physician wants to test the residual. After waiting the prescribed amount of time, aspirate all the stomach contents again and place them in a specimen container that has been properly labeled, dated, and numbered. Send the container to the laboratory. You will probably do this three or four more times at 15-minute intervals. Depending on the type of test prescribed, you may be required to repeat the procedure after administering subcutaneous histamine to the client. Histamine not only stimulates acid secretion, it rapidly dilates capillaries as well, resulting in a potential drop in blood pressure, increased pulse rate, and headache. Assess and document the client's pulse and blood pressure immediately after the histamine administration.

Managing Intestinal Tubes

NURSING GUIDELINES: MANAGING INTESTINAL TUBES

Single-Lumen Tube

Description

91–300 cm (36 in–10 ft); made of silicone, rubber, or polyurethane. Most are mercury-weighted at the distal end and have centimeter markings at 25, 50, and 75.

Sizes

Decompression tubes usually 16–18F
Feeders usually 8–16F

Uses

Gavage, decompression, medication instillation, splinting of the small bowel after anastomosis

Nursing Considerations

- The tube is usually inserted by the physician.

- The insertion of the tube into the stomach is similar to that of the nasogastric tube.

- For decompression, connect the tube to intermittent suction.

- Ensure intestinal placement by checking pH of aspirate: a reading greater than 7 indicates intestinal contents; one less than 7 indicates gastric contents.

- Tube feedings are usually begun with water, advanced to half-strength of the formula, and finally to full strength, according to client tolerance.

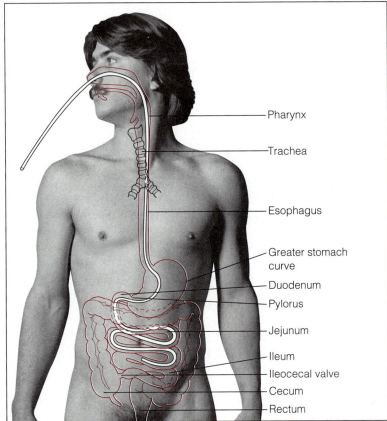

Pharynx

Trachea

Esophagus

Greater stomach curve

Duodenum

Pylorus

Jejunum

Ileum

Ileocecal valve

Cecum

Rectum

- Reposition the client frequently when the tube is in place to facilitate drainage.

- Use infusion pumps to deliver feedings if continuous feedings are prescribed.

- Provide oral and nasal hygiene at least three to four times daily.

NURSING GUIDELINES: MANAGING INTESTINAL TUBES *(continued)*

Double-Lumen Tube

Description

180–300 cm (72 in–10 ft) in length; rubber or plastic material; one outlet is for suction, and the other is for balloon inflation with air, water, saline, or mercury.

Size

12–18F

Uses

Decompression, gavage, diagnostic testing

Nursing Considerations

- The tube is usually inserted by the physician.
- The insertion to the stomach is similar to the insertion of a naso-gastric tube.
- This tube is most often used for clients with bowel obstructions.
- It is usually attached to intermittent suction.
- In the Hodge tube, only air is injected into the pigtail port.
- Assess the client frequently for the need for oral and nasal hygiene.
- Frequently reposition the client to facilitate drainage.

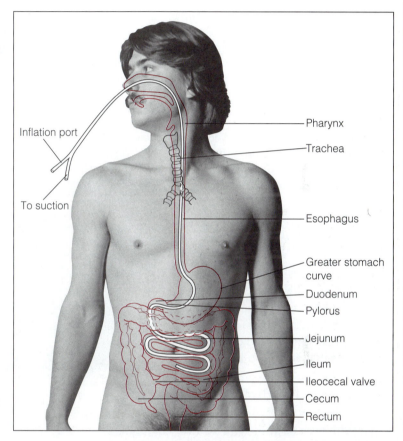

Inflation port

To suction

Pharynx

Trachea

Esophagus

Greater stomach curve

Duodenum

Pylorus

Jejunum

Ileum

Ileocecal valve

Cecum

Rectum

- Ensure correct intestinal placement by checking pH of aspirated intestinal contents: a reading greater than 7 indicates intestinal contents; one less than 7 indicates gastric contents.

NURSING GUIDELINES: MANAGING INTESTINAL TUBES (continued)

Jejunostomy Tube

Description and Sizes

May use larger-lumen tube, similar to gastrostomy tube (see description, page 248); or smaller-lumen tube, 35 cm (14 in), made of silicone or plastic; 8F.

Use

Usually gavage only

Nursing Considerations

- The tube is surgically inserted into the jejunum and sutured into place; after 2 weeks, it usually can be removed and reinserted as necessary for feedings.

- It is often inserted to feed clients after upper gastrointestinal and abdominal surgery because the jejunum can accommodate larger-volume feedings.

- The feedings are begun with water or weak concentrations of formula, advancing to full strength usually after 24 hours.

- Assess for "dumping syndrome" and diarrhea due to high osmolarity of formula.

- Perform tests for urine glucose every 6–8 hours when giving high-carbohydrate formulas.

- Frequently inspect abdominal exit site for indications of skin breakdown potentially caused by leaking intestinal contents.

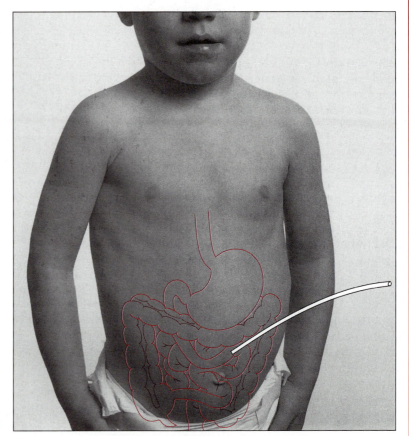

- If necessary, use skin barriers to protect the skin from the highly caustic intestinal contents (see "Managing Stoma Care," pages 286–301).

- Change postoperative dressing as prescribed, using aseptic technique.

- Involve parents in their children's tube feedings.

- Infants should be given nipples to satisfy sucking needs.

Managing Rectal Elimination and Distention

ADMINISTERING A NONRETENTION ENEMA

Assessing and Planning

1 Describe the procedure to the client and explain why it has been prescribed. Gather the following information: the time, amount, and character of the last stool; an evaluation of sphincter control; and the ability to ambulate to the bathroom. This information will assist you in your evaluation of the return and enable you to assemble the appropriate equipment.

2 Assemble the following equipment:

☐ a container and tubing with a clamp for delivering the enema solution

☐ a bed-saver pad

☐ water-soluble lubricant

☐ toilet paper

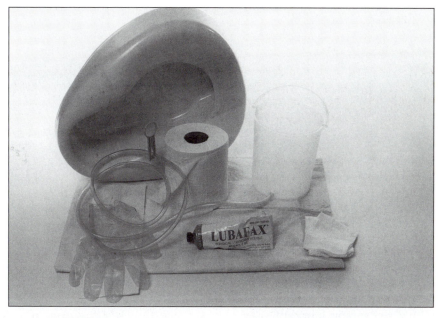

☐ disposable gloves

☐ 4 X 4 gauze pads

☐ a bedpan if the client has limited sphincter control or is nonambulatory

Prepare the prescribed amount of enema solution and warm it to 40.5 C (105 F) or as prescribed. You can either hang the solution container on an IV pole or place it on a bedside stand elevated 30–45 cm (12–18 in) above the client's abdomen.

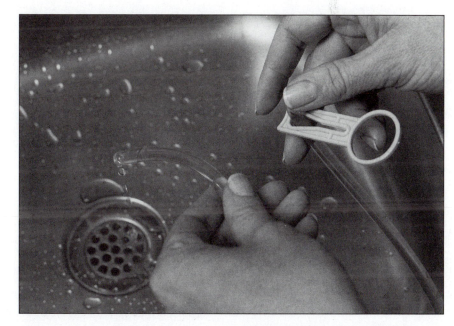

3 Flush air from the tubing by opening the tube clamp and allowing the solution to flow to the end of the tubing. Then reclamp the tube.

➤

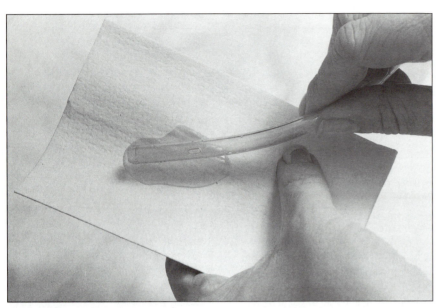

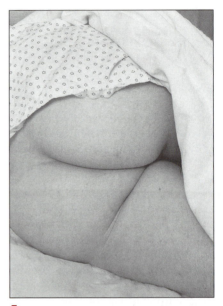

4 Lubricate the tip of the tube with water-soluble lubricant, usually around 5 cm (2 in) for the adult and 2.5 cm (1 in) for the child.

5 Pull the curtain to ensure privacy, and assist the client into a left side-lying position with the right knee flexed (Sims' position). This position will promote the flow of enema solution into the client's sigmoid colon. Place a bed-saver pad under the hips and expose the buttocks. For optimal hydrostatic pressure, suspend the enema solution 30–45 cm (12–18 in) above the client's abdomen. If the client has poor sphincter tone, place her on a bedpan in a supine position.

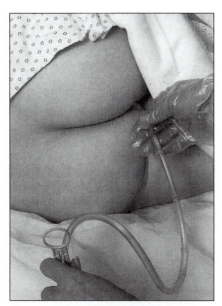 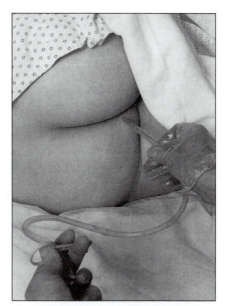 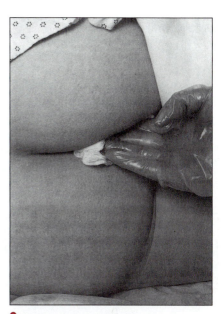

6 Apply a clean glove and separate the client's buttocks. Insert the tube 5–10 cm (2–4 in) toward the umbilicus, past both the external and internal sphincters. For infants and small children, insert the tube 2.5–7.5 cm (1–3 in). Be sure to avoid external hemorrhoids, and be very gentle if the client has internal hemorrhoids. Let the solution flow slowly to prevent cramping. Advise the client to breathe in deeply through her mouth if she experiences discomfort. If cramps occur, stop the flow until the cramps subside; then start the flow again, slowly.

7 When the solution has been instilled, clamp and then gently remove the tube.

8 If the client has difficulty retaining the solution for the usual 5- to 10-minute period, press the anus firmly with tissues or gauze, and encourage her to keep her upper body flat until she is allowed to expel the solution. Then either assist the client into the bathroom or, if she cannot ambulate, assist her onto a bedpan in Fowler's position. If indicated, instruct the client not to flush the toilet so that you can inspect the returns. Provide her with materials for perianal cleansing after the solution has been expelled, as well as a washcloth for handwashing if she is on bed rest.

Evaluating

9 Evaluate the return, and document the procedure.

ADMINISTERING A RETENTION ENEMA

Assessing and Planning

1 Familiarize yourself with the steps for giving a nonretention enema in the preceding procedure. Explain the procedure and position the client accordingly.

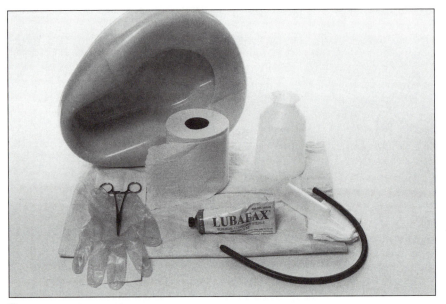

2 Assemble the following materials:

- ☐ 50 mL syringe barrel
- ☐ rectal tube or a catheter (20–22F for an adult or 12–18F for a child)
- ☐ tubing clamp or hemostat
- ☐ water-soluble lubricant
- ☐ toilet paper
- ☐ 4 X 4 gauze pads

- ☐ bed-saver pad
- ☐ bedpan (optional, depending on the client's sphincter tone and ability to ambulate to the bathroom)
- ☐ clean gloves
- ☐ prescribed enema solution warmed to no more than 40.5 C (105 F) to minimize the stimulation of peristalsis—or obtain a commercially prepared enema such as a Fleets

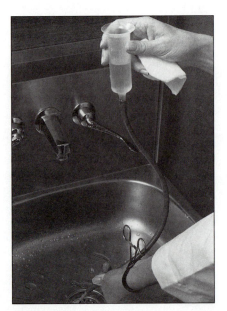

3 To avoid instilling air into the client's rectum, pour a small amount of solution into the syringe barrel and slowly flush the solution through the tubing just until it begins to drain out the distal end. When the solution reaches the end of the tube, pinch the tubing or clamp it. Do not allow the solution to drain out of the tubing because a loss of solution volume could diminish its desired therapeutic effect.

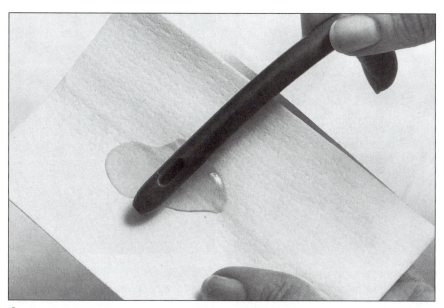

4 Lubricate the tip of the tubing with a water-soluble lubricant.

Implementing

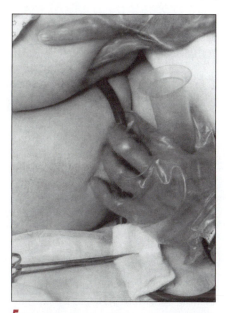

5 Apply gloves. Then separate the client's buttocks, and gently insert the tube toward the umbilicus, past both the external and internal sphincters. Use care to avoid traumatizing external and internal hemorrhoids if they are present.

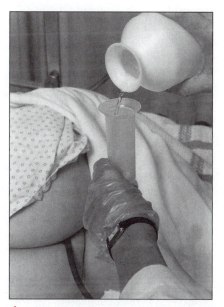

6 Fill the barrel of the syringe with the remaining solution.

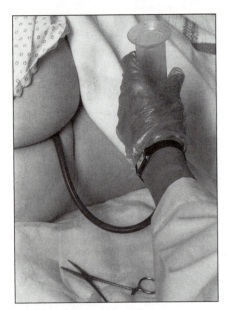

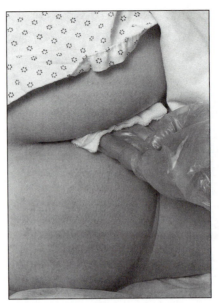

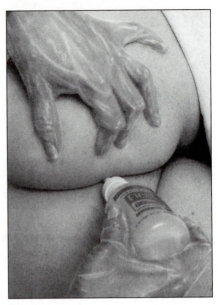

7 Then unclamp the tubing and raise the level of the barrel to achieve adequate hydrostatic pressure. The solution should be instilled slowly to avoid stimulating peristalsis because the client will need to retain the enema for at least 1 hour.

8 When the solution has been instilled, gently remove the tube and press firmly on the client's anus for a few moments, using a gauze pad or toilet paper (or the client may wish to do this herself). Advise the client to lie flat to help prevent the stimulation of peristalsis. Before leaving the room, be sure a call light and bedpan are within reach in case she is unable to retain the solution. When the prescribed retention time has elapsed, assist the client into the bathroom or onto a bedpan as indicated. *Note: If the client is unable to retain an enema solution, a Foley catheter can be inserted, following the steps for inserting a rectal tube in the next procedure. After insertion past the external and internal sphincters, inflate the balloon with the designated amount of air. Then pull the balloon gently against the anal sphincter to seal the rectum. Deflate the balloon and remove the Foley as soon as the retention time has passed. An inflated balloon can impede circulation in the rectal mucosa.*

9 If a Fleets enema has been prescribed, separate the client's buttocks, and gently insert the pre-lubricated tip into the anus. Then raise the base of the container to avoid instilling air into the rectum, and squeeze the container to instill the solution.

Evaluating

10 If the procedure necessitates your observation of the return, do so at this time. If an oil-based retention enema was instilled, determine whether a cleansing enema needs to be instilled next. Document the procedure.

INSERTING A RECTAL TUBE

Assessing and Planning

1 A rectal tube can be inserted to relieve gastric distention when the distention is caused by flatus. However, you should first auscultate the client's abdomen for bowel sounds. An absence of bowel sounds in a rigid abdomen can mean that an obstruction or paralytic ileus, rather than flatus, is causing the distention; either condition necessitates immediate medical intervention.

2 Assemble the following materials:

☐ rectal tube or a catheter (22–24F for adults or 12–18F for children)

☐ water-soluble lubricant

☐ hypoallergenic tape

☐ bed-saver pad

☐ clean gloves

☐ flatus bag or receptacle for collecting fecal discharge, such as a specimen container (as an alternative, gauze and tape may be used to wrap the draining end of the tube or catheter)

Explain the procedure to the client and provide privacy.

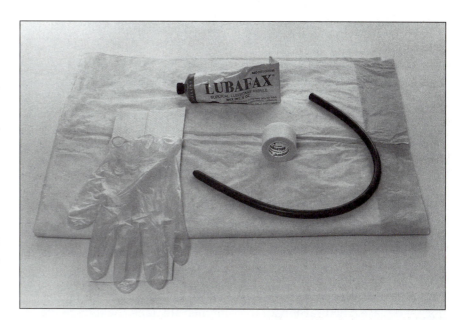

Implementing

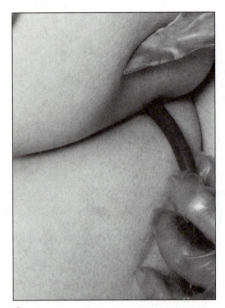

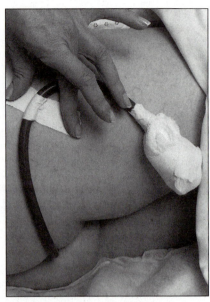

Evaluating

5 Continue to assess the client for distention, and intervene accordingly.

3 Assist the client into Sims' position, and place a bed-saver pad under the buttocks. Lubricate the tip of the tube with water-soluble lubricant, apply gloves, and insert the tube into the rectum 7.5–10 cm (3–4 in), past both the external and internal sphincters. (For a child, insert the tube 2.5–7.5 cm [1–3 in].)

4 If relief from distention is not immediate, tape the tube to the thigh so that the client can have mobility without dislodging the tube. *Caution: To minimize the potential for rectal irritation or a loss in sphincter tone, do not leave the tube indwelling for longer than 20–30 minutes.* At the appropriate time, remove the tube and clean or discard it, depending on agency policy. Wash your hands, and document the procedure.

TESTING STOOL FOR OCCULT BLOOD

If possible, advise the client not to eat red meat for 24 hours prior to testing. Obtain a stool specimen, using gloves while handling the feces. If the client is unable to defecate, you might need to obtain the specimen during a digital rectal exam. Note the presence of hemorrhoids, which if present, may give a false-positive reading.

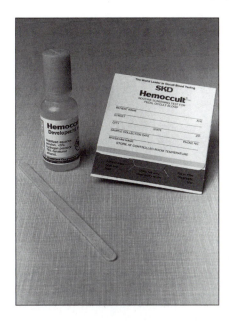

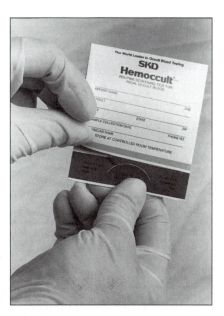

1 Apply clean gloves. Open the front side of the slide.

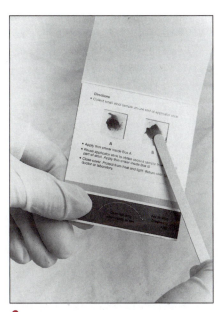

2 Smear the stool onto the filter paper in both windows with a wooden stick or with your gloved finger if you have performed a digital exam. Close the cover.

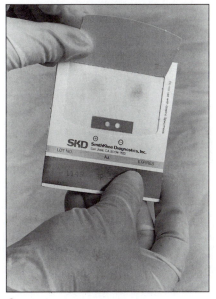

3 Turn the slide over and open the back flap.

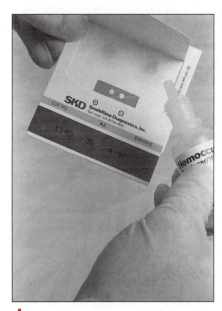

4 Apply 1–2 drops of the developer solution directly over the stool on this reverse side of the filter paper. Also apply the developer solution to the control dots at the bottom of the slide.

Finally, observe the filter paper for color changes. In many tests, the filter paper will turn blue if the stool contains blood. Discard the used slide according to agency policy. Remove your gloves, wash your hands, and record the procedure and its results.

HOME HEALTH CARE CONSIDERATIONS

For at-home use, clients follow steps 1 and 2 only and then mail or deliver the slide to their physician as directed.

Managing Stoma Care

NURSING GUIDELINES: MANAGING OSTOMIES

Ascending Colostomy

Surgical Indications

Perforating diverticulitis, Hirschsprung's disease, obstructed colon, trauma (for example, gunshot or stab wounds), rectovaginal fistula, and inoperable tumors in the colon.

Nursing Considerations

- This is the least common colostomy.
- The surgery is performed on clients of all ages.
- The stoma location is on the right upper quadrant or right lumbar area of the abdomen, and it usually protrudes.
- This ostomy is managed as if it were an ileostomy (see page 292).
- The client will have liquid or pasty stools that flow almost continually.
- The effluent contains digestive enzymes that are damaging to the skin.
- Peristomal skin assessment, skin care, and a properly fitting appliance are essential for preventing skin breakdown.
- Full-time use of an appliance (usually a drainable pouch) with a skin barrier is necessary.

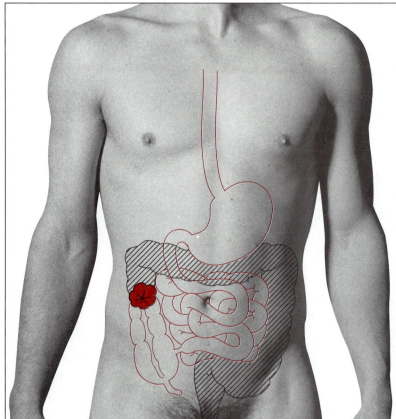

- Irrigation is contraindicated.
- Odor control is usually not a major problem because most appliances are odorproof.

NURSING GUIDELINES: MANAGING OSTOMIES (continued)

Transverse Colostomies

Surgical Indications

Same as ascending colostomies. These ostomies are usually temporary and are the most frequently performed fecal diversions for relief of bowel obstruction and colon perforation secondary to trauma.

Nursing Considerations for the Single-Barrel Colostomy

- The surgery is performed on clients of all ages.

- The stoma location is usually high on the abdomen, at waist level, and near the midline. It usually protrudes.

- The stools are usually semisolid, although formed stools are possible.

- A drainable pouch is recommended.

- The enzymatic, watery stools can lead to peristomal skin irritation.

- The rectum is not removed, so the client occasionally may defecate from the rectum.

- Although this ostomy is not controllable, it is more predictable than an ascending colostomy as to when it will function.

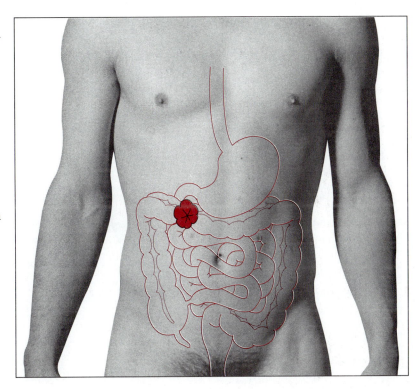

NURSING GUIDELINES: MANAGING OSTOMIES (continued)

Nursing Considerations for the Double-Barrel Colostomy

- This is often a temporary intervention for resting the colon, with a possible anastomosis at a later date.

- The client has two stomas: the proximal stoma is active and discharges feces; the distal stoma is inactive and discharges mucus. The inactive stoma may be covered eventually with a gauze pad to absorb mucus.

- Postoperatively, the client may use a loop ostomy appliance or an open-end drain with a skin barrier.

- The client may experience occasional rectal drainage of stool or mucus.

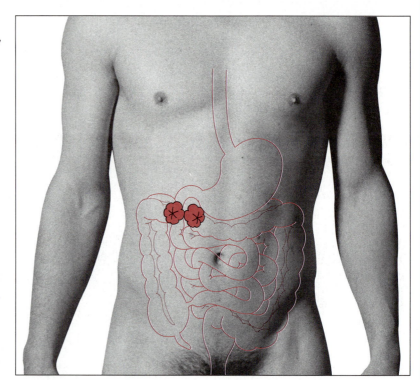

NURSING GUIDELINES: MANAGING OSTOMIES (continued)

Nursing Considerations for the Loop Colostomy

- An intact segment of the colon is looped through the abdomen rather than severed.

- The loop is held exterior to the body and stabilized with a plastic bridge or glass rod for 7–10 days postoperatively.

- Fecal material is released through an incision on the anterior section of the loop.

- This type of fecal diversion is usually performed in emergency situations; therefore the client is often ill-prepared both physiologically and psychologically.

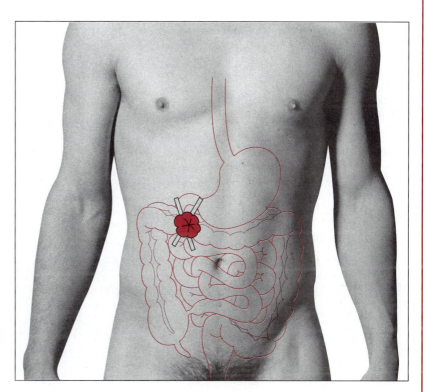

NURSING GUIDELINES: MANAGING OSTOMIES (continued)

Nursing Considerations for the Pediatric Colostomate

- For the child, a pediatric postoperative pouch and skin barrier are used during the first 3–5 postoperative days. Thereafter pediatric drainable pouches are frequently used.

- The use of skin barriers and close observation of peristomal skin is crucial because of the watery, enzymatic feces.

- For the infant, a diaper alone might be used until discharge from the hospital. Follow agency protocol.

- Closely monitor the infant and child for weight loss and indications of dehydration.

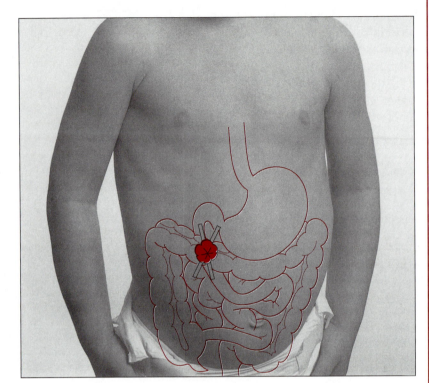

NURSING GUIDELINES: MANAGING OSTOMIES *(continued)*

Descending or Sigmoid Colostomy

Surgical Indications

Cancer of the sigmoid colon or rectum, chronic diverticulitis, congenital anomaly, or trauma.

Nursing Considerations

- This is the most commonly performed fecal diversion.

- The surgery may be performed on clients of all ages, but most clients are 40 years of age or older.

- The stoma is located in the left lower quadrant, and it might be either flush or protruded.

- After recovery, clients may wear either a closed nondrainable pouch or an open drainable pouch, depending on whether or not they will be irrigating their colostomies.

- After the initial postoperative period, the stools may be pasty to semisolid.

- Elimination may be regulated by irrigation and diet.

- Teach the client how to manage elimination by increasing intake of foods high in bulk and

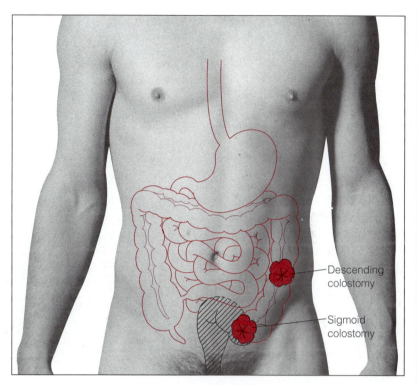

decreasing intake of foods known to give the individual loose stools, flatus, and odor. Increase the intake of fluids as well.

- Encourage the intake of parsley, yogurt, and cranberry juice to decrease fecal odor.

NURSING GUIDELINES: MANAGING OSTOMIES (continued)

Ileostomy

Surgical Indications

Ulcerative colitis (80%), Crohn's disease, cancer, trauma, familial polyposis.

Nursing Considerations for the Brooke Ileostomy

- This procedure is performed most frequently on adolescent to middle-aged clients, with 40 years as the average age.

- The stoma is located in the right lower quadrant, and it usually protrudes.

- The pouch must fit properly to prevent skin breakdown caused by the enzymatic effluent.

- Change the pouch immediately if leakage occurs at the peristomal area or if the client complains of itching or burning around the stoma.

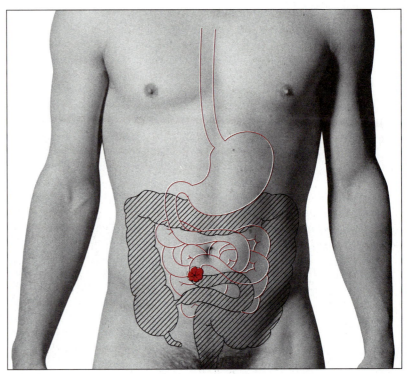

- Because of a potential fluid volume deficit from colon loss, encourage a fluid intake of 2–3 L/day.

- Because of electrolyte loss, increase the client's intake of sodium and potassium through foods, fluids, and supplements.

- Instruct the client to decrease roughage in the diet, which can cause a blockage, and to chew food thoroughly.

- Change the appliance when the ileostomy is more quiescent, for example, in the morning before eating or 2–4 hours after meals.

- The maximum wearing time for the pouch is 7 days, although some clients change their pouches as frequently as every 3 days, and others change them every 5 days.

NURSING GUIDELINES: MANAGING OSTOMIES (continued)

Nursing Considerations for the Pediatric Ileostomate

- Care of these children is similar to that given to children with pediatric transverse loops.

- The fecal output is high in digestive enzymes, and therefore the use of skin barriers and close observation of the peristomal skin are essential.

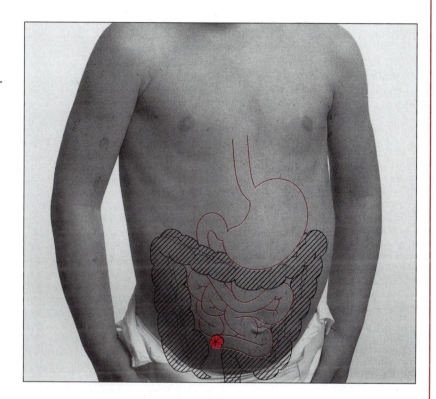

NURSING GUIDELINES: MANAGING OSTOMIES (continued)

Continent Ileostomy

Surgical Indications

Ulcerative colitis and familial polyposis. It is often contraindicated for clients with Crohn's disease because of the potential for recurrence of the disease, which could necessitate reservoir removal.

Nursing Considerations

- The age group involved is the same as that for the ileostomy.

- The stoma is located on the right lower quadrant, and it is flush with the skin.

- The intra-abdominal reservoir is created from the looped ileum. It collects feces, making external collection pouches unnecessary.

- A gastrostomy tube is often sutured into the stomach during surgery for decompression.

- A 28F catheter is inserted into the reservoir and sutured to the peristomal skin during surgery; it remains in place for 14–21 days to provide decompression. Maintain catheter on low, continuous suction or on gravity drainage. It is irrigated with 30 mL normal saline every 4–6 hours, or as prescribed.

- At 14–21 days postoperatively, the reservoir is intubated and drained every 3–4 hours with a lubricated silastic catheter. This is decreased to every 6 hours by week 8 or 9.

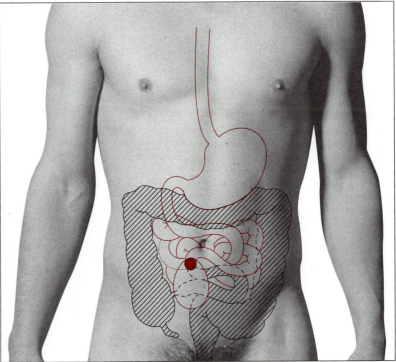

- The stoma is covered with a bandage or a gauze pad between intubations to absorb leaks or mucus.

- Instruct the client to avoid gas-forming foods, decrease roughage, and chew food thoroughly to prevent clogging the silastic catheter.

- The adjustment to the body change is usually less traumatic for these clients than for those with conventional ileostomies.

- The reservoir gradually increases in size and may attain a capacity of 500 mL.

NURSING GUIDELINES: MANAGING OSTOMIES (continued)

Ileoanal Reservoir

Surgical Indications

Clients with ulcerative colitis or familial polyposis who normally would require a total colectomy have an option for preserving fecal continence by having an ileoanal reservoir. It is done in two stages. The first stage, which follows total colectomy and removal of the anal lining (with preservation of the anal sphincter), involves construction of an ileal reservoir from the small bowel. The reservoir's ileal outlet is brought down through the cuff of the rectal muscle and anastomosed to the anal canal. The reservoir stores the feces. A temporary ileostomy is performed to enable healing of the anastomosis. During the second stage (after 2–3 months), the temporary ileostomy is taken down, and fecal continence is restored.

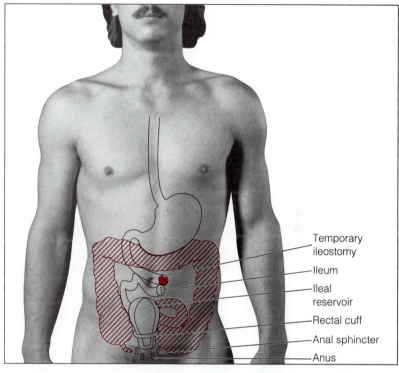

Temporary ileostomy

Ileum

Ileal reservoir

Rectal cuff

Anal sphincter

Anus

Nursing Considerations

- The ideal client for this procedure is 20–40 years of age, has good sphincter control, is physically fit enough to endure a full year of recovery, and is very motivated not to have a permanent ileostomy.

- For care of the temporary ileostomy during the first stage of this procedure, see discussion on page 292 for nursing care considerations for the client with an ileostomy.

- There are more surgical complications with this procedure than with a permanent ileostomy.

- To prevent fluid and electrolyte imbalance caused by the colectomy, encourage clients to increase their fluid intake to 8–10 glasses/day.

- Following the first stage of this procedure, the client will experience mucus production through the anus. The ileostomy takedown is scheduled following a normal healing process.

- During the period of mucus incontinence, irrigate the mucus out of the reservoir daily using 60 mL water. Cleanse the perineal area with water and cotton balls, avoiding soap and toilet paper, which can cause irritation and itching.

- Following the second stage of this procedure, the client may experience incontinence of feces and 10 or more bowel movements per day. This will decrease in frequency after 3–6 months as the reservoir expands and absorbs fluids, with 4–8 bowel movements per day and increased ability to control stool. Suggest that the client wear a small pad to protect clothing. Antidiarrheals, bulk-forming diet, and dietary changes may be necessary to control this problem.

- Suggest that the client avoid foods that cause liquid stools, such as spinach, highly seasoned foods, raw fruit, and broccoli, and to increase intake of the foods that cause thickened stools, such as bananas, jello, pasta, cheese, and apples.

- Although this procedure enables evacuation of feces through the anus and appears to restore normal functioning, it is important to note that anatomic structure of the colon and rectum has changed.

NURSING GUIDELINES: MANAGING OSTOMIES (continued)

- Perineal skin care is essential following the second stage of this procedure because of irritation caused by enzymes in the stool. Cleansing gently with a soft tissue or spraying water with a squirt bottle will help protect the skin. Following cleansing and drying, apply an occlusive protective skin sealant or ointment to nonirritated skin. Sitz baths may be recommended for clients whose skin irritation worsens or fails to heal.

- Teach the client that the following foods may promote perineal irritation: nuts, popcorn, stir-fried vegetables, and raw fruits and vegetables (eg, oranges, corn, and celery).

- Some clients may benefit from exercising the anal sphincter and deep pelvic muscles to promote bowel function control. These exercises are not begun until a minimum of 2 weeks following surgery. As appropriate, teach the client the following:

—Anal sphincter toning: Squeeze and hold the anal muscles to a slow count of three; release. Repeat this exercise 10–20 times a day.

—Deep pelvic muscle toning: Pull in your abdomen as though you are flattening your stomach. Hold for a slow count of 3; release. Repeat this exercise 10–20 times a day.

PATCH TESTING THE CLIENT'S SKIN

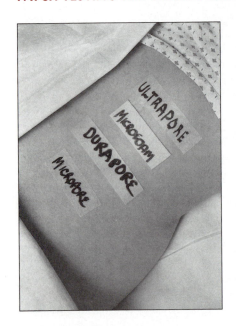

At least 24 hours prior to ostomy surgery, perform skin patch testing to assess for allergies your client might have to tape that may be used to adhere the ostomy appliance to the abdominal skin. Test the abdomen on the nonoperative side, rather than testing the inner arm. The inner arm is not as sensitive as the abdomen, and the test results may not be as accurate.

Test at least four different types of tape that are used by your agency. This will provide you with more options should the client be allergic to more than one type. The photo depicts the testing of foam, silk, and two types of paper tape on the client's abdomen. If you are patch testing skin on a client with abdominal hair, clip the hair with scissors as close to the follicle as possible before applying the tape. Unless the client complains of itching and burning before the 24-hour period has elapsed, remove the tape at the scheduled time, using a tape solvent if necessary. Thoroughly cleanse the area with water and a gentle soap or skin cleanser; assess for redness, swelling, and other indications of an allergic reaction. Document the test's results in the chart. If your client does have an allergic reaction to any of the tapes, note the type(s) on the front of the chart, stating "Allergic to _____ Tape." This will alert both the surgical team before their application of the postoperative pouch and the nursing staff during follow-up care.

APPLYING A DRAINABLE POUCH

A drainable pouch is typically worn during the early part of the hospital stay. It is usually clear to facilitate observation of fecal drainage.

Assessing and Planning

1 To apply a drainable pouch, assemble the following materials:

- [ ] the postoperative pouch
- [ ] pectin wafer skin barrier
- [ ] straight scissors
- [ ] curved scissors (optional)
- [ ] pouch closure clip
- [ ] skin cleanser (optional)
- [ ] stomal measurement guide
- [ ] skin barrier paste
- [ ] 4 X 4 gauze pads
- [ ] skin preparation wipes (optional) for protecting the skin if you plan to reinforce the seal of the pouch to the client's skin with tape

In addition, keep a supply of bed-saver pads and gloves at the client's bedside.

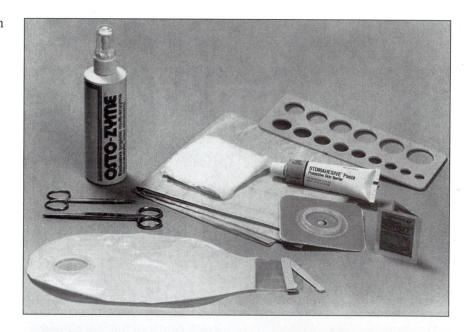

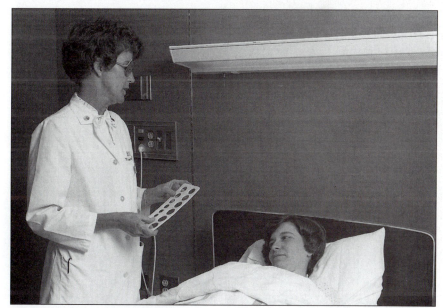

2 Explain the procedure to the client, and lower the head of the bed to decrease the angle at the peristomal area. Assess the client's reaction to her stoma, and let her know that you have as much time as she needs for answering her questions and assisting her with future pouch applications. If she is psychologically ready, encourage her to inspect and touch her stoma so that she can begin to develop a realistic appraisal of her altered appearance and body function. It is essential that you project a positive reaction to the client's ostomy.

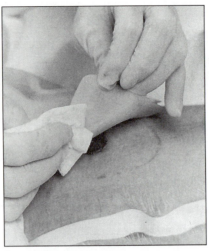 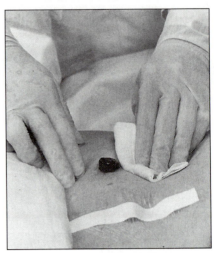

3 To protect the client's gown and bed from fecal drainage, place a bed-saver pad under the pouch. Then, apply gloves and moisten a 4 X 4 gauze pad or cloth with warm water and lift up the uppermost inside corner of the skin barrier. Position the moistened gauze pad at the loosened corner, and gently depress the skin as you peel back the adhesive material. This method will facilitate the removal of the appliance as quickly and painlessly as possible.

4 After removing the appliance, assess the color of the stoma. It should be a healthy red, similar in color to the mucosal lining of the inner cheek. Report immediately a darker, purplish cast or a very pale stoma, which could suggest impaired blood circulation to the area. Also assess for impaired peristomal skin integrity potentially caused by leakage of fecal effluent, an allergic reaction to the tape or skin barrier, or infected hair follicles (folliculitis). Plan skin care or appliance changes accordingly.

Implementing

5 Cleanse the peristomal area with warm water and a skin cleanser (as shown) or a nonoily soap such as Ivory. Be sure to avoid using soaps that contain creams or lanolin because the residue left on the skin could prevent the appliance from adhering properly. Rinse and dry the skin thoroughly.

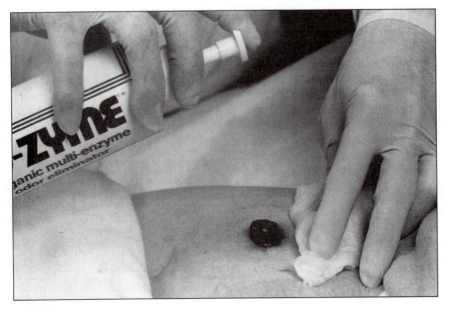

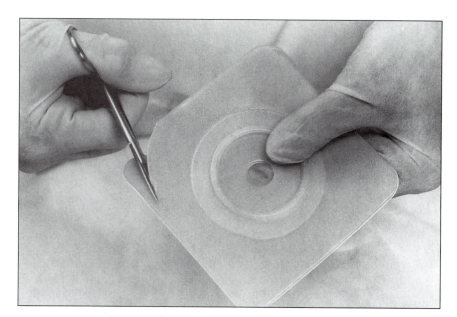

6 A pectin wafer skin barrier protects the client's peristomal skin from contact with the effluent and pouch adhesive. If you are using a pectin wafer with squared edges, curve the edges (as shown) to prevent them from jabbing your client's skin. Set the skin barrier aside.

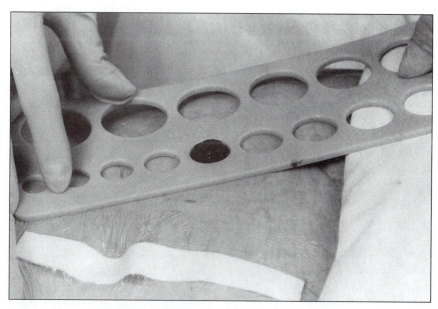

7 Measure the stoma with a stomal measuring guide. You will need to measure the stoma frequently during the postoperative period because the stoma will continue to shrink in size, with the majority of the shrinkage occurring during the first 2–3 months.

8 Trace the exact measurement of the stoma on the back and in the center of the skin barrier.

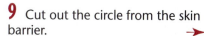

9 Cut out the circle from the skin barrier.

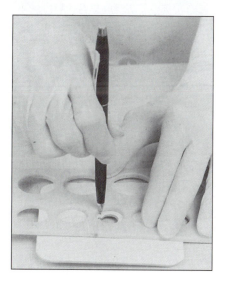

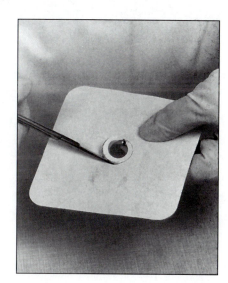

➤

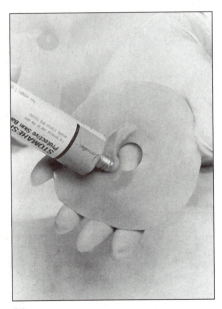

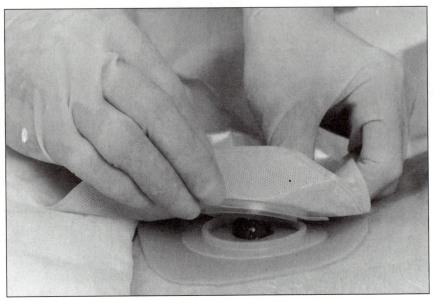

10 Remove the adhesive backing from the pectin wafer skin barrier. After removing the adhesive backing, apply a thin layer of protective skin barrier paste to the adhesive side of the pectin wafer along the periphery of the circle you cut out (as shown). This will help protect the client's peristomal skin from effluent drainage.

11 Apply the pectin wafer, adhesive side down, over the client's stoma. Then attach the pouch to the pectin wafer by gently snapping the back of the pouch onto the lip of the pectin wafer, as shown.

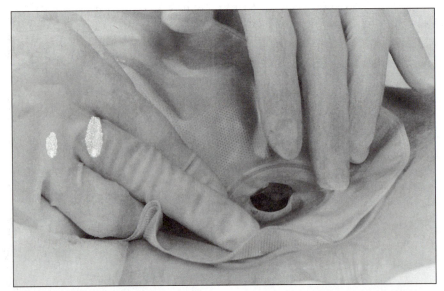

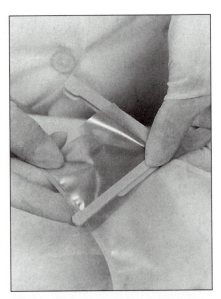

12 Continue snapping the pouch to the pectin wafer in a circular fashion. Note that the pouch angles toward the side of the bed. This facilitates emptying the pouch into a basin or bedpan during the early postoperative period. It should be angled in this manner only during the period of time the client is on bed rest. If you will be taping the pouch to the client's skin to reinforce the seal, see procedure in Chapter 8.

13 Open and position the tail closure device (clamp) 4 cm (1½ in) from the bottom of the pouch tail.

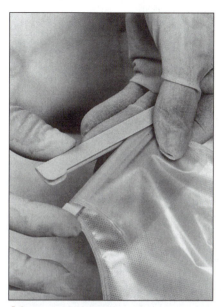

14 Fold the end of the pouch tail over the clamp, as shown. Then snap the clamp together. You will hear or feel it snap.

Evaluating

15 Continue to monitor the client for alterations in fluid and electrolyte balance, impairment of stomal and peristomal skin, alterations in nutrition, and daily changes in body weight. In addition, it is especially important in the early postoperative period to be alert to indications of paralytic ileus or peritonitis. Inspect and palpate the abdomen for the presence of distention or rigidity, and auscultate the abdomen to ensure that there are bowel sounds. Although an absence of fecal output is one indicator of ileus, an ileostomy usually does not function until the first 12–24 hours; a lack of fecal output during the first 24–36 hours is often normal for a colostomy. Keep accurate daily records of the amount, color, and consistency of fecal output, and compare the output to the client's intake.

When the pouch becomes one-third full, detach the closure clip and empty the pouch into a basin or bedpan. If the pouch is allowed to become full of effluent, its seal with the skin can break, resulting in leakage of effluent onto the client's abdomen.

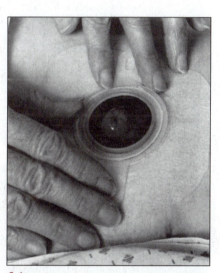

16 The top portion of a disposable pouch has been cut away to show you a correct fit.

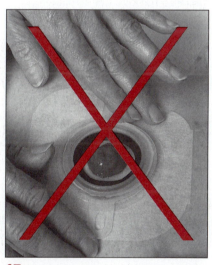

17 The top portion of a disposable pouch that no longer fits because of typical stomal shrinkage during the postoperative period has been cut away. Because the exposed peristomal skin can readily become excoriated after contact with caustic fecal effluent, it is essential that the appliance be changed as soon as stomal shrinkage occurs and the skin is exposed. Similarly, if your client has an irregularly shaped stoma, you should use karaya paste to fill in the exposed area, or cut a pectin wafer skin barrier to fit the stoma.

DILATING A STOMA

Stoma dilation is performed to stretch and relax the stomal sphincter and to assess the direction of the proximal colon prior to a colostomy irrigation. Check for a physician's prescription before dilating a client's stoma, because the procedure is not done for all colostomates.

Assessing and Planning

1 Assemble the following materials:

☐ gauze pads

☐ water-soluble lubricant

☐ a clean glove

Be sure that you also have bed-saver pads on hand. Then ask the client to remove her appliance.

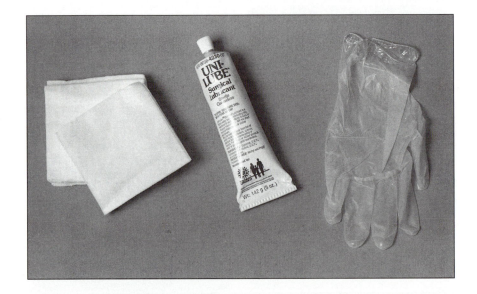

2 Instruct the client to put on the disposable glove and generously lubricate the small and index fingers of her gloved hand with the water-soluble lubricant.

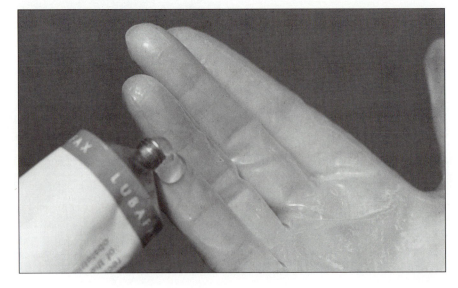

Implementing

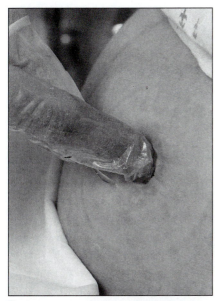

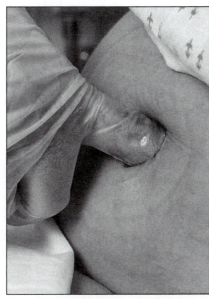

Evaluating

5 Because the stoma comprises a vast number of capillaries, there may be slight bleeding from this procedure; however, copious bleeding is abnormal and should be reported immediately. Document the procedure and your client's performance.

3 Drape the client's lap with a bed-saver pad, and position a gauze pad under the stoma to collect drainage. Instruct the client to introduce her small finger gently into the stoma and to maintain the position for 1 minute to relax the sphincter.

4 She may then insert her index finger, gently rotating the finger to midknuckle or 5 cm (2 in) to assess the direction of the proximal colon. This assessment will enable her to position the tip of the irrigation cone correctly.

IRRIGATING A COLOSTOMY

Colostomy irrigations are performed to evacuate the bowel of stored fecal content, potentially enabling clients to regulate their fecal elimination. They are most appropriate for clients with ostomies of the descending or sigmoid colon. Check for a physician's prescription before performing this procedure. Irrigations are not performed for all colostomates; and they are contraindicated for infants, for clients with diarrhea, or for those receiving radiation therapy.

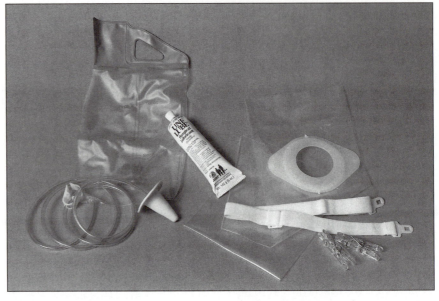

Assessing

1 To ensure that your client does not have an obstruction or paralytic ileus, assess the client's abdomen before initiating the procedure by palpating for distention and auscultating to determine the presence of bowel sounds.

Planning

2 Assemble the following equipment:

- ☐ irrigation bag with tubing and a cone
- ☐ irrigation sleeve and belt
- ☐ water-soluble lubricant
- ☐ closure clamps

You will also need an IV pole or a bathroom hook and the prescribed amount of irrigant, which is usually warm tap water. Unless otherwise prescribed, the amount of the first postoperative irrigation is 500 mL, and it is gradually increased by 250 mL up to 1000 mL until the effective amount is determined by a complete and comfortable evacuation.

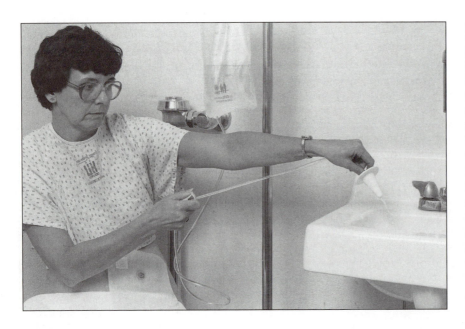

3 Although the procedure can be performed in bed, if the client is ambulatory, set up the equipment in the bathroom. Ideally, at this stage in the client's recovery, she should perform as much self-care as possible, with your assistance. This photo shows 750 mL or warm tap water hung on an IV pole. The bottom of the irrigation bag should be positioned at shoulder level to ensure an effective rate of flow. Instruct the client to open the clamp on the irrigation tubing, and allow the irrigant to flow through the tubing and irrigation cone to remove the air from the irrigation set (as shown). She should then remove her used appliance and perform stomal dilation (if prescribed) to relax the sphincter and to assess the direction of the proximal colon (see steps in preceding procedure).

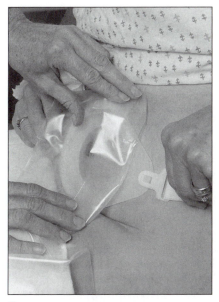

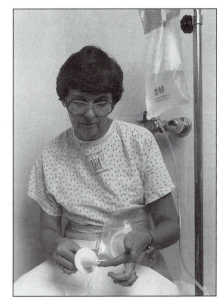

4 Assist the client with applying the irrigation sleeve and belt, and instruct her to place the tail of the sleeve between her legs so that the irrigation return can drain directly into the toilet. If the client is in bed, the tail of the sleeve can be placed into a bedpan.

5 Squeeze some water-soluble lubricant onto a paper towel and have the client generously lubricate the tip of the irrigation cone. An irrigation cone is preferred to a straight catheter as a means of delivering the irrigant because the latter has a greater potential for perforating the bowel.

Implementing

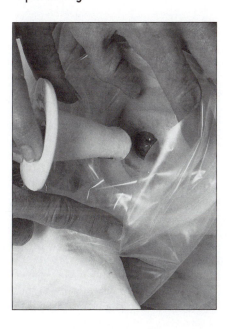

6 Assist the client with placing the cone into the proximal end of the irrigation sleeve and gently centering the tip of the cone into the stoma until it fits snugly, facing the direction of the proximal colon. ←

7 Control the speed of the irrigational flow by adjusting the regulator. Instruct the client to stop the flow if she begins cramping. Once the cramps have subsided, she can slowly restart the flow. However, if the cramps continue, the irrigation should be discontinued. →

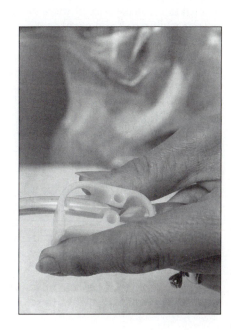

➤

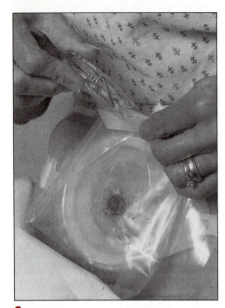

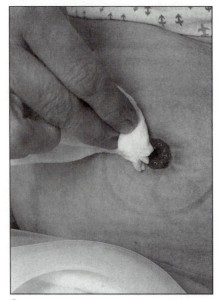

8 When the irrigant has finished draining, instruct the client to fold the top end of the irrigation sleeve twice and to secure it with a closure clamp. This will protect her from the forceful rush of the return. It will usually take around 45 minutes for a complete evacuation, with the initial return occurring within the first 15–20 minutes. During the final 15–20 minutes, the client should be encouraged to ambulate to facilitate evacuation. If there is no return, instruct the client to massage her abdomen or drink warm fluids to stimulate peristalsis. *Note: If you are keeping output records, you will need to measure the return. To do this, either fold up the tail of the irrigation sleeve and secure it with the other closure clamp or allow the return to flow directly into a bedpan. Subtract the amount of irrigant from the return.*

9 When a complete evacuation has been achieved, the client should remove the irrigation equipment and clean the peristomal skin with water and cleanser or a gentle soap. The stoma may be lightly patted with a soft cloth. When the peristomal skin has been rinsed and dried, the client may then obtain a drainable pouch or the appliance appropriate for her needs.

Evaluating

10 Inspect and palpate the client's abdomen to assess for gastric distention, which can be indicative of an incomplete evacuation. Assess the stoma and peristomal skin for color and integrity. Document the procedure, noting the amount of irrigant and the character and amount of the return. If client teaching took place, document the client's performance.

DRAINING A CONTINENT ILEOSTOMY

Assessing

1 To assess the need for draining the internal reservoir, inspect the client's abdomen and gently palpate the abdomen exterior to the reservoir to determine the amount of fecal content. Assess the client's knowledge of the procedure, and explain why it is performed.

Planning

2 Assemble the following materials and equipment:

- ☐ irrigation set with a 50-mL syringe
- ☐ 30–40 mL warm water
- ☐ #28 silastic or teflon-coated catheter
- ☐ water-soluble lubricant
- ☐ stoma cap (as shown) or bandage (depending on your client's need for drainage absorption)

If the client is ambulatory, perform the procedure in the bathroom.

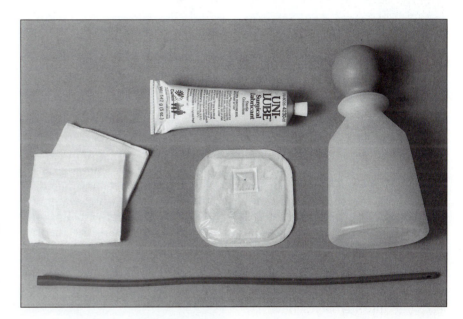

3 Squeeze some water-soluble lubricant onto a gauze pad or paper towel, and instruct the client to lubricate 7.5 cm (3 in) of the catheter's tip.

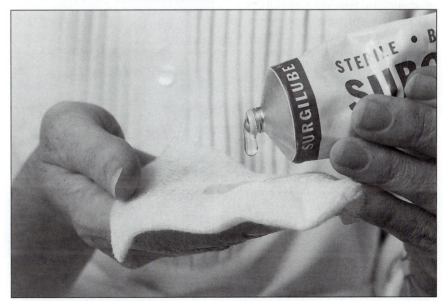

➤

Implementing

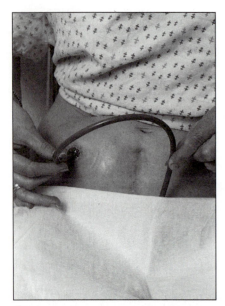

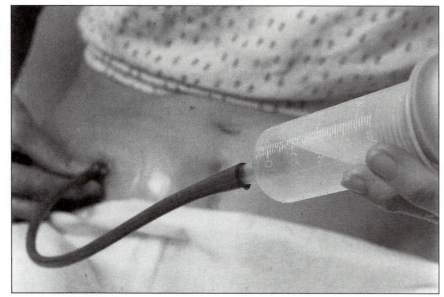

4 The client should next place the draining end of the catheter between her legs so that the fecal material can empty into the toilet (or into a 500-mL bedpan if she is performing the procedure in bed). She should then carefully insert the catheter's lubricated tip into the stoma, angling downward so that it can enter the nipple valve that leads into the internal reservoir. At approximately 5–7.5 cm (2–3 in) when the client feels resistance, the catheter has entered the nipple valve. Instruct her to use gentle pressure as she enters the reservoir via the nipple valve. If the client has difficulty entering the reservoir, she should take deep breaths and press gently with the catheter during exhalations.

5 If fecal contents do not drain easily through the catheter after the reservoir has been intubated, instill 30–50 mL of warm water through the catheter with a 50-mL syringe, and try again. The client also may try bearing down with her abdominal muscles, pressing gently on the abdomen exterior to the reservoir, or moving the catheter gently in and out of the reservoir. *Note: The reservoir should be flushed with water on a daily basis to remove the fecal residue.*

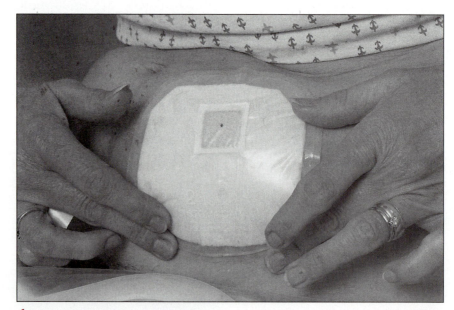

6 When the ileostomy has been drained, have the client remove the catheter, clean the peristomal skin, and apply a stoma cap (as shown) or a bandage.

Evaluating

7 Observe for stomal bleeding. Slight bleeding is normal, but report large amounts immediately. Monitor the client for indications of fluid volume deficit, and increase the fluid intake to 8 to 10 glasses per day if indicated. Also, continue to assess the client for the following indicators of peritonitis, the most frequently occurring complication of this surgery in the early postoperative stage: fever, abdominal tenderness, elevated pulse, and an absence of bowel sounds. Document the procedure and your observations.

REFERENCES

Beck M, Evans N (eds): *Gastroenterology Nursing: A Core Curriculum.* St Louis: Mosby, 1993.

Bockus S: Troubleshooting your tube feedings. *Am J Nurs* 91(5):24–30, 1991.

Bockus S: When your patient needs tube feedings: Making the right decisions. *Nursing 93* 23(7):34–43, 1993.

Bowers AC, Thompson JM: *Clinical Manual of Health Assessment,* ed 4. St Louis: Mosby, 1992.

Doughty DD, Jackson DB: *Gastrointestinal Disorders.* St Louis: Mosby, 1993.

Faller N, Lawrence K: Comparing low-profile gastrostomy buttons. *Nursing 93* 23(12):46–48, 1993.

Indiana University Hospitals: *Nursing Procedures and Policies.* Indianapolis, 1994.

Keen JH: Gastrointestinal dysfunctions. In Swearingen PL, Keen JH (eds): *Manual of Critical Care Nursing,* ed 3. St Louis: Mosby, 1995.

Kozier B, Erb G: *Techniques in Clinical Nursing,* ed 4. Redwood City, CA: Addison-Wesley, 1993.

Krasner D: What's wrong with this stoma? *Am J Nurs* 90(4):46–47, 1990.

Long L: Ileostomy care: Overcoming the obstacles. *Nursing 91* 21(10):73–75, 1991.

Paulford-Lecher N: Teaching your patient stoma care. *Nursing 93* 23(9):47–49, 1993.

Rice R: *Handbook of Home Health Nursing Procedures.* St Louis: Mosby, 1995.

Sims LK et al: *Health Assessment in Nursing.* Redwood City, CA: Addison-Wesley, 1994.

Society of Gastroenterology Nurses and Associates, Core Curriculum Committee: *Gastroenterology Nursing: A Core Curriculum.* St Louis: Mosby, 1993.

Spence AP: *Basic Human Anatomy,* ed 3. Redwood City, CA: Addison-Wesley, 1991.

Thompson JM: *Mosby's Manual of Clinical Nursing,* ed 3. St Louis: Mosby, 1993.

Van Niel J: What's wrong with this peristomal skin? *Am J Nurs* 91(12):44–45, 1991.

Young C, White S: Preparing patients for tube feeding at home. *Am J Nurs* 92(4):46–53, 1992.

CHAPTER 6

Managing Respiratory Procedures

CHAPTER OUTLINE

ASSESSING THE RESPIRATORY SYSTEM

The Respiratory System

Nursing Assessment Guidelines

Examining the Thorax

Inspecting

Palpating for Thoracic Expansion

Palpating for Fremitus and Crepitation (Subcutaneous Emphysema)

Percussing

Auscultating

MAINTAINING PATENT AIRWAYS

Nursing Guidelines: Artificial Airways

   Oropharyngeal Tube

   Nasopharyngeal Tube

   Endotracheal Tube

   Tracheostomy Tube

   Tracheostomy Button

Inserting Artificial Airways

Inserting an Oropharyngeal Airway

Inserting a Nasopharyngeal Airway

Performing Mouth-to-Mask Ventilation

Managing Routine Tracheostomy Care

Suctioning the Client with a Tracheostomy

Managing Tracheostomy Cuffs

Providing Tracheostomy Hygiene

Replacing a Disposable Inner Cannula

MANAGING RESPIRATORY THERAPY

Administering Oxygen, Humidity, and Aerosol Therapy

Nursing Guidelines: Devices Used in the Delivery of Oxygen, Humidity, and Aerosols

   Simple Face Mask (Low-Flow System)

   Nasal Cannula (Low-Flow System)

   Partial Rebreathing Mask (Low-Flow System)

   Nonrebreathing Mask (Low-Flow/High-Flow System)

   Venturi (Air Entrainment) Mask (High-Flow System)

   CPAP Mask

   Oxygen Hood

   Incubator (Isolette)

   Oxygen Analyzer

   Aerosol Face Mask

   Tracheostomy Collar

   T-Piece

Monitoring Oxygen Saturation Using Pulse Oximetry

Converting a Nonrebreathing Mask to a Partial Rebreathing Mask

Assembling a Venturi Delivery System

Setting Up an Oxygen System with Humidification

Delivering Heated Humidity

Assembling a Nebulizer

Employing Techniques for Lung Inflation

Instructing Clients in Deep-Breathing Exercises

Assisting with Coughing

Using Incentive Spirometers

Assisting with IPPB

Performing Chest Physiotherapy

Percussing, Vibrating, and Draining the Adult

Percussing, Vibrating, and Draining the Infant or Small Child

MANAGING THE CLIENT WITH A CHEST TUBE

Nursing Guidelines: Disposable Closed Chest Drainage System

   Suction Control Chamber

   Water Seal Chamber

   Collection Chamber

Monitoring the Client with a Chest Tube

Assisting with the Removal of a Chest Tube

Assessing the Respiratory System

THE RESPIRATORY SYSTEM

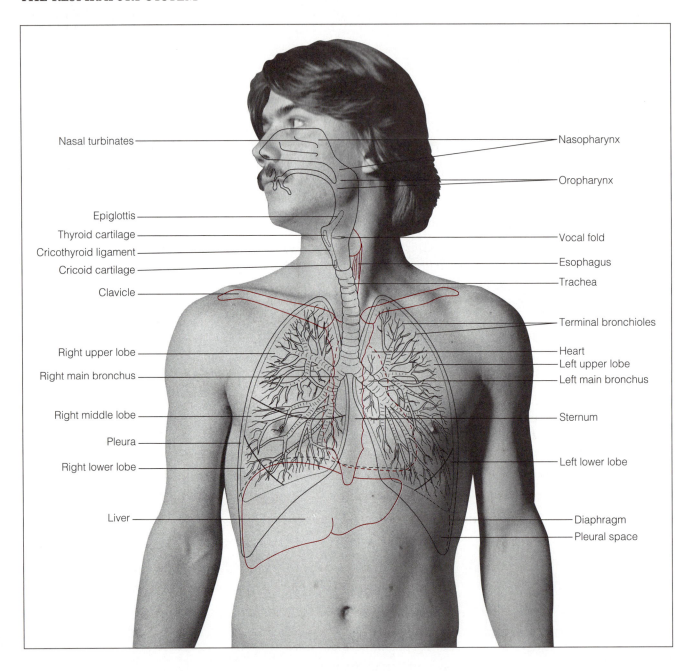

Nasal turbinates

Nasopharynx

Oropharynx

Epiglottis

Thyroid cartilage

Cricothyroid ligament

Cricoid cartilage

Vocal fold

Esophagus

Trachea

Clavicle

Terminal bronchioles

Right upper lobe

Right main bronchus

Heart

Left upper lobe

Left main bronchus

Right middle lobe

Sternum

Pleura

Right lower lobe

Left lower lobe

Liver

Diaphragm

Pleural space

NURSING ASSESSMENT GUIDELINES

To assess your client's respiratory system, you need to interview him or her for subjective data, take vital signs, and examine the thorax. A comprehensive nursing care plan includes a complete evaluation for the following subjective data:

Personal factors: age; occupation—for example, coal mining or history of working with chemicals or other toxins; geographic history

History or family history of: bronchitis, tuberculosis, pneumonia, lung cancer, emphysema, asthma, allergies, surgery for lung or breathing disorders

Smoking: history, past and present; amount; live or work with smokers

Pollutants: environmental or occupational

Psychologic stressors

History or presence of: colds, respiratory infections, cough; frequency of same

Medications: for example, flu vaccine, pneumococcal pneumonia vaccine, dates of same; over-the-counter or prescription; use of vaporizer or nebulizer; oxygen

Chest x-ray film: frequency, date of most recent

Pulmonary function test: frequency, date of most recent

Presence of: fever/chills, diaphoresis, fatigue, postnasal drip, chest pain

Activity intolerance

Recent weight loss/gain

Peripheral edema

Alterations in breathing: painful, labored, oral, noisy, wheezing, shortness of breath, paroxysmal nocturnal dyspnea, relation to activity

Cough: duration, frequency, character, productive or nonproductive, activated by which factors

Sputum: color, frequency, odor, amount, consistency, hemoptysis

EXAMINING THE THORAX

INSPECTING

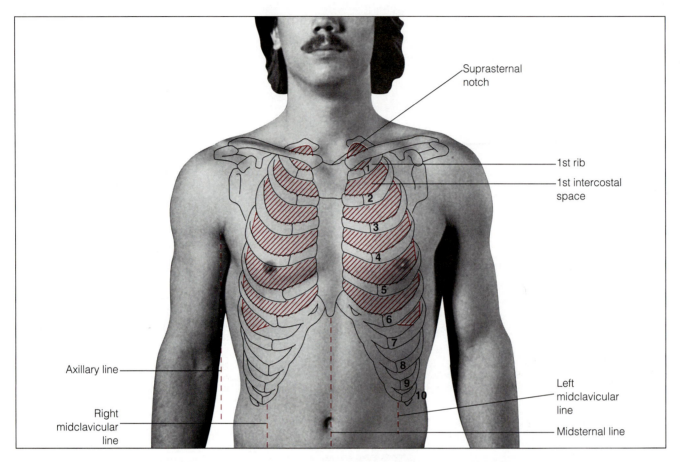

Suprasternal notch

1st rib

1st intercostal space

Axillary line

Right midclavicular line

Left midclavicular line

Midsternal line

Familiarize yourself with these overlays so that you can identify thoracic locations by intercostal space and anatomic landmark. Explain the assessment procedure to the client and ask him to lower his gown to the waist. Be sure to provide the client with a towel or bath blanket for warmth and privacy. If possible, the client should sit on the edge of the bed and dangle his legs to promote optimal chest excursion. Inspect the anterior, lateral, and posterior chest, noting anteroposterior diameter and the symmetry of chest movement. An increased anteroposterior diameter, "barrel chest," is often found in clients with emphysema. The client also might have deformities, such as scoliosis or kyphosis, that can alter aeration. Observe for scarring from trauma or previous surgeries. Also inspect the extremities and note the temperature and texture of the skin. Does the client have digital clubbing, a swelling or "drumstick" appearance of the extremity tips frequently found in clients with pulmonary disease? Also observe for the presence of cyanosis in the distal extremities, nailbeds, conjunctiva, lips, tips of the ears, or nose. Assess the rate, depth, and rhythm of the respirations while the client is unaware that you are doing so and therefore will be less likely to alter them. The healthy adult will have a rate

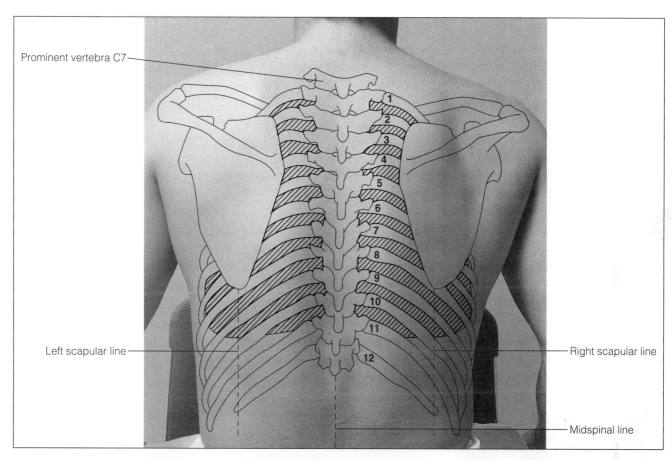

Prominent vertebra C7

1
2
3
4
5
6
7
8
9
10
11
12

Left scapular line

Right scapular line

Midspinal line

of 12–20 even and moderate breaths per minute; the young child will have 20–25; and the infant can have 40 or more. Children younger than age 6 or 7 breathe using their abdominal muscles. Individuals older than age 6 or 7 who use their abdominal muscles for respirations may have thoracic problems. Preview Table 10.2 to help you determine your client's respiratory pattern. Note the client's ratio of inspiration to expiration, which normally is 1:1–1:2. With chronic obstructive pulmonary disease (COPD), the expiration is prolonged, for example, 1:3–1:4. Also listen to the respirations to detect labored breathing (increased work of breathing) or congestion. Observe for indications of labored breathing, such as the use of accessory muscles while breathing (for example, neck or shoulder muscles), flared nostrils, or bulging of intercostal spaces during expiration. Clients with breathing difficulties might sit up and lean forward to facilitate respirations. Finally, note the position of the trachea, which is normally at the midline. Record any deviation and the side to which it deviates. With pneumothorax and pleural effusion, the trachea might deviate away from the affected side; with atelectasis, it can deviate toward the affected side.

PALPATING FOR THORACIC EXPANSION

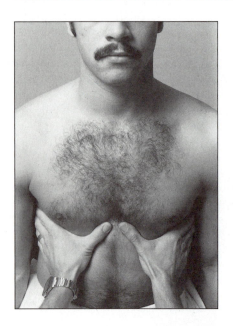

Place your hands together at the base of the sternum so that your thumbs meet (as shown).

Instruct the client to inhale deeply. Observe the quality and symmetry of the expansion. If one side moves more than the other, there might be a lung pathology, pneumothorax, an obstruction of a major bronchus, or the client might be protecting a fractured rib or avoiding discomfort. In the healthy adult, your thumbs should separate 5.0–7.5 cm (2–3 in). Repeat the assessment posteriorly.

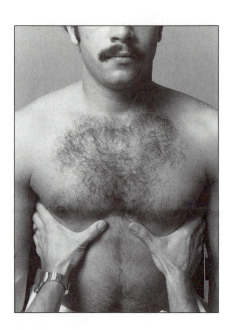

PALPATING FOR FREMITUS AND CREPITATION (SUBCUTANEOUS EMPHYSEMA)

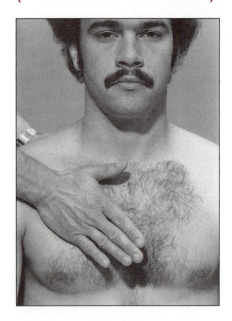

Fremitus is the vibration of the thoracic wall that is felt over the chest when a person speaks. Position your hand over a lung segment as shown, and instruct the client to say "ninety-nine" so that you can feel the vibration on the palmar surface of your hand. Continue the assessment over the lung segments, progressing from right to left (or vice versa), and from the top of the chest to the bottom, repeating the assessment on the posterior chest. The response normally should be equal when comparing one side of the chest to the symmetric area on the opposite side. An increase in fremitus is often found in clients with lung abscesses or with consolidation, as in the case of pneumonia, because the density of the tissues will increase the transmission of the vibrations. A decrease or absence in fremitus will be found in clients with COPD, pneumothorax, or pleural effusion when additional air or fluid or a fibrous thickening creates an additional layer through which the vibrations must be transmitted. Fremitus is normally greater at parasternal or intrascapular areas.

Palpation also can be performed to assess for crepitation (subcutaneous emphysema), a crackling sound or sensation felt in the subcutaneous tissues. It is usually caused by the presence of foreign body, such as a tracheostomy tube or chest tube that allows air to leak into subcutaneous tissue, and it is located in the area around the foreign body.

PERCUSSING

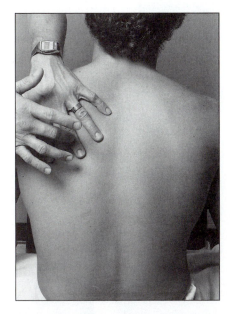

AUSCULTATING

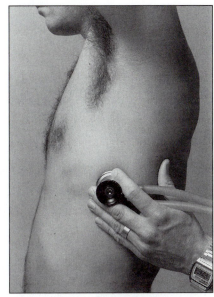

Percussion will help you determine whether underlying structures are solid or filled with air or fluid. Percussion of the thorax is performed by placing a middle finger over an intercostal space and sharply striking that finger with the opposite middle finger to elicit sounds. Hollow sounds, referred to as resonance, mostly will be heard over the greater portions of the healthy lung. Hyperresonance, which is booming and low in pitch, normally may be heard in children with thin chest walls. It also will be found in clients with hyperinflated lungs or where there is an increase in pleural air, for example in clients with emphysema or a pneumothorax. Dullness will be elicited over dense lung areas in clients with pneumonia or atelectasis, but it is normally heard over the heart and liver. When percussing, you can follow the same pattern used for auscultating (see page 318). The assessment should progress down one side of the chest, going from right to left (or vice versa) so that each side is checked against the symmetrical area on the opposite side, and repeated on the posterior (or anterior) chest.

Warm the diaphragm of the stethoscope between your hands before placing it on the client's skin. Instruct the client to breathe through his mouth, more slowly and deeply than usual. Listen to at least one full breath in each position, comparing one side of the chest to the symmetrical area on the opposite side of the chest. (See next page for auscultation patterns.)

Follow the pattern in these photos for auscultating your client's chest. Listen for normal breath sounds (see Table 6.1), which include vesicular, bronchial, and bronchovesicular sounds; note their intensity, decrease in intensity, or absence from one auscultation site when compared to its symmetrical opposite. Vesicular sounds are soft and swishing and are considered normal when heard over the peripheral lung, but they are abnormal when heard over the large airways. A decrease in their sound over a segment of the peripheral lung might be found with emphysema, in the presence of pleural fluid, or with a pneumothorax. Bronchial sounds are louder, coarser, and of longer duration, and they can be heard over the trachea and bronchi during inhalation and exhalation. They should not be heard over the normal peripheral lung, but they may be elicited over lungs of clients with some type of consolidation, such as a lung tumor or atelectasis. Bronchovesicular sounds are moderate in both pitch and intensity and are heard at the sternal borders of the major bronchi. Assume there is an abnormality if they are heard over the peripheral lung, which can occur with consolidation.

Review Table 6.2 to help you identify adventitious (added or abnormal) breath sounds. Regardless of the terminology used in your agency to describe adventitious sounds, it is important that you determine whether the added sounds you hear are continuous or discontinuous, low or high in pitch, fine or coarse, and whether they are heard during inhalation or exhalation. Coarse crackles (rales), associated with resolving pneumonia or pulmonary edema, are often heard during inhalation and may be eliminated by coughing when they are caused by secretions in the airway. Fine crackles, found in interstitial lung disease or heart failure, are heard late during

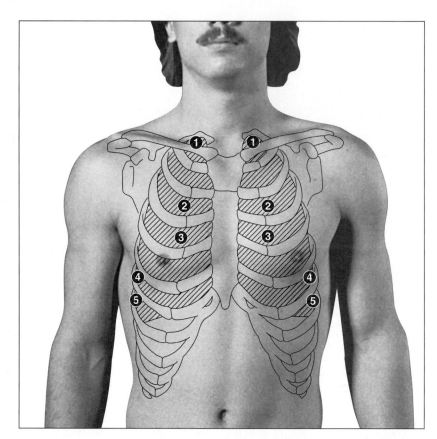

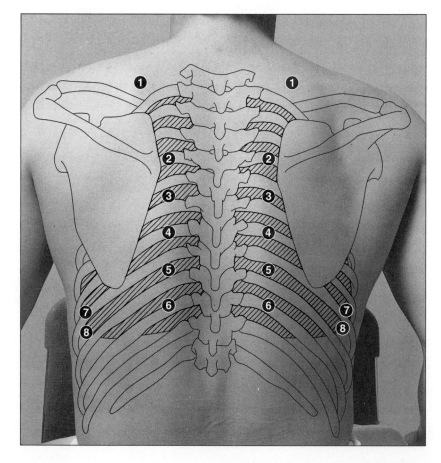

inspiration, usually over lung bases, and are rarely cleared by coughing. Wheezes (sibilant rhonchi) are musical and high in pitch and are most often associated with bronchial asthma or COPD. They are best heard over the larynx during exhalation; however, wheezes of different pitches and sounds might at times be heard simultaneously over all lung fields. Rhonchi occur with increased sputum production and are most often heard during exhalation as air passes through passages narrowed by mucosal swelling or secretions. They are usually cleared or lessened by coughing.

A pleural friction rub, which sounds like two pieces of sandpaper rubbing together, is typically heard over the anterolateral chest. It is caused by the loss of normal pleural lubrication, for example, with pleurisy.

Table 6.1   Assessing Normal Breath Sounds

Type	Normal site	Duration	Characteristics
Vesicular	Peripheral lung	I > E	Soft and swishing sounds. Abnormal when heard over the large airways.
Bronchial	Trachea and bronchi	E > I	Louder, coarser, and of longer duration than vesicular. Abnormal if heard over peripheral lung.
Bronchovesicular	Sternal border of the major bronchi	E = I	Moderate in pitch and intensity. Abnormal if heard over peripheral lung.

I = inspiration; E = expiration

From: Swearingen PL: Heart and breath sounds. In Swearingen PL, Keen JH: *Manual of Critical Care Nursing,* ed 3. St Louis: Mosby, 1995. Used with permission from Mosby-Yearbook.

Table 6.2   Assessing Adventitious Breath Sounds

Type	Waveform	Characteristics	Possible clinical condition
Coarse crackle		Discontinuous, explosive, interrupted. Loud; low in pitch.	Pulmonary edema; pneumonia in resolution stage.
Fine crackle		Discontinuous, explosive, interrupted. Less loud than coarse crackles, lower in pitch, and of shorter duration.	Interstitial lung disease; heart failure; atelectasis.
Wheeze		Continuous, of long duration, high pitched, musical, hissing.	Narrowing of airway; bronchial asthma; COPD.
Rhonchus		Continuous, of long duration, low pitched, snoring.	Production of sputum (usually cleared or lessened by coughing or suctioning).
Pleural friction rub		Grating, rasping noise.	Rubbing together of inflamed parietal linings; loss of normal pleural lubrication.

From: Swearingen PL: Heart and breath sounds. In Swearingen PL, Keen JH: *Manual of Critical Care Nursing,* ed 3. St Louis: Mosby, 1995. Used with permission from Mosby-Yearbook.

NURSING GUIDELINES: ARTIFICIAL AIRWAYS

Oropharyngeal Tube

Description

S-shaped plastic device that fits over the tongue and extends into the posterior pharynx. Available in infant, child, and adult sizes.

Uses

For clients requiring an assisted airway immediately postanesthesia, or for those who are semiconscious and in danger of obstructing their own airways with a displaced tongue. It also can be used when suctioning is required on a short-term basis or as a bite blocker when used with an endotracheal tube.

Nursing Considerations

- To facilitate insertion and to keep the client's tongue from falling back into the pharynx, the client should be supine with a hyperextended neck unless it is contraindicated by head and neck injuries.

- After insertion, keep the client's head turned to the side to prevent aspiration of vomitus and secretions.

- Remove the airway every 4 hours and provide oral hygiene.

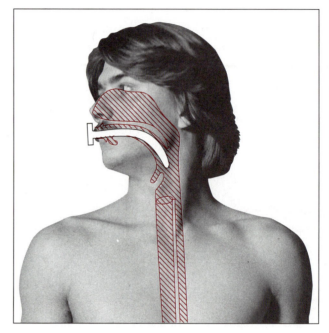

- The airway should not be discontinued until the client is conscious, can swallow on his own, and his gag and cough reflexes have returned.

- This airway is contraindicated in the conscious client because it stimulates the gag reflex.

NURSING GUIDELINES: ARTIFICIAL AIRWAYS (continued)

Nasopharyngeal Tube

Description

Rubber or latex tube (also called trumpet) that extends from the naris to the hypopharynx. Large variation in sizes accommodates the infant to the adult.

Uses

For clients requiring short-term airway management when the oral route is contraindicated, or for those with a sensitive gag reflex. Also inserted to protect the nasal mucosa during nasopharyngeal or nasotracheal suctioning.

Nursing Considerations

- Prior to insertion, lubricate the tube with water-soluble lubricant, or topical anesthetic, if prescribed.

- For optimal fit, the diameter of the tube should be only slightly smaller than the diameter of the naris.

- To prevent pressure areas, rotate the tube to the alternate naris at least every 8 hours.

- Provide nasal hygiene to both nares.

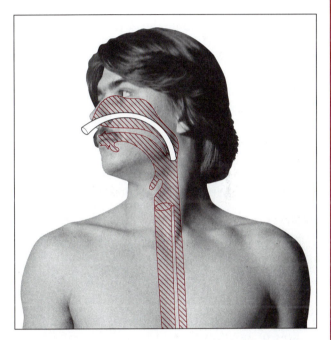

- Nasotracheal suctioning should be done only when necessary because it can stimulate the vagus nerve and potentially lead to bradycardia and cardiac arrest.

Endotracheal Tube

Description

Polyvinyl chloride curved tube that extends from the mouth or nose to just above the bifurcation of the trachea (carina). Inner and outer diameters of the tube are measured in millimeters; the length, in centimeters. Sized to accommodate the newborn to the adult, with cuffed tubes available in adolescent and adult sizes. Has universal adaptors for use with mechanical ventilation.

Uses

Most commonly for clients receiving general anesthesia or in short-term emergency situations to provide a patent airway, facilitate suctioning, or provide a means for mechanical ventilation.

Nursing Considerations

- Turn the client to the side to prevent aspiration of vomitus and secretions.

- Keep the airway taped securely in place. Accidental extubation can be life threatening.

- To monitor tube slippage, mark the tube at the nose or mouth with indelible ink.

- Provide frequent oral and nasal hygiene.

- Oral tubes should be repositioned to the opposite side of the mouth at least daily to prevent pressure areas in the mouth. With nasal tubes, the nares should be evaluated frequently for breakdown.

- Hyperinflate the client's lungs with high concentrations of oxygen before, during, and after suctioning (see page 332) to minimize hypoxemia.

- Because there is the risk of this tube slipping into the right main stem bronchus, monitor for symmetry of respiratory movement and the presence of bilateral breath sounds.

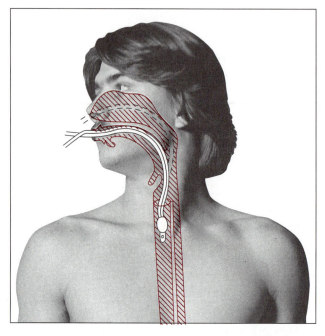

- To prevent unconscious clients from biting down on oral tubes, a bite block can be inserted to keep the jaws apart.

- Provide means for communication; keep the call light within the client's reach.

- Frequently monitor cuff pressure to prevent tracheal necrosis. It should not be greater than 25 mm Hg.

- Continuous humidification or aerosol therapy is mandatory to prevent drying of respiratory mucosa.

- Review Nursing Considerations for the tracheostomy tube (see page 323). The nursing care plan is basically the same.

NURSING GUIDELINES: ARTIFICIAL AIRWAYS (continued)

Tracheostomy Tube

Description

Plastic or metal tube that extends from an incision in the anterior neck directly into the trachea. Available in infant to adult sizes, but smaller sizes generally come without cuffs. Single-cannula tubes are indicated for short-term use; tubes with both inner and outer cannulas are most often used in long-term care. Can attach to mechanical ventilator with an adaptor.

Nursing Considerations

- To assess need for suctioning and patency of airway, frequently auscultate lung fields and trachea for breath sounds.

- To minimize the potential for infection and for client comfort, change the dressing around the tracheostomy as soon as blood and secretions collect.

- Hyperinflate the client's lungs with high concentrations of oxygen before, during, and after suctioning to minimize hypoxemia.

- Encourage turning, coughing, deep breathing, and range of motion exercises to help mobilize secretions.

- Continuous humidification or aerosol therapy is necessary to prevent drying of respiratory mucosa.

- If heated humidity is delivered, monitor the temperature frequently to prevent injury to the trachea. Keep it within 34–36 C.

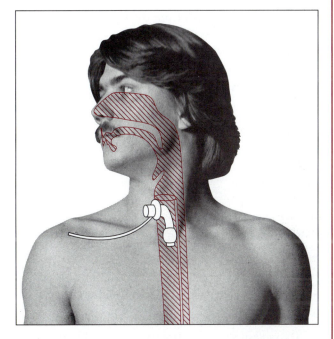

- Inflate cuffed tracheostomy tubes during eating, intermittent positive pressure breathing (IPPB), and mechanical ventilation.

- Provide a means for communication, and keep the call light within reach.

- Secure the tube carefully to prevent accidental dislodgement.

- Keep an identical, spare tracheostomy tube and obturator at the client's bed.

NURSING GUIDELINES: ARTIFICIAL AIRWAYS (continued)

Tracheostomy Button

Description

Short tube that extends from the tracheal stoma to just inside the tracheal wall. Most come with adapters for use with IPPB and manual resuscitator, and plugs for closing the button.

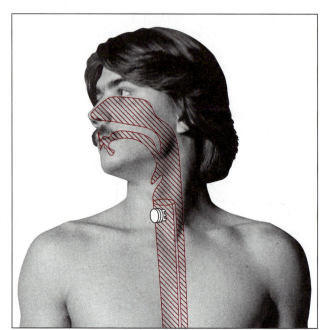

Uses

Maintains stoma for emergency airway management after the tracheostomy tube has been removed. It also can be used to wean client from ventilatory support.

Nursing Considerations

- The button allows the client to cough and breathe more easily than does a tracheostomy tube.

- Remove closure plug for suctioning and/or ventilating.

- Insert IPPB adapter plug for ventilating.

- The client can speak when the button is plugged.

- To prevent skin irritation, keep stomal area clean with hydrogen peroxide. Dry thoroughly after rinsing with sterile water.

- Clean the cannula often, according to agency protocol, by immersing in hydrogen peroxide solution and rinsing with sterile water.

INSERTING ARTIFICIAL AIRWAYS

INSERTING AN OROPHARYNGEAL AIRWAY

Assessing and Planning

1 Choose the correct airway size. Generally, they are available in infant, child, and adult sizes. Wash your hands and explain the procedure to the client, even though she is semiconscious. Position her so that her neck is hyperextended, unless this position is contraindicated by a head or neck injury. You also can roll a large towel or small pillow and place it under the client's shoulders to increase the angle of the head tilt. Positioning her in this manner will open her airway and help keep the tongue away from the pharynx. Push up on the client's mandible (as shown) to prevent obstruction of the oral pharynx by her tongue.

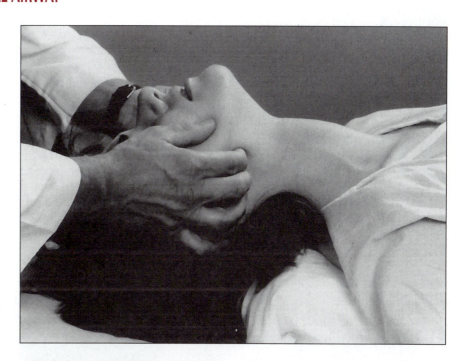

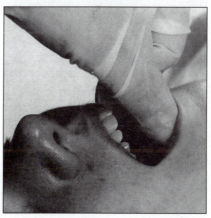

2 To open her mouth, apply gloves and employ the crossed-finger technique (as shown). In this position, your fingers will pop out of her mouth should she have a seizure or clamp down with her teeth. *Note: If you use a tongue blade instead, depress the tongue and place the airway directly over the tongue and into the back of the mouth.* Before inserting the artificial airway, make sure the client's airway is clear of obstructions.

Implementing

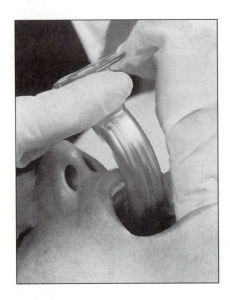

3 With your other hand, position the airway so that it is upside down, with the tip pointing upward toward the roof of the mouth. Insert it into the back of the mouth. Positioning it in this manner will depress the tongue and prevent tongue displacement into the posterior pharynx.

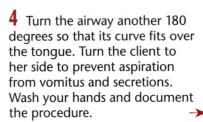

4 Turn the airway another 180 degrees so that its curve fits over the tongue. Turn the client to her side to prevent aspiration from vomitus and secretions. Wash your hands and document the procedure.

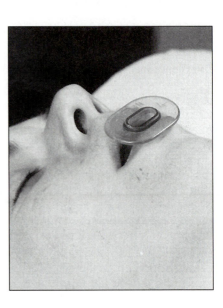

Evaluating

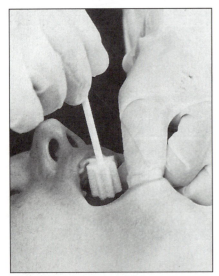

5 At least every 4 hours, remove the airway by gently pulling it downward and outward following the natural curve of the mouth. Use a gauze-covered tongue depressor or employ the crossed-finger technique to keep the client's mouth open while assessing the oral cavity and providing hygiene. The photo illustrates swabbing the mouth with a Toothette.

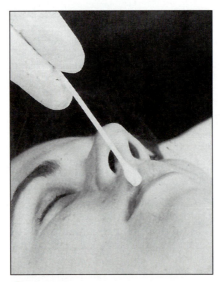

6 Moisturize the client's lips to prevent cracking and breakdown from the pressure of the airway's flange. The photograph illustrates the use of a cotton-tipped applicator saturated with a water-soluble lubricant. Following mouth care, reinsert the airway following the steps outlined above. Before discontinuing the airway, ensure that the client is at least semiconscious, that she can swallow on her own, and that gag and cough reflexes have returned.

INSERTING A NASOPHARYNGEAL AIRWAY

Assessing and Planning

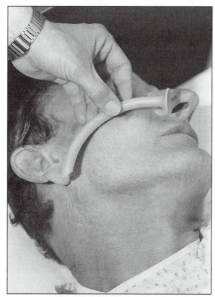

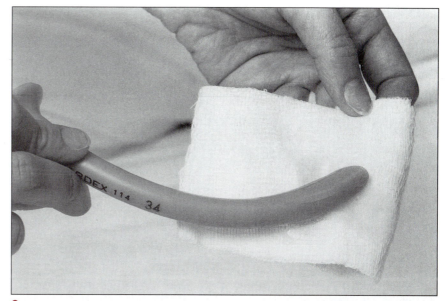

1 Explain the procedure to your client. Place him in semi-Fowler's to Fowler's position to enhance his respirations unless this position is contraindicated. Select an airway that extends from the earlobe to the naris. For optimal fit, the outer diameter of the airway should be only slightly smaller than that of the naris.

2 If you have a prescription for an anesthetic jelly, lubricate the entire length of the airway with the topical anesthetic. Otherwise, lubricate the airway with a water-soluble lubricant to facilitate its insertion.

➤**327**

Implementing

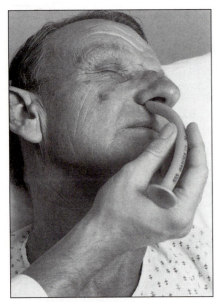

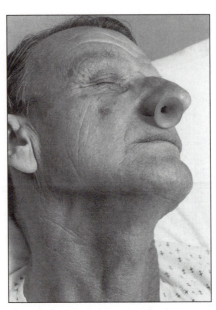

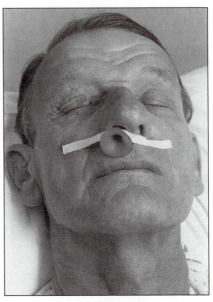

3 Select the naris that looks more patent; gently insert the airway while pushing up the tip of the nose so that the tube follows the curve of the nasopharynx. If the naris you selected proves to be obstructed, intubate the other.

4 When the flange of the airway reaches the naris, the distal end of the airway should be correctly positioned in the hypopharynx.

5 To prevent its expulsion, tape the airway in place by looping 1.25 cm (½ in) of hypoallergenic tape over the area of the airway that is distal to the flange and adhering the rest of the tape to the skin above the client's upper lip. Use a skin preparation first if your client has sensitive skin. Wash your hands and document the procedure.

Evaluating

6 Prior to its removal, suction down the airway (see page 330) to remove the secretions. Be sure to rotate the airway to the other naris at least every 8 hours. Assess the naris for breakdown and provide materials for cleansing the naris and moisturizing the nasal mucosa.

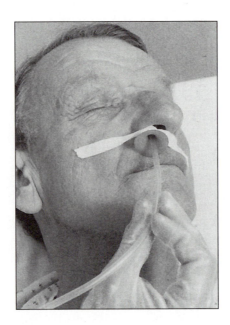

PERFORMING MOUTH-TO-MASK VENTILATION

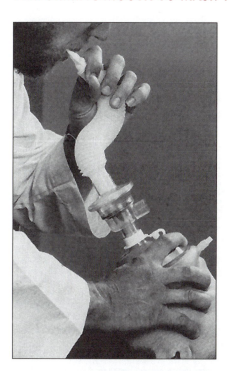

Mouth-to-mask ventilation is the only method that is recommended to prevent the health care worker's mouth from coming into direct contact with the client's oral secretions. To position the client's head and neck appropriately, see photo and review the procedure on page 325. Position the mask over the client's mouth, keeping the mask in place with your index finger and thumb and extending your other fingers over the client's jawline. Take a deep breath and position your mouth over the mouthpiece.

Exhale and watch the client's chest rise and fall or listen for breath sounds. Continue until one of the following occurs:

- The client's spontaneous ventilations return.
- You are relieved by an individual trained in the procedure.
- Adjunct equipment arrives (eg, mask and self-inflating bag or endotracheal tube).
- The attending physician arrives and requests that you stop.

MANAGING ROUTINE TRACHEOSTOMY CARE
SUCTIONING THE CLIENT WITH A TRACHEOSTOMY

Assessing and Planning

1 Evaluate the client's need for suctioning by bilaterally auscultating the lung fields to identify and locate secretions. If suctioning is needed, explain the procedure to the client and place her in Fowler's position unless it is contraindicated. Remember that suctioning is always done as needed rather than as a standard order; therefore, frequent client assessment is crucial. Frequent suctioning may cause airway irritation, resulting in more secretions.

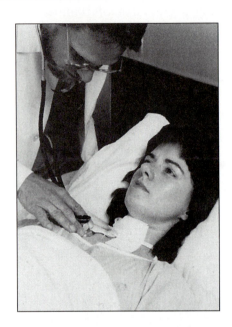

2 Assemble the following materials:

☐ suction kit containing the following sterile supplies:

— suction catheter of the appropriate size*

— gloves

— basin

☐ sterile solution (usually normal saline)

☐ manual resuscitator with appropriate adapter for client-resuscitator connection and an attached oxygen reservoir for delivering higher oxygen concentrations

The use of two gloves (one designated sterile to protect the client and one designated clean to protect the nurse's other hand) is required.

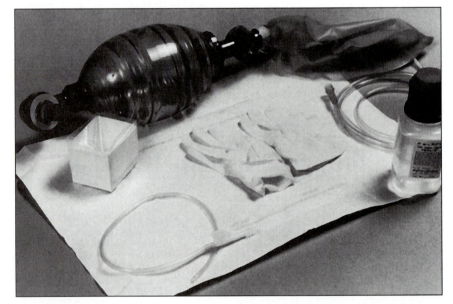

* To minimize the potential for atelectasis, make sure the outer diameter of the suction catheter is no greater than half of the inner diameter of the tracheostomy tube.

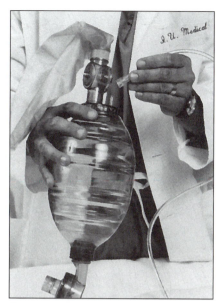

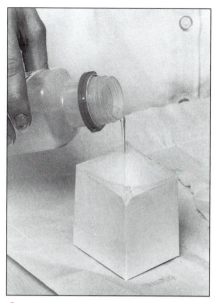

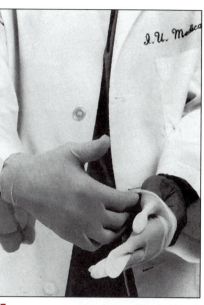

3 Attach the resuscitator to source oxygen (as shown). When hyperinflating the client (using the "sigh maneuver"), you will need to adjust the oxygen flowmeter to deliver 12–15 L/min or enough to ensure that the reservoir bag remains inflated during manual ventilation. This will provide the necessary oxygen concentration.

4 Wash your hands and loosen the cap on the sterile solution bottle. Open the sterile suction kit on a clean surface, using the internal wrapping as a sterile field, and fill the sterile basin with the sterile solution.

5 Put on sterile gloves, following the procedure in Chapter 1.

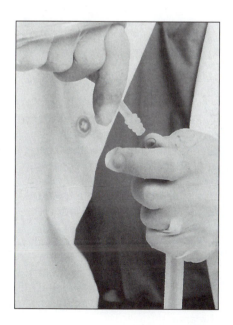

6 Attach the suction catheter to the suction tubing, holding the sterile catheter in your dominant hand (which will remain sterile) and the suction tubing in your nondominant hand (which will be contaminated from touching nonsterile equipment). *Note: The same catheter can be used during the entire procedure provided it does not become contaminated, and it is not used to suction the oropharynx or nasopharynx before suctioning or resuctioning the trachea. If either of these situations occurs, replace the contaminated catheter with a sterile one to prevent contaminating the respiratory tract.*

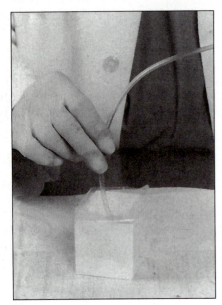

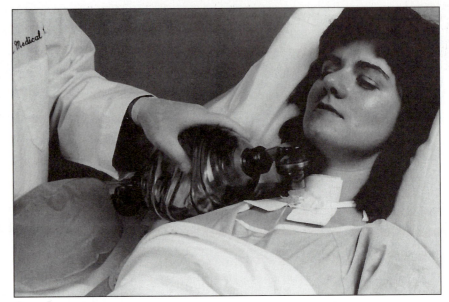

7 Set the suction regulator dial at 80–120 mm Hg. Submerge the tip of the catheter into the sterile solution, and briefly place your nondominant thumb over the suction port to produce suction. This not only tests the efficiency of the suction apparatus but also lubricates the catheter to facilitate its insertion into the trachea. In addition, it lubricates the inside of the catheter, which helps to prevent tenacious secretions from sticking to the tubing.

8 Using your nondominant hand, oxygenate your client with three to five deep lung inflations to help compensate for the oxygen you will remove during the suctioning process. To do this, turn the oxygen on, connect the tracheostomy adapter of the manual resuscitator to the tracheostomy tube, and compress the bag to deliver the oxygen. Wait for the client to exhale before administering each

successive ventilation. Ideally, a second person should "sigh" the client. Because the second person can place both hands firmly around the resuscitation bag, there is less potential for trauma from manipulation of the bag. In addition, the second person can provide greater volume with two hands than that which can be provided with one hand.

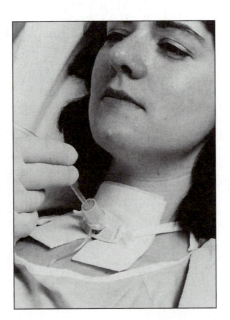

Implementing

9 Remove the oxygen device and position it on the bed or on the client's chest, with the tracheostomy adapter facing up. With your dominant (sterile) hand, gently insert the catheter into the tracheostomy, keeping your nondominant thumb off the suction port. Insert the catheter as far as it will go, but do not use force. When you reach the carina or bronchial wall, withdraw the catheter 1–2 cm (⅓–¾ in) to prevent damaging the area.

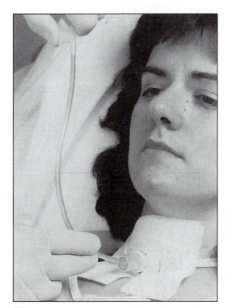

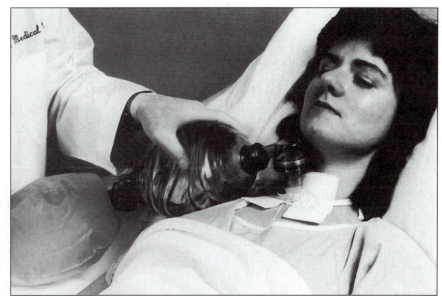

10 Place your nondominant thumb over the suction port to produce suction. Rotate the catheter between your dominant thumb and forefinger, gradually withdrawing the catheter as you apply intermittent suction by moving your nondominant thumb up and down on the suction port. This should prevent the catheter from adhering to the mucosa and damaging the bronchial wall. To minimize hypoxemia, do not suction for longer than 10–15 seconds during each suction attempt. Some experts suggest having the client turn the head to the right while you attempt to suction the left tracheobronchial tree, and the head to the left while you attempt to suction the right tracheobronchial tree. Although this technique is recommended, its efficacy has not been proved.

11 To prevent suction-induced hypoxemia, reoxygenate the client after every suction attempt, following the technique outlined in step 8.

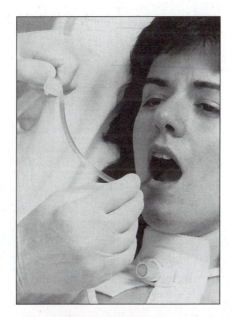

12 If your client has a tracheostomy tube with an inflated cuff, before deflating the cuff (see page 335), you will need to suction above the cuff to ensure removal of the secretions in the upper respiratory tract. First reoxygenate the client and rinse the catheter in the sterile solution. Suction the mouth and pharynx by employing the same technique used for suctioning the tracheostomy. When suctioning the pharynx, instruct the client to extend her tongue so that you can suction the area more readily.

HOME HEALTH CARE CONSIDERATIONS

- In most instances, clean, rather than sterile, technique can be used in the home setting. Caregivers can use clean gloves when suctioning. Sterile gloves usually are not required.

- Suctioning catheters may be reused until they are no longer pliable.

- After each use, catheters can be cleaned with warm, soapy water; rinsed well; and allowed to dry thoroughly. They can be stored in clean plastic bags between uses.

- Tap water may be used to clear the catheter of secretions during and after suctioning.

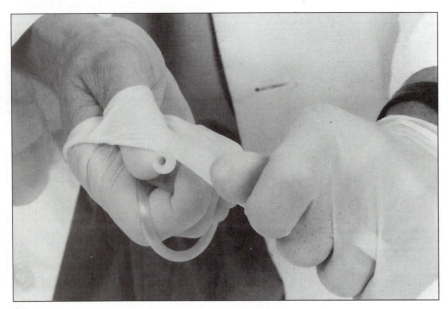

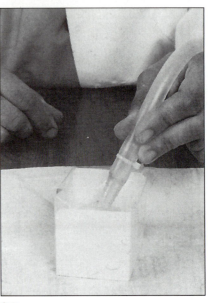

13 Dispose of the contaminated catheter by pulling your glove inside out over the catheter and depositing both into a waste container. Again, reoxygenate the client or attach her own delivery system, increasing the liter flow for a few minutes. *Note: Remember to turn the oxygen flow back to the regular prescribed rate.*

14 Flush the suction tubing by applying suction while submerging the tubing in the same solution you used to rinse the sterile catheter.

Evaluating

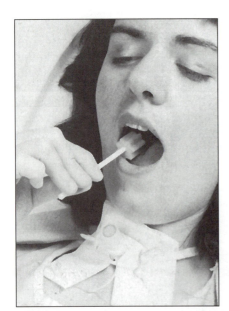

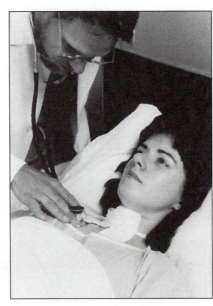

15 Provide your client with materials for oral hygiene. A Toothette, for example, is a convenient way to refresh the mouth.

16 Again auscultate the lung fields to evaluate the results of the suctioning. Optimally, the client will have absent or greatly diminished adventitious sounds and should exhibit nonlabored respirations. In addition, the apical pulse will be within her normal rate, indicating that suctioning has not stimulated the vagus nerve and slowed the heart rate. Document the procedure: note the amount, color, odor, and consistency of the secretions and your client's response to the procedure. If secretions are tenacious, the physician might prescribe continuous aerosol or humidity via a T-piece or tracheostomy mask. Augment fluid intake unless it is medically contraindicated.

MANAGING TRACHEOSTOMY CUFFS

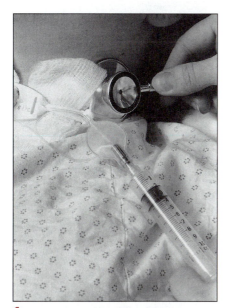

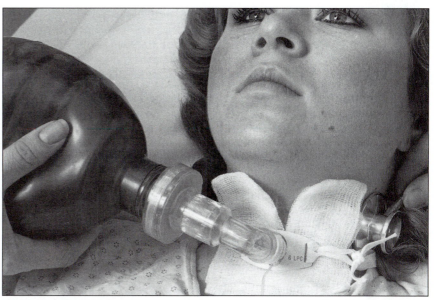

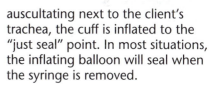

1 When properly using a high-volume/low-pressure (floppy) cuff, it is not necessary to deflate the cuff hourly, but it is important to inflate the cuff correctly when necessary, for example, when the client receives intermittent positive pressure breathing (IPPB) or if mechanical ventilation is used. With the aid of an assistant you can easily inflate the cuff. Attach a calibrated 10-mL syringe to the distal end of the cuff (the inflating balloon).

2 Have your assistant hyperinflate the client with a manual resuscitator as you slowly inject air into the cuff. At the point that air movement is no longer heard when auscultating next to the client's trachea, the cuff is inflated to the "just seal" point. In most situations, the inflating balloon will seal when the syringe is removed.

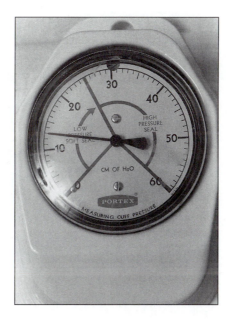

3 When a manometer (such as the one shown) is available, you can inflate the cuff on your own. In addition to the calibrated syringe, you will also need a three-way stopcock.

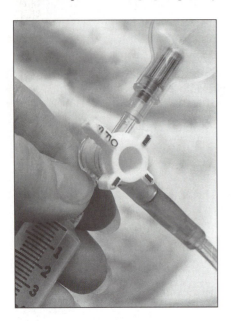

4 Attach the three ends of the stopcock to the inflating balloon, the manometer tubing, and the syringe. Open the stopcock to all ports (as shown). Inject air into the inflating balloon until the manometer reads 25 cm H_2O, or until it reaches the prescribed pressure. Always use the smallest amount of pressure to achieve minimal occluding volume (see step 2). The cuff should now be properly inflated.

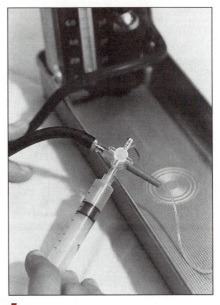

5 You also may use a blood pressure manometer in the same way. Inject air into the inflating balloon until the manometer reads 15 mm Hg or the prescribed pressure.

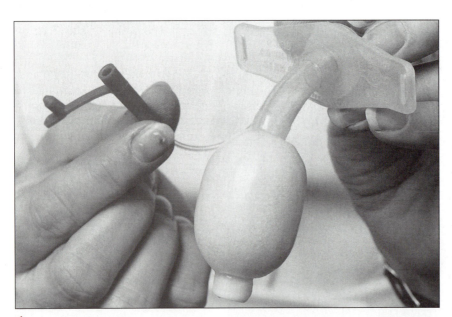

6 *Variation for Foam Cuffs:* If your client has a foam cuff, you will not inject air into the cuff to inflate it. Instead, when the port is open, ambient air will enter the balloon and conform it to the client's trachea.

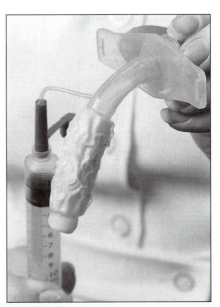

7 The physician will aspirate air from the foam cuff prior to intubation or extubation, but it might be your responsibility to assess the cuff's proper functioning before the procedure.

PROVIDING TRACHEOSTOMY HYGIENE

1 Wash your hands and obtain:

☐ tracheostomy tray that contains the following sterile supplies:

—two soaking trays (bowls)

—gloves

—plastic forceps

—gauze sponges

—unfilled gauze tracheostomy dressing

—pipe cleaner or brush

—twill tape

—cotton-tipped applicator

—overwrap for establishing a sterile field

☐ impervious plastic bag for disposal of used dressing and supplies

☐ sterile normal saline and hydrogen peroxide

Pour the hydrogen peroxide and normal saline into each of the sterile bowls. Apply the sterile gloves and remove the soiled tracheostomy dressing using the forceps. Avoid touching the dressing with your gloved hands. Deposit the dressing into the impervious plastic bag.

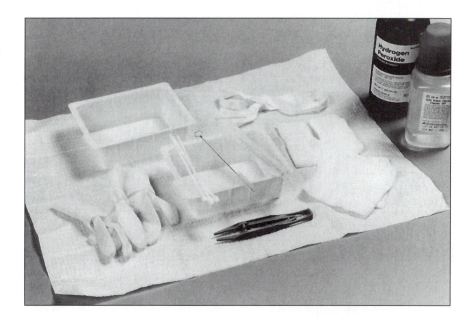

HOME HEALTH CARE CONSIDERATIONS

- In many instances, the caregiver may use clean, rather than sterile, gloves.

- For clients whose tracheostomy is well-healed, warm soapy water may be used to clean the stoma.

- Caregivers routinely should look for areas of excoriation or skin breakdown around the stoma or under the tracheostomy ties.

- Clean nondisposable cannulas at least daily using hot, soapy water. Rinse well, air dry, and store in a clean plastic bag for the next cannula change.

- For cleaning encrustations, the cannula may be soaked in a hydrogen peroxide solution. The inside of the cannula may be scrubbed with a pipe cleaner or brush, followed by a tap water rinse. Hydrogen peroxide is contraindicated for metal cannulas, however.

- The suction collection container should be emptied and washed daily with hot, soapy water. The suction tubing may be washed in the same manner and hung for air drying.

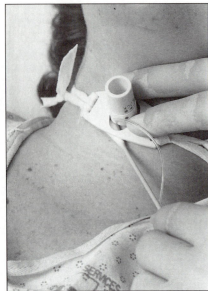

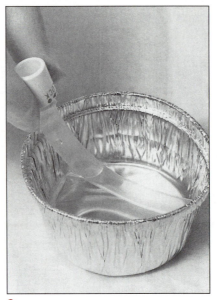

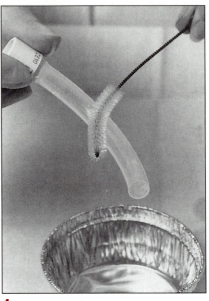

2   *Cleansing the Stoma Site:*
Cleanse the stoma with a sterile cotton-tipped applicator that has been moistened with hydrogen peroxide. After you have cleansed the stomal site, swab the tube's flange. Rinse the stomal site with another sterile cotton-tipped applicator that has been moistened with sterile normal saline, and dry the area with sterile gauze pads. Be sure to record the condition of the stoma at least once per shift.

3   *Cleaning the Inner Cannula:*
Note: *Not all tracheostomy tubes have an inner cannula.* During each suctioning and as necessary (or at least once during each shift), remove the inner cannula and immerse it in a solution of hydrogen peroxide.

4   With a sterile test-tube brush, clean the cannula on both the outside and the inside, being certain to remove all the encrustations.

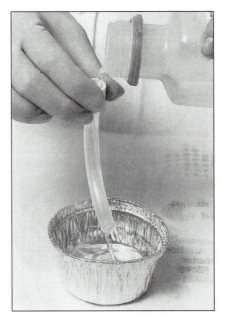

5   Rinse the cannula thoroughly with sterile saline. Suction the outer cannula and reinsert the inner cannula and lock it into position. *Caution: To prevent the formation of crusts in the outer cannula, the inner cannula should not be removed for longer than 5 minutes; if the client is on oxygen therapy or a respirator, the inner cannula must be replaced as soon as possible. Always have a sterile spare available at the bedside.*

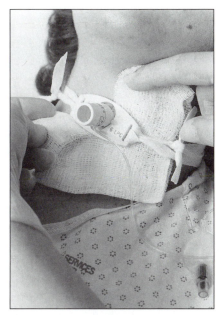

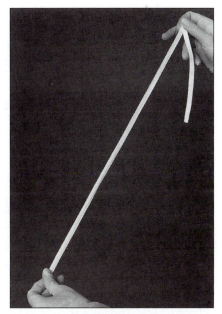

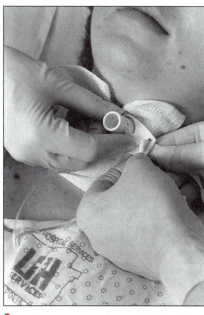

6 *Changing the Tracheostomy Dressing:* Insert the tracheostomy dressing so that the slit encircles the tracheostomy tube (as shown). If the client has a copious amount of drainage, it is a good idea to position the dressing with the slit side up, which will provide more surface area on the lower portion of the dressing to absorb the moisture. Although the dressing should be changed at least once per shift, more frequent changes are necessary if blood and secretions collect at the site.

7 *Changing Tracheostomy Ties:* For your client's safety, ask another caregiver to assist you by holding the tracheostomy tube in place as you change the ties. Begin by cutting two pieces of twill tape, each approximately 45 cm (18 in) in length. Fold over a quarter of each tape and pinch the creases to facilitate their insertion into the flange of the tube.

8 Insert the folded end of one of the twill tapes through the slot in the flange.

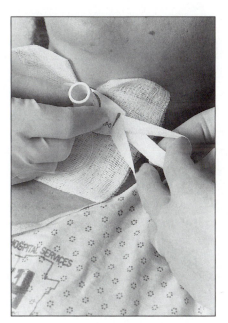

9 Tie a slipknot by pulling the folded end through the slot approximately 5 cm (2 in) and forming a loop. Pull the longer end of the tape through the center of the loop (as shown).

←

10 Pull the longer end snugly to complete the slipknot. Do the same on the other side, or ask your assistant to do this as you hold the tracheostomy tube in place.

→

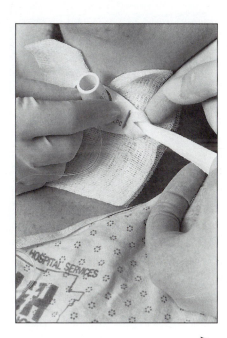

→

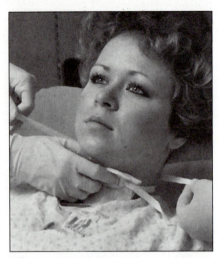

11 Pass the long end of the tape behind the client's head as your assistant does the same; exchange the ends.

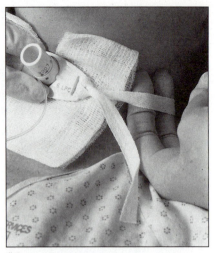

12 Before tying a square knot, ensure that one or two fingers can fit between the tape and the client's neck. The tape should fit snugly enough to prevent the tracheostomy tube's expulsion, but not so tightly that it is uncomfortable for the client.

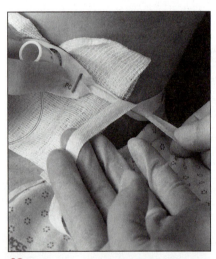

13 Tie the two ends of the tape together.

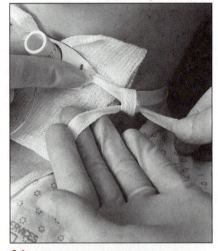

14 Make a square knot, tying the knot on the side of the client's neck to prevent pressure to areas on the back of the neck. As an extra precaution, tie another square knot over the original to make a double square knot. Repeat on the other side.

REPLACING A DISPOSABLE INNER CANNULA

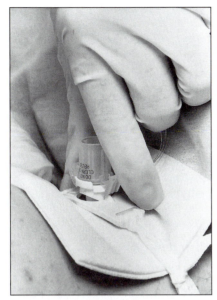

1 Wash your hands. Obtain a disposable inner cannula of the appropriate size for your client. Apply clean gloves. Pinch the connecting wings together on the cannula you will remove from your client.

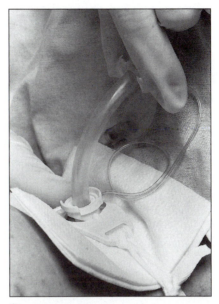

2 Slowly remove the cannula from the tracheostomy tube, noting any evidence of secretions or bleeding. Dispose of the cannula according to your agency's policy.

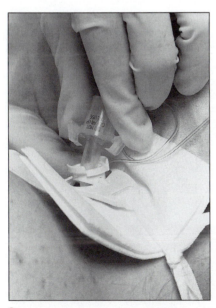

3 Pinch together the wings of the clean cannula, and insert the cannula slowly into the tracheostomy tube.

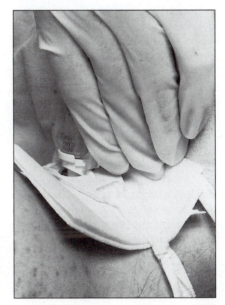

4 Continue inserting the cannula until you hear or feel the "click" of the inner cannula wings attaching to the tracheostomy tube. Visually assess the connection to ensure that it is secure. Remove and dispose of your gloves. Wash your hands.

Managing Respiratory Therapy

ADMINISTERING OXYGEN, HUMIDITY, AND AEROSOL THERAPY

NURSING GUIDELINES: DEVICES USED IN THE DELIVERY OF OXYGEN, HUMIDITY, AND AEROSOLS

Low-Flow System

A method of oxygen delivery that does not supply all of the inspired gas needs; thus, room air is inhaled along with oxygen. The fraction of inspired oxygen (FiO_2) will vary, depending on respiratory rate, tidal volume, and liter flow. It is contraindicated for clients requiring carefully gauged concentrations of oxygen.

High-Flow System

A method of oxygen delivery that supplies all of the inspired gas needs regardless of the client's rate, volume, and flow. This system is a precise and consistent method for controlling the client's FiO_2.

Both high-flow and low-flow systems can deliver a variety of oxygen concentrations.

Devices Used in the Administration of Supplemental and Environmental Therapy

Simple Face Mask (Low-Flow System)

Description

Clear plastic device with exhalation ports, which covers the nose and mouth. It can deliver 35%–60% oxygen concentrations.

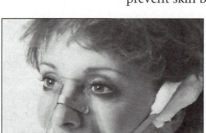

Uses

Short-term therapy when moderate concentrations of oxygen are desired, but it must be used cautiously on clients who potentially may vomit and aspirate.

Nursing Considerations

- The recommended liter flow is 5–8 L/min.
- Use with a humidifier prevents drying of nasal and oral mucosa.
- To prevent skin irritation, keep the face as dry as possible.
- Ensure a tight fit so that the mask will yield maximum oxygen concentration.
- Pad behind ears and over bony prominences to prevent skin breakdown.
- Frequently monitor client's vital signs, arterial blood gas (ABG) values, O_2 saturation, breath sounds, and level of consciousness to evaluate respiratory status.
- Clean mask with warm, soapy water as needed.

HOME HEALTH CARE CONSIDERATIONS

- Avoid use of gas or electric appliances (eg, heaters, razors) near oxygen source.
- Maintain the oxygen container in a stable and sturdy stand to minimize the risk of it accidentally falling over.
- Keep the oxygen tank well away from heat and direct sunlight.

NURSING GUIDELINES: DEVICES USED IN THE DELIVERY OF OXYGEN, HUMIDITY, AND AEROSOLS (continued)

Nasal Cannula (Low-Flow System)

Description
Plastic tubing with two short prongs through which oxygen is administered into the nares. It can achieve up to a 50% oxygen concentration.

Uses
Clients without nasal obstructions for whom simple, comfortable, long-term therapy is desired. For example, it is frequently used for clients with myocardial infarctions and to deliver maintenance oxygen to clients with COPD.

Nursing Considerations
- The recommended liter flow is 1–6 L/min. Increased rates can cause client discomfort, such as headaches.

- It is more comfortable and convenient than most other oxygen administration devices, especially the nasal catheter.

- Some cannulas are adjusted and tightened under the chin; others are secured with an elastic strap at the back of the head.

- Pad behind ears and over bony prominences to prevent skin breakdown.

- At flows greater than 3 L/min, use of a humidifier will prevent drying of nasal mucosa.

- For client comfort, frequently provide nasal and oral hygiene.

- When administering oxygen to clients with COPD, observe for signs of oxygen-induced hypoventilation: shallow respirations, dyspnea, confusion/restlessness, and tremors.

- Monitor the client's vital signs, breath sounds, ABG values, O_2 saturation, and level of consciousness to evaluate respiratory status.

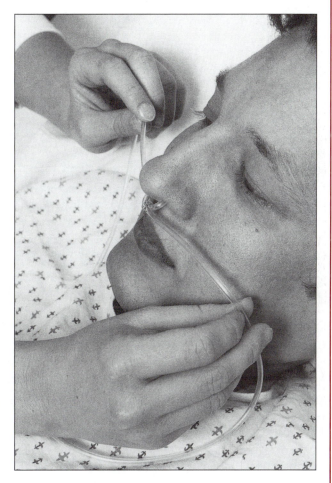

NURSING GUIDELINES: DEVICES USED IN THE DELIVERY OF OXYGEN, HUMIDITY, AND AEROSOLS *(continued)*

Partial Rebreathing Mask (Low-Flow System)

Description

Clear plastic face mask with exhalation ports, which attaches to a reservoir bag, allowing client to rebreathe one third of his exhaled air in conjunction with source oxygen. It can deliver oxygen concentrations up to 60%.

Uses

Short-term treatment for clients having increased FiO_2 demands in such conditions as cardiac or pulmonary disease. It is usually contraindicated for clients with COPD.

Nursing Considerations

- Occlude reservoir bag at the bedside to test for leaks and patency before applying to client.

- To prevent carbon dioxide buildup, the liter flow must be adequate (greater than 6 L/min) to ensure that the reservoir bag does not totally deflate during inspiration. Increase the liter flow as needed.

- When delivering higher oxygen concentrations, observe for signs of oxygen toxicity: cough, dyspnea, substernal pain and burning, and nausea.

- Mask requires tight fit to enhance oxygen delivery.

- To prevent skin irritation, pad behind ears and over bony prominences.

- Monitor the client's vital signs, ABG values, oxygen saturation via pulse oximetry, breath sounds, and level of consciousness to evaluate respiratory status.

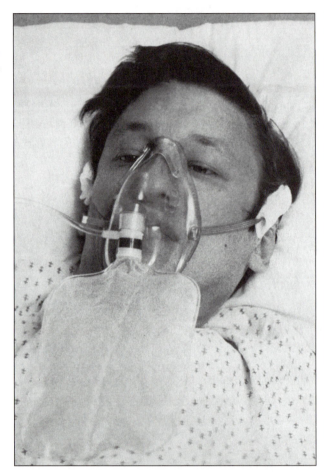

- Mask can easily convert to nonrebreathing mask by inserting rubber disks at the port between reservoir bag and mask, and at one of the exhalation ports.

- Clean mask with warm, soapy water as needed.

Nonrebreathing Mask
(Low-Flow/High-Flow System)

Description

Similar to partial rebreathing mask, except that it has two rubber disks. One disk occludes the port between the reservoir bag and the mask, and the other disk occludes one of the exhalation ports. To achieve higher concentrations of oxygen, this system allows exhaled gas to leave the mask while at the same time preventing inhalation of room air. It can deliver up to 80%–95% oxygen concentrations.

Uses

To increase client's Fio_2 on a short-term basis in such conditions as cardiac failure or pulmonary disease. It is usually contraindicated for clients with COPD.

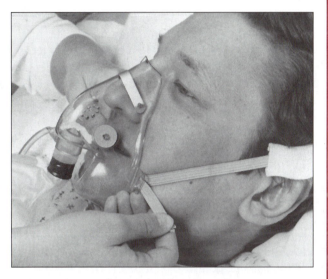

Nursing Considerations

- Occlude reservoir bag at the bedside to test for leaks and patency before applying to client.

- To prevent carbon dioxide buildup, liter flow must be adequate (greater than 6 L/min) so that reservoir bag does not totally deflate during inspiration. Increase the liter flow as needed.

- Use with humidifier will prevent drying of nasal and oral mucosa.

- To function properly, mask should fit client's face snugly with no audible leaks.

- Pad behind ears and over bony prominences to prevent skin breakdown.

- When delivering high oxygen concentrations, observe for signs of oxygen toxicity: coughing, substernal pain and burning, dyspnea, and nausea.

- The mask can convert to a partial rebreather (see page 355) or simple face mask.

- Frequently monitor the client's vital signs, ABG values, oxygen saturation via pulse oximetry, breath sounds, and level of consciousness to evaluate respiratory status.

- If the oxygen is turned off, the client has only one small exhalation port through which to breathe.

- Clean mask with warm, soapy water as needed.

NURSING GUIDELINES: DEVICES USED IN THE DELIVERY OF OXYGEN, HUMIDITY, AND AEROSOLS (continued)

Venturi (Air-Entrainment) Mask (High-Flow System)

Description

Different brands of masks may vary in design, but it is the size of the opening in the adapter or jet that determines the delivered percentage of oxygen concentration. It can deliver 24%–50% oxygen concentration.

Uses

For clients requiring reliable, precise, and controlled concentrations of oxygen; for example, those with COPD.

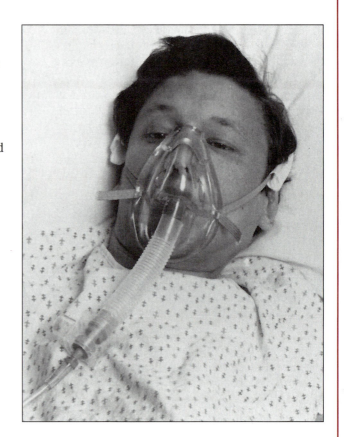

Nursing Considerations

- Explain to client that if his oxygen concentrations are increased, the total liter flow delivered to him will decrease, resulting in a reduced gas flow (velocity).

- To function efficiently, the mask should fit snugly, with no audible leaks.

- Pad areas behind ears and over bony prominences to prevent skin breakdown.

- When administering oxygen to clients with COPD, observe for signs of oxygen-induced hypoventilation: shallow respirations, dyspnea, confusion/restlessness, tremors.

- When using mask without humidity, keep humidity adapter attached to prevent air entrainment ports from being occluded by blanket or body weight.

- For humidity, each mask comes with special humidity adapters that can be attached to appropriate humidification devices.

- Clean mask with warm, soapy water as needed.

NURSING GUIDELINES: DEVICES USED IN THE DELIVERY OF OXYGEN, HUMIDITY, AND AEROSOLS (continued)

CPAP Mask

Description

Cushioned mask with harness-type headgear that can be used to create a seal on the client's face, enabling exhalation against pressure, which maintains alveolar patency during exhalation.

Uses

For clients requiring constant positive airway pressure (CPAP) in the treatment of oxygen deficiencies, such as in preventing or treating atelectasis. Clients in critical care areas with signs of early adult respiratory distress syndrome (ARDS) also may benefit from this mask.

Nursing Considerations

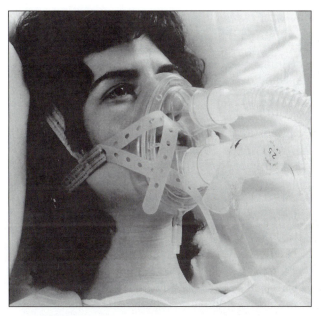

- This mask is indicated for clients who are severely hypoxemic (PaO_2 <60 mm Hg) on high concentrations of oxygen.

- This mask is contraindicated for clients with COPD and hypotension caused by hypovolemia.

- Potential side effects of positive end expiratory pressure can include fluid retention, decreased cardiac output, pneumothorax, and gastric distention.

- Benefits of this mask are lost after 1 hour following every removal because the alveoli will collapse in the susceptible client after this amount of time has lapsed. Do not discontinue this mask for anything less than an urgent matter (eg, removal of sputum or vomitus).

- Careful monitoring of the client's PaO_2 via arterial blood gases (ABGs) or oxygen saturation via pulse oximetry is critical for clients who are treated with CPAP.

  —This client's $PaCO_2$ must remain in the "normal" range (30–50 mm Hg), and the pH must remain in the "normal" range (7.30–7.50).

  —If the client's $PaCO_2$ is greater than "normal" and the pH is less than "normal," mechanical ventilation may be necessary due to acute ventilatory failure.

- The client's risk of aspiration is markedly increased should vomiting occur with this mask in place. Monitor the client at frequent intervals.

- Clients who cough spontaneously may experience difficulty handling secretions. Remove the mask, as necessary, to facilitate sputum removal.

- The necessary snug fit of the mask to the face is uncomfortable for most clients.

- Provide writing materials for this client, whose verbal communication will be impaired by this mask.

- A humidifier chamber can be used to deliver warmed gas to the CPAP mask. Attach wide-bore tubing to the outlet port of the humidifier reservoir, as shown in the photo on page 360, to deliver the gas to the mask. Fill the reservoir with sterile water.

- Adjust the head strap, as needed, to ensure that the two latex straps remain positioned 1¼ cm (½ in) in front of the ears, level with the earlobes.

➤

Oxygen Hood

Description

Rigid dome of clear plastic with inlet ports through which low or high concentrations of oxygen can be delivered. It covers just the head of the infant, and it is similar to the oxygen hut, which is cubic in shape and designed for the older child.

Uses

For infants in cribs or incubators or under radiant warmers, when controlled concentrations of oxygen, temperature, and humidity are desired.

Nursing Considerations

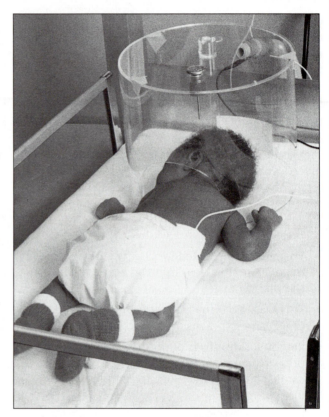

- When removing hood during suctioning or feeding, direct oxygen source toward child's airway to prevent a drastic reduction of his Fio_2.

- Keep neck opening from being obstructed with towels, toys, and blankets so that gas flow can flush carbon dioxide from the hood.

- When an outside heating source is not used, the temperature is usually kept at 29–34 C, and this range produces a small amount of condensation.

- Observe for buildup of condensation in the delivery tubing and empty as needed.

- To prevent an increase in oxygen consumption, the gas should be warmed and humidified when it is delivered to the neonate.

- When a heated humidifier is used with the hood, check the hood temperature frequently and maintain the range between 34 and 36 C, or as prescribed. For premature infants, keep the hood as close to body temperature as possible.

- Add sterile solution to the humidifier or nebulizer as necessary.

- Keep tubing free of condensation buildup.

- Use an oxygen analyzer (see page 350) to ensure that oxygen concentrations are within the prescribed range.

Incubator (Isolette)

Description

Self-contained, clear unit with access portholes for giving nursing care. Can deliver up to 40%–60% concentrations of oxygen.

Uses

For newborn, especially premature, infants for whom oxygen therapy, controlled temperature, and humidity are desired. Can also provide infant isolation.

Nursing Considerations

- When portholes are open, oxygen concentration can drop drastically. Open portholes only as necessary.

- Use oxygen analyzer (see page 350) to assess concentrations of oxygen.

- To be assured of delivering oxygen concentrations greater than 40%, oxygen hoods must be used in conjunction with the unit.

- When humidity is used, change sheets often. Dampness contributes to respiratory complications and bacterial growth.

- Monitor incubator temperature to keep within 34–36 C, or as prescribed. Attach temperature probe to infant with hypoallergenic tape.

- When the incubator is unplugged, keep the portholes open to prevent buildup of carbon dioxide, and provide external oxygen.

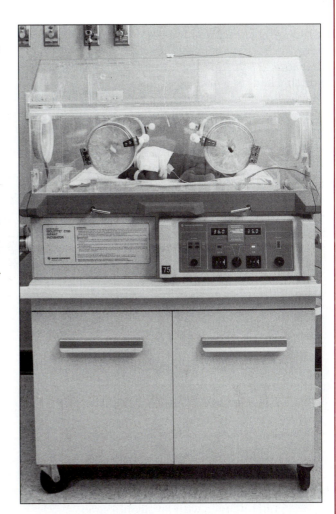

NURSING GUIDELINES: DEVICES USED IN THE DELIVERY OF OXYGEN, HUMIDITY, AND AEROSOLS (continued)

Oxygen Analyzer

Description

Although there are many types of units that vary in design and operational principle, each is portable and used at the bedside to draw in the client's environmental oxygen via a sampling tube.

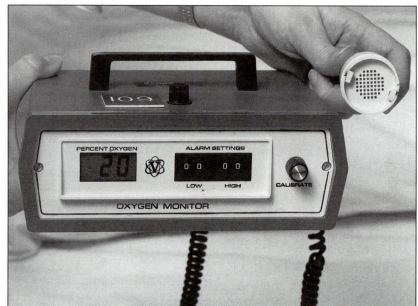

Uses

Each unit measures the concentration of oxygen being delivered in such devices as tents, hoods, and incubators to ensure that the client is receiving the prescribed FiO_2.

Nursing Considerations

- Before monitoring the client's oxygen concentration, measure the room air to ensure that the unit calibrates to 0.21 (21%). Adjust the dial, if necessary, to achieve this reading.

- When measuring oxygen concentrations with the device described in this section, position the sampling tube next to the client's nose.

- If necessary, adjust the flow rate to achieve the prescribed FiO_2.

- When the unit is used from client to client, clean the sampling tube with an alcohol swab.

NURSING GUIDELINES: DEVICES USED IN THE DELIVERY OF OXYGEN, HUMIDITY, AND AEROSOLS (continued)

Attachments and Devices Used to Administer Aerosol Therapy

Aerosol Face Mask

Description

Plastic face mask with two large exhalation ports, which connects the client to a humidifier or nebulizer.

Uses

Supplies client with warmed and moistened room air or oxygen, which prevents drying of tracheal secretions and liquefies thickened secretions.

Nursing Considerations

- Observe for visible and constant mist or vapor, which indicates adequate humidification is being delivered. Increase the flow rate if mist disappears during inspiration.

- Observe for condensation buildup in the tubing and empty as necessary.

- Keep nebulizer or humidifier supplied with adequate levels of sterile solution. Discard residual solution before replenishing the fluid reservoir.

- If using heated humidity, check the temperature frequently to prevent injury to the respiratory tract. Keep within 34–36 C, or as prescribed.

- Assess for increased secretion production and encourage coughing. Suction as necessary.

- Pad bony prominences and behind ears to prevent skin breakdown.

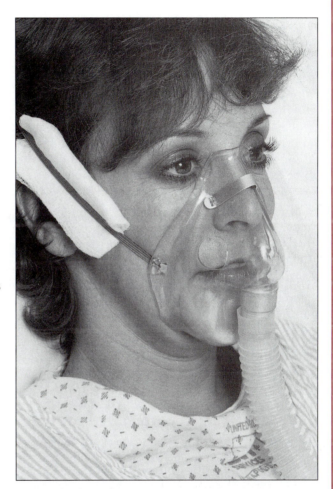

- To ensure adequate delivery of aerosol, mask should fit snugly.

- Clean mask with warm, soapy water as needed.

→

NURSING GUIDELINES: DEVICES USED IN THE DELIVERY OF OXYGEN, HUMIDITY, AND AEROSOLS (continued)

Tracheostomy Collar

Description

Lightweight plastic device that connects the client's tracheostomy to a humidification source. It is positioned directly over the tracheostomy and secured in place with an elastic strap.

Uses

Supplies client with warmed and moistened room air or oxygen, which prevents drying of tracheal secretions and liquefies thickened secretions. It also can be used to deliver aerosolized medications.

Nursing Considerations

- Observe for visible and constant mist or vapor, which indicates adequate humidification is being delivered.

- Observe for condensation buildup in tubing and empty prn or at least q2h and as necessary, especially before turning the client.

- The trachea can be suctioned directly through the frontal port.

- Keep humidification source supplied with adequate levels of sterile solution. Discard residual fluid before replenishing the fluid reservoir.

- When using heated humidity, check the temperature frequently to prevent injury to the trachea. Keep within range of 34–36 C, or as prescribed.

- Assess for increased secretion production and encourage coughing. Suction as necessary.

- Clean collar with warm, soapy water as needed.

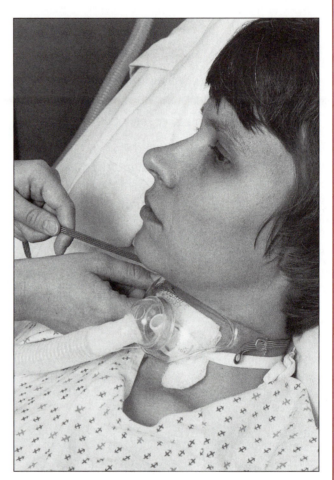

NURSING GUIDELINES: DEVICES USED IN THE DELIVERY OF OXYGEN, HUMIDITY, AND AEROSOLS (continued)

T-Piece

Description

Lightweight plastic tube that connects the client's tracheostomy or endotracheal tube to a humidification or oxygen source via a center connection.

Uses

Same as tracheostomy collar, but also can be connected to an endotracheal tube.

Nursing Considerations

* The reservoir tube on the downstream side of the T-piece allows for the accumulation of oxygen so that the client receives a consistent oxygen concentration with each inspiration.

* Keep T-piece in proper alignment to prevent undue pressure on the stoma.

* Keep exhalation (downstream) end of tube unobstructed.

* Visible and constant mist produced in the device indicates adequate humidification.

* Observe for condensation buildup in tubing and empty frequently, especially before turning the client.

* If attached to a Venturi, it can function as high-flow system.

* Clean the center connection as necessary with hydrogen peroxide to prevent it from sticking to the tracheostomy.

* Keep humidification source supplied with a sterile solution. Discard residual fluid before replenishing fluid reservoir.

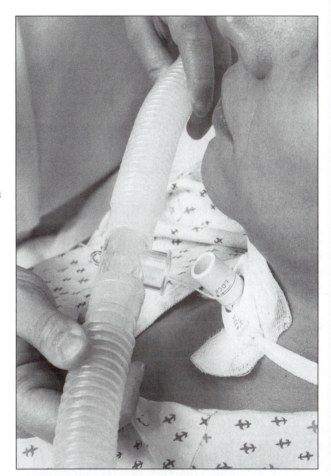

* When using heated humidity, monitor temperature frequently to prevent damage to trachea. Keep within 34–36 C, or as prescribed.

* Assess for increased secretion production and encourage coughing. Suction as necessary.

MONITORING OXYGEN SATURATION USING PULSE OXIMETRY

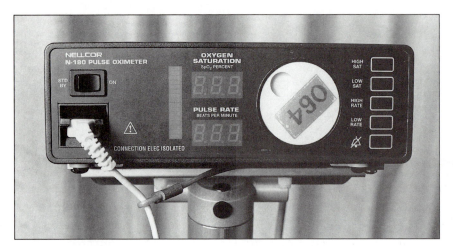

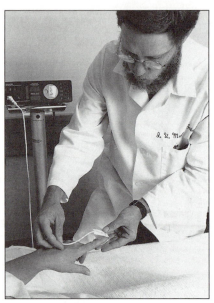

Pulse oximetry (abbreviated SpO_2) is a safe, noninvasive diagnostic tool that measures and continuously displays the oxygen saturation of arterial blood on a monitor. A probe, which is generally attached to the client's finger, measures red and infrared wavelengths of light to calculate oxygen saturation, using the difference between the light that is transmitted and the light that is absorbed by the client's red blood cells.

A normal reading is greater than or equal to 90%. Factors that can influence accuracy of this reading include altered body temperature, anemia, cigarette and cigar smoking, and smoke inhalation injury. The physician may prescribe ABG measurement when initiating pulse oximetry for baseline comparison. Arterial saturation values via ABG analysis should be within 2% of the oxygen saturation value obtained with pulse oximetry.

1 Before initiating pulse oximetry, select a finger that is warm and has brisk capillary refill (less than 2 seconds). Remove nail polish if indicated. Detach the backing from the self-adhesive probe and attach the probe to the client's finger with the wire positioned uppermost (as shown). *Note: The probe also may be attached to a toe (particularly in the pediatric population) or earlobe (eg, with the burn clients).*

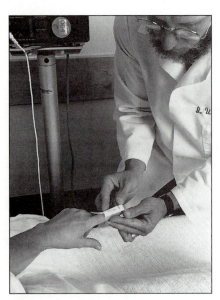

2 Secure the probe snugly to the finger to prevent ambient light from affecting the readings.

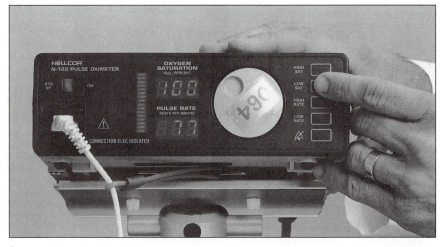

3 Turn the monitor on. Set high and low saturation alarm limits as prescribed and high and low heart rate alarm limits 10% above and below your client's baseline heart rate.

Remove the probe at least daily to assess the underlying skin for redness caused by exposure to the infrared lights. Change the site accordingly.

CONVERTING A NONREBREATHING MASK TO A PARTIAL REBREATHING MASK

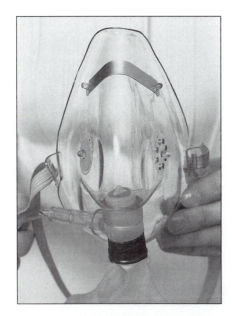 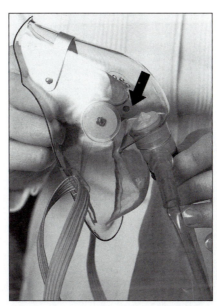 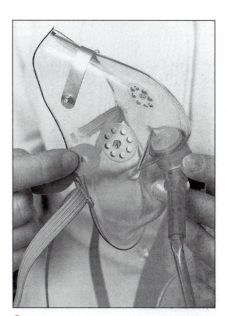

The difference between a nonrebreathing mask and a partial rebreathing mask is that the former has two rubber disks. One disk occludes one of the exhalation ports, and the other occludes the port between the mask and the reservoir bag. These disks allow for the exhalation of gas while also minimizing the inhalation of room air. When it is no longer necessary for the client to receive the higher concentration of oxygen that is provided by the nonrebreathing mask, the physician might prescribe a partial rebreathing mask. You can easily convert the client's existing mask to a partial rebreather.

1 Begin by removing the rubber disk at the port between the mask and the reservoir bag.

2 Remove the rubber disk at the exhalation port. Save the disks in the event your client might again need the higher oxygen concentrations that require reconversion to a nonrebreathing mask.

ASSEMBLING A VENTURI DELIVERY SYSTEM

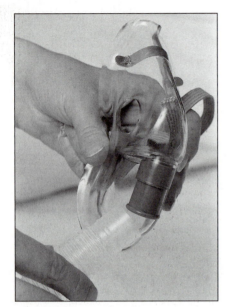

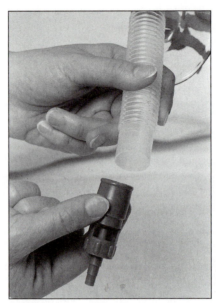

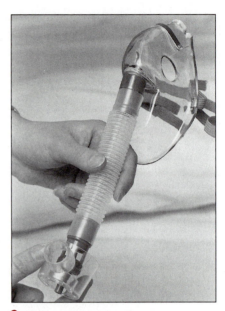

1 A Venturi mask comes prepackaged with a 15- to 20-cm (6- to 8-in) wide-bore tube, a humidification adapter, and a variety of jets or adapters that are usually color-coded to coincide with the prescribed concentration of oxygen. To assemble a Venturi mask, attach the wide-bore tubing to the mask's adapter.

2 The lower hand in the photograph holds the jet adapter. The size of the jet's opening determines the delivered concentration of oxygen. Slide the jet into the open end of the wide-bore tubing. Keep the remaining jets at your client's bedside in case the physician prescribes a different oxygen concentration at a later time. Most manufacturers imprint the adapters with concentration and recommended liter flow, for example, 24% (4–6 L/min).

3 Attach the humidity adapter to the jet, regardless of whether or not humidity has been prescribed. The adapter will prevent the jet adapter's air entrainment ports from becoming occluded by blankets or the client's body.

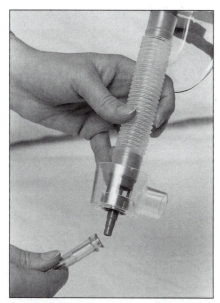

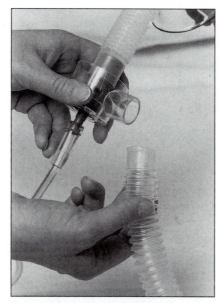

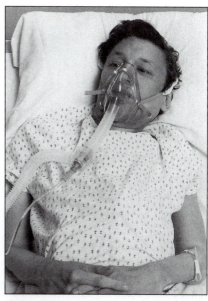

4 Attach the oxygen tubing to the jet's nipple, and the other end of the tubing to the oxygen flowmeter. Adjust the flowmeter to the level prescribed on the nipple.

5 If humidification has been prescribed, attach one end of the wide-bore tubing to the humidity adapter, and the other end to the humidifier or nebulizer.

6 Apply the Venturi mask to your client. The client in this photograph is wearing a Venturi mask that is attached to humidity. The system also can attach to a T-piece for a client with a tracheostomy.

SETTING UP AN OXYGEN SYSTEM WITH HUMIDIFICATION

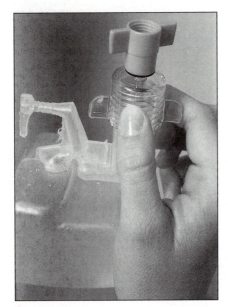

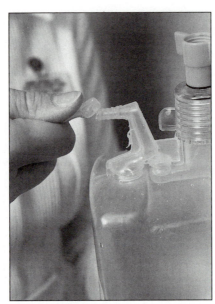

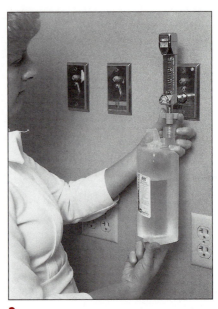

1 Follow these steps to deliver humidified oxygen to your client. A disposable humidifier is used here, but the principles are basically the same if you are using a reusable humidifier. Attach the adapter to the humidifier. The adapter is usually packaged with the disposable humidifier.

2 Snap off the seal from the outlet port of the humidifier.

3 Connect the humidifier to the flowmeter via the adapter, being careful not to cross-thread the connection.

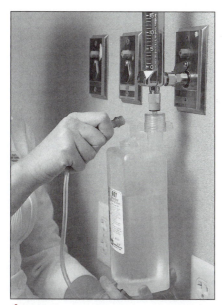

4 Connect small-bore oxygen tubing to the outlet port of the humidifier bottle.

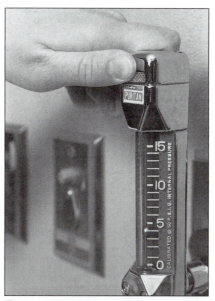

5 Adjust the flowmeter to the prescribed number of liters of oxygen per minute.

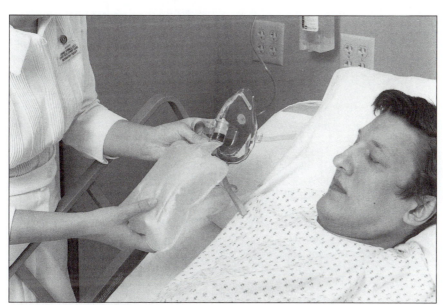

6 You are now ready to attach the distal end of the oxygen tubing to one of the following: simple oxygen mask, nasal cannula, partial rebreathing mask, or to a nonrebreathing mask as shown here.

DELIVERING HEATED HUMIDITY

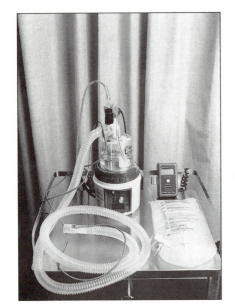

1 A heated servo-controlled humidifier can be used to deliver heated humidity with or without oxygen. In this photo, wide-bore tubing is attached to deliver the humidity. In addition, the reservoir is filled with sterile water. If oxygen also has been prescribed for your client, you will need to attach one end of the small-bore oxygen tubing to the oxygen flowmeter and the other end to the oxygen port of the system. Remember to adjust the flowmeter to achieve the prescribed Fio$_2$.

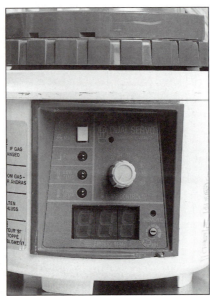

2 Set the temperature control dial to the prescribed temperature (usually as close to body temperature as possible).

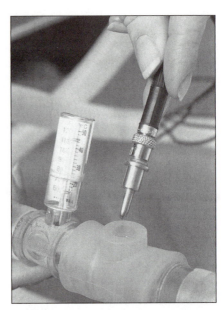

3 The other end of the probe attaches to a rubber adapter, as close to the client's airway as is feasible. The unit will automatically heat and turn off, as needed, to maintain the preset temperature. If the heat surpasses that which you have set on the temperature-control dial, or in the event of an equipment malfunction, an alarm will sound. You can now attach the free end of the wide-bore tubing to an oxygen hood, tracheostomy collar, or T-piece.

ASSEMBLING A NEBULIZER

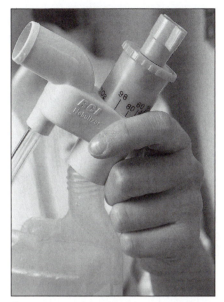

1 A common method for the delivery of aerosol therapy is the use of a pneumatic (jet) nebulizer as outlined in these steps. The first step is to attach a Venturi adapter to the nebulizer bottle.

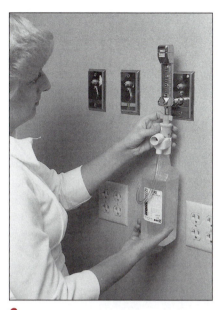

2 Attach the assembled nebulizer to the flowmeter, which is plugged into compressed air.

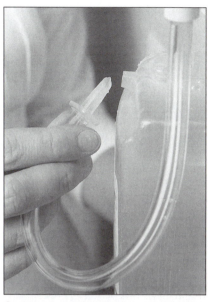

3 This Venturi adapter has a small tube that collects condensation. Connect it to the small outlet on the front of the nebulizer, after first snapping off the outlet's seal.

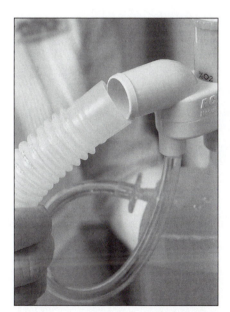

4 Attach wide-bore tubing to the outlet of the Venturi adapter.

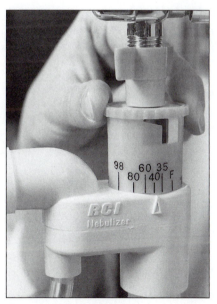

5 If you also will be delivering oxygen, adjust the Venturi dial to the prescribed oxygen concentration. If oxygen has not been prescribed, set the dial to "F" (for flush).

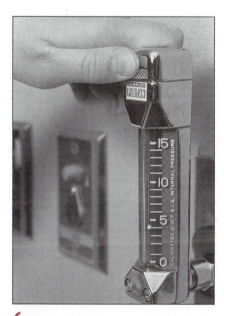

6 Adjust the flowmeter until a visible mist is produced at the distal end of the tubing. The flowmeter is usually turned to its maximum level to ensure adequate gas flow to the client.

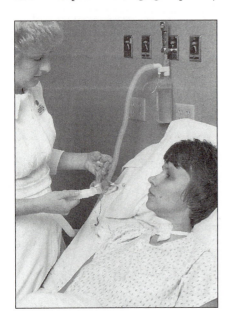

7 Connect the distal end of the tubing to an aerosol mask, to a T-piece, or to a tracheostomy collar (as shown).

←

8 The tubing also can be connected to the high humidity adapter of a Venturi mask. Check to make sure the client is receiving adequate gas flow from the nebulizer. Mist should be visible from the delivery device during inspiration and exhalation. If mist is not visible, increase the liter flow by adjusting the flowmeter.

→

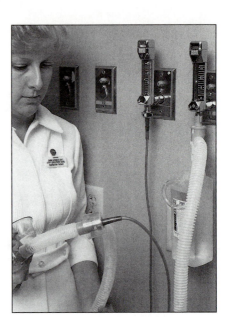

EMPLOYING TECHNIQUES FOR LUNG INFLATION

INSTRUCTING CLIENTS IN DEEP-BREATHING EXERCISES

Teaching Apical Expansion Exercises: Clients who will benefit from this exercise are those who might be restricting their upper chest movement because of splinting from pain—for example, clients who have had a lobectomy, mastectomy, or gross pleural effusion. Position your fingers below the clavicles and apply moderate pressure. Instruct the client to inhale while pushing his chest upward and forward, expanding against your finger pressure. Encourage him to retain the expansion for a few moments and then exhale quietly and passively. Once you have taught him the technique, he can perform the exercise on his own by positioning his fingers over the same area. When done correctly and frequently, apical expansion will help reexpand remaining lung tissue, eliminate secretions, and minimize flattening of the upper chest wall.

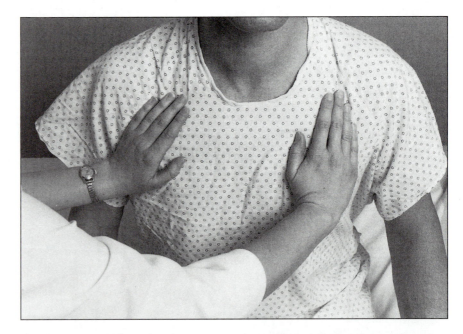

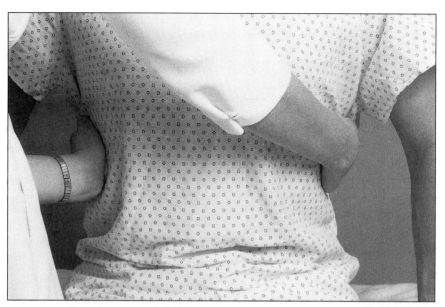

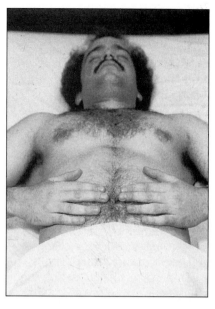

Teaching Basal Expansion Exercises:
Lower thoracic exercises are frequently indicated for clients recovering from chest surgery, for whom pain on the affected side inhibits bilateral chest movement. Position your hands on the midaxillary lines in the area of the eighth ribs, and apply moderate pressure as the client inhales. Instruct the client to attempt to move your hands outward as he expands his lower ribs. He should retain his maximum inhalation for 1 or 2 seconds to help promote aeration of his alveoli, and then exhale in a relaxed, passive manner. Clients with COPD, especially, should be closely observed for both a slow, relaxed exhalation and a relaxed upper chest. Encourage clients to perform the exercise on their own by using the palms of their hands. When practiced frequently and correctly, this technique will promote and maintain lower chest wall mobility.

Teaching Diaphragmatic Breathing:
Your clients will breathe more efficiently and obtain better lung function when correctly using their abdominal muscles and diaphragms.

To instruct the client in diaphragmatic breathing, have him assume a supine position and flex his knees to relax the abdominal wall. He should then place his hands over his abdomen and breathe in deeply and slowly through his nose as he pushes his abdomen outward. If he does this correctly, his hands will rise during the inspiration. The exhalation should be quiet and passive, with the lower ribs and abdomen sinking downward as the abdomen relaxes. Once the client has been taught diaphragmatic breathing while supine, he may then assume other positions for practicing this technique. Emphasize the need for frequent and regular practice until breathing in this manner becomes automatic and no longer requires a conscious effort. *Note: Clients with COPD should be taught to inhale through the nose and exhale slowly through pursed (puckered) lips. This will help to minimize small airway collapse.*

ASSISTING WITH COUGHING

Teaching clients an effective, controlled cough is essential in the management of bronchial secretions, and it should be taught to all clients before surgery. Instruct the client to sit with her upper body flexed slightly forward. If this position is contraindicated, she can assume a lateral position, with flexed knees and hips. Either position will promote a forceful cough, while also minimizing strain in the lower back. First, instruct the client to take two or three deep breaths with passive exhalation. She should then take a deep breath, hold it briefly, and cough forcefully.

An alternative method is the "double cough" technique, which is especially recommended for clients with COPD in whom one very forceful cough could cause small airway collapse. The client is instructed to cough from the midinspiratory point rather than from the point of deep inspiration. The client exhales in a rapid

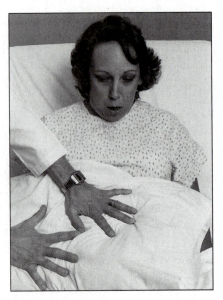 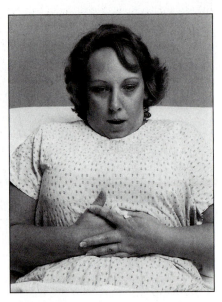

succession of two or more abrupt, sharp coughs. The first cough loosens secretions, and the following cough or coughs facilitate the movement of the secretions toward the upper airway.

To minimize pain, a postoperative client will require splinting over her incisional area during the coughing process. A pillow can be pressed over the affected area (left), or you can show the client how to splint her own incision by pressing the arm and hand of the unaffected side against the site (right).

USING INCENTIVE SPIROMETERS

Assessing

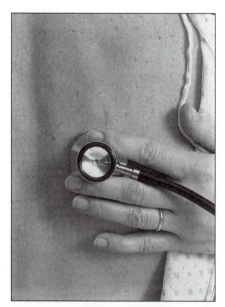

1 Auscultate the client's lung fields to establish a baseline for post-exercise comparison. Explain the procedure in detail. Many clients incorrectly exhale rather than inhale during the exercise. Incentive spirometry is a goal-oriented and measurable breathing exercise that helps clients increase their inspiratory volume while also inflating their alveoli.

Planning and Implementing

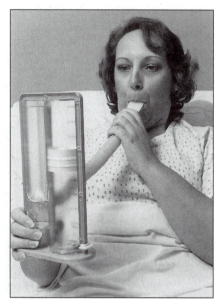

2 Many disposable incentive spirometers have pointers that you can slide to the prescribed inspiratory volume level. Check the operating instructions on the unit used by your agency. Instruct the client to hold the unit upright because tilting it will make the exercise less challenging. She should complete a normal exhalation and then seal her lips tightly around the mouthpiece while inhaling slowly and deeply until the desired volume is reached. Encourage the client to sustain the inspiration for at least 3 seconds. Optimum results can be achieved if the client uses incentive spirometry at least hourly while awake for 10–20 breaths and over a 72-hour period.

Evaluating

3 Auscultate the client's lung fields for postexercise breath sounds, and compare them to your earlier assessment. Compare inspired volumes to previous measured volumes, and document the procedure and the client's response.

ASSISTING WITH IPPB

Assessing and Planning

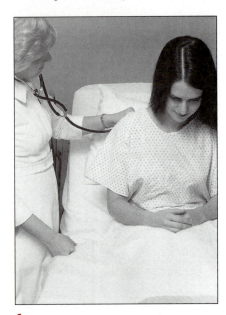 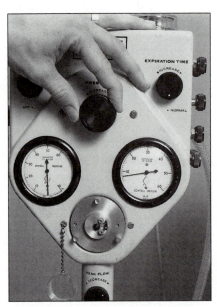 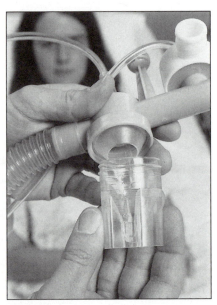

1 If IPPB has been prescribed for your client, explain to the client that this treatment will assist her in achieving deep lung inflation while also promoting expectoration of secretions. To facilitate lung expansion, assist her into Fowler's position, unless it is contraindicated. If a pain medication has been prescribed to precede the therapy, begin the procedure 30 minutes after administering the drug. Assess the baseline status of the client's respiratory system before initiating the therapy.

2 Turn the pressure control knob to achieve the prescribed amount of tidal volume or pressure.

3 Fill the nebulizer with the prescribed medication with diluent, and reattach it. *Note: Some bronchodilators, such as metaproterenol, significantly alter the heart rate. Monitor the client's pulse rate frequently throughout the therapy and record the pretreatment and posttreatment measurements. Stay with the client throughout the treatment.*

Implementing

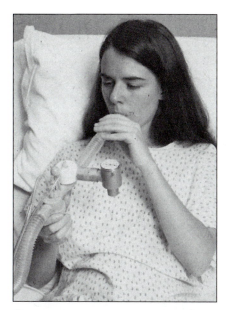

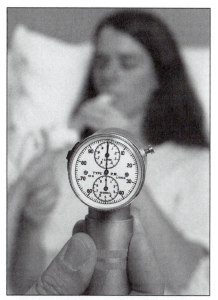

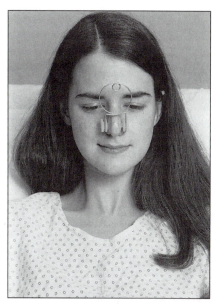

4 Instruct the client to place her lips tightly around the mouthpiece and inhale to cycle the unit on. The client should breathe with the machine until it cycles off. At that time she should hold her breath for 3–5 seconds and then exhale passively through the mouthpiece. Observe for adequate chest expansion with each inhalation, and make sure the exhalations are relaxed and passive. Forced exhalations can further increase small airway obstruction. Encourage both diaphragmatic breathing and coughing during the treatment. Treatment continues until all medication is delivered (10–20 breaths).

5 To determine whether your client is receiving adequate deep lung inflations during the therapy, a measuring device such as the Wright respirometer will measure the index of her expired tidal volume. It connects to the expiratory port of the IPPB manifold. (See its attachment to the manifold in the preceding photograph.)

6 If your client cannot avoid breathing through her nose during the treatment, have her hold her nose or provide her with nose clips. However, once she becomes accustomed to the therapy and no longer breathes through her nose, she might no longer need them.

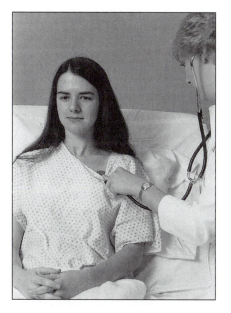

Evaluating

7 When the treatment has been completed, auscultate the lung fields to assess for improved aeration and absent or diminished adventitious sounds. Document the procedure, noting the client's response to the therapy, as well as the amount and character of the expectorated secretions.

PERFORMING CHEST PHYSIOTHERAPY

PERCUSSING, VIBRATING, AND DRAINING THE ADULT

Assessing and Planning

1 Auscultate your client's lung fields to assess breath sounds and monitor the rate and depth of the respirations to provide a baseline for posttreatment assessment. Note the presence and location of retained secretions. Be especially alert to diminished, absent, or bronchial breath sounds, which are indicative of obstructed airways and reduced airflow caused by retained sections. Then palpate for bilateral thoracic expansion and percuss for areas of dullness. Thoroughly explain each step, and demonstrate the techniques you will use during the procedure. Clients with chronic lung diseases may need to perform the procedure on their own after discharge. Therefore, they should be able to demonstrate the process to you prior to discharge. Provide an

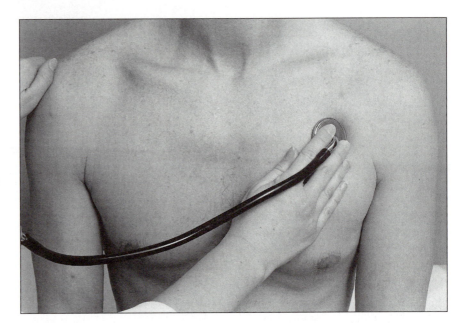

emesis basin and tissues for expectoration of secretions. To minimize the potential for vomiting and discomfort, the procedure should be performed either before meals or at least 1 hour after eating. Ensure that you percuss and vibrate over a thin layer of clothing or a towel to avoid traumatizing the skin.

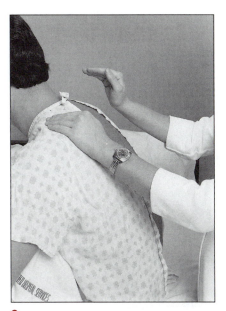 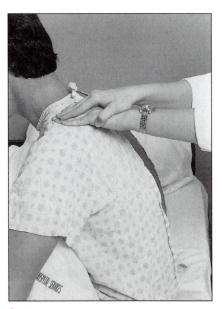 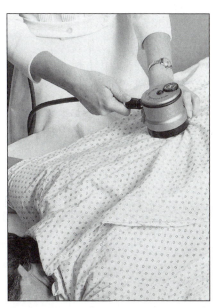

2 *Understanding Percussion (Clapping):* Percussion is performed by clapping cupped hands alternately and in rapid sequence over a lung segment. Cupping the hand provides a trapped pocket of air that will transmit vibrations through the chest wall to the secretions, thereby loosening or dislodging them. Your elbows should be flexed and the wrists relaxed to achieve a rapid, popping action. Although percussion is a noisy procedure, it should not be painful to the client. It is performed during inhalation and exhalation while the client deep breathes.

3 *Understanding Vibration:* Vibration or shaking is often performed in conjunction with percussion as an aid to segmental drainage by loosening secretions and propelling them into the larger bronchi. Flatten your hands, and position them one on top of the other over a lung segment. With straight arms, lean into the client's chest, using moderate pressure. Alternately contract and relax your shoulder and upper arm muscles to produce a vibratory shaking. Vibrate for approximately 10 seconds per exhalation as the client exhales slowly and completely.

4 *Using Mechanical Percussors/Vibrators:* The use of a mechanical percussor is often indicated for clients in critical care areas who are connected to external equipment or for whom hand percussion is intolerable or too painful.

Implementing

Positioning Your Client for Segmental Bronchial Drainage: The physician might prescribe some or all of the following positions, with or without percussion and vibration, to drain the loosened secretions out of the client's lung, preventing them from repooling or draining into healthy lung segments. Many of the positions will need modification for clients with compromised cardiac, neurologic, or pulmonary conditions. A complete sequence for percussion, vibration, and drainage, however, will consist of the following: (1) Have the client assume the prescribed position(s) for 5–15 minutes, or until secretions can be expectorated; (2) percuss the involved lung segments for 2–3 minutes each; (3) vibrate for at least two or three exhalations, depending on the client's secretion viscosity; (4) encourage coughing and expectoration or suction as needed; (5) change to the next position, if others have been prescribed.

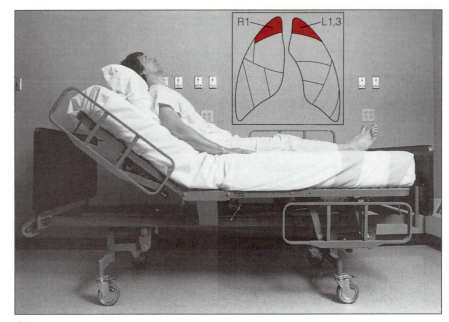

5 To drain the apical segments of the upper lobes, position your client so that he is reclining at a 30-degree angle. Percuss and vibrate the segments between the clavicles and the scapulae.

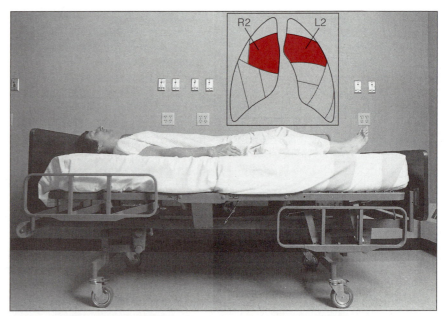

6 To drain the anterior segments of the upper lobes, the client should be supine, with knees flexed for comfort and effective breathing. Percuss and vibrate the segments between the clavicles and nipples.

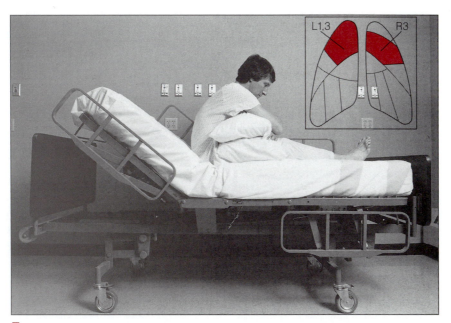

7 To drain the posterior segments of the upper lobes, instruct the client to lean forward over two pillows to achieve a 30-degree angle. Percuss and vibrate over the upper back, near but not over the scapulae.

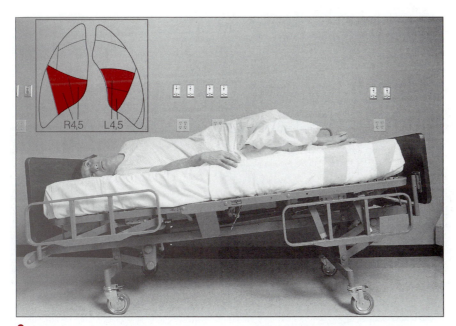

8 To drain the lateral and medial segments of the right middle lobe, raise the foot of the bed around 15 degrees. The client should lie on his left side and then rotate a quarter turn toward his back. Place a pillow under his back to support his position. Percuss and vibrate over the uppermost nipple. If your client is a female, cup your hand under the axilla and extend your fingers forward, beneath her breast. Repeat after having the client lie on the right side and rotate a quarter turn toward the back (as shown). This drains the lingular segments of the left upper lobe. *Caution: A head-down position is usually contraindicated for clients with increased intracranial pressure, known intracranial disease, hypertension, and hemodynamic instability.*

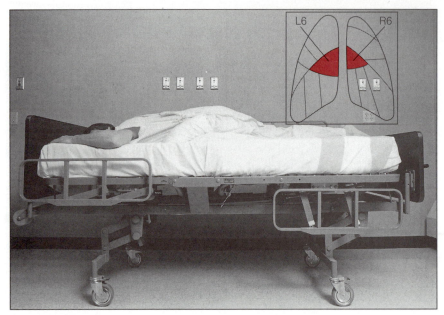

9 To drain the superior segments of both lower lobes, the client should assume a prone position, with two pillows under the hips. Percuss and vibrate over the middle of his back at the tips of the scapulae.

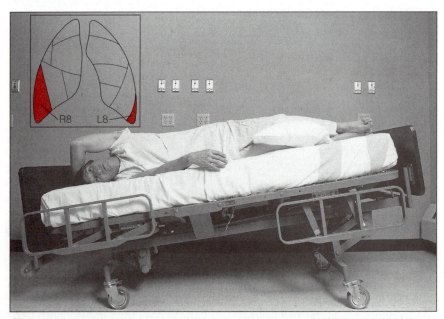

10 To drain the anterior basal segments of the lower lobes, raise the foot of the bed approximately 30 degrees. Instruct the client to lie on his side with a pillow between his knees and to place his upper arm over his head. Percuss and vibrate under the axillae over the lower ribs. The photograph depicts the position for draining the left anterior basal segment.

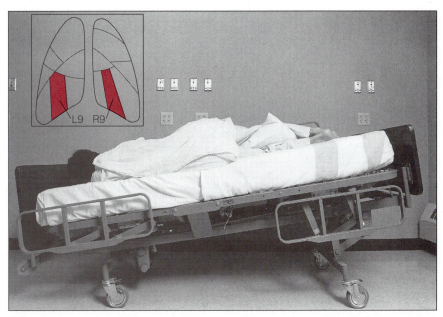

11 To drain the lateral basal segments of the lower lobes, raise the foot of the bed approximately 30 degrees. Have the client lie on his abdomen and rotate the upper half of his body a quarter turn toward his side. Percuss and vibrate over the lower ribs on his lateral chest. After he assumes the corresponding position on his opposite side, percuss and vibrate that segment. The photograph depicts the position for draining the right lateral segment.

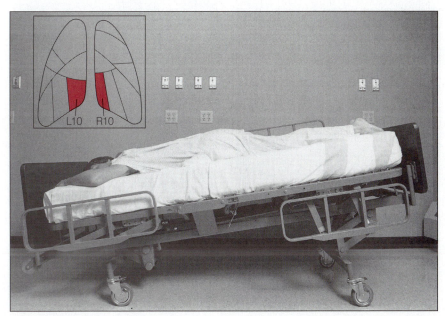

12 To drain the posterior basal segments of the lower lobes, raise the foot of the bed around 30 degrees. Have the client lie on his abdomen with two pillows under his hips. Percuss and vibrate the segment over the lower ribs on both sides of his spine, but avoid the area over the kidneys.

Evaluating

13 Auscultate the client's lung fields and monitor the rate and depth of his respirations to evaluate the results of the treatment. Optimally, improved aeration will result in improved breath sounds and a respiratory rate within normal limits. Document the procedure and the client's response. Note the amount, color, and character of his expectoration. Provide him with mouthwash or other oral hygiene.

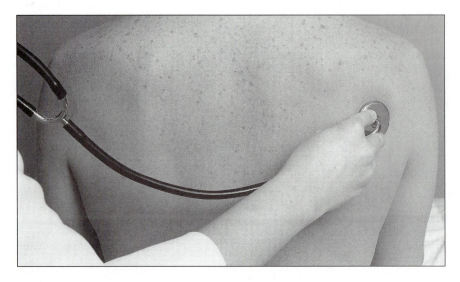

PERCUSSING, VIBRATING, AND DRAINING THE INFANT OR SMALL CHILD

Assessing and Planning

1 Review the process for percussing, vibrating, and draining the adult, but follow these variations for the infant or small child. Infants will better tolerate the procedure just prior to feeding. Before initiating the therapy, hold and comfort the infant for a while. At all times, speak reassuringly to help minimize the fear and anxiety he will experience, especially during percussion and while in head-down positions. Develop a rapport with the small child, and if possible, first demonstrate the procedure on one of his favorite dolls or stuffed animals. Percussion and vibration, if prescribed, should be less forceful and vigorous for infants and children than for adults.

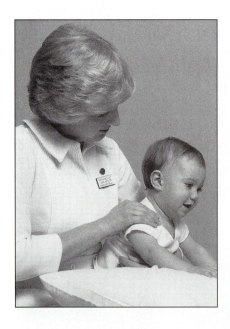

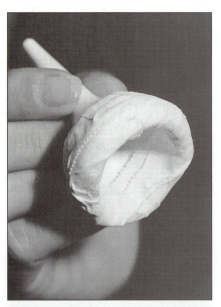

2 If a child is too small for hand percussion, consider cutting a bulb syringe in half, dissecting as if you were slicing a globe at the equator, and taping the cut surfaces to make it smooth (shown). Percuss while holding onto the nozzle. To make an infant's vibrator, remove the toothbrush from a portable electric toothbrush and tape padding over its vibrating surface.

Implementing

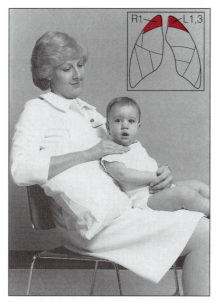

3 To drain the apical segments of the upper lobes, position the child so that he is reclining at a 30-degree angle, and place a pillow between the two of you. Percuss and vibrate the segments between the clavicles and scapulae.

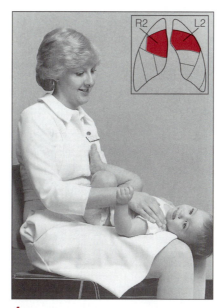

4 To drain the anterior segments of the upper lobes, position the child so that he is supine. Then percuss and vibrate the segments between the clavicles and nipples. If you have determined the need for suctioning, use a bulb syringe as demonstrated on page 231.

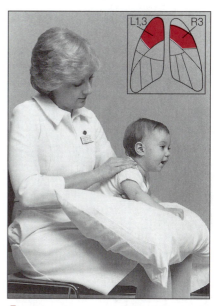

5 To drain the posterior segments of the upper lobes, lean the child forward at about a 30-degree angle; percuss and vibrate the upper back on both sides.

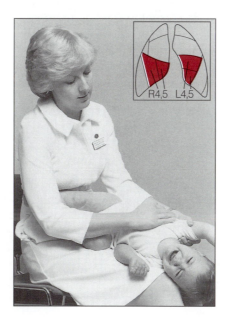

6 To drain the lateral and medial segments of the right middle lobe, position the child as shown so that he is on the left side, with his head down at 15-degree angle. Then rotate the child toward his back a quarter turn and percuss and vibrate over the uppermost nipple. Turn the child to the corresponding position on the opposite side to drain the lingular segments of the left upper lobe.

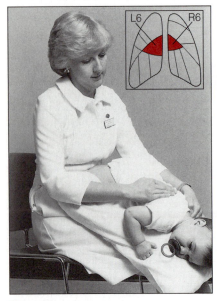

7 To drain the superior segments of the lower lobes, position the child on his abdomen, over a pillow. Percuss and vibrate on each side of the spine, below the tips of the scapulae.

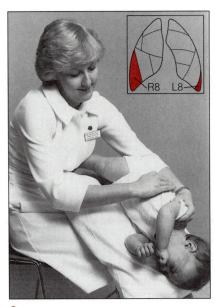

8 To drain the anterior basal segments of the lower lobes, extend your legs and position the child on a pillow so that his head is down approximately 30 degrees and he is on his side. Percuss and vibrate the segments over the lower ribs beneath the axillae. Turn the child to the opposite side, and repeat the procedure.

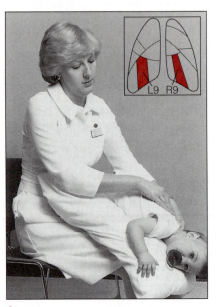

9 To drain the lateral basal segments of the lower lobes, place the child in a prone position, with his head down approximately 30 degrees. Rotate the upper half of the body a quarter turn toward the side. Percuss and vibrate over the lower ribs. Repeat the procedure after rotating the child to the opposite side.

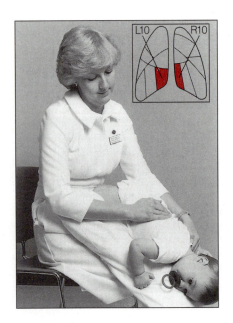

10 To drain the posterior basal segments of the lower lobes, position the child so that he is prone, with his head lowered 30 degrees. Percuss and vibrate over the lower ribs on each side of the spine, avoiding the area over the kidneys.

11 *Evaluating:* See step 13, page 374.

Managing the Client with a Chest Tube

NURSING GUIDELINES: DISPOSABLE CLOSED CHEST DRAINAGE SYSTEM

A disposable closed chest drainage system attaches to a chest tube to relieve pressure from a buildup of air or fluid in the pleural space. For example, clients who have had thoracic trauma with concomitant pleural tears, a spontaneous pneumothorax, or a hemothorax will require a chest tube and closed chest drainage. In this section we are showing a Pleur-evac® dry suction control system.

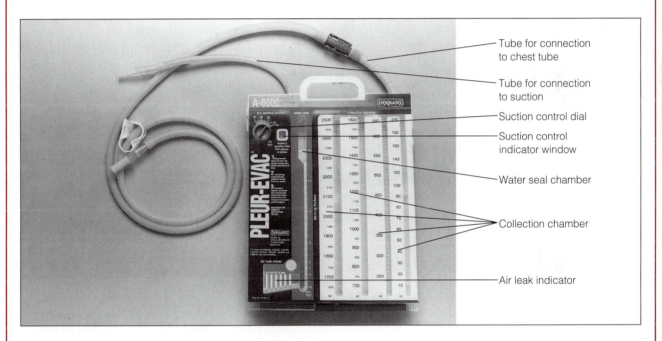

Tube for connection to chest tube

Tube for connection to suction

Suction control dial

Suction control indicator window

Water seal chamber

Collection chamber

Air leak indicator

Suction Control

- Attach the closed chest drainage system to the suction source using the short tubing.

- Set the suction control dial to the prescribed setting, usually 20–25 cm for the adult and 10–20 cm for the pediatric population.

- Turn on the suction source and increase the suction until the orange float appears in the suction control indicator window. ***Note:*** *The suction con-trol dial, not the suction source, controls the amount of suction.*

- If the system is attached to dry suction, be sure the suction control dial is set at the prescribed level. The suction is working appropriately when the float is visible in the suction control indicator window.

➤

NURSING GUIDELINES: DISPOSABLE CLOSED CHEST DRAINAGE SYSTEM (continued)

Water Seal Chamber

- Fluctuations (tidaling) in this chamber occur normally during inhalation and exhalation until the lung reexpands and the client no longer requires chest drainage.

- Fluctuations in water level greater than 6 cm per respiration could mean the client has copious secretions or increased work of breathing due to low compliance. Assess the client for indicators of increased work of breathing and auscultate the lung fields for breath sounds. If congestion is noted, encourage coughing, turning, and deep breathing to facilitate secretion expectoration, and suction if necessary.

- A cessation in water level fluctuations prior to lung reexpansion could mean the tubing is either kinked or occluded, or that one of the connection sites is loose. Ask the client to cough and change positions. Check for kinks, and inspect the connection sites for integrity.

- Bubbling in the chamber labeled air leak indicator is normal if the client has an air leak, for example, from a pneumothorax. However, once the tear in the client's lung tissue begins to seal over, the bubbling should lessen. If continuous bubbling occurs in the chamber after it has had only occasional bubbling, assess the client's respiratory status. If the client's respirations and lung sounds are normal for the client, follow these steps to find the leak:

  1. Squeeze the chest tube at the insertion site, but for no longer than a second or two to prevent pressure buildup in the chest. If the bubbling stops, air may be entering the chest from the insertion site. Palpate around the insertion site, and if leakage is noted, apply tape to the area to reinforce the air-occlusive seal.

  2. If the bubbling continues as you squeeze the chest tube, the leak is in the tubing or within the drainage system itself. Squeeze the connection between the chest tube and the long rubber tube. If the bubbling stops, reinforce the juncture with tape or replace the tubing.

  3. Bubbling that continues means the fault is within the drainage system itself, and it should be replaced with a new system.

Collection Chamber

- Monitor the drainage every 30 minutes for the first 2 hours after chest tube insertion, then hourly for the next 24 hours, and every 2 hours thereafter.

- Mark the level of drainage directly on the chamber every 8 hours with the time and date.

- Drainage greater than 100 mL/hour is considered excessive, and the physician should be alerted immediately.

- Cessation in drainage can mean either the client's lung has reexpanded or the tubing is kinked or occluded with tissue or blood.

MONITORING THE CLIENT WITH A CHEST TUBE

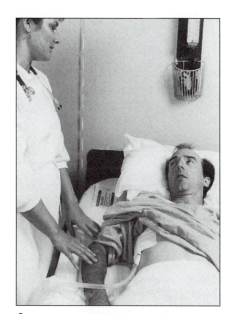

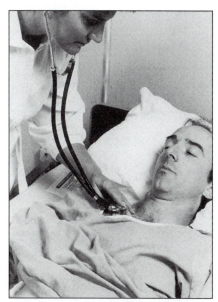

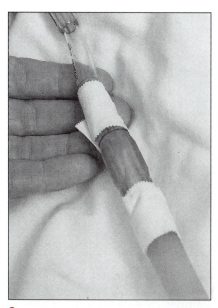

1 Assess the client for comfort, and administer pain medications as prescribed. Keep a petrolatum gauze pad within easy reach so that you can apply pressure with an air-occlusive material in case the chest tube becomes dislodged from the client's chest. Unless contraindicated, keep the client in semi-Fowler's position for his comfort and to facilitate drainage. Monitor the closed chest drainage system by following the guidelines on pages 377–378.

Know your agency's policy regarding clamping a chest tube. Some specialists say the chest tube should not be clamped for any reason until the client's condition has improved enough for the tube to be removed; others believe there are special indications for clamping, such as a disconnection between the chest tube and the drainage tubing.

2 Auscultate your client's lung fields for breath sounds and monitor the vital signs to assess for signs of respiratory distress. Recognize the indications of acute pneumothorax: sharp, stabbing pain on the affected side; shortness of breath; and cyanosis. A physical assessment during pneumothorax might reveal diminished or absent breath sounds on the affected side, as well as a decrease in chest expansion and tactile fremitus. You might also note hyperresonance in the affected lung while percussing over that area. Deviation of the trachea toward the unaffected side indicates a tension pneumothorax. This is life threatening and requires immediate treatment.

3 Ensure that the system is airtight by checking to see that the chest tube is securely connected to the drainage chamber and that all connection sites are secure.

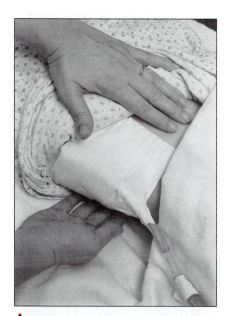

4 Palpate around the dressing site to assess for crepitation (subcutaneous emphysema). Also, inspect the dressing for abnormal drainage. Any sudden change in amount, odor, or appearance of the drainage should be documented, and the physician should be notified.

➡

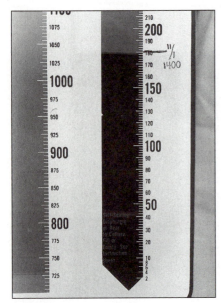

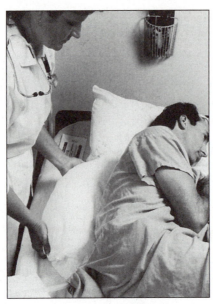

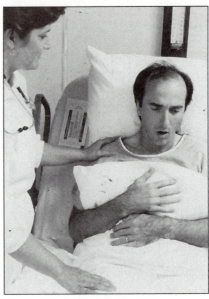

5 Check the amount, color, and character of the drainage in the drainage collection chamber at least every 30 minutes during the first 2 hours after chest tube insertion. Do this hourly during the next 24 hours and every 2 hours thereafter. Every 8 hours, mark the time and date directly on the chamber at the level of the drainage.

6 Unless it is contraindicated, reposition the client every 2 hours to provide comfort and to facilitate drainage. Place a pillow at the back to support his position. Also, assist the client with range of motion exercises on the affected shoulder. These should be performed a minimum of three times per day.

7 Encourage deep breathing and coughing exercises to facilitate drainage and help remove accumulations from the pleural space and tracheobronchial tree. This will help the lung to reexpand. Splint the insertion site with a pillow or with your hand to minimize discomfort. ***Note:*** *To ensure that the client is achieving adequate thoracic expansion, palpate for thoracic expansion, following the procedure on page 316. Your thumbs should separate at least 2.5–5 cm (1–2 in) as the client inhales.*

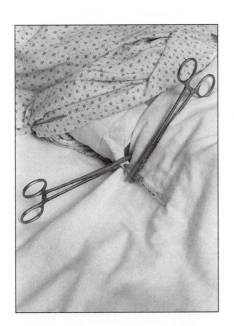

8 If your client does not have an air leak, if chest tube clamping is approved by your agency, and if the chest tube becomes accidentally disconnected from the drainage system but you are unable to reconnect it immediately, clamp the chest tube close to the insertion site with a rubber-shod clamp. Immediate action is necessary to prevent a pneumothorax. Be certain to have the client exhale fully

before clamping the tube to prevent an air buildup in the pleural space. Attach a second clamp distal to the first as a precautionary measure. ***Caution:*** *To prevent a tension pneumothorax, the tube should not be clamped for longer than a minute or two while you change the drainage system or reattach the chest tube to the rubber tubing of the drainage system.*

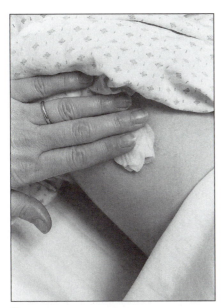

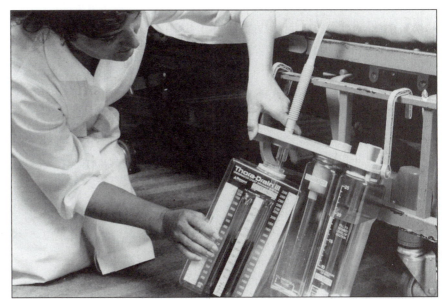

9 If the chest tube should be accidentally pulled out from the insertion site, remove the dressing and immediately apply pressure with the petrolatum gauze to prevent a pneumothorax. If petrolatum gauze is not available, apply pressure with a towel or a gloved hand. Have a coworker notify a physician immediately. If the client already has a pneumothorax, this is a life-threatening situation.

10 Some closed chest drainage systems have drainage collection chambers that can be removed and replaced without disrupting the closed system. Follow agency and system manufacturer's guidelines for changing the collection chamber.

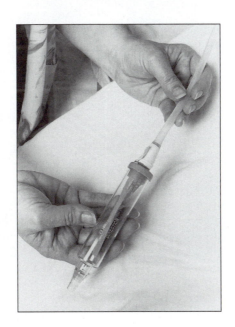

Understanding the Heimlich Valve: A Heimlich valve is a one-way device that is attached to the end of a small-bore chest tube to evacuate air from a smaller pneumothorax. While air can escape through the end of the tube, it cannot enter the pleural space.

Never occlude the exit end of the Heimlich valve, because air will accumulate in the pleural space, potentially resulting in a tension pneumothorax.

➤

ASSISTING WITH THE REMOVAL OF A CHEST TUBE

Assessing

1 Assess your client's respiratory status by auscultating the lung fields for the presence of normal breath sounds and palpating to ensure that improved bilateral chest expansion has occurred. Determine the need for a pain medication. If one has been prescribed, administer it 30 minutes prior to the removal of the chest tube. In many instances, the chest tube will have been clamped for a period of time (1–2 days before removal) to evaluate the client's tolerance.

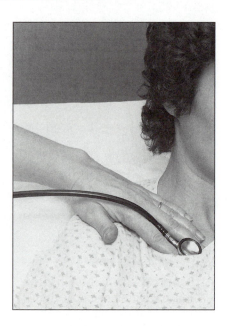

Planning

2 You will need to assemble:

☐ a suture-removal kit

☐ sterile 4 X 4 gauze pads

☐ 3-inch tape

☐ a petrolatum gauze pad

☐ sterile gloves

☐ tincture of benzoin for tape adherence

An impervious drape should be placed under the client's chest to protect the bed from drainage.

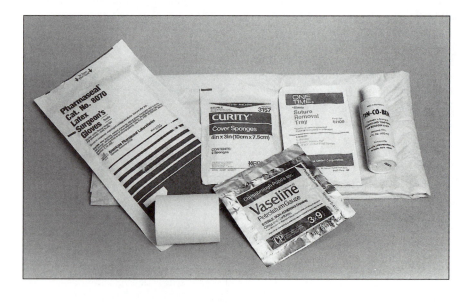

3 Explain the procedure to your client. Instruct her in Valsalva's maneuver so that she can hold her breath and bear down as the physician removes the tube. This will increase intrathoracic pressure, thereby lessening the potential for air or drainage to enter the pleural space. In addition, Valsalva's maneuver may decrease the pain response.

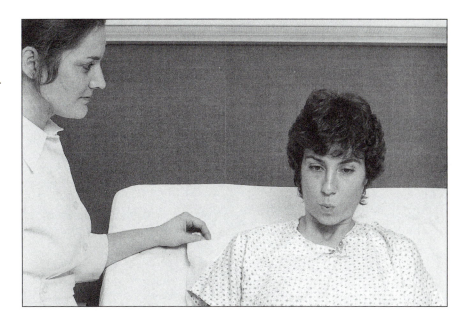

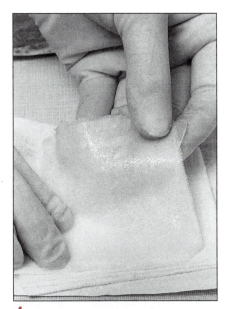

4 Before chest tube removal, prepare the dressing by applying sterile gloves and placing the petrolatum gauze pad on top of the sterile 4 X 4. The physician will then apply the dressing to the insertion site immediately after removing the chest tube. This will minimize the potential for air to enter the chest wall.

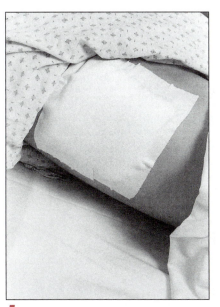

5 Tape the dressing in place. To seal the site from inrushing air, cover the entire dressing with wide strips of air-occlusive tape. Label the dressing with the date and time.

Evaluating

6 Continue to monitor your client's respiratory status. Observe for indications of a pneumothorax or for the condition that necessitated the chest tube's insertion. Assess the dressing for copious drainage, and document the procedure and your assessments.

REFERENCES

Barnes TA (ed): *Core Textbook of Respiratory Care Practice,* ed 2. St Louis: Mosby, 1994.

Bowers AC, Thompson JM: *Clinical Manual of Health Assessment,* ed 4. St Louis: Mosby, 1992.

Burton GG, Hodgkin JE, Ward JJ (eds): *Respiratory Care: A Guide to Clinical Practice,* ed 3. Philadelphia: Lippincott, 1991.

Ehrhardt B, Graham M: Pulse oximetry: An easy way to check oxygen saturation. *Nursing 90* 20(3):50–54, 1990.

Howard C: Respiratory disorders. In Swearingen PL (ed): *Manual of Medical-Surgical Nursing Care,* ed 3. St Louis: Mosby, 1994.

Howard C: Respiratory dysfunctions. In Swearingen PL, Keen JH (eds): *Manual of Critical Care Nursing,* ed 3. St Louis: Mosby, 1995.

Indiana University Hospitals: *Nursing Procedures and Policies.* Indianapolis, 1994.

Kozier B, Erb G: *Techniques in Clinical Nursing,* ed 4. Redwood City, CA: Addison-Wesley, 1993.

McPherson SP, Spearman CB: *Respiratory Therapy Equipment,* ed 4. St Louis: Mosby, 1990.

Rice R: *Handbook of Home Health Nursing Procedures.* St Louis: Mosby, 1995.

Seidel HM: *Mosby's Guide to Physical Examination,* ed 2. St Louis: Mosby, 1991.

Shapiro BA: *Clinical Application of Respiratory Care,* ed 4. St Louis: Mosby, 1991.

Sims LK et al: *Health Assessment in Nursing.* Redwood City, CA: Addison-Wesley, 1994.

Sonnesso G: Are you ready to use pulse oximetry? *Nursing 91* 21(8):60–64, 1991.

Spence AP: *Basic Human Anatomy,* ed 3. Redwood City, CA: Addison-Wesley, 1991.

Swearingen PL: Heart and breath sounds. In Swearingen PL, Keen JH (eds): *Manual of Critical Care Nursing,* ed 3. St Louis: Mosby, 1995.

Thompson JM: *Mosby's Manual of Clinical Nursing,* ed 3. St Louis: Mosby, 1993.

CHAPTER 7

Managing Cardiovascular Procedures

CHAPTER OUTLINE

ASSESSING THE CARDIOVASCULAR SYSTEM

The Cardiovascular System

Nursing Assessment Guidelines

Examining the Cardiac Area (Precordium)

Inspecting and Palpating

Auscultating

Palpating Arterial Pulses

MONITORING THE CARDIOVASCULAR SYSTEM

Inspecting the Jugular Veins

Measuring Blood Pressure

Obtaining the Ankle-Brachial Pressure Ratio (A/B Ratio)

Measuring Paradoxical Pulse

Nursing Guidelines: Identifying Common Telemetry Lead Sites

Applying Disposable Electrodes for Telemetry Monitoring

Positioning Electrodes for a 12-Lead EKG

Assessing the Postcardiac Catheterization Client

Measuring Central Venous Pressure (CVP)

CARING FOR CLIENTS WITH VASCULAR DISORDERS

Applying Elastic (Antiembolic) Stockings

Applying Pneumatic Sequential Compression Devices

Using a Foot Pump

Employing Buerger-Allen Exercises

Assessing the Cardiovascular System

THE CARDIOVASCULAR SYSTEM

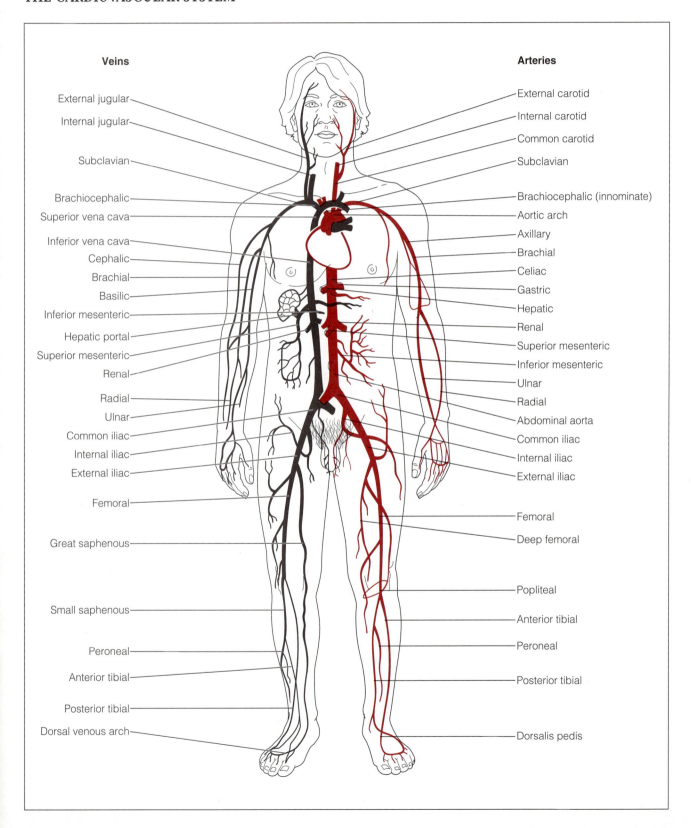

Veins

External jugular

Internal jugular

Subclavian

Brachiocephalic

Superior vena cava

Inferior vena cava

Cephalic

Brachial

Basilic

Inferior mesenteric

Hepatic portal

Superior mesenteric

Renal

Radial

Ulnar

Common iliac

Internal iliac

External iliac

Femoral

Great saphenous

Small saphenous

Peroneal

Anterior tibial

Posterior tibial

Dorsal venous arch

Arteries

External carotid

Internal carotid

Common carotid

Subclavian

Brachiocephalic (innominate)

Aortic arch

Axillary

Brachial

Celiac

Gastric

Hepatic

Renal

Superior mesenteric

Inferior mesenteric

Ulnar

Radial

Abdominal aorta

Common iliac

Internal iliac

External iliac

Femoral

Deep femoral

Popliteal

Anterior tibial

Peroneal

Posterior tibial

Dorsalis pedis

NURSING ASSESSMENT GUIDELINES

To assess your client's cardiovascular system, you need to interview him or her for subjective data, take vital signs, examine the cardiac area (precordium), and monitor pulses. A comprehensive assessment includes a complete evaluation for the following subjective data:

Personal factors: age, sex, race, nationality, occupation, marital status

History or family history of: cardiac or coronary artery disease (especially prior to the age of 60), myocardial infarction (MI), diabetes mellitus, gout, hypertension, cerebrovascular accident (CVA), congenital heart defects, rheumatic heart disease, angina, congestive heart failure

Risk factors: hypercholesterolemia, smoking, type A personality, major life change units, excessive stress response, obesity, lack of exercise

Dietary habits: intake in approximate amounts of calories, cholesterol, sodium, fluids, "fast foods," alcohol; food allergies

Medications: for example, nitroglycerin, diuretics, cardiotonics (such as digoxin), quinidine, antiarrhythmics, beta blockers, antihypertensives, calcium channel blockers; over-the-counter; drug allergies; recreational drugs; substance abuse

Pain: location, intensity, duration, character, frequency of onset, precipitating factors, methods of alleviation

Cyanosis: precipitating factors, sites

Peripheral vascular alterations: coldness, numbness, discolorations, blanching, edema, sites

Limitations of activities: exercise intolerance, dyspnea on exertion, precipitating factors

Sleep patterns: need for pillows (orthopnea), nocturia, night sweats

Miscellaneous: diaphoresis, syncope, dizziness, palpitations, nausea, vomiting, edema, digital clubbing, headaches

Client's knowledge level: disease, risk factors, medications, general health

EXAMINING THE CARDIAC AREA (PRECORDIUM)

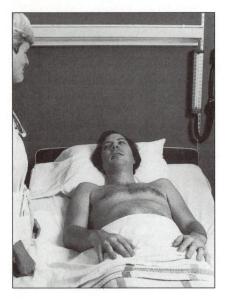

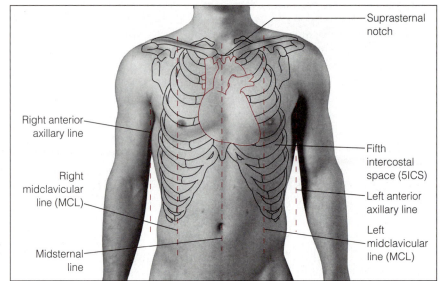

Explain the procedure to your client and examine him in a warm, quiet, and private environment. Good lighting is essential. Assist the client into a supine position, with his head slightly elevated. Ask him to uncover his chest, but provide a robe or blanket for warmth and privacy. For optimal inspection and to facilitate palpation of the cardiac area, approach the client on his right side.

To assist you with your examination and documentation of sites, familiarize yourself with these anatomic landmarks.

INSPECTING AND PALPATING

1 Identify these areas for cardiac palpation on your client's chest. Begin by inspecting the apical area for the point of maximal impulse (PMI) at the fifth intercostal space, near the left midclavicular line. Normally, it is seen in the male client as a pulsation covering an area no greater than 2 cm. If the PMI is not observable—for example, in clients with barrel chests, in obese males, and in females—you may need to palpate for it. A pulsation that covers a larger area may indicate left ventricular hypertrophy, a recent MI, or an aneurysm. Erb's point is the site at which small aortic murmurs or a friction rub may be auscultated.

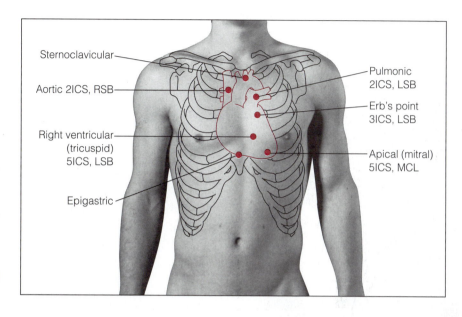

2 Palpate the apical area to assess duration and strength of the beat. An abnormally strong and sustained pulsation is often found in clients with left ventricular hypertrophy. However, anemia, fever, or hyperthyroidism can produce moderately strong pulsations. Also, palpate for thrills by using the palmar surface of your hand (as shown). Thrills give the sensation of water running through a hose. They are most often indicative of ventricular or atrial septal defects. If you are able to palpate a thrill, you will probably also detect a murmur over the same area during auscultation.

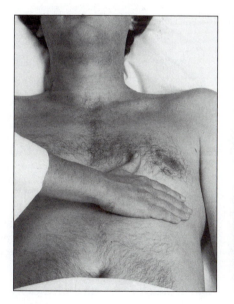

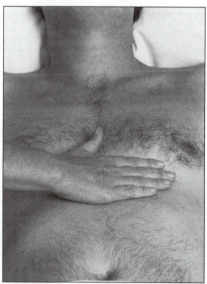

3 Palpate these areas using the palmar surface of your hand and the fat pads of your fingers: right ventricular, aortic, pulmonic, Erb's point, sternoclavicular, and epigastric (as shown). Note the presence or absence of pulsations. In addition to the apical area, they may be felt over the aortic and right ventricular areas; you might detect a light pulsation at the sternoclavicular area. Bounding pulsations at the epigastric or sternoclavicular areas, however, could be indicative of an aortic aneurysm.

AUSCULTATING

1 Familiarize yourself with these areas for cardiac auscultation. Remember that a valve's sound is heard better in the direction of its blood flow rather than directly over the valve itself. Use this guideline as you develop your own pattern for cardiac auscultation.

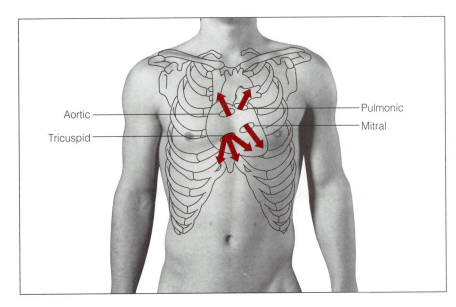

Table 7.1   Assessing Heart Sounds

Sound	Auscultation site	Timing	Pitch	Clinical occurrence	End-piece/patient position
S_1 (M_1 T_1)	Apex	Beginning of systole	High	Closing of mitral and tricuspid valves. Normal sound.	Diaphragm/patient supine.
S_1 split	Apex	Beginning of systole	High	Ventricles contracting at different times due to electrical or mechanical problems. For example, a longer time span between M_1 T_1 caused by right bundle-branch heart block, or reversal (T_1 M_1) caused by mitral stenosis.	Same as S_1.
S_2 (A_2 P_2)	A_2 at 2nd ICS, RSB; P_2 at 2nd ICS, LSB	End of systole	High	Closing of aortic and pulmonic valves. Normal sound.	Diaphragm/patient supine.
S_2 physiologic split	2nd ICS, LSB	End of systole	High	Accentuated by inspiration; disappears on expiration. Sound that corresponds with the respiratory cycle due to normal delay in closure of pulmonic valve during inspiration. It is accentuated during exercise or in individuals with thin chest walls; heard most often in children and young adults.	Same as S_2.

Table 7.1   Assessing Heart Sounds *(continued)*

Sound	Auscultation site	Timing	Pitch	Clinical occurrence	End-piece/patient position
S_2 persistent (wide) split	2nd ICS, LSB	End of systole	High	Heard throughout the respiratory cycle; caused by late closure of pulmonic valve or early closure of aortic valve. Occurs in atrial septal defect, right ventricular failure, pulmonic stenosis, hypertension, or right bundle-branch heart block.	Same as S_2.
S_2 paradoxic (reversed) split ($P_2 A_2$)	2nd ICS, LSB	End of systole	High	Because of delayed left ventricular systole, the aortic valve closes after the pulmonic valve rather than before it. (Normally during expiration the two sounds merge.) Causes may include left bundle-branch heart block, aortic stenosis, severe left ventricular failure, MI, and severe hypertension.	Same as S_2.
S_2 fixed split	2nd ICS, LSB	End of systole	High	Heard with equal intensity during inspiration and expiration due to split of pulmonic and aortic components, which are unaffected by blood volume or respiratory changes. May be heard in pulmonary stenosis or atrial septal defect.	Same as S_2.
S_3 (ventricular gallop)	Apex	Early diastole just after S_2	Dull, low	Early and rapid filling of ventricle, as in early ventricular failure, CHF; common in children, during last trimester of pregnancy, and possibly in healthy adults over age 50.	Bell/patient in left lateral or supine position.
S_4 (atrial gallop)	Apex	Late in diastole just before S_1	Low	Atrium filling against increased resistance of stiff ventricle, as in CHF, coronary artery disease, cardiomyopathy, pulmonary artery hypertension, ventricular failure. May be normal in infants, children, and athletes.	Same as S_3.

ICS = intercostal space; RSB = right sternal border; LSB = left sternal border

Source: Swearingen PL: Heart and breath sounds. In Swearingen PL, Keen JH (eds): *Manual of Critical Care Nursing,* ed 3. St. Louis: Mosby, 1995. Reprinted with permission from Mosby-Yearbook.

➤

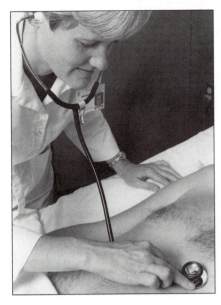

2 Review Table 7.1. Use the diaphragm of the stethoscope to auscultate normal heart sounds, S_1 and S_2. S_1 ("lub") is heard best over mitral and tricuspid areas (apex), and S_2 ("dub") is heard best over aortic and pulmonic areas (base). Both sounds are more easily heard when the client is supine. If the heart sounds are distant, for example, in clients who are obese or who have large thoraxes, ask the client to turn slightly toward his left side so the heart is closer to the chest wall.

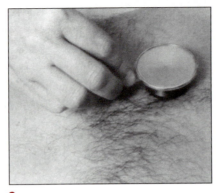

3 Lightly position the bell side of the stethoscope against the client's chest to detect adventitious heart sounds such as murmurs and gallops (see Table 7.2). Follow the guideline, page 390, for auscultating normal heart sounds. Murmurs may be heard during systole (between S_1 and S_2) at the pulmonic and mitral area, or during diastole (between S_2 and S_1) over most of the precordium, but the latter are more often pathologic and are found in heart disease or congenital defects. Murmurs may be palpated as thrills over the same area. Note the timing, location, intensity, and pitch of murmurs when recording your findings. S_3 (ventricular gallop) is a dull and low-pitched sound, "lub-dub-dee" (S_1-S_2-S_3), and it is best heard over the apical and right ventricular areas during exhalation when the client lies on his left side. In this position, gravity enhances ventricular filling and thereby exaggerates the sound. Because a ventricular gallop is one of the first clinical signs of congestive heart failure (CHF), early detection can avert advancing cardiac failure. Normally it may be heard in children and in young adults. S_4 (atrial gallop) has a higher pitch, and if present, it is elicited in the mitral area (apex). It sounds like "dee-lub-dub" (S_4-S_1-S_2). Clients with congestive heart failure might have both S_3 and S_4 (sounding like a galloping horse in the chest), as well as an increased heart rate. A pericardial friction rub might be heard in postmyocardial infarction clients and sounds like two pieces of sandpaper rubbing against each other. A pericardial rub can best be heard when the client leans forward and exhales, whereas a pleural rub (see page 319) is heard only on inspiration and disappears if the client is asked to hold his breath.

Table 7.2   Commonly Occurring Heart Murmurs

Type	Timing	Pitch	Quality	Auscultation site	Radiation
Pulmonic stenosis	Systolic ejection	Medium-high	Harsh	2nd ICS, LSB	Toward left shoulder, back
Aortic stenosis	Midsystolic	Medium-high	Harsh	2nd ICS, RSB	Toward carotid arteries
Ventricular septal defect	Late systolic	High	Blowing	4th ICS, LSB	Toward right sternal border
Mitral insufficiency	Holosystolic	High	Blowing	5–6th ICS, left MCL	Toward left axilla
Tricuspid insufficiency	Holosystolic	High	Blowing	4th ICS, LSB	Toward apex
Aortic insufficiency	Early diastolic	High	Blowing	2nd ICS, RSB	Toward sternum
Pulmonary insufficiency	Early diastolic	High	Blowing	2nd ICS, LSB	Toward sternum
Mitral stenosis	Mid–late diastolic	Low	Rumbling	5th ICS, left MCL	Usually none
Tricuspid stenosis	Mid–late diastolic	Low	Rumbling	4th ICS, LSB	Usually none

ICS = intercostal space; RSB = right sternal border; LSB = left sternal border; MCL = midclavicular line

Source: Swearingen PL: Heart and breath sounds. In Swearingen PL, Keen JH (eds): *Manual of Critical Care Nursing,* ed 3. St. Louis: Mosby, 1995. Reprinted by permission from Mosby-Yearbook.

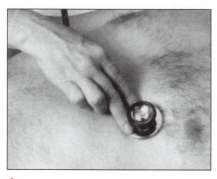

4 Auscultate the chest for the apical pulse (as shown) for 1 minute to determine the rate and rhythm of the heart. Irregular rhythms, bradycardia (less than 60 beats per minute) in nonathletes, or tachycardia (greater than 100 beats per minute) are considered abnormal in adults. Palpate the brachial or radial pulse as you auscultate the apical pulse to assess for a potential pulse deficit in the peripheral artery. A peripheral pulse deficit occurs when the cardiac systole is not strong enough to produce a palpable arterial pulse. It can occur with atrial fibrillation. If a pulse deficit is found, ask an associate to count peripheral pulsations while you auscultate the apical pulse. Document both pulse rates.

PALPATING ARTERIAL PULSES

1 Review these anatomic landmarks to assist you in locating the arterial pulse points. For infants, pulses can range between 80 and 180 beats per minute. At 4 years old, children can have pulses ranging from 80 to 120, and at age 10, pulses range from 70 to 110. From 14 years on, pulses can range from 50 to 100, with women averaging a slightly faster pulse than men.

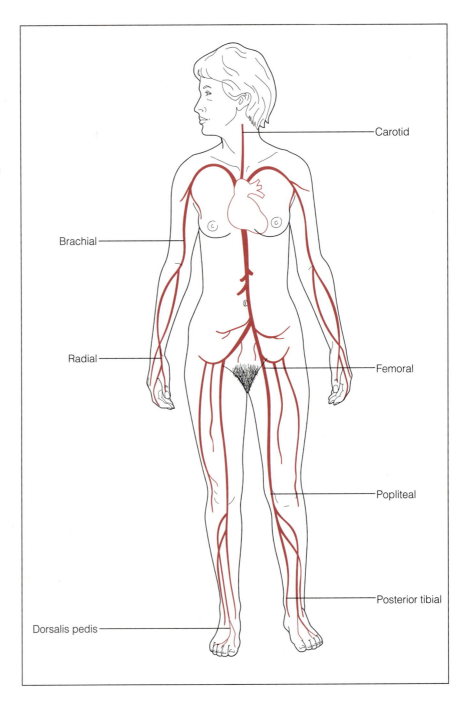

Carotid

Brachial

Radial

Femoral

Popliteal

Posterior tibial

Dorsalis pedis

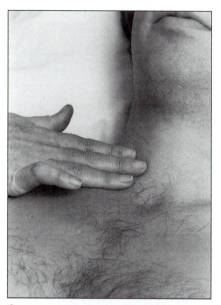

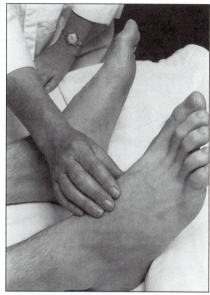

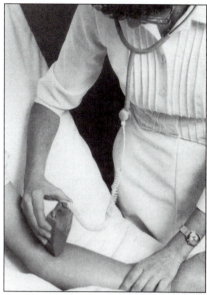

2 Begin your assessment of the arterial pulses by palpating the carotid artery to evaluate rate, rhythm, and amplitude of the pulse. Use a light touch to avoid arterial occlusion and the precipitation of bradycardia by carotid sinus massage. Palpate only one artery at a time to ensure adequate cerebral blood flow. The artery should feel soft and pliant to the touch, but clients with atherosclerosis may have cordlike arteries. Palpate the opposite artery and compare the two pulses. An abrupt cessation of one pulse with accompanying chest or back pain suggests an aortic aneurysm.

3 Palpate the peripheral pulses for rate, rhythm, and amplitude; compare each pulse to its corresponding pulse on the opposite side. Begin by palpating the brachial arteries, and then palpate the radial arteries. Palpate the femoral and popliteal arteries and complete the assessment with the arteries farthest from the heart: posterior tibial and dorsalis pedis (as shown). The posterior tibial pulse can be palpated behind and slightly inferior to the medial malleolus; the dorsalis pedis pulse is best palpated over the dorsum of the foot, with the foot slightly dorsiflexed. Document your client's pulses using Table 7.3.

4 *Using A Doppler Ultrasonic Probe:* If you are unable to palpate peripheral arterial pulses, a Doppler ultrasonic probe may be used to elicit sounds that will identify the flow of arterial blood. In this photo, the nurse has positioned the probe's transducer over the client's brachial pulse site, which she has lubricated with a conducting gel. The earphones enable her to hear wavelike "whooshing" sounds, which are produced by the reflection of red blood cells as they flow through the artery. The Doppler also can be used to evaluate the patency of veins and arteries for clients with a potential for thrombus or embolus, or those who have undergone vein grafts. After using the Doppler, record either the presence or the absence of pulsations. Be sure to describe the rate and character of the sound you hear, including its intensity and frequency.

Table 7.3 Scale for Pulse Palpation

0	Pulse not palpable
1[+]	Pulse weak
2[+]	Pulse obliterated easily with slight digital pressure
3[+]	Pulse easily palpable; considered normal
4[+]	Pulse strong and bounding; considered hyperdynamic

Monitoring the Cardiovascular System

INSPECTING THE JUGULAR VEINS

To inspect the jugular veins, elevate the head of the client's bed to a 45-degree angle. Assess and record the highest level of distention and pulsation in the interior jugular vein in centimeters, using the sternal angle (the point at which the clavicles meet) as a reference point.
If you find the level to be 3 cm (1.2 in) above the sternal angle, the client's central venous pressure is probably elevated. The client in the photo does not have a distended jugular vein. Normal findings are as follows: When the client is lying flat, the jugular vein will be slightly distended; when the client is in Fowler's position, the vein will be flat.

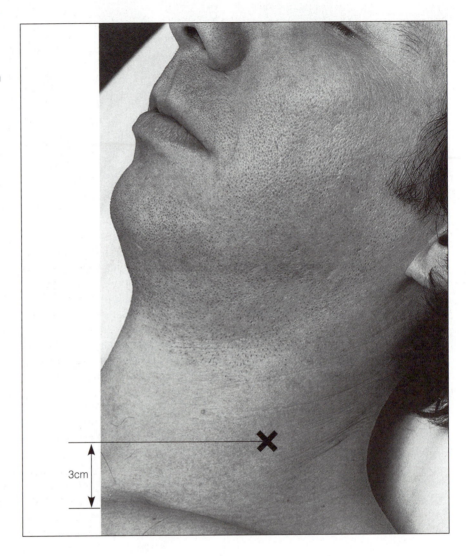

3cm

MEASURING BLOOD PRESSURE

Assessing and Planning

1 Assess your client's knowledge of the procedure and follow up accordingly, stressing the importance of regular blood pressure monitoring. Determine whether the client has exercised, eaten, drunk, or smoked within the last 30 minutes. These activities, in addition to pain, urinary bladder distention, or merely having the blood pressure measured, can alter the reading. It is also important that you have the correct bladder and cuff size. The bladder from an adult-sized cuff has been removed here to help you envision its width and length. To ensure an accurate reading, the width of the bladder should be 40% of the circumference of the midpoint of the limb on which it is used (or approximately 20% wider than the diameter of the same site). The length of the bladder should be equal to 80% of the limb's midpoint circumference. For the average adult arm, bladder widths of 12–14 cm (4¾ in–5½ in) are recommended, but remember, it is the circumference of the limb, not the client's age, that determines cuff size.

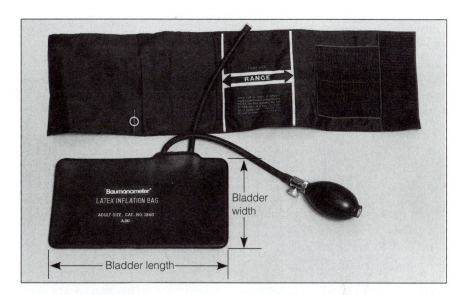

Bladder width

Bladder length

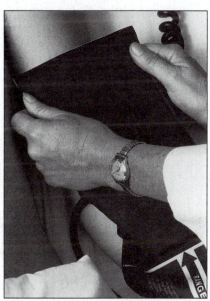

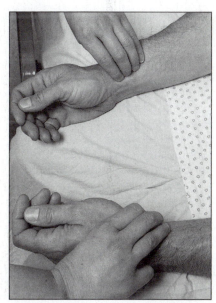

2 For example, in this photo the width of the cuff is being compared to the diameter of the client's upper arm to ensure that the cuff's bladder is 20% wider than the arm's diameter. If the bladder is too narrow, the blood pressure reading may be falsely high; if it is too wide, the reading may be falsely low.

3 If this is an initial screening, you should measure the blood pressure in both arms; if it is a routine assessment, first compare the quality of the pulses in both arms by palpating both radial pulses simultaneously (as shown). Measure the blood pressure in the arm with the stronger pulse if the pulses are unequal; if they are equal, measure the pressure on the right arm if you are right-handed or on the left arm if you are left-handed. This is recommended for your comfort and convenience to facilitate the procedure.

➤

Implementing

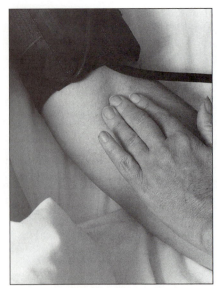

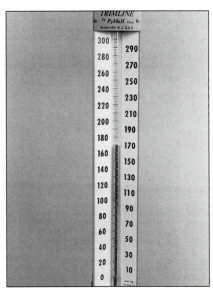

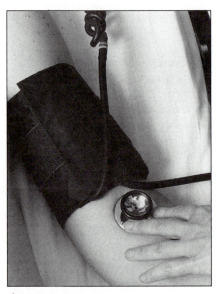

4 Support and position the client's arm at his heart level, and place the center of the cuff's bladder over the brachial artery. Wrap the cuff snugly around the upper arm 2.5 cm (1 in) above the antecubital space to allow room for the diaphragm of the stethoscope. While you palpate the brachial (or radial) artery, inflate the cuff until you feel the pulse disappear.

5 When you feel the pulse disappear, immediately note the reading on the manometer. This is the palpated systolic blood pressure. Read the gauge at eye level to ensure a correct reading. Then rapidly deflate the cuff and wait 30 seconds to allow for a decrease in venous congestion. A failure to do so could cause an alteration in the reading.

6 Place the stethoscope over the brachial artery, and rapidly reinflate the cuff to a point 30 mm Hg above the palpated systolic pressure, which is referred to as the point of maximum inflation. You must inflate to this point to ensure that the first sound (systolic pressure or Korotkoff I) is heard and that you have inflated above the auscultatory gap that occasionally occurs in hypertensive clients. *Note: To minimize extraneous sounds, the diaphragm of the stethoscope should contact neither the cuff nor any clothing.*

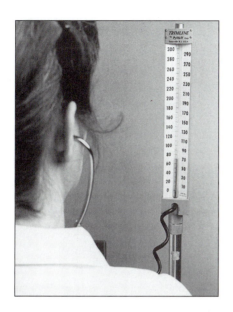

7 Slowly deflate the cuff at a rate of 2–4 mm Hg per heartbeat, and note the systolic pressure when the first sound is heard (Korotkoff I) for both adults and children. To be sure that the first sound you hear is not an extraneous noise, make sure the initial sound is accompanied by at least one other consecutive beat. The diastolic pressure is recorded for children when the sound muffles (Korotkoff IV), and for both children and adults when the sound disappears and silence begins (Korotkoff V). Thus, for children, three numbers should be recorded: Korotkoff I, Korotkoff IV, and Korotkoff V; for adults, only Korotkoff I and Korotkoff V are recorded, unless sounds are heard all the way down to zero. If this occurs, record three numbers: systolic, muffled sound, and the disappearance (zero); for example, 100/40/0. After completely deflating the cuff, wait 2 minutes for venous congestion to decrease and repeat the procedure in the same arm to verify the reading. If this is the initial screening, measure the blood pressure three times in both arms, averaging each of the last two readings.

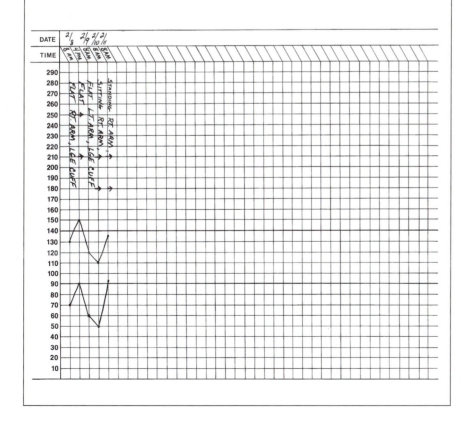

Evaluating

8 Document your client's blood pressure, noting the limb(s) on which the blood pressure was taken, the client's position during the reading, and the cuff size. If you have been the first to detect hypertension or related significant findings, refer the client for further evaluation. See Table 7.4 for details.

For children, the following systolic/diastolic blood pressure values are considered significantly hypertensive (Report of the Second Task Force on Blood Pressure Control in Children—1987).

- ages 3–5 ≥116/76 mm Hg
- ages 6–9 ≥122/78 mm Hg
- ages 10–12 ≥126/82 mm Hg
- ages 13–15 ≥136/86 mm Hg
- ages 16–18 ≥142/92 mm Hg

Table 7.4   Classification of Blood Pressure for Adults and Recommendations for Follow Up

Category	Systolic pressure (mm Hg)	Diastolic pressure (mm Hg)	Follow up
Normal	<130	<85	Recheck in two years.
High normal	130–139	85–89	Recheck in one year.*
Hypertension:			
Stage I (mild)	140–159	90–99	Confirm within two months.
Stage II (moderate)	160–179	100–109	Evaluate or refer to source of care within one month.
Stage III (severe)	180–209	110–119	Evaluate or refer to source of care within one week.
Stage IV (very severe)	≥210	≥120	Evaluate or refer to source of treatment immediately.

* Begin instructions on lifestyle modification. This includes:
- Lose weight if overweight.
- Limit alcohol intake to <1 oz ethanol/day (24 oz beer, 8 oz wine, or 2 oz whiskey)
- Reduce sodium intake to <100 mmol/d (2.3 gm sodium or 6 gm sodium chloride)
- Maintain adequate dietary potassium, calcium, and magnesium intake.
- Stop smoking.
- Reduce dietary saturated fat and cholesterol intake for general cardiovascular health.

Source: Joint National Committee: The fifth report of the Joint National Committee on Detection, Evaluation, and Treatment of High Blood Pressure (JNC V), *Archives of Internal Medicine* 153:154–183, 1993.

Source: Baas LS: Cardiovascular dysfunctions. In Swearingen PL, Keen JH (eds): *Manual of Critical Care Nursing,* ed 3. St Louis: Mosby, 1995. Reprinted with permission from Mosby-Yearbook.

Clients with systolic pressures less than 90 mm Hg and diastolic pressures less than 60 mm Hg may be considered hypotensive if illness or medications are the cause, and you should evaluate and follow up accordingly. However, if it is your client's typical pattern, low pressure readings are considered to be both normal and desirable. Establish your client's baseline blood pressure status early on admission so that you will have an adequate database from which to evaluate the integrity of each body system.

OBTAINING THE ANKLE-BRACHIAL PRESSURE RATIO (A/B RATIO)

A/B ratios are obtained to evaluate the patency of the vascular system in the lower extremities following vascular surgery or in the presence of vascular insufficiency.

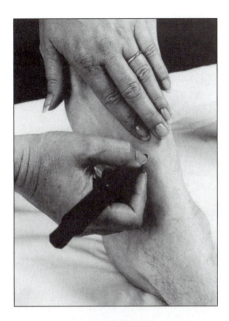

Assessing and Planning

1 Explain the procedure to the client. Review anatomic landmarks of pedal pulses (dorsalis pedis and posterior tibial), page 394. Locate and mark sites of pedal pulses with indelible ink.

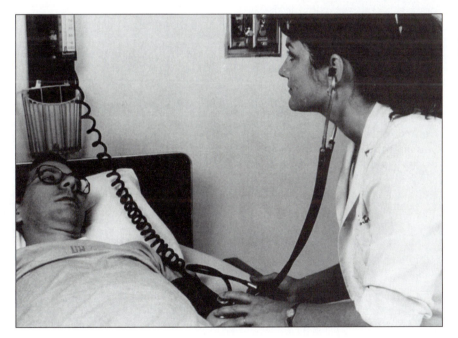

Implementing

2 Measure the systolic brachial pressure on the client's operative or involved side and record.

→

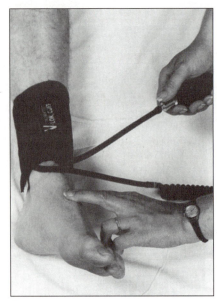

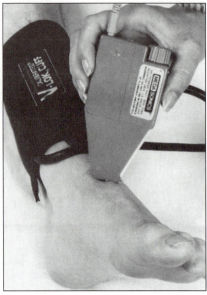

3 With the client maintaining the same position to prevent a false reading, wrap an appropriately sized blood pressure cuff around the client's ankle above the malleolus. If possible, avoid placing the cuff on any new incisions, lesions, or skin grafts. If pedal pulses were palpable, position your finger over the marked site as shown.

4 If pulses are not palpable, assess pulses with a Doppler probe (review procedure, page 395). Regardless of the method used to assess the pulse, inflate the cuff until the pulse is no longer palpable (or audible if using a Doppler probe), and then continue to inflate 20 mm Hg higher than this number. Slowly deflate the cuff until the pulse returns. Record this measurement. Next, measure the pressure over the site of the other pedal pulse (for example, the posterior tibial if you already have palpated the dorsalis pedis). Repeat on the opposite extremity if measurements are to be obtained on both sides.

Evaluating

5 Divide the highest of the two ankle (pedal) pressures on one foot by the brachial systolic pressure:

$$\frac{\text{ankle pressure}}{\text{brachial pressure}} = \text{A/B ratio.}$$

Repeat for the opposite foot, if applicable, and record.

Notify physician of a ratio less than that specified on physician's prescription. Clinical significance for ankle/brachial ratio is as follows (Cudworth-Bergin, 1984).

Ankle/brachial ratio	Clinical significance
1 to 0.75	Mild vascular insufficiency
0.75 to 0.5	Claudication
0.5 to 0.25	Pain at rest
0.25 to 0	Pregangrene

MEASURING PARADOXICAL PULSE

A paradoxical pulse refers to a decrease of ≤10 mm Hg in the systolic blood pressure during inspiration. If present, paradoxical pulse can signal pericardial disease, such as cardiac tamponade.

Assessing, Planning, and Implementing

1 Explain the procedure to the client. Measure the client's systolic blood pressure (see procedure, page 397) with him inhaling and holding a deep breath. Record the client's systolic pressure, noting that it was measured with the client holding his breath.

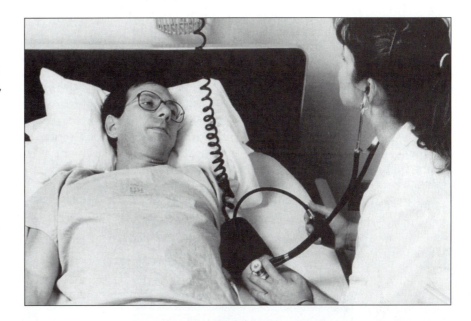

2 Have the client take a deep breath and then exhale. As the client exhales, measure his systolic blood pressure and record, noting that it was measured with the client exhaling his breath.

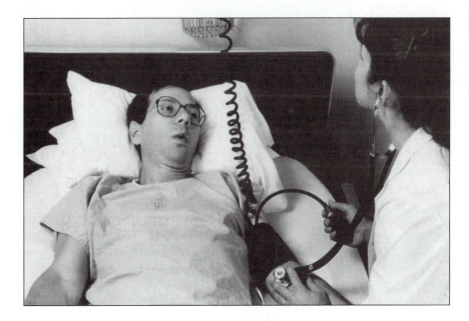

Evaluating

3 Compare the systolic blood pressure readings from steps 1 and 2, noting the difference in mm Hg. If the difference is ≥10 mm Hg, the client has a paradoxical pulse (pulsus paradoxus). Record the readings, and notify the physician accordingly.

NURSING GUIDELINES: IDENTIFYING COMMON TELEMETRY LEAD SITES

If your agency uses telemetry monitoring, probably it employs a three-electrode monitor. Review these common lead sites to assist you with electrode placement. Negative, positive, and ground lead positions will vary, depending on the telemetry unit you will use; however, the electrode placement will be the same, regardless of the telemetry unit. Position the upper electrodes just under the clavicular hollows at the mid-clavicular line. This will minimize artifact from muscles and arm movement. Lower electrodes are placed at the intercostal spaces, either at the right sternal border (fourth or fifth intercostal space) or at the left midclavicular line (sixth or seventh intercostal space). If necessary, vary the electrode placement slightly to accommodate your client's anatomy. For example, obese clients may require electrode placement over bony surfaces to decrease artifact from adipose tissue.

MCL$_1$

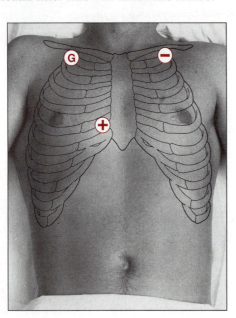

Lead II

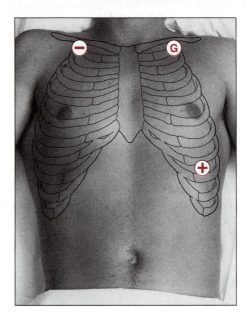

APPLYING DISPOSABLE ELECTRODES FOR TELEMETRY MONITORING

Assessing and Planning

1 The procedure for applying disposable electrodes is the same, regardless of the type of cardiac monitoring equipment that is used. In these photos the steps for initiating telemetry monitoring are also included. If the physician prescribes telemetry for your client, study the operational guidelines for the telemetry unit your agency employs. Determine the prescribed lead site position, and familiarize yourself with the guidelines for identifying common telemetry lead sites, page 404.

Assemble the following:

☐ scissors for clipping hair (optional)

☐ alcohol pad to remove skin oils (optional)

☐ electrodes

☐ electrode wires

☐ telemetry unit

☐ tincture of benzoin

☐ gauze pads

☐ telemetry carrying pouch

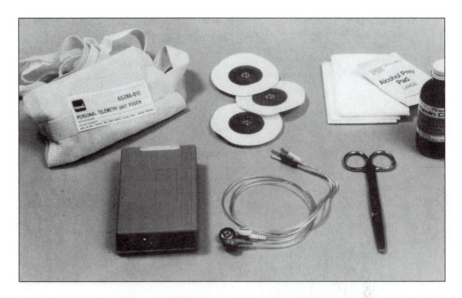

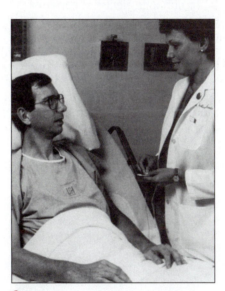

2 Assess your client's knowledge of the procedure and its purpose, and intervene accordingly.

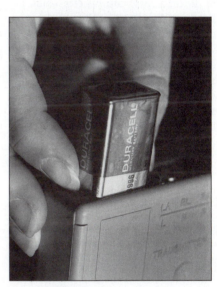

3 Insert the battery into the transmitter. *Note: Many transmitters have a test light on the back that lights up when pressed if the battery is functioning.*

Implementing

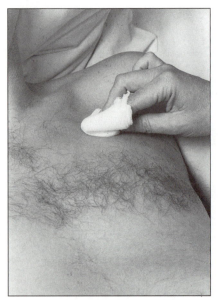

4 If necessary, clip his chest hair at the lead sites to allow for better conductivity. Briskly rub the sites with a dry 4 X 4 gauze pad to produce erythema and to remove the skin oils that can interfere with electrical conductivity. A gauze pad saturated with alcohol also can be used to remove the skin oils.

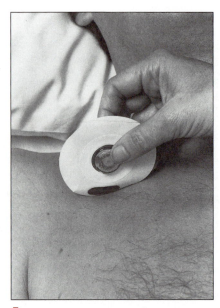

5 To enhance electrical conductivity, some disposable electrodes have rough patches for slightly abrading the skin at the lead site. If your client's electrode does not have this feature, you may instead lightly scrape the skin with a tongue blade.

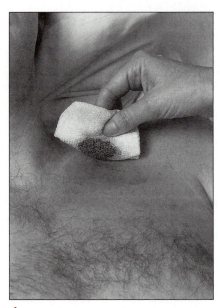

6 If your client is not allergic to tincture of benzoin, apply a small amount to the lead sites with a clean gauze pad. This will facilitate electrode adherence and inhibit skin breakdown. Let it dry thoroughly.

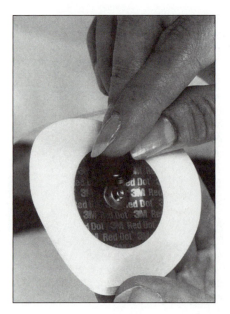

7 Attach lead wires to the appropriate electrodes. The monitoring system your agency employs will identify the positive, negative, and ground lead sites. The lead wires will be coded by color, by symbols, or by initials.

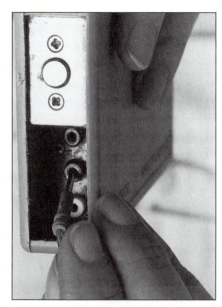

8 Ensure that the lead wires are securely connected to the telemetry transmitter.

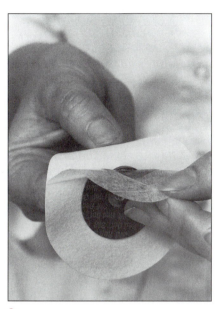

9 Remove the electrode's paper backing, but touch the adhesive surface only minimally.

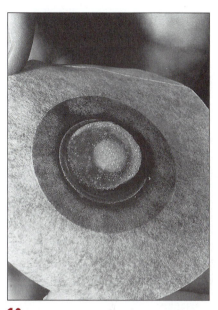

10 Inspect the spongy center of the electrode's adhesive surface. If it is not covered with a moist gel, replace the electrode with a new one.

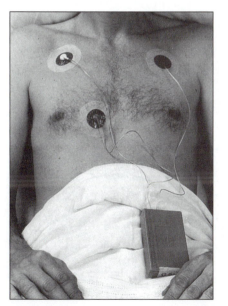

11 Position the electrodes to form the desired pattern. Electrodes should be placed near but not over bony surfaces unless the client is obese. In that case, you may place them over bones to minimize artifact from adipose tissue. And, to minimize artifact from muscles or arm movement, position the upper electrodes just below the clavicular hollows at the midclavicular line.

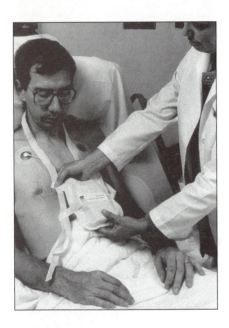

12 Insert the transmitter into a cloth carrying pouch. Attach the telemetry pouch to the client, either by wrapping both straps around the client's neck or by wrapping the interior strap around the client's neck and the exterior strap around the client's abdomen. Secure the straps to the pouch with Velcro™ if it is used by the pouch manufacturer. Another option is to place the telemetry pouch in a pajama top pocket. Make sure the pouch is in a comfortable position for the client and that it does not obstruct the electrodes.

Evaluating

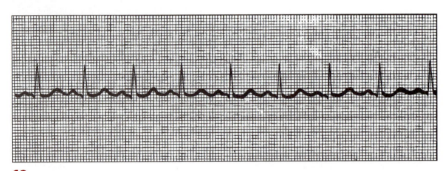

13 At the central console, press the record button on the unit reserved for your client. When the waveform has been printed, tear off the printout sheet. Evaluate the waveform, and file a 6-second printout in your client's chart as a baseline for future readings. Set the alarm's limits to those prescribed by the physician—for example, at a low of 50 beats per minute and a high of 120 beats per minute.

POSITIONING ELECTRODES FOR A 12-LEAD EKG

Assessing and Planning

1 Assemble the appropriate electrodes, indelible pen to mark anatomic sites (optional), and scissors for clipping hair (optional). Plug in the EKG machine, and turn it on to allow it to warm up, if this is appropriate for the machine used by your agency. ***Note:*** *For our purposes, we will demonstrate placement of the electrodes only. Refer to specialized texts for evaluation of lead tracings or interpretation of EKG strips.* Place the client no higher than semi-Fowler's position to ensure proper heart position.

Implementing

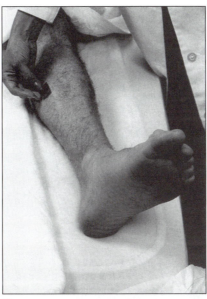

2 Attach the appropriate electrode to the client's medial calf, as shown. Repeat on the opposite limb. Place the electrodes on a smooth and fleshy part of each extremity to ensure optimal conduction.

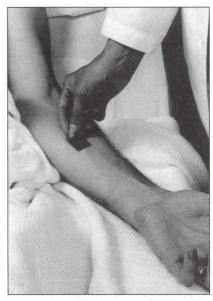

3 Attach the appropriate electrode to the inner aspect of the forearm, as shown. Repeat on the opposite limb.

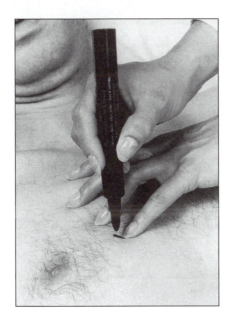

4 Begin to identify chest lead sites, using indelible ink to mark the sites. First, position your fingers to identify the fourth intercostal space at the right sternal border for V-1.

➡

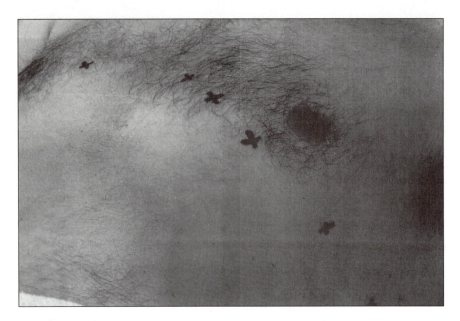

5 Continue to mark the remaining chest sites, as shown. As necessary, review anatomic landmarks on page 388. V-2: fourth intercostal space at the left sternal border; V-3: site midway between V-2 and V-4; V-4: fifth intercostal space at the midclavicular line; V-5: fifth intercostal space at the anterior axillary line (horizontal with V-4); V-6: fifth intercostal space at the mid-axillary line.

Evaluating

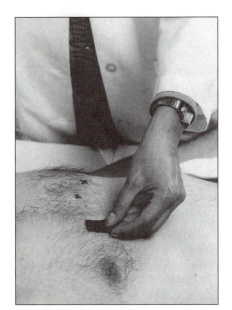

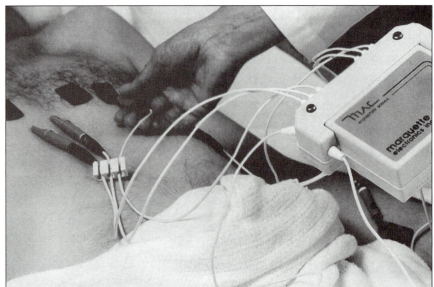

6 Attach electrodes to the lead sites, as shown.

7 Next, attach the appropriate lead wires to the electrodes. Lead wires are usually labeled with an identifying landmark, for example, "RL" (right leg), "V-6," and so on.

Follow agency and manufacturer's guidelines for running the EKG machine and recording the limb and chest lead tracings.

ASSESSING THE POSTCARDIAC CATHETERIZATION CLIENT

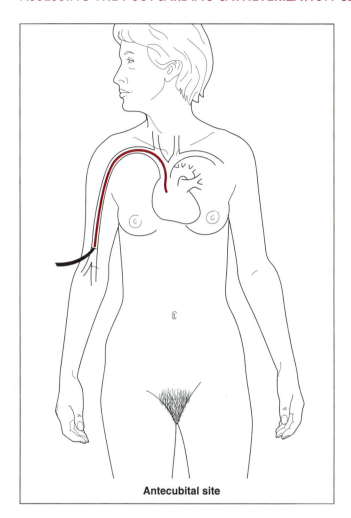

Antecubital site

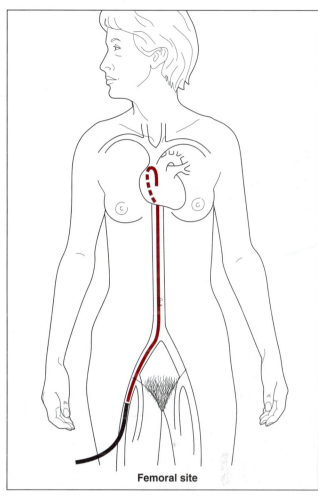

Femoral site

A cardiac catheterization is an invasive procedure performed to assess cardiac anatomy and function. It frequently is performed for clients with chest pain of unknown origin, congenital heart disease, pulmonary hypertension, dysrhythmias, congestive heart failure, and postmyocardial infarction to determine ventricular function. It is a valuable diagnostic tool for the preoperative cardiac client, and it is performed postoperatively, as well, to assess the results of cardiac surgery. It is usually performed in conjunction with angiography, during which a contrast medium is injected for visualizing the ventricle, aorta, and coronary arteries.

In order to visualize and measure the mechanical, structural, and hemodynamic integrity of the heart, both venous and arterial approaches are used. After a local anesthetic is given, a radiopaque catheter is introduced into the venous system via an antecubital, basilic, or femoral approach. Measurements of right atrial, right ventricular, and pulmonary arterial vasculature may be obtained. To visualize the coronary arteries and identify the location and severity of any stenotic lesions, another catheter is introduced into the arterial system and fed through the aorta into the coronary arteries. The entire procedure usually lasts 2–4 hours.

When the client has been returned to your care after cardiac catheterization, make her as comfortable as possible; explain that routine assessments will be performed frequently over the next 24 hours so that she does not become unnecessarily alarmed, thinking her condition has deteriorated. The protocol for assessment will vary from agency to agency. The following are general procedures for assessment and its frequency. Be sure to follow the protocol outlined by your agency.

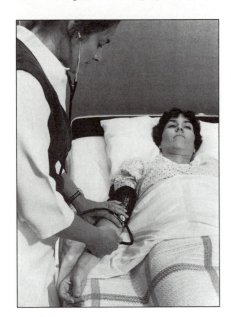

1 Measure and record the blood pressure every 15 minutes until it is stable on at least three successive checks. Once it is stable, measure it every 2 hours for the next 12 hours, and every 4 hours thereafter. *Caution: If the catheterization site was the antecubital area, be sure to measure the blood pressure in the opposite arm.* Notify the physician and lower the head of the bed if the client's systolic pressure drops 20 mm Hg lower than that already recorded. Hypotension can be a result of cardiac tamponade, vagal response, hematoma at the catheterization site, or hypovolemia. The hypertonic dye used during the catheterization can cause osmotic diuresis, so be sure to monitor the urinary output carefully. In addition to diuresis, also be alert to hypotension and bradycardia, which occur with dye reaction. If you suspect that the client is having a dye reaction, place her in Trendelenburg's position, administer fluid boluses per agency protocol, and notify the cardiologist immediately. In clients with heart disease, the hypotension caused by a dye reaction can precipitate angina and even myocardial infarction. With fluid replacement this situation usually resolves quickly.

If the client is not being monitored continuously on a cardiac monitor, auscultate the apical pulse with each blood pressure check. Be alert to an irregular pulse rate, which could be indicative of dysrhythmias. Remember that an acute myocardial infarction can occur as a complication of cardiac catheterization; therefore, you must monitor the client closely for dysrhythmias, as well as for diaphoresis, a thready pulse, and complaints of chest pain.

Encourage increased fluid intake (or increase IV drip rates as prescribed) to assist in flushing the dye from the client's system. Be alert to signs of fluid overload, which can occur in response to the increased intake: tachypnea, tachycardia, shortness of breath, crackles, rhonchi, increased CVP, gallop rhythm, and increased BP.

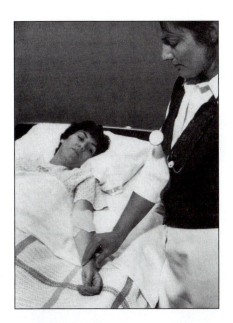

2 Assess the limb distal to the catheterization site to ensure that the color, temperature, sensation, capillary refill, and pulse(s) are adequate. Compare these assessments to the uninvolved limb. If the catheterization site was in the upper extremities, palpate the radial pulse. Palpate the popliteal, dorsalis pedis, and posterior tibial pulses if the site was in the lower extremities. In addition, the client should be able to move her fingers or toes easily. A faint pulse; pain at the catheterization site; or coolness, numbness, or tingling at the distal extremity can be indicative of an embolus, thrombus, or arterial insufficiency in the involved limb and should be reported to the attending physician immediately. Instruct the client to alert you if any of these conditions occur.

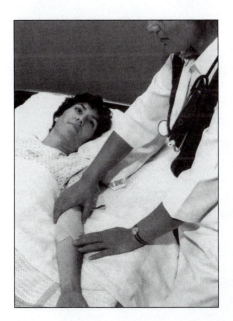

3 Inspect the pressure dressing over the catheterization site for the presence of bleeding. Ask the client about pain or tenderness at the site, which could be indicative of hematoma formation. If bleeding occurs, apply pressure to the site. Then recheck vital signs and notify the cardiologist. Be especially alert to (and palpate for) hematoma formation in the anatomic sites that were catheterized. The arterial catheterization site is more vulnerable to bleeding than the venous catheterization site because of the higher pressures that are present in the arterial system. Bleeding at the femoral arterial site may place the patient at risk for hemodynamic demise because significant blood loss into the peritoneum and abdominal cavity may occur. The peritoneum and abdominal cavity can hold significant blood volume, thus masking the true extent of blood loss until significant bleeding has occurred. Monitor for signs of bleeding (hematoma) when the client returns from the catheterization laboratory, and reassess frequently per agency protocol or as prescribed. If there are signs of bleeding (hematoma), mark the borders. If the hematoma enlarges, mark the new borders and inform the cardiologist promptly.

Keep the limb in extension to prevent bleeding, and encourage the client to keep it immobile for approximately 6 hours or per agency protocol. Movement may cause the clot to dislodge and bleeding to occur. Use sandbags, as necessary, to keep the limb immobile and in extension. Some agencies apply sandbags directly to the insertion site to provide pressure as a further deterrent against bleeding. Instruct the client to apply pressure to the site and alert you immediately if she detects bleeding. In many instances, the client will be on bed rest until the next morning. Check the orders for ambulation and follow through accordingly. Carefully document every assessment.

MEASURING CENTRAL VENOUS PRESSURE (CVP)

Assessing and Planning

1 Explain the procedure to your client. Check the intake and output record, measure his pulse and blood pressure, and auscultate his precordium for heart sounds. This assessment will provide you with a baseline from which to evaluate his CVP. Normal CVP values are as follows: 2–6 mm Hg or 5–12 cm H_2O.

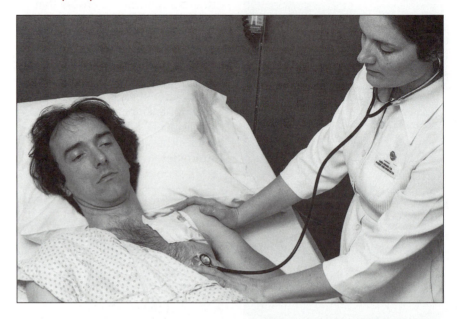

2 To minimize inaccuracies, the client should neither cough nor strain, and he must be in the same position for every reading. If the supine position is not contraindicated (and if previous readings were taken with the client in this position), place him flat in bed and remove his pillow. This will increase intrathoracic venous pressure and minimize the risk of an air embolism during the negative phase of inspiration. Make sure the IV solution is running well, and, to minimize the potential for an air embolism, ensure that all IV connections are securely attached.

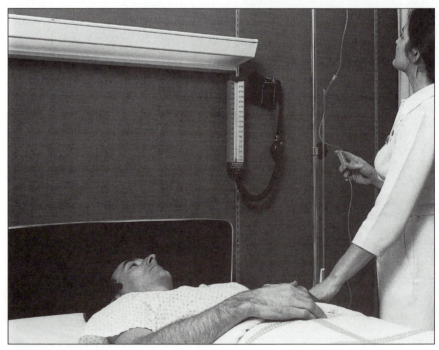

Implementing

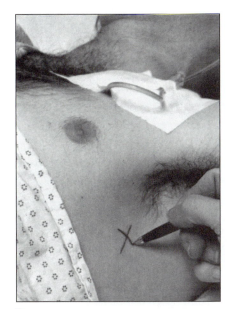

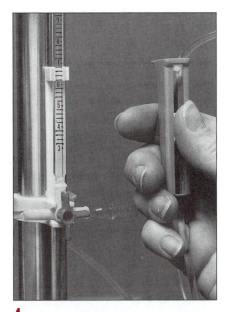

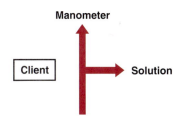

3 Locate the level of the client's right atrium at the fourth or fifth intercostal space of his midaxillary line (phlebostatic axis). Mark the site with indelible ink to ensure that the pressure is always measured from this point. Align the stopcock at the end of the disposable manometer with the phlebostatic axis.

4 If your client's IV connects to an infusion pump, turn the pump off at this time. Rotate the stopcock so that the solution is off to the client, open to the manometer, and open to the solution to allow the solution to enter the manometer. Let the manometer fill slowly to the 25-cm mark, or 10–20 cm above the expected pressure reading. Because a CVP normally will calibrate between 5 and 15 cm H_2O, filling the scale to at least 10 cm above the expected norm will ensure calibration of most readings.

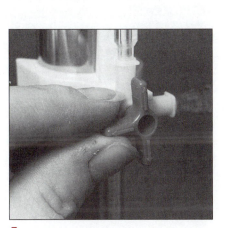

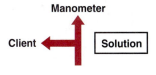

5 Rotate the stopcock so that it is open to the manometer, open to the client, and off to the solution. This will allow the solution to enter the client.

6 Observe the height of the fluid in the manometer at eye level to make sure the reading is not distorted. The level should fall as the solution flows into the client and adjusts to the pressure level of the right atrium. It will then fluctuate in response to the client's respirations. Record the measurement when the level is at the lowest point.

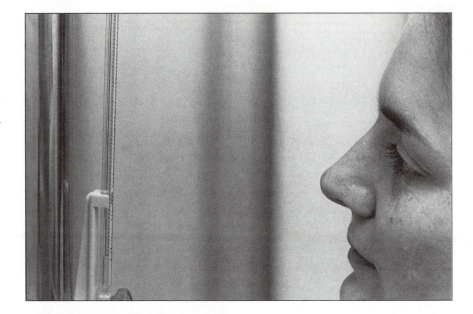

7 Adjust the stopcock so that it is open to the solution, open to the client, and off to the manometer. Adjust the flow rate to the prescribed rate, and return the client to a comfortable position.

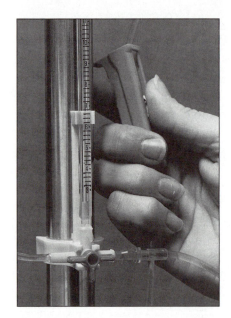

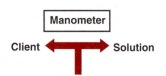

Evaluating

8 Compare the client's CVP to his baseline to ensure that it is within his normal range. Consider also his cardiac assessment, blood pressure, level of consciousness, skin turgor, diagnosis, fluid intake, and hourly urine output. Review the parameters the physician has established for reporting CVP readings, and follow up accordingly. Rates near zero may indicate hypovolemic shock, and rates above 15 cm H_2O may indicate hypervolemia or poor cardiac contractility. Both extremes necessitate further assessment and evaluation. Document the procedure, the CVP reading, and the client's position during the procedure.

Caring for Clients with Vascular Disorders

In general, there are two systems of compression that are used to promote circulation and prevent stasis: elastic stockings and pneumatic sequential compression devices.

APPLYING ELASTIC (ANTIEMBOLIC) STOCKINGS

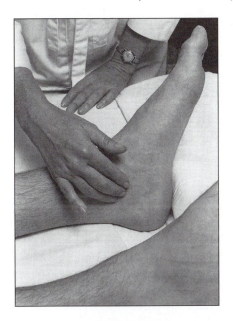

Assessing and Planning

1 The best time for applying elastic stockings is early in the morning before swelling has occurred in your client's legs and feet. Determine the type of stockings the physician has prescribed, either thigh-high stockings or below-the-knee stockings. Explain the procedure to your client. Drape his thighs as you remove the top linen. Assess both legs and feet for ulcers or infections, the absence of peripheral pulses below the femoral artery, or unequal pulses. These conditions, in addition to severe peripheral edema secondary to congestive heart failure, are contraindications for applying these hose. Also, evaluate the color and temperature of both extremities. If you find them cool or cyanotic, alert the physician. *Note: The stockings can be applied easily if talc or cornstarch is sprinkled on the legs and feet first to absorb perspiration.*

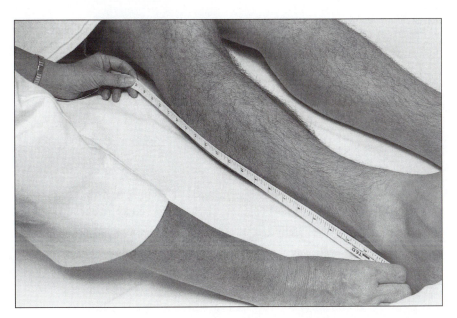

2 To ensure a correct fit, measure the leg from the Achilles tendon to the popliteal fold (as shown) for the below-the-knee stockings, or from the Achilles tendon to the gluteal furrow for thigh-high stockings. A tape measure is usually included with each package.

Implementing

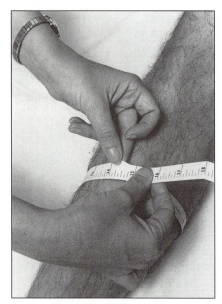

3 Measure the circumference of the midcalf (and the midthigh for the thigh-high stocking). Compare your measurements to the manufacturer's guidelines to make sure you have the correct size.

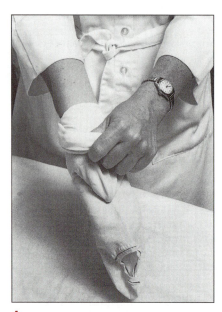

4 Make sure the stockings are "inside out." The manufacturer often packages them that way. Insert your hand through the top of the stocking deeply enough to grasp the stockings.

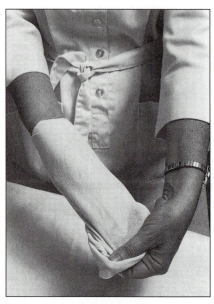

5 With your free hand, invert the stocking to its heel by pulling the stocking over the hand that is inside the stocking. Remove your hand from the inside of the stocking.

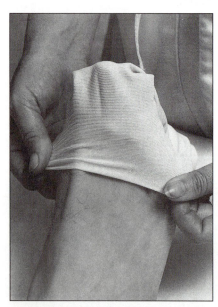

6 Grasp each side of the stocking and pull the inverted stocking foot over your client's toes.

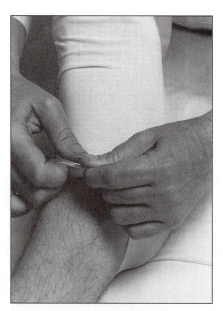

7 In one motion, pull the stocking past the client's heel so that the stocking will be anchored and not slip back.

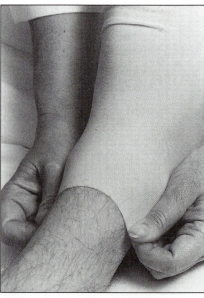

8 Grasp the fabric by the sides as you pull it up past the ankle.

Evaluating

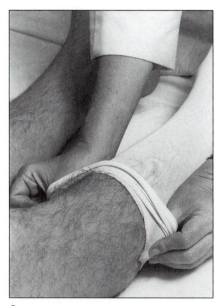

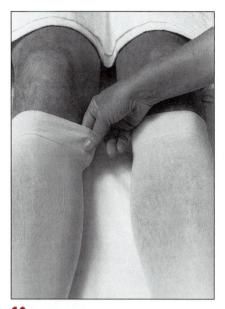

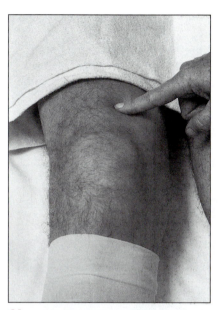

9 In increments of 5 cm (2 in) at a time, continue to pull the stocking up in this manner until you reach the premeasured area. Apply the other stocking in the same way. Because wrinkles can cause pressure areas, both stockings must fit smoothly.

10 Periodically check that the stocking does not roll at the top. Alert your client to watch for this, if he is able, explaining that rolling can produce a tourniquet effect. This can cause stasis to occur, predisposing thrombus formation and increasing edema.

11 Monitor the client frequently for swelling proximal to the stocking top. To do this, press a finger into the flesh above the stocking. If you can see a dent after removing your finger, swelling has occurred, and the stockings should be removed.

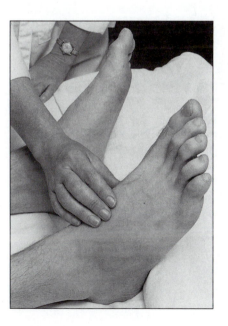

12 To minimize swelling proximal to the hose, and for client comfort, remove the stockings at least twice a day for 30 minutes at a time. Wash and dry the legs (or provide the client with the materials to do so), and reapply talc or corn starch. Always palpate peripheral pulses in the legs and feet before reapplying the hose, and observe for improvement or for an alteration in his circulatory system, such as swelling and color changes. Wash the hose with detergent and water. It is a good idea for the client to have two pairs of hose so that one pair can be worn while the other is being washed and dried.

APPLYING PNEUMATIC SEQUENTIAL COMPRESSION DEVICES

Clients who are immobile for an extended period of time are at risk of developing deep venous thrombosis due to stasis in the lower extremities. Intermittent calf compression via sequential pressure cuffs can be employed to empty the calf veins, thereby minimizing venous stasis. By allowing better drainage of the veins, the fibrinolytic (anticlotting) system is improved, as well. Because the cuffs work on the principle of compression, they are contraindicated in disorders associated with venous thrombosis or arterial insufficiency.

Assessing and Planning

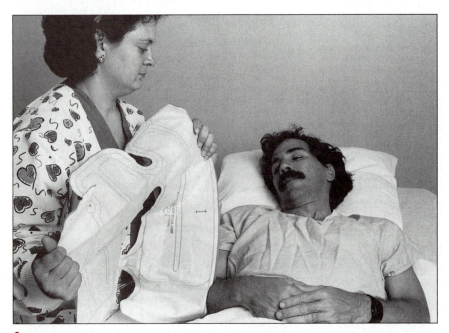

1 Assemble the equipment and explain the procedure to your client. Let him know that the cuffs are quite comfortable and that they will be worn during the period of time he is on bed rest. Be aware that if your client is wearing elastic stockings at the same time, the function of the compression device will be enhanced. Using the proper size of cuffs is important, so be sure to measure your client's extremities and use the appropriate cuffs according to manufacturer's recommendations.

2 Palpate both pedal pulses (as shown) and popliteal pulses, and perform baseline neurovascular assessments in both feet (review the procedure in Chapter 9) before applying the cuffs. If the client shows evidence of marked arterial insufficiency (diminished or absent pedal and popliteal pulses, loss of sensation in the lower extremities, leg pallor and numbness, loss of hair on the legs, sharp and cramping pain during exercise or at night), skin irritation or breakdown, ulcerations, or signs of infection, notify the physician because the application of the cuffs might be contraindicated.

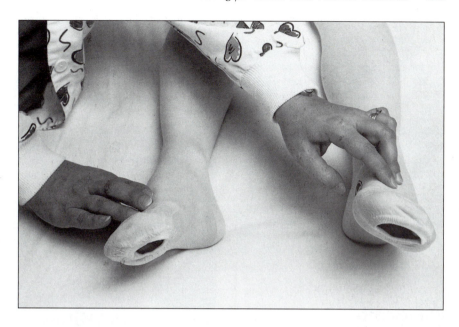

Implementing

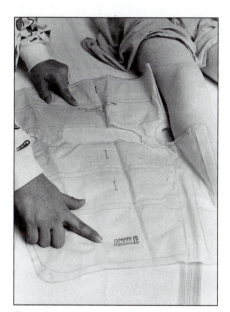

3 Position the cuff flat on the client's bed next to the leg. Note the positions of the ankle and popliteal markings on the cuff and align them with the appropriate areas on the client's legs.

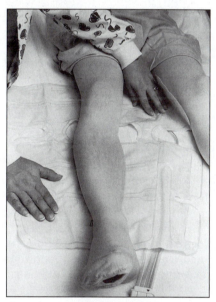

4 Place the client's leg directly in the center of the cuff, aligning the back of the knee with the opening in the back of the cuff.

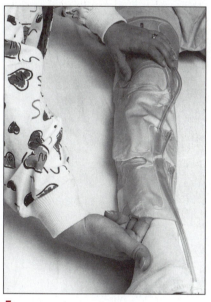

5 Wrap the cuff around the client's leg, making sure the opening in the front of the cuff is over the client's knee. Ensure that two fingers fit between the client's leg and the cuff at both the ankle and the knee before turning on the unit. This will ensure proper slack in the cuff to enable adequate expansion during inflation.

Evaluating

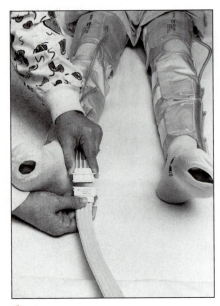

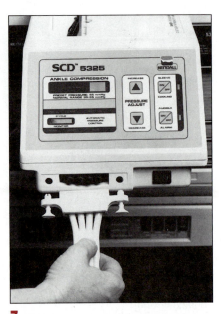

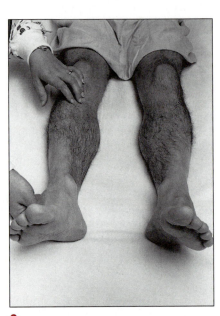

6 Attach the connectors between the cuff and the compression pump. This unit has one connector for each leg.

7 Plug the connector from the leg cuffs into the compression unit and press the button to turn on the device. Observe each cuff for at least two cycles to be sure the cuffs are functioning properly. Only one cuff should inflate at a time. The ankle cell should fill first, followed by the inflation of the second, third, and the thigh cells. All the cells will remain inflated until the system vents, at which time all the cells should deflate. The cuff on the opposite leg should then begin its cycle in the same manner. Document the procedure, being certain to note the client's baseline neurovascular assessment and the condition of the skin on both legs.

8 At prescribed intervals, unplug the unit and remove the cuffs after they have deflated (and the elastic stocking if they are worn). Inspect the skin and provide skin care. However, avoid massaging the skin because vigorous rubbing can dislodge a thrombus. Perform a neurovascular assessment (see Chapter 9) to evaluate the color, temperature, sensation, pulses, and capillary refill of the distal extremities, and compare the assessment to the baseline assessment.

USING A FOOT PUMP

During the weight-bearing phase of normal ambulation, a plexus of veins in the foot acts as a powerful venous pump sending blood back to the heart. The system pictured below mimics the natural circulatory process inherent in ambulation by compressing the venous plexus, thereby stimulating it to empty and minimizing venous stasis. If the client wears elastic stockings at the same time, this will enhance the function of the foot pump.

Assessing and Planning

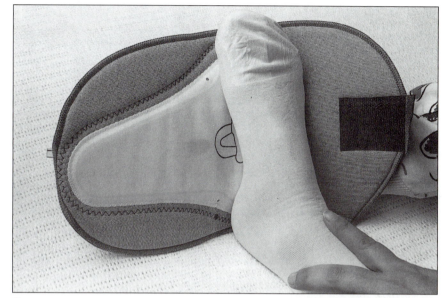

1 Explain the procedure to your client. Be sure that the client knows that he should not walk with the foot pad in place.

Refer to the manufacturer's chart for the correct size of the pneumatic inflation foot pad. Position the foot so that it is in the center of the pad (as shown).

Implementing

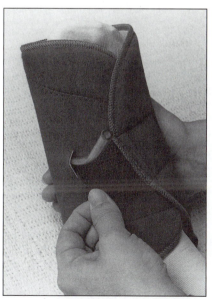

2 Wrap the foot pad from side to side so that it fits snugly around the foot.

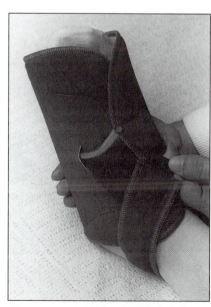

3 Wrap the Velcro™ strap snugly around the ankle.

➤

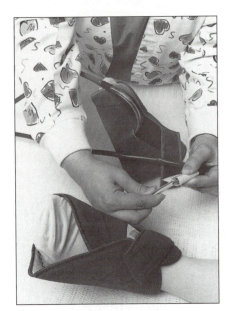

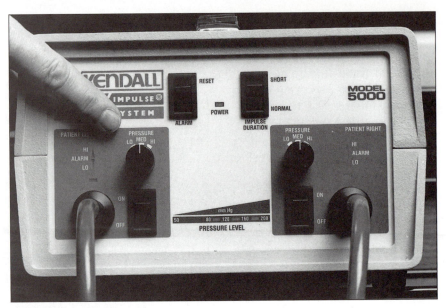

4 Attach the cords to the foot pads, being certain to match the right and left tubing to the appropriate foot pad.

5 Set the impulse duration (the range is short to normal) for client comfort.

Evaluating

6 Remove the foot pads at least once per shift to provide skin assessment and skin care. Be alert to skin redness or rash.

EMPLOYING BUERGER-ALLEN EXERCISES

Assessing and Planning

Implementing

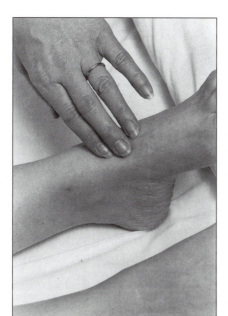

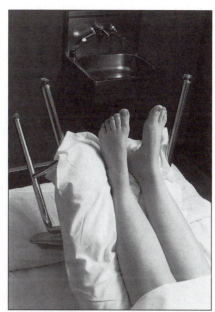

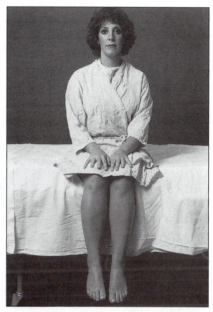

1 Buerger-Allen exercises may be prescribed for clients with occlusive arterial disorders—for example, arteriosclerosis obliterans, Buerger's disease, or Raynaud's disease. Explain to your client that these exercises will promote circulation in the lower extremities by the gravitational filling and emptying of the blood vessels. To evaluate the effectiveness of the exercises, you must first perform a baseline assessment of your client's legs and feet. While your client lies flat, palpate the femoral, popliteal, posterior tibial, and pedal pulses. Then assess for the presence or absence of pain and ulcerations and the temperature and color of the extremities.

2 Initially, the client should recline with her legs elevated above the level of her heart for a minute, or until blanching occurs in the legs and feet. You may raise the foot of the hospital bed, but it is a good idea to show the client how to implement the procedure at home. In this photo, the back of a straight-back chair is cushioned with a pillow so that the chair's back supports the client's legs. Make sure you keep the client warm, because chilling will further diminish arterial circulation.

3 Once blanching has occurred, have the client sit on the side of the bed and plantarflex her feet. This is the first of six leg-stretching positions that are employed to promote blood flow and minimize stasis. This and the following five positions should be maintained for 30 seconds each. *Note: Instead of the six leg-stretching positions, the physician may prescribe one in which the client's legs dangle over the side of the bed for 3 minutes, or until they are pink.*

➡

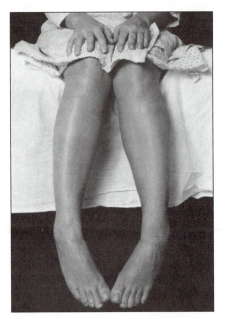

4 For the second position, the client plantarflexes and inverts her feet.

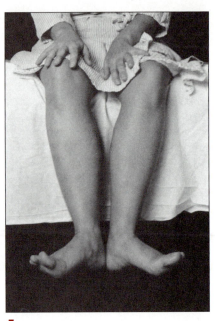

5 For the third position, the client dorsiflexes and everts her feet.

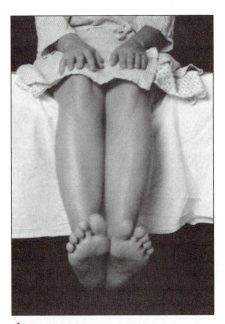

6 For the fourth position, the client dorsiflexes her feet.

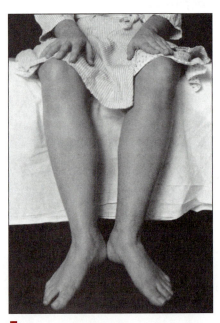

7 For the fifth position, the client plantarflexes and everts her feet.

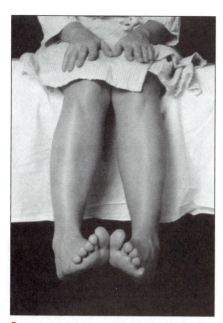

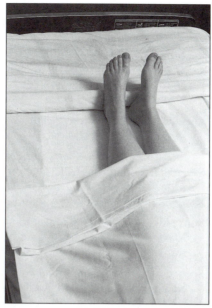

Evaluating

10 When the exercise has been completed, evaluate its effectiveness by comparing the color, temperature, and pulsations of the legs and feet to your initial assessment; document accordingly. Note whether the skin is mottled, blanched, red, black, gray, or blue. Determine whether a foot cradle is needed to keep the bed covers off the affected skin. To enhance arterial circulation, ensure that the client and the environment are kept warm.

8 For the sixth position, she dorsiflexes and inverts her feet. Observe her feet and legs at this time. Optimally, they will be red or pink to indicate that adequate circulation has occurred.

9 Finally, the client should lie flat in a supine position. Usually, this position is maintained for 3–5 minutes. Depending on the physician's directions, the set may be repeated another four or five times. Buerger-Allen exercises are usually prescribed for three or four times daily.

REFERENCES

Baas L, Steuble BT: Cardiovascular dysfunctions. In Swearingen PL, Keen JH (eds): *Manual of Critical Care Nursing,* ed 3. St Louis: Mosby, 1995.

Bowers AV, Thompson JM: *Clinical Manual of Health Assessment,* ed 4. St Louis: Mosby, 1992.

Cudworth-Bergin K: Detecting arterial problems with a Doppler probe. *RN* 47(1):38–41, 1984.

Drew B: Using cardiac leads the right way. *Nursing 92* 22(5):50–54, 1992.

Hill M, Grim C: How to take a precise blood pressure. *Am J Nurs* 91(2):38–42, 1991.

Holloway NM: *Nursing the Critically Ill Adult,* ed 4. Redwood City, CA: Addison-Wesley, 1993.

Hutchins LN: Drug therapy for hypertension and hyperlipidemia. *J Cardiovascular Nurs* 9(2):37–53, 1995.

Indiana University Hospitals: *Nursing Procedures and Policies.* Indianapolis, 1994.

Joint National Committee: The fifth report of the Joint National Committee on detection, evaluation, and treatment of high blood pressure (JNC V). *Archives of Internal Medicine* 153:154–183, 1993.

Keen JH: Coronary artery thrombolysis. In Swearingen PL, Keen JH (eds): *Manual of Critical Care Nursing,* ed 3. St Louis: Mosby, 1995.

Kinney M: *Comprehensive Cardiac Care,* ed 7. St Louis: Mosby, 1991.

Kozier B, Erb G: *Techniques in Clinical Nursing,* ed 4. Redwood City, CA: Addison-Wesley, 1993.

Report of the second task force on blood pressure control in children—1987. *Pediatrics* 79:1–25, 1987.

Rice R: *Handbook of Home Health Nursing Procedures.* St Louis: Mosby, 1995.

Saver C: Decoding the ACLS algorithms. *Am J Nurs* 94(1):27–35, 1994.

Sims LK et al: *Health Assessment in Nursing.* Redwood City, CA: Addison-Wesley, 1994.

Spence AP: *Basic Human Anatomy,* ed 3. Redwood City, CA: Addison-Wesley, 1991.

Swearingen PL: Heart and breath sounds. In Swearingen PL, Keen JH (eds): *Manual of Critical Care Nursing,* ed 3. St Louis: Mosby, 1995.

Thompson JM: *Mosby's Manual of Clinical Nursing,* ed 3. St Louis: Mosby, 1993.

Woods SL, Underhill SL et al: *Cardiac Nursing,* ed 3. Philadelphia: Lippincott, 1995.

CHAPTER 8

Managing Renal-Urinary Procedures

CHAPTER OUTLINE

ASSESSING THE RENAL-URINARY SYSTEM

The Renal-Urinary System

Nursing Assessment Guidelines

Assessing the Bladder

Inspecting

Palpating

Percussing

Palpating the Kidneys

Assessing Skin Turgor

Weighing the Client on a Bed Scale

Collecting a Timed Urine Specimen

CATHETERIZING AND MANAGING CATHETER CARE

Performing Intermittent Catheterization

Inserting a Robinson (Straight) Catheter into a Female

Inserting a Robinson (Straight) Catheter into a Male

Managing a Foley Catheter

Performing a Catheterization with a Foley (Indwelling) Catheter

Nursing Guidelines: Foley Catheter Management

Making a Catheter Strap

Obtaining a Urine Specimen

Emptying the Drainage Bag

Using a Urine Meter

Irrigating the Catheter

Removing a Foley Catheter

CARING FOR CLIENTS WITH RENAL-URINARY DISORDERS

Applying an External Urinary Device (with a Leg Drainage System)

Monitoring the Client Receiving Continuous Bladder Irrigation (CBI)

Establishing CBI

Nursing Guidelines: Care of the Client with CBI

Nursing Guidelines: Care of the Client with a Suprapubic Catheter

Nursing Guidelines: Care of the Client with a Nephrostomy Tube and Ureteral Stents

Administering a Sodium Polystyrene Sulfonate (Kayexalate) Enema

Performing Credé's Maneuver

CARING FOR CLIENTS UNDERGOING DIALYSIS

Nursing Guidelines: Quinton and Permcath Dialysis Accesses

Administering an Exchange for a Client with Chronic Ambulatory Peritoneal Dialysis

CARING FOR CLIENTS WITH URINARY DIVERSIONS

Nursing Guidelines: Common Types of Urinary Diversions

Ileal Conduit

Cutaneous Ureterostomy

Continent Urinary Diversion

Performing a Postoperative Assessment

Managing Appliance Care

Applying a Postoperative (Disposable) Pouch

Picture Framing the Pouch

Connecting the Pouch to a Urinary Drainage System

Assessing the Renal-Urinary System

THE RENAL-URINARY SYSTEM

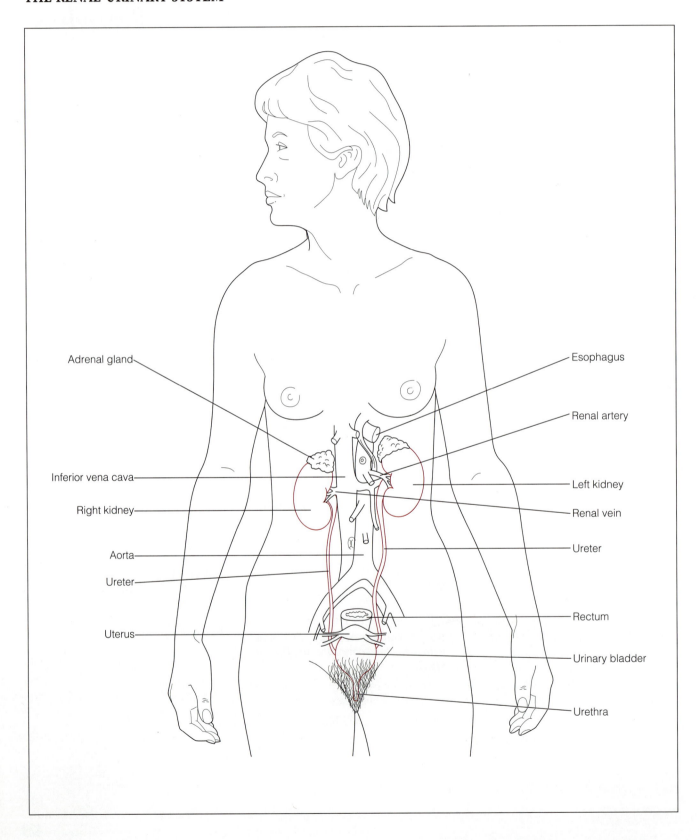

Adrenal gland

Inferior vena cava

Right kidney

Aorta

Ureter

Uterus

Esophagus

Renal artery

Left kidney

Renal vein

Ureter

Rectum

Urinary bladder

Urethra

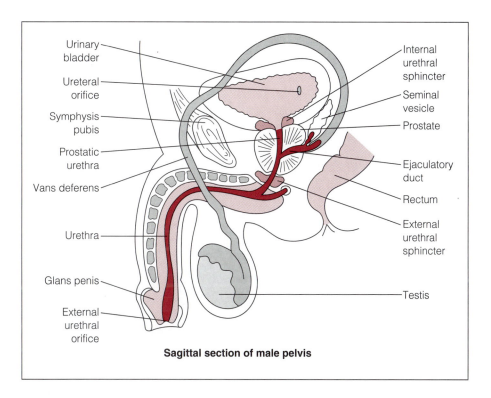

Urinary bladder
Ureteral orifice
Symphysis pubis
Prostatic urethra
Vans deferens
Urethra
Glans penis
External urethral orifice

Internal urethral sphincter
Seminal vesicle
Prostate
Ejaculatory duct
Rectum
External urethral sphincter
Testis

Sagittal section of male pelvis

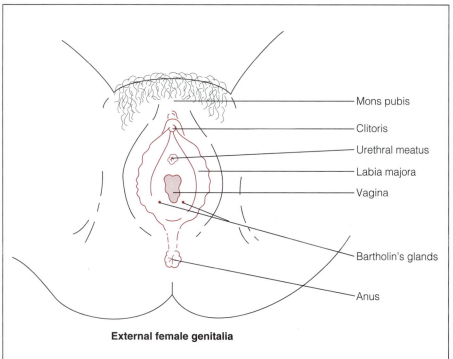

Mons pubis
Clitoris
Urethral meatus
Labia majora
Vagina
Bartholin's glands
Anus

External female genitalia

NURSING ASSESSMENT GUIDELINES

To assess your client's renal-urinary system, you need to interview him or her for subjective data, take vital signs, assess the bladder and kidneys, and obtain a urine specimen. A comprehensive nursing care plan includes a complete evaluation for the following subjective data.

Personal factors: for example, age, marital status, occupation, continued exposure to nephrotoxic substances such as carbon tetrachloride or lead or use of recreational drugs

History or family history of: renal calculi, strictures, urinary tract disease or infections, polyuria, incontinence, diabetes mellitus, polycystic kidney disease, renal transplant, dialysis, cardiac disease, cancer, or endocrine disorders such as diabetes insipidus

History of: bladder infection, renal/urinary trauma or surgery, blood transfusions, glomerulonephritis, autoimmune diseases

Dietary habits: intake in approximate amounts of sodium, calcium, protein, purines, potassium, phosphates, or acids; amounts consumed of coffee, tea, or alcoholic beverages; presence or history of polydipsia and polyphagia; food allergies

Risk factors: psychologic stressors, hypertension, pregnancy, smoking, kidney stones, prostatic hypertrophy, diabetes mellitus

Medications: aminoglycosides, NSAIDs, chemotherapy, diuretics, antispasmotics, anticholinergics, aspirin or acetaminophen; presence of drug allergies; exposure to dyes. In addition, obtain a list of all medications recently or currently taken by client, inasmuch as many drugs have the potential for nephrotoxicity.

Alterations in urinary elimination: frequency, urgency, retention, nocturia, dysuria, residual urine, hesitancy, burning during voiding, stress incontinence, dribbling, hematuria, proteinuria; presence of an ostomy or stent

Amount and character of urine: polyuria, oliguria, anuria; changes in color, odor, clarity

Flow of urinary stream: high/low pressure, change in size of stream, ability to maintain stream

Fluid status: fluid volume deficit or excess; thirst; presence of peripheral, periorbital, sacral, or pulmonary edema; increase or decrease in weight

Pain: location—for example, lower back, flank, perineum, testicular area, suprapubic area, inner thigh, groin; intensity; relieved by; intensified by

Urethral discharge: amount and character

Presence of genital sores or ulcers

ASSESSING THE BLADDER

INSPECTING

Routine assessment of the bladder is essential when you are caring for clients with urinary tract disorders, as well as for those who have indwelling catheters. Be sure that you provide warmth and privacy for your client, and that you have washed your hands and explained the reason for the assessment. To facilitate the procedure, the client's gown should be raised to the umbilicus and the sheet or drape lowered to the symphysis pubis. Unless your client is obese, a distended bladder usually can be assessed visually while you are at eye level to the lower abdomen. Often you will be able to see a swollen mound just proximal to the symphysis pubis and distal to the umbilicus.

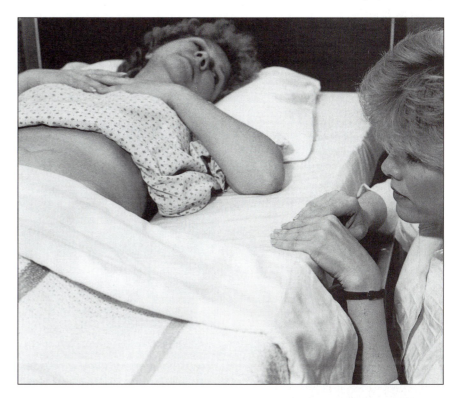

PALPATING

If your client is oliguric or anuric and you need to assess for bladder retention to ensure that catheterization is indicated; if you are assessing your client for a potential catheter obstruction; or if you are assessing for residual urine in clients with neurogenic bladders, light palpation of the bladder can be employed to help determine bladder size. Palpate at the midline, approximately 5 cm (2 in) above the symphysis pubis. If the bladder is distended, you should be able to feel its firm, rounded contour. *Note: For routine assessment, the client should void prior to bladder palpation to minimize the potential for discomfort.*

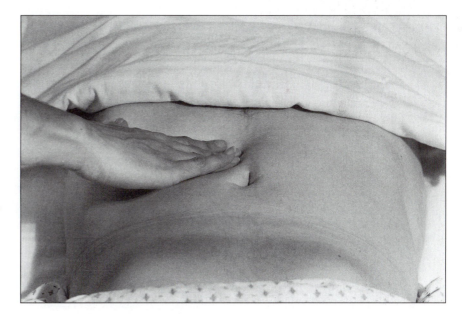

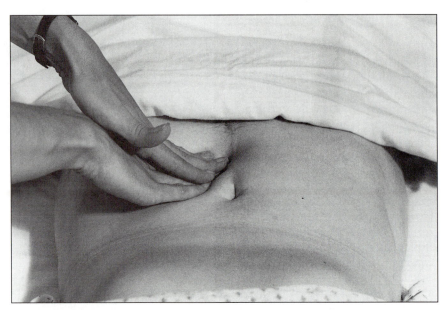

Deep Palpation: When the bladder is not distended, it may be necessary to palpate deeply to assess for location and size. To do this, press with the fingertips of both hands approximately 2.5–5 cm (1–2 in) proximal to the symphysis pubis, near the midline. Assess for size and location of the bladder and for the presence of any masses. Be sure to note indications of client discomfort, as well.

PERCUSSING

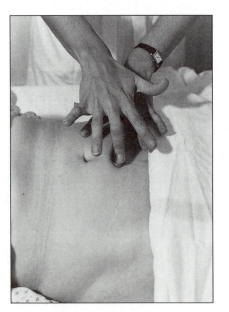

Percussion is another assessment tool that will help you determine whether the bladder is empty or if it contains urine. Place a middle finger at the midline, approximately 5 cm (2 in) above the symphysis pubis. To elicit sounds, sharply strike that finger with the opposite middle finger. If the bladder contains urine, you should hear dull sounds as you continue to percuss downward toward the symphysis pubis. However, an empty bladder should produce tympanic (hollow) sounds.

PALPATING THE KIDNEYS

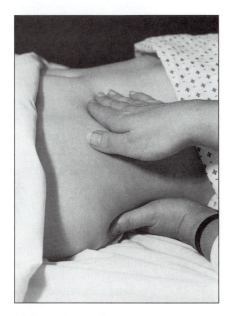

ASSESSING SKIN TURGOR

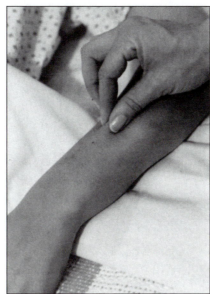

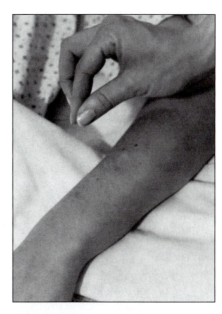

Although not always a routine assessment for the hospitalized urologic client, kidney palpation can be incorporated into a comprehensive assessment. Position your hands on both sides of the client's flank at the area between the iliac crest and lower costal margins (as shown). Instruct the client to inhale, and increase the pressure between your hands with each inhalation until you feel you have achieved the maximum depth. As the client inhales deeply a final time, you should be able to feel the lower edge of the kidney between your hands. This will be more difficult if your client is obese. Compare your assessment of the left kidney to that of the right kidney. Assess and document differences in size, absence of a kidney, masses, nodules, and discomfort from the assessment. *Caution: Kidney palpation is contraindicated in clients in whom neuroblastoma or Wilms' tumor is suspected.*

If your client is dehydrated, the suppleness of the skin will be diminished because of moisture loss. To assess skin turgor, lift a section of skin along an area in which there is adequate subcutaneous tissue—for example, the forearm, lower abdomen, or calf. Release the skin (far right) and observe its return to the original position. If the client has good turgor, the skin will return quickly to its original position. For clients with poor turgor, the skin will remain in the lifted position (tenting) and return slowly to the original position. Document your findings in the client's medical record.

WEIGHING THE CLIENT ON A BED SCALE

To monitor hydration status more precisely, for example in clients with nephrotic syndrome, it may be necessary to weigh your clients at the same time every day. If your client is immobile or restricted to bed rest, a prescription for a bed scale should be obtained to facilitate the process. Ensure that the client wears the same amount of clothing and that the bed linen is comparable from one weighing to the next.

Be certain to balance the scale first, by following the manufacturer's instructions. Lock the attached weighing platform securely in place, and then lock the wheels on the bed. To provide warmth and to prevent the potential for cross-contamination, cover the platform with a drape before moving the client. It is important that

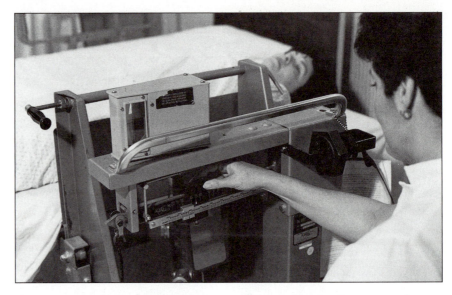

the same type of drape be used consistently with each weighing to prevent miscalculations of the client's weight. In addition, be aware of any prosthetic or treatment device worn by the client, eg, artificial limb, splint/cast, or peritoneal dialysis fluid in the peritoneal cavity. Ensure consistency for each weighing. If your client is immobile, follow the procedure in Chapter 2 for transferring the immobile client. Weigh the client, return her to her bed, and document the weight on the appropriate records.

COLLECTING A TIMED URINE SPECIMEN

If a timed urine specimen has been prescribed for your client, explain the procedure and point out the proper container and storage area for the urine. Some agencies require the refrigeration of all specimens; others advocate that the urine container be kept on ice.

To begin the test, have the client void. *Discard* the urine, and record the time. This is the starting time for the collection. *All* urine must be collected during the prescribed period, and the final specimen should be obtained as close as possible to the termination of the collection period.

During the collection period, post signs on the client's door, bathroom door, and near the bed to remind personnel and the client about the need to save all urine. If the timed collection is for the testing of creatinine clearance, ensure that the serum creatinine is drawn

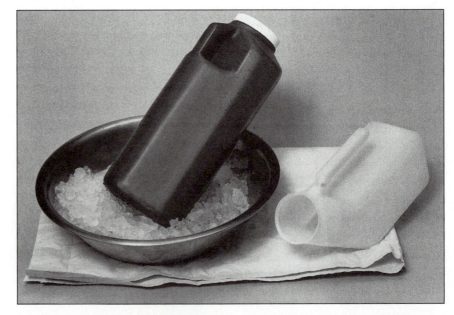

during the collection period. After obtaining the final specimen, record the time again on the laboratory slip (and on other appropriate records) and arrange for its delivery to the laboratory. If the client is menstruating, be sure to note it on the laboratory slip. Also be certain to note or mark any amount of urine lost during the test.

Catheterizing and Managing Catheter Care

PERFORMING INTERMITTENT CATHETERIZATION

INSERTING A ROBINSON (STRAIGHT) CATHETER INTO A FEMALE

Unless catheterization has been specifically prescribed, avoid this procedure if other measures can be taken to achieve the same outcome. For example, many experts believe that a midstream urine catch is as dependable a specimen as that obtained via an invasive catheterization. Often, clients who have urine retention can void after the stimulus of hearing running water or submerging their hands in a basin of warm water. Other clients respond to the sensation of warm water being poured over the perineum.

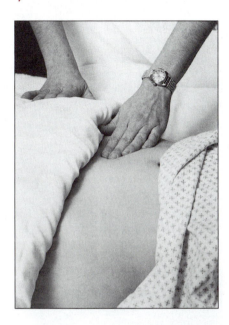

Assessing

1 Inspect the lower abdomen and palpate or percuss the bladder to determine the need for catheterization or the degree of distention. If intermittent catheterization is indicated, explain the procedure to your client and arrange for a private and warm environment.

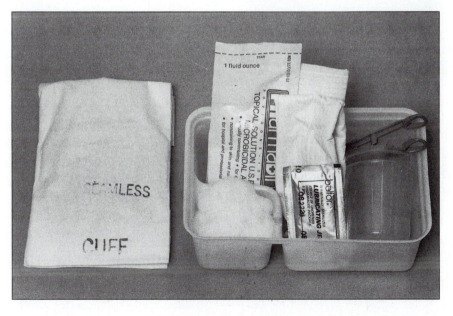

Planning

2 Obtain a urethral catheterization kit or assemble the following sterile materials for urethral catheterization:

- ☐ sterile underpad and fenestrated drape
- ☐ sterile rayon or cotton balls
- ☐ sterile gloves
- ☐ sterile forceps
- ☐ sterile specimen container
- ☐ sterile water-soluble lubricant
- ☐ sterile antiseptic solution

3 In addition, assemble the following:

☐ extra pair of sterile gloves

☐ two straight Robinson catheters of a size appropriate for your client (from 16F to 22F) (catheters for females tend to be shorter than those for males because of the shorter distance to the bladder for women)

Although the extra gloves and catheter may not be necessary during the procedure, they will be readily available at the bedside in the event of contamination of the original catheter or gloves.

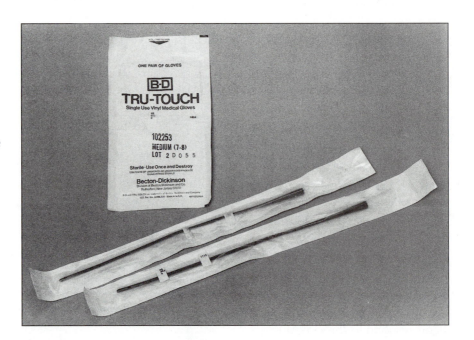

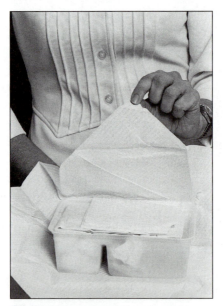

4 Wash your hands and open the catheter kit on a clean, dry surface, using aseptic technique.

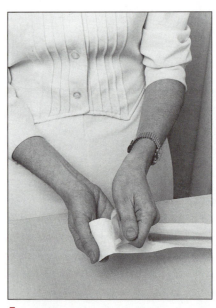

5 Using aseptic technique, open an end of one of the catheter packages and drop the catheter into the opened catheterization kit.

Implementing

6 Assist your client into a dorsal recumbent position, and instruct her to flex her knees. To ensure her warmth and protect her privacy, place a folded bath blanket, sheet, or towel over her abdomen and upper thighs until it is time to cover the perineum with a sterile drape. Grasp the sterile underpad, which is the uppermost drape in the catheterization kit. Hold it by a small section at two corners and wrap the undersurface around your hands (as shown) so that you can insert it under the client's buttocks with minimal contamination. Instruct the client to raise her buttocks so that you can position the underpad (far right).

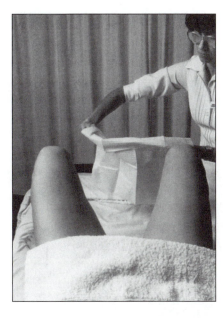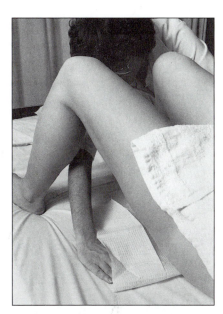

7 Put on sterile gloves, following aseptic technique as detailed in Chapter 1.

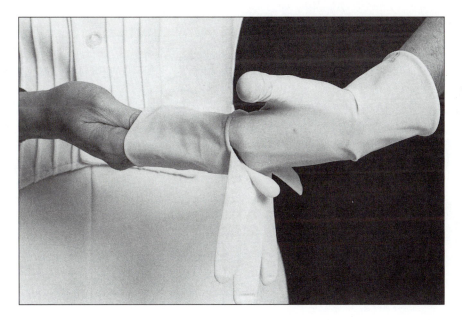

8 Instruct the client to abduct her legs and pull up on the sheet or towel as you place the fenestrated sterile drape over her perineum. Move the sterile catheterization kit to the sterile field between her legs.

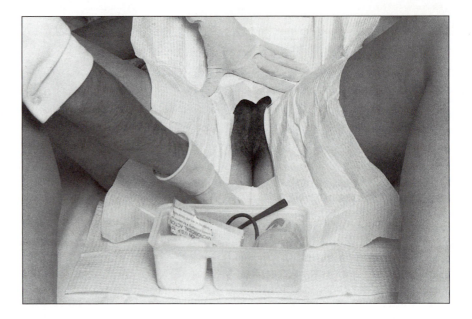

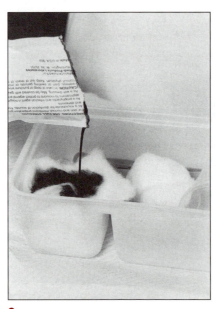

9 Set one or two of the cotton balls aside, and pour the antimicrobial solution over the others.

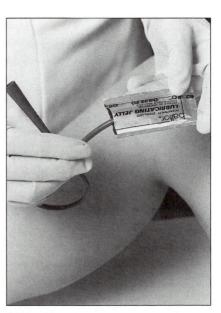

10 Open the sterile lubricant and either place the catheter's tip into the package (as shown) or squeeze the lubricant onto the sterile field and generously lubricate the tip of the catheter.

11 You are ready to prepare the urethral meatus and its surrounding area. With your nondominant hand, separate the labia to expose the urethral meatus. Use your thumb and index finger to apply slight upward and backward tension. This hand is now considered contaminated.

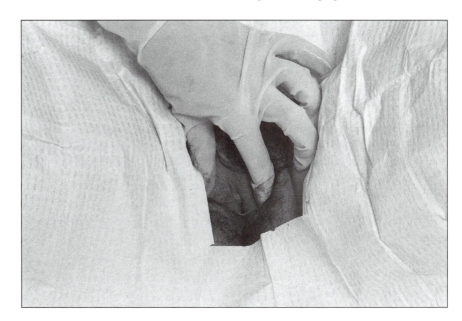

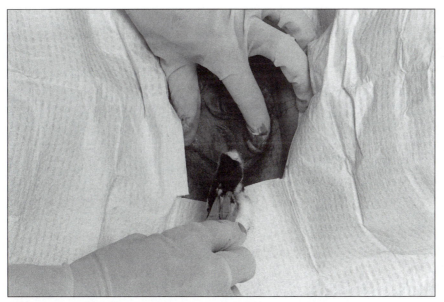

12 With your dominant hand, grasp a saturated cotton ball with the sterile forceps. With one downward stroke per cotton ball, cleanse on each side of the meatus. After each stroke, discard the used cotton ball into a waste container.

Cleanse the meatus (as shown) with one downward stroke. Continue to separate the labia until you have completed the catheterization. *Note: If the labia are allowed to fall together, repeat the cleansing process.*

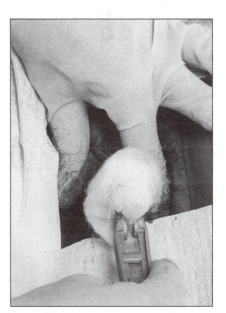

13 After preparing the area, wipe the meatus with a dry cotton ball, using one downward stroke. Discard the cotton ball.

➤

14 Gently insert the catheter into the meatus, and ask the client to breathe deeply and slowly and to bear down with her pelvic muscles. If you meet resistance, slightly angle the catheter toward her symphysis pubis, but do not force the catheter. If urine has not returned after you have inserted the catheter 7.5–10 cm (3–4 in) (adjust the insertion length accordingly in the pediatric population), it is possible that your client is dehydrated or has recently voided. It is more likely, however, that you have inserted the catheter into the vagina, rather than into the urethra. Use the extra pair of sterile gloves and a new catheter and repeat the catheterization. Keep the original catheter in place to avoid making the same mistake.

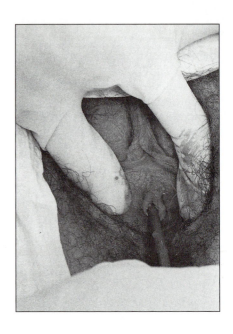

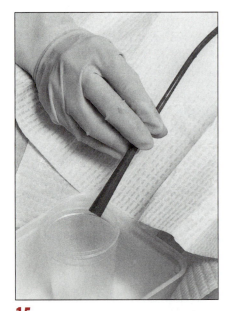

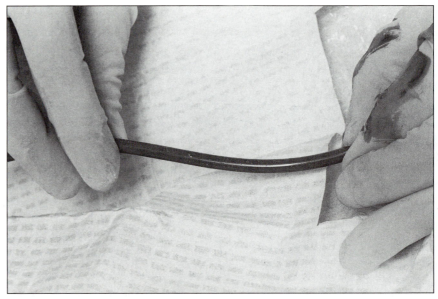

15 When you have catheterized the client successfully, obtain a urine specimen if one has been requested. Place the sterile specimen cup at the distal end of the catheter. After obtaining the specimen, allow the urine to drain into the empty catheterization tray. Follow agency policy regarding the amount of urine you should allow to drain.

16 After emptying the bladder, squeeze the catheter between your thumb and index finger to prevent urine from filling the urethra. Gently remove the catheter. Remove the catheterization materials from the bedside, and assist your client into a comfortable position.

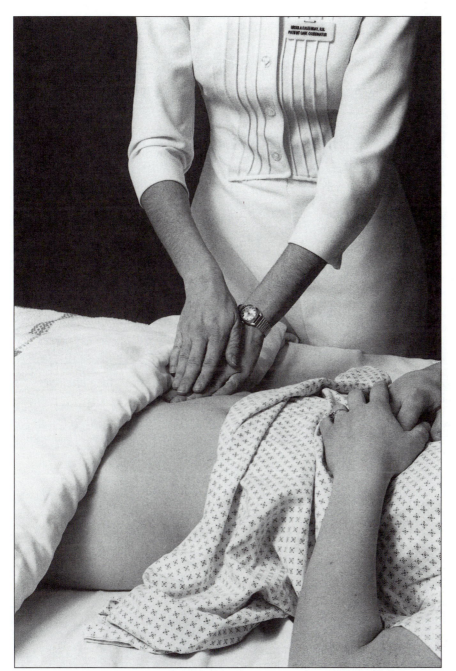

Evaluating

17 Measure the urine; document the procedure, noting the amount, color, and character of the urine. If the catheterization was prescribed for urinary retention, assess your client periodically for her ability to void and for a distended bladder.

HOME HEALTH CARE CONSIDERATIONS

- Caregivers and clients may use clean technique for catheterization.

- Catheters may be reused until they are no longer pliable.

- Catheters and supplies usually are washed in warm, soapy water after each use.

INSERTING A ROBINSON (STRAIGHT) CATHETER INTO A MALE

Implementing

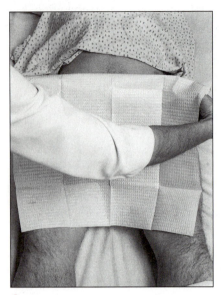

1 For the male client, first follow steps 1–5 in the preceding technique. The male client should assume a dorsal recumbent position with his legs extended. Hold the sterile underpad so that the undersurface of the two corners encircles your hands. Ask the client to raise his gown as you position the pad over his thighs and under his penis.

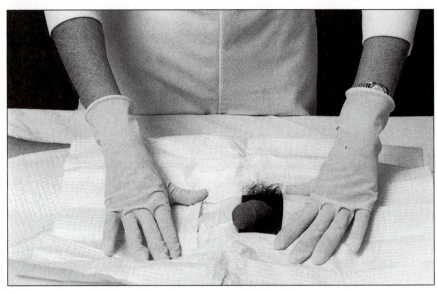

2 After putting on sterile gloves, position the fenestrated drape so that its open surface encircles the penis.

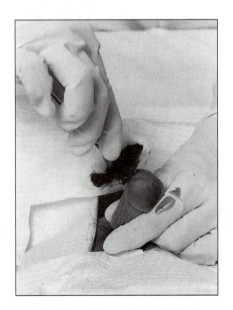

3 Prepare the cotton balls with the antimicrobial solution, following step 9 in the preceding technique. Hold the penis upright with your nondominant hand, and prepare the glans and meatus with your dominant hand, being certain to keep this hand sterile. Hold the cotton balls with the sterile forceps, and cleanse the penis from the meatus toward the shaft, using a circular motion. If your client is uncircumcised, maintain a gentle retraction on the foreskin throughout the procedure. Use fresh cotton balls and repeat the cleansing process at least three more times, disposing of each used cotton ball outside of the sterile field or in a trash can.

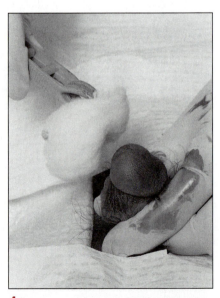

4 After a thorough cleansing, wipe the glans with a dry cotton ball.

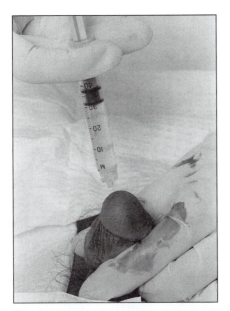

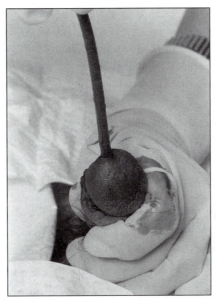

6 Continue to hold the shaft of the penis at a 90-degree angle to the client's abdomen. Apply gentle traction to straighten the urethra, and ask the client to bear down as if to urinate (ask the pediatric client to blow out air) so that the sphincters will relax and allow an easier entry into the urethra. Gently insert the catheter approximately 15–20 cm (6–8 in) until the tip enters the bladder and urine is returned. Adjust the insertion length accordingly in the pediatric population. If you feel resistance, increase the traction on the penis and apply a little more pressure with the catheter, but do not use force. This will enable you to advance the catheter beyond the many folds in the urethra.

5 If the catheterization kit contains a premeasured, lubricant-filled syringe, you can inject the lubricant directly into the urethra of an adult. Otherwise, lubricate the tip of the catheter at least 17.5 cm (7 in) following step 10 in the preceding technique. Adjust the insertion length accordingly in the pediatric population.

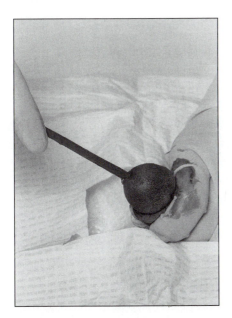

7 If you continue to feel resistance, change the angle of the penis, and use short, rotating movements as you advance the catheter. Continue the insertion until urine begins to flow. Once the catheter has entered the bladder, reposition the foreskin for clients who are uncircumcised. ***Caution:*** *For clients with prostatic hypertrophy, it may be difficult to pass the catheter beyond the prostate. In that situation you may need a special urologic coudé catheter (12–16F) for the adult client. For the pediatric client, notify the physician for insertion.*

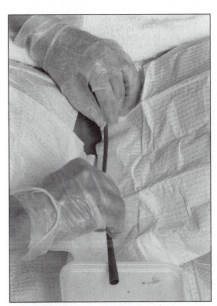

8 Obtain a urine specimen or empty the bladder, following steps 15–17 in the preceding technique.

MANAGING A FOLEY CATHETER

PERFORMING A CATHETERIZATION WITH A FOLEY (INDWELLING) CATHETER

Assessing and Planning

1 Follow the steps for assessing and planning in the procedure for performing intermittent catheterization on pages 437–438. In addition to the catheterization kit, you also will need the following sterile supplies:

☐ drainage collection bag with tubing

☐ syringe and sterile water for inflating the catheter balloon

☐ two Foley catheters (the extra one will be at the bedside in the event that the original is contaminated)

☐ extra pair of sterile gloves in the event the original pair becomes contaminated

☐ extra drainage tubing protector (optional) to keep at the bedside

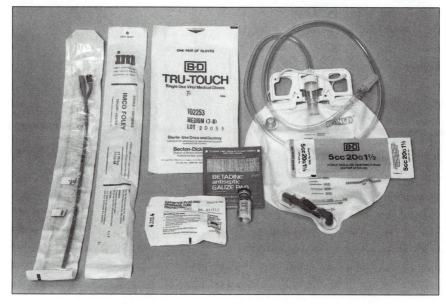

☐ extra antiseptic wipe (optional) to keep at the bedside for subsequent openings of the system (eg, during irrigations or instillations)

☐ tape of an appropriate width for securing the drainage tubing to the client

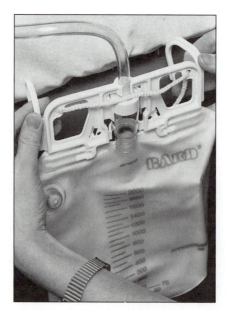

2 Attach the drainage collection bag to the bed frame, and bring the drainage tubing up onto the bed so that it will be readily accessible. Make sure the end of the tubing remains covered by the drainage tubing protector.

Implementing

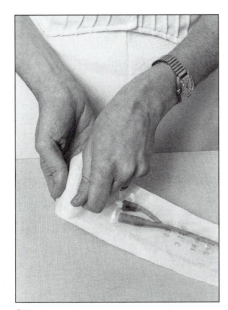 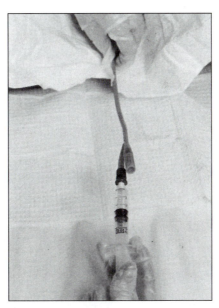 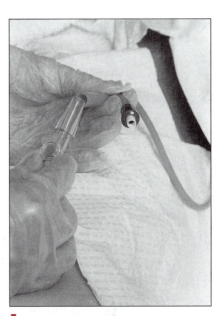

3 After opening the sterile catheterization kit, aseptically open one of the sterile packages containing the Foley and drop the catheter onto the sterile field. Do the same for the sterile syringe if it is not prepackaged with the catheterization kit. Cleanse the urethral meatus and surrounding area, following the appropriate steps for preparing the female or the male. These steps were described in the preceding procedures.

4 Following the steps in the previous two procedures for intermittent catheterization of the male or the female, insert the catheter.

To make sure the catheter is in the bladder, advance it another 2.5 cm (1 in) beyond the distance at which urine begins to flow. For the adult female, the total distance of the insertion will be approximately 7.5–10 cm (3–4 in). The total distance for the adult male, however, can be as much as 25 cm (10 in), and the bifurcation of the catheter might be quite close to the urethral meatus. If the syringe for balloon inflation does not already contain the sterile water, aspirate the appropriate amount. The usual amount is 5 mL, but this can vary depending on the brand and size of catheter used. The appropriate amount is always stamped on the lumen of the balloon portal. Slowly inject the water as you assess the client for discomfort. If the client complains of pain, immediately aspirate the water because the balloon may be incorrectly positioned in the urethra. After inflating the balloon, pull back gently on the catheter to check for resistance, a sign that the balloon is correctly positioned against the proximal wall of the bladder.

5 If the catheter, tubing, and bag are not preconnected, remove the drainage tubing protector and connect the drainage tubing to the open lumen of the catheter. This often requires manipulation, and because your gloves no longer can be considered sterile, it might be necessary to use the antimicrobial wipe at the connection site. Secure the tubing to the bed linen with the attached clip (bottom photo). Be certain to keep the tubing looped on the bed rather than hanging on the floor.

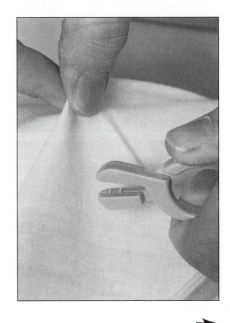

Evaluating

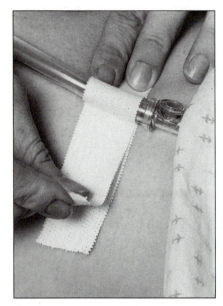 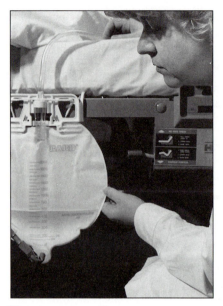 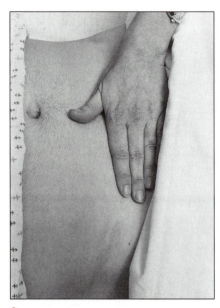

6 Tape the drainage tubing to your client to help prevent it from becoming dislodged. For female clients, tape the tubing to the medial thigh. For the male client, tape the tubing either to the anterior thigh or to the lower abdomen. It is believed that the latter position especially minimizes urethral pressure that would occur at the normal penoscrotal angle. For more secure taping, place a strip of tape on your client's skin; then tape the catheter to the tape (as shown). Allow some slack in the tubing. If the catheter will be left indwelling for an extended period of time, protect your client's skin by making a dressing similar to a Montgomery strap (see the next procedure). Label the drainage bag with the time and date.

7 Document the procedure, noting the time and date of catheterization as well as the size and type of catheter used. Periodically check the drainage tubing for patency and ensure that the output of urine is adequate when compared to the client's intake. Assess the urine for the presence of blood, cloudiness, or a foul odor, which are indications that the client may have a urinary tract infection.

8 If the client has a diminished urinary output, inspect the lower abdomen and palpate or percuss the bladder to assess for urine retention, which can occur with an occluded catheter. Obtain a prescription for an irrigation, if indicated. Also, assess the client for the presence of fever, chills, or discomfort, which are indicators of a urinary tract infection. Ensure that the perineum is washed daily.

HOME HEALTH CARE CONSIDERATIONS

- Change the collection bag and drainage tubing when they are soiled. It may be helpful to set an arbitrary interval of once per month for consistency.

- Change the Foley catheter when it feels gritty when it is rolled between the fingers, using the same sterile technique discussed in this procedure.

- Before changing the Foley, the caregiver should position a towel under the client to protect the bedding.

- For home use, the client may desire to change to a leg bag or to a larger drainage collection bag.

NURSING GUIDELINES: FOLEY CATHETER MANAGEMENT

- Coil and secure the drainage tubing to the bed linen to prevent looping below the drainage bag, which can promote urine stasis and bacterial growth.

- To prevent urinary tract infections caused by urinary reflux, always keep the drainage bag below the level of the client's bladder.
  — Instruct ambulatory clients to carry the drainage bag below the level of their bladders.
  — Instruct transport personnel to keep the drainage bag below the client's bladder.

- To reduce the risk of transferring organisms from one client's urinary drainage container to another client's urinary drainage container, the Centers for Disease Control and Prevention recommends that no more than one client in a room have an indwelling urethral catheter.

- Unless it is contraindicated, as, for example, in cardiac and renal failure clients, encourage a fluid intake of at least 2–3 L/day to dilute the urine and maximize urinary flow. It is believed that this will help reduce the risk of urinary tract infections.

- Unless it has been specifically prescribed, hand irrigate the catheter only when it is obstructed.

- Assess for indications of a urinary tract infection: chills, increased temperature, flank/suprapubic pain, hematuria, and cloudy or foul-smelling urine.

- Inspect and cleanse the perineal area with soap and warm water during the client's daily bath.

- Be alert to meatal swelling, discharge, and erythema, which are indicators of infection. For clients performing self-care, remind them of the importance of daily perineal cleansing.

- Evaluate the need for an indwelling drainage device on a daily basis. Collaborate with the physician to remove the device as soon as possible to reduce the risk of the client developing a urinary tract infection. The longer the catheter remains in the bladder, the greater the risk of urinary tract infection to the client.

- Label and keep a separate graduated measuring container for each client with a urinary drainage device. Use this container only for emptying the client's urinary drainage bag; rinse it and allow it to dry between uses. This practice reduces the risk of transferring organisms from one client's drainage bag to another client's drainage bag via a shared graduate that may be contaminated.

MAKING A CATHETER STRAP

Instead of using tape to anchor your client's Foley catheter, consider making a catheter strap, which is similar to a Montgomery strap. This will eliminate the need for repeated removal and reapplication of tape when frequent repositioning of the Foley is necessary. To make the catheter strap, you will need two pieces of tape 10 X 10 cm (4 X 4 in) and a 25-cm (10-in) piece of twill tape.

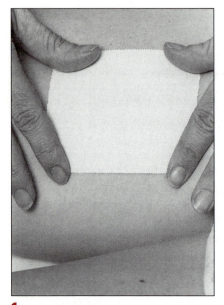

1 For female clients, adhere one of the tape squares to the medial thigh. For male clients, attach the tape to the anterior thigh or lower abdomen. Shave the site first, if necessary.

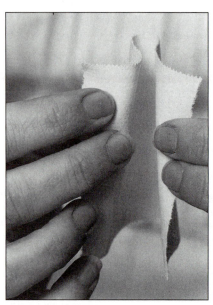

2 Fold the other square in half, so that the nonadhering surfaces face one another.

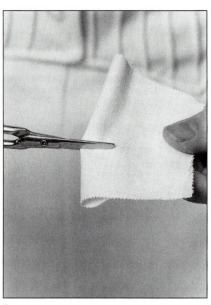

3 Cut two slits along the folded edge, 6 mm (¼ in) in width and approximately 2.5 cm (1 in) apart.

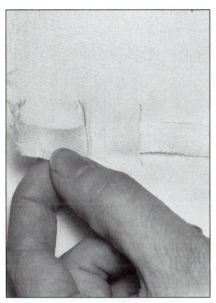

4 Unfold the tape and pull the twill tape through the slits.

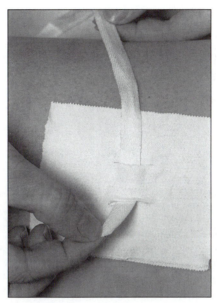

5 Adhere the second tape to the first, and pull the twill tape until it is at equal lengths on each side.

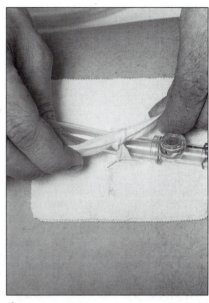

6 Position the drainage tubing over the twill tape, and tie the tape around the tubing. When the outer tape square becomes soiled, you can easily replace it without removing the inner square, thus saving your client discomfort.

OBTAINING A URINE SPECIMEN

As you know, urine in the drainage bag is considered contaminated; and disconnecting the catheter from the drainage tubing opens the system and increases the potential for infection. Therefore, urine samples for diagnostic testing must be obtained through a closed system, either through a sampling port or directly through the urinary catheter.

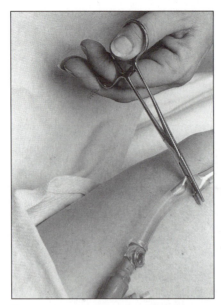

1 To obtain the specimen, you will need to clamp the drainage tubing for a few minutes (usually around 15) to allow the urine to collect in the catheter. Clamp at a point directly below the sampling port where the tubing is flexible.

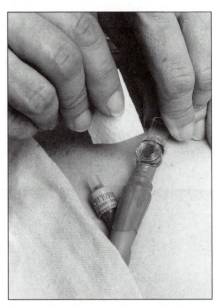

2 Wash your hands and cleanse the sampling port with an antimicrobial wipe such as an alcohol sponge. Allow it to dry.

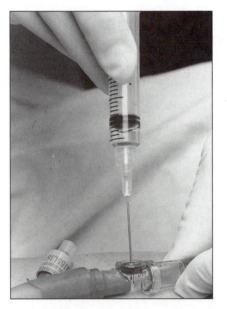

3 Apply clean gloves. Aspirate the urine directly through the port, using a sterile needle and syringe. Usually 2–3 mL will be adequate for a diagnostic test. Remove the needle and syringe, and cleanse the sampling port again with an antimicrobial wipe.

4 If the catheter does not have a sampling port, cleanse the catheter just distal to the bifurcation.

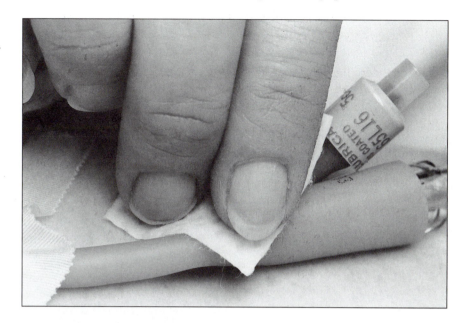

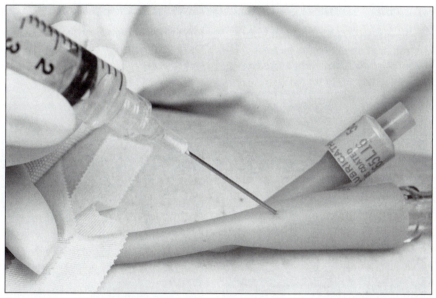

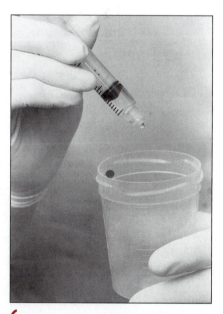

5 Apply clean gloves. Using a 21- to 25-gauge needle and a sterile syringe, aspirate the urine through the catheter wall. Point the needle away from the bifurcation to prevent puncturing the balloon port and aspirating the balloon's contents. Remove the needle and cleanse the site again.

6 Inject the urine into a sterile specimen cup unless the syringe itself is to be sent to the laboratory. As indicated, dispose of the needle and syringe in a sharps container following agency protocol. Remove your gloves. Label the specimen with the client's name, the time and date of collection, and note that it was obtained from the catheter. If you cannot send the specimen to the laboratory immediately, refrigerate it (contraindicated for urine cultures). Be sure that you have unclamped the catheter. Wash your hands.

EMPTYING THE DRAINAGE BAG

The urinary drainage bag should be emptied every 8 hours, or more frequently during periods of large urinary output. This is essential in reducing the infection risk because urine that is allowed to stagnate is an excellent medium for bacterial growth.

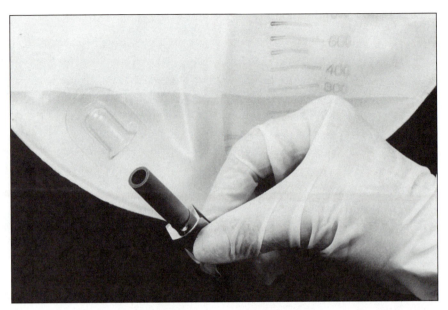

1 To empty the bag, wash your hands and apply clean gloves; then position the client's measuring container under the spout. Detach the spout from its protective sleeve.

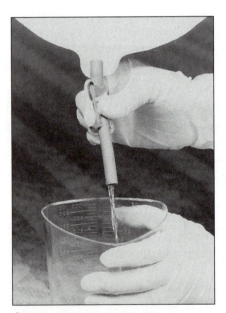

2 Open the clamp, allowing the entire contents to drain into the measuring container. To prevent contamination, do not allow the spout to touch the measuring container.

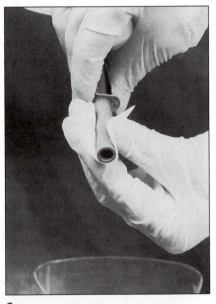

3 After emptying the drainage bag, clean the spout with an antiseptic wipe and reinsert it into its sleeve on the drainage bag. Measure and record the amount of urine. Empty and wash the measuring container. Remove your gloves and wash your hands.

USING A URINE METER

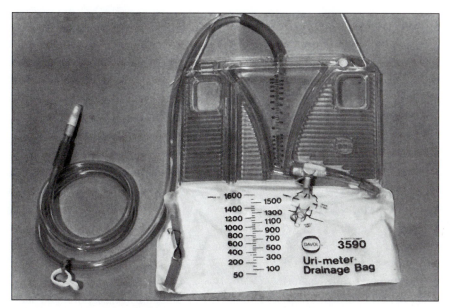

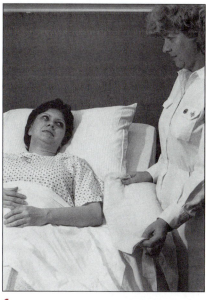

When accurate monitoring of urinary output is necessary, for example, for clients in acute renal failure, obtain a urine meter with a drainage bag and attach it to your client's Foley catheter. The urine meter will enable you to measure minute quantities of urine, either hourly or during specified time intervals.

1 Wash your hands and explain the procedure to your client. Place a bed-saver pad under the catheter, and attach the urine meter to the bedside frame next to the Foley drainage bag. Secure the drainage tubing to the bed linen so that it will be readily accessible.

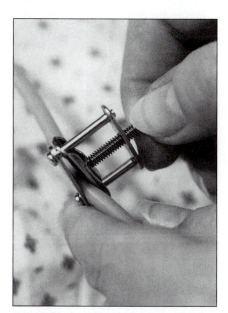

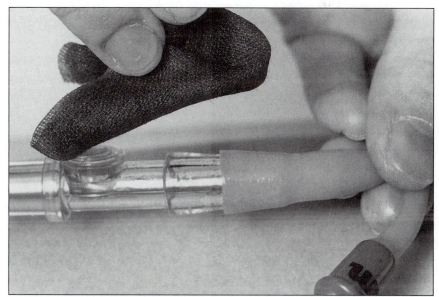

2 Straighten the drainage tubing to drain the urine into the drainage bag, and then clamp the catheter.

3 Thoroughly cleanse the connection site of the catheter and drainage tubing with an antiseptic wipe. Because it is sometimes difficult to manipulate the tubing without touching the ends, it may be a good idea to apply sterile gloves.

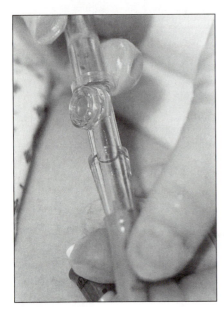

4 Aseptically detach the Foley drainage tubing from the catheter.

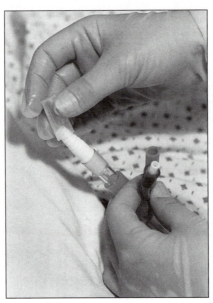

5 Remove the protective cap on the end of the urine meter drainage tubing, and aseptically insert the tubing into the catheter lumen. Unclamp the catheter and tape the drainage tubing to your client's thigh or abdomen. After measuring the output, discard the Foley drainage system.

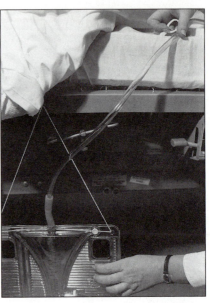

6 Hourly, or during specified time intervals, straighten the drainage tubing and inspect the collection chamber to assess the amount of urine that has collected. Record the amount and open the stopcock to allow the urine to drain into the drainage bag. When the client no longer requires hourly urine checks, just keep the stopcock open to allow the urine to drain into the drainage bag. This will prevent reopening the system to attach a regular drainage bag, which potentially could contaminate both the system and the client's urinary tract.

IRRIGATING THE CATHETER

Assessing

1 Because irrigating a catheter can greatly increase the risk of infection by opening a closed system, irrigation should not be performed unless you are certain the catheter is obstructed. Diminished urinary output is an unacceptable rationale for irrigation, unless it is accompanied by additional indications of obstruction (see step 2, below). Evaluate the integrity of the collection system by inspecting the drainage tubing for kinks or exterior obstructions. Evaluate your client's intake and compare it to the output. If you assess that your client might be dehydrated, increase the fluid intake and reevaluate the output

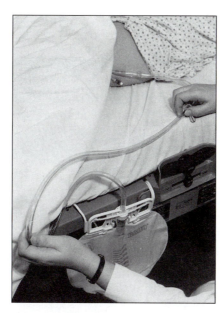

after 30–45 minutes. Because hypotension also can reduce urinary output, be sure to check the client's blood pressure.

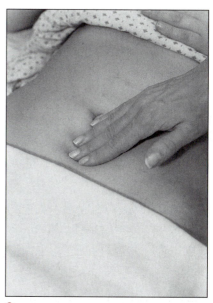

2 Inspect the suprapubic area and palpate or percuss your client's bladder. If the bladder is distended, the urinary output is minimal (less than 30 mL/hr or 0.5 mL/kg/hr), blood clots are noted, urine is leaking around the catheter, or the client is experiencing bladder spasms, obtain a prescription for an irrigation.

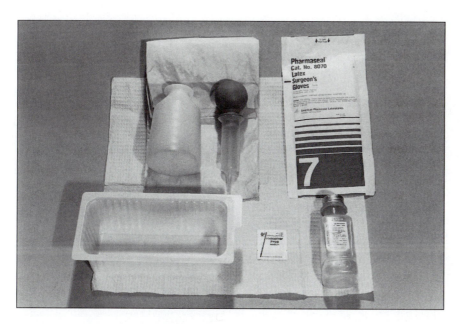

Planning

3 Obtain a catheter irrigation kit or assemble the following materials:

- ☐ sterile underpad for use as a sterile field and bed protector
- ☐ sterile drainage tray
- ☐ sterile graduated container with a 50–60 mL bulb (not piston) syringe
- ☐ sterile gloves
- ☐ antiseptic wipe
- ☐ sterile normal saline or the prescribed irrigant warmed to room temperature
- ☐ bed-saver pad

Remember to keep the following items sterile at all times: the open ends of both the drainage tubing and the catheter, the irrigant, and the syringe.

Implementing

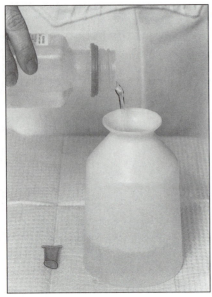

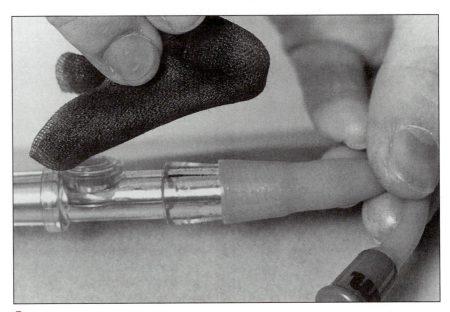

4 Wash your hands and explain the procedure to your client. After the client assumes a dorsal recumbent position, place a bed-saver pad under the Foley catheter. Aseptically open the irrigation tray, and place the underpad over a clean, dry surface to make a sterile field. Pour the sterile irrigant into the graduated container, and position the empty tray close to the client's perineum.

5 Clean the connection of the drainage tubing and catheter with an antiseptic wipe.

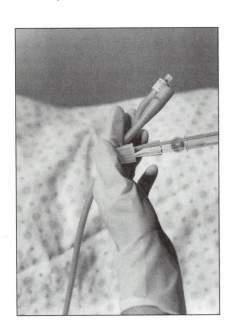

6 Put on a clean glove. Disconnect the drainage tubing from the Foley. Keep the end of the drainage tubing sterile by capping it with a tube protector (as shown) or by attaching a sterile gauze pad and securing it with a rubber band. To keep the end of the catheter sterile, place it over the drainage tray so that it will be protected as you apply sterile gloves.

7 Put on sterile gloves and aspirate 30–50 mL of the sterile irrigant into the bulb syringe. Attach the syringe to the end of the catheter, and inject the irrigant gently by slowly squeezing the bulb of the syringe.

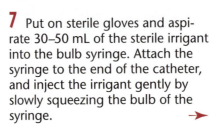

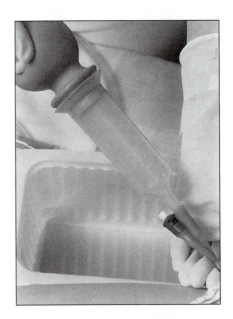

Evaluating

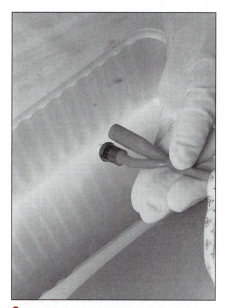

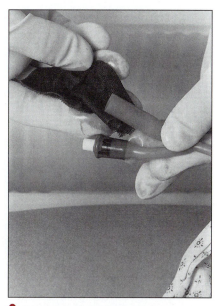

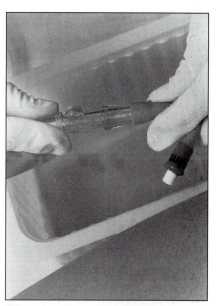

8 Remove the syringe and allow the irrigant to return into the drainage tray by gravity. After the irrigant has returned, and if it is indicated, repeat the irrigation process until the returns are clear.

If the fluid fails to return, gently rotate the catheter between your fingers, press gently on the suprapubic area, or ask the client to perform Valsalva's maneuver or turn from side to side. If these measures fail to return the irrigant, apply gentle suction with the bulb. This might be necessary if blood clots are obstructing the catheter.

Unless absolutely necessary, avoid aspiration with a piston syringe because vigorous suctioning can damage the bladder wall. Follow agency protocol for further intervention if you still are unable to return the irrigant. It may be necessary to reconnect the drainage tubing and observe the client closely for the next hour or two, assessing for continued indications of obstruction as well as for eventual gravity drainage, which may occur once bladder spasms cease. If the obstruction continues, notify the physician for further intervention, such as changing the catheter.

9 After completing the irrigation, clean the open end of the catheter with an antiseptic wipe.

10 Grasp the drainage tubing, remove the protective cover, and aseptically connect the drainage tubing to the open end of the catheter. Remove the used equipment from the bedside. Measure the amount of the return and compare it to the amount that was instilled. Remove your gloves, wash your hands, and assist the client into a position of comfort. Document the procedure, noting the amount and character of the return. Be certain to note the amount of residual irrigant on the intake and output record, as well. Continue to assess the client to ensure that there are no indications of bladder distention, spasms, or diminished urinary output.

REMOVING A FOLEY CATHETER

When the physician has requested the discontinuation of your client's Foley catheter, you first will need to deflate the balloon to allow the catheter to pass through the urethra.

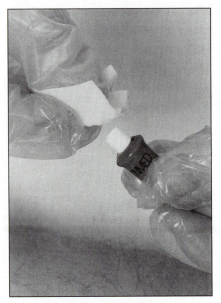

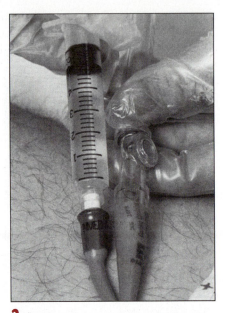

1 Apply clean gloves. Place a bed-saver pad under your client's catheter, and cleanse the balloon port with an antiseptic wipe. Untape the catheter from your client's thigh or abdomen.

2 Depending on the type of catheter used, either cut the balloon port or attach a sterile syringe to the balloon port (some catheters may require both a syringe and a needle), and aspirate the water. The amount required to inflate the balloon should be imprinted on the lumen of the balloon port. Be certain to aspirate the same amount of water that was injected after the catheter's insertion. When the water has been aspirated, pinch the catheter between your thumb and index finger to prevent urine from filling the urethra during the removal. Gently pull on the catheter to remove it from your client's bladder and urethra. If you are unable to withdraw the catheter, do not use force. Notify the physician, instead, for further intervention. Remove the catheter and drainage bag from the bedside, and provide your client with soap and water for cleansing the meatus and perineum. Measure and document the output and record the procedure. During the first 24 hours following the removal of the Foley catheter, or according to agency protocol, document the time, amount, and character of each voiding.

Caring for Clients with Renal-Urinary Disorder

APPLYING AN EXTERNAL URINARY DEVICE (WITH A LEG DRAINAGE SYSTEM)

Assessing and Planning

When caring for male clients for whom the prolonged use of indwelling catheters may be contraindicated, you might assess the need for an external collection device such as the Hollister™ Male Urinary Collection System. Exdwelling catheters, also known as condom and Texas catheters, usually require a physician's prescription. Be sure to read manufacturer's instructions carefully before applying the exdwelling catheter used by your agency.

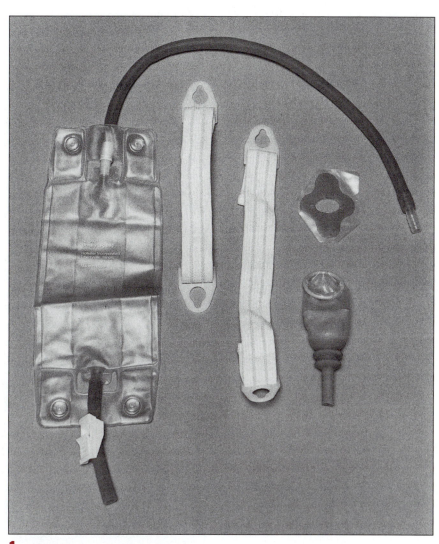

1 If an external urinary device has been prescribed for your client, explain the procedure and, if appropriate, prepare to instruct him in the application technique. Assemble the following equipment:

- [ ] leg drainage bag
- [ ] extension tubing
- [ ] leg straps
- [ ] skin protector
- [ ] exdwelling (condom) catheter

Implementing

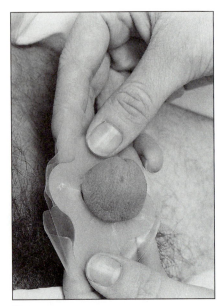

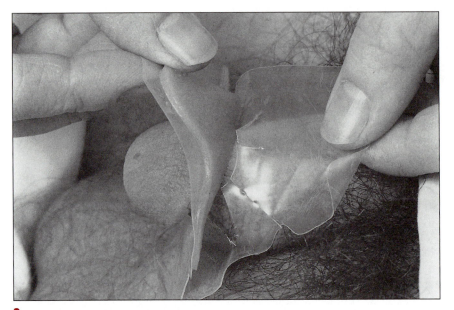

2 Wash your hands and begin the procedure by trimming or pushing the pubic hair away from the penis. It is seldom necessary to shave the hair because hair that adheres to the sticky surface of the adhesive skin protector can be pulled away carefully. Gently pull the glans penis through the opening of the skin protector. The skin protector will stretch and yet rapidly return to its original shape without constricting the penis or losing its elasticity.

3 Pull off the protective film on the underside of the skin protector. Adhere the posterior surface of the skin protector to the shaft of the penis. Be certain that the pubic hair is pushed away first.

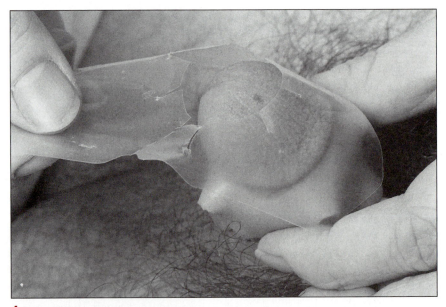

4 Remove the protective film from the anterior surface of the skin protector.

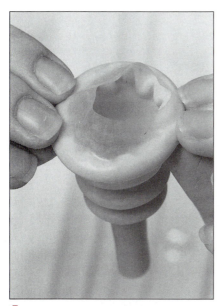

5 Roll the catheter until the inner flap is exposed. This is important because it is this flap that prevents the reflux of urine.

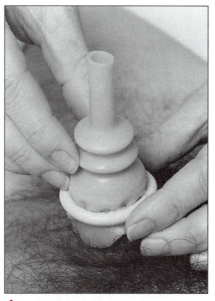

6 Position the catheter over the glans penis so that the opening of the inner flap surrounds the urethral meatus.

Assembling the Leg Drainage Bag

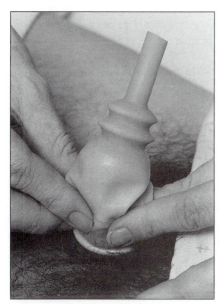

7 Carefully unroll the catheter with as little wrinkling as possible until it covers the skin protector. Gently press along the exterior of the catheter to adhere it to the skin protector. If more than a few wrinkles occur, do not attempt to reposition the catheter on the skin protector. See step 11 for removal instructions.

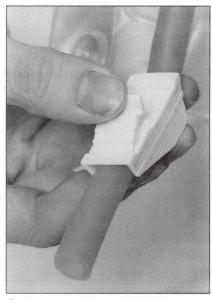

8 After removing the drainage bag from its container, close the drain clamp at the bottom of the bag.

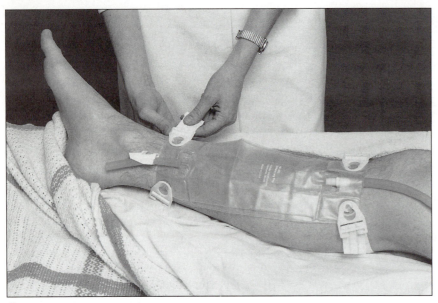

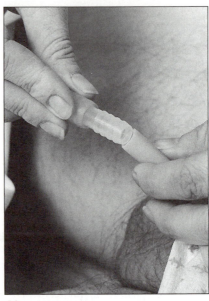

9 Position the bag at the medial aspect of the lower leg, and bring each strap around the leg, attaching the straps to the buttons on the drainage bag. Adjust each strap so that it securely attaches the drainage bag to the leg yet does not constrict circulation.

10 Attach the extension tubing to the external urinary device via the connector. The tubing should have enough slack so that it does not tug on the external catheter. For shorter clients, the tubing can be cut to ensure a good fit. Explain to the client that the drainage bag can be emptied by opening the drain clamp. Wash your hands and document the procedure. ***Note:*** *For nonambulatory clients, a closed drainage collection bag can be used instead.*

Evaluating

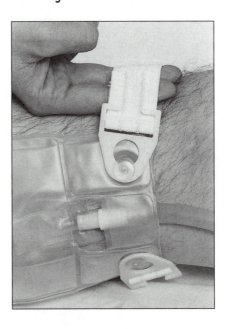

11 Periodically assess the skin under the straps for pressure areas, irritation, or skin breakdown, and ensure that the straps are not too tight by placing two fingers between the client's skin and the straps (as shown). Alert, mobile clients should be shown how to adjust the straps and to assess for the presence of leakage or irritation.

It is recommended that the catheter be changed daily. To remove the catheter, roll it off the penis together with the skin protector. After removal, warm water can be used to remove any residue left by the skin protector.

MONITORING THE CLIENT RECEIVING CONTINUOUS BLADDER IRRIGATION (CBI)

ESTABLISHING CBI

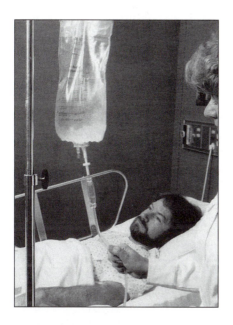

1 If your client has had a transurethral prostatectomy, he might return from surgery with a three-way Foley catheter, which allows closed continuous bladder irrigation. The irrigation is usually performed for a 24-hour period, during which the client remains on bed rest. If the irrigation solution and drainage bag were not already connected in surgery, it might be your responsibility to assemble the equipment and establish the irrigation. Explain the procedure to your client, and wash your hands. Obtain the prescribed irrigation solution (usually a glycine preparation), its special irrigation tubing, and a large (3,000–4,000 mL) collection bag (optional). Spike the solution container, hang it on an IV pole, and prime the tubing as you would an intravenous infusion set. Be certain to flush out all the air, and then clamp off the tubing.

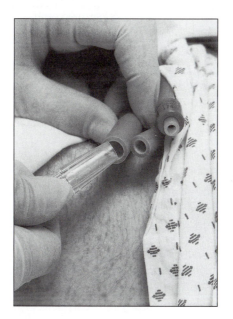

2 If the three-way catheter is not already attached to a large collection bag, you may need to detach the regular-sized collection bag and replace it with the large bag. To do this, briefly clamp the catheter, apply sterile gloves, cleanse the large outflow lumen with an antiseptic wipe, and aseptically attach the tubing for the large collection bag (as shown). Unclamp the catheter.

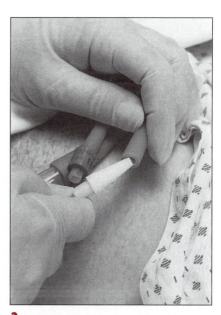

3 Cleanse the inflow lumen with an antiseptic wipe, and aseptically insert the connector for the primed infusion tubing. Establish the prescribed flow rate and refer to the following guidelines for client care. Document the procedure.

NURSING GUIDELINES: CARE OF THE CLIENT WITH CBI

- Unless prescribed, keep the client on bed rest during CBI (usually 24 hours).

- Moderate bleeding (pink to deep-pink returns) is normal. Bright red returns containing numerous blood clots are indicative of hemorrhage, and the physician should be alerted immediately.

- With normal hematuria, maintain the infusion rate of the irrigant at 40–60 drops/min. Increase the rate if the returns are a brighter red, and decrease the rate when the returns become clearer.

- Monitor vital signs at least every 4 hours during the irrigation (every 15 minutes if they are unstable). Assess for these indicators of impending shock if the returns are bright red: hypotension, pallor, diaphoresis, and rapid pulse and respirations.

- To ensure that there is no obstruction, which can occur with blood clots, inspect the catheter for patency and assess the client's suprapubic area for distention. In addition, question the client regarding the presence of severe discomfort or recurring bladder spasms.

- Keep careful records of intake and output, subtracting the amount of irrigation solution from the total output to determine the true amount of urine production.

- Irrigate *only* if the catheter is obstructed and if you have a physician's prescription to do so.

- If the physician requests traction on the balloon portion of the catheter, maintain traction with tape or a gauze strip. The traction will keep the balloon wedged against the prostatic fossa to minimize bleeding.

- If it is not contraindicated, encourage a fluid intake of 2–3 L/day. Dilute urine has less potential for the growth of bacteria and the formation of encrustations.

- When a glycine irrigating solution is used, assess for these signs of hyponatremia: muscle twitching, confusion, convulsions.

NURSING GUIDELINES: CARE OF THE CLIENT WITH A SUPRAPUBIC CATHETER

If your client is having bladder or prostatic surgery or a vaginal hysterectomy, or if the urethra is impassable, the physician might drain the bladder via an incision through the suprapubic area into the bladder. The catheter is then attached to a closed drainage collection container.

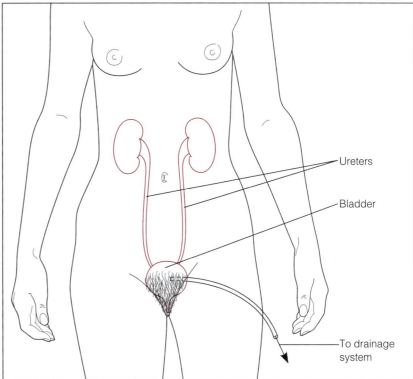

- To prevent dislodging, tape the tubing securely to the lateral abdomen.

- Should the catheter become dislodged, cover the site with a sterile dressing, and inform the physician at once for immediate replacement.

- To prevent contamination from the backflow of urine, keep the drainage collection container below the level of the client's bladder.

- Slight hematuria is normal during the first 24–48 hours postinsertion. Bright red drainage is abnormal and should be reported immediately. Be sure to document the character and amount of drainage. It should have a characteristic urine odor. Foul-smelling, cloudy urine or drainage is indicative of an infection.

- Keep drainage records from the suprapubic catheter separate from those of other indwelling catheters or tubes.

- Inspect the catheter for patency, and prevent external obstruction. Irrigate only if an internal obstruction is noted, following the procedure on pages 457–459.

- Assess the dressing for drainage, and change it as soon as it becomes wet, using aseptic technique. Because it contains urine, a saturated dressing can lead to skin breakdown. Consider applying a pectin wafer skin barrier around the catheter insertion site to protect the skin.

- Encourage a fluid intake of at least 2–3 L/day. Dilute urine minimizes the potential for infection and encrustations.

- Prior to removal, the physician may prescribe catheter clamping for 3–4 hours at a time to test the client's ability to void spontaneously. After the client has voided, unclamp the catheter and measure the residual urine in the collection container. Notify the physician for removal when the residual urine is less than 100 mL after each of two successive voidings. Usually the catheter can be removed safely at that time.

Nursing Guidelines: Care of the Client with a Nephrostomy Tube and Ureteral Stents

A percutaneous nephrostomy tube might be inserted for the client who has a ureteral obstruction, such as nephrolithiasis. The tube is inserted directly into the renal pelvis via an incision in the flank (below the posterior ribs and above the ilium) and anchored in place with one or more sutures or an inflated balloon. The tube is then connected to a closed drainage collection container. Ureteral catheters (stents) and drains also might be inserted (as shown).

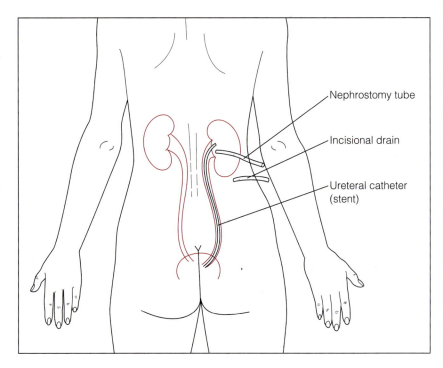

Nephrostomy tube

Incisional drain

Ureteral catheter (stent)

- To prevent the nephrostomy tube from becoming dislodged, tape it securely to the client's flank. Elastic tape works especially well. Unless otherwise prescribed, keep the client on bed rest.

- Should the tube become dislodged, cover the site with a sterile dressing and notify the physician at once for immediate replacement.

- To prevent infection from reflux, keep the drainage collection container below the level of the client's kidney at all times.

- Clients also will have an indwelling bladder catheter to measure urine from the functioning kidney.

- A ureteral stent may be placed for a client with nephrolithiasis to help locate the stones.

- Monitor and record the character and amount of drainage in the collection container every hour. Some hematuria is normal during the first and second day postinsertion; bright red drainage is abnormal and should be reported to the physician immediately. An abrupt cessation in urine is often indicative of a dislodged or obstructed catheter. Copious amounts of drainage, however (eg, 2,000 mL or more during an 8-hour period), can signal postobstructive diuresis, which can cause fluid and electrolyte disturbances. Differentiate and record the amounts for each tube or

NURSING GUIDELINES: CARE OF THE CLIENT WITH A NEPHROSTOMY TUBE AND URETERAL STENTS (continued)

catheter, and add the total together for total output.

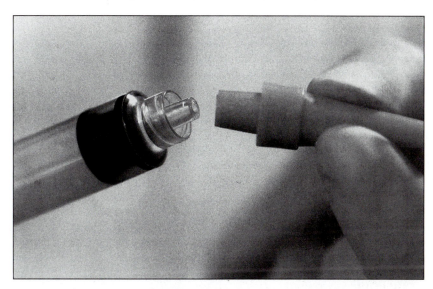

- During the first 24 hours postinsertion, monitor the client for indications of hemorrhage: decrease in blood pressure, rapid pulse and respirations, and copious amounts of bright red drainage. Also be alert to swelling or bruising in the affected flank, which can signal internal bleeding. Also assess for these indicators of infection: increase in temperature, chills, and foul-smelling and cloudy urine in the collection container. Also monitor the insertion site for erythema, swelling, and purulent drainage.

- To reduce the risk of infection, keep the drainage system closed at all times unless you have a physician's specific prescription for irrigation.

- If irrigation has been prescribed, instill a maximum of 5 mL of irrigant at one time into the nephrostomy tube. Greater amounts, resulting in overdistention, can damage the kidney. To instill the irrigant into the tube, it may be necessary to attach a male adaptor to a 5-mL syringe (as shown).

- Assess the dressing for excessive drainage and the insertion site for leakage around the tube. Either problem is indicative of a tube that is dislodged or obstructed. To prevent skin breakdown from the highly irritating urine, change the dressing before it becomes saturated.

- Because pyelonephritis can result from an infection, always use aseptic technique for dressing changes and irrigation.

- To minimize the potential for infection and the formation of calculi, encourage a fluid intake of at least 2–3 L/day.

- Once ureteral patency has been determined, the physician might request that the nephrostomy tube be clamped before removal to ensure client tolerance. During the clamping period, assess the client for the presence of flank pain or fever, or for a diminished urinary output. These are indications of ureteral obstruction.

ADMINISTERING A SODIUM POLYSTYRENE SULFONATE (KAYEXALATE) ENEMA

Sodium polystyrene sulfonate is a sodium resin, which exchanges sodium for potassium in the gastrointestinal tract for clients with hyperkalemia. It frequently is given with sorbitol, which because of its hypertonicity induces diarrhea. This facilitates expulsion and prevents reabsorption of the potassium.

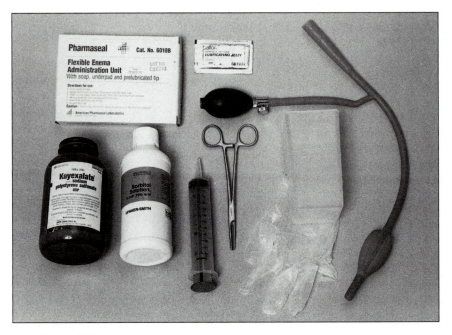

Assessing and Planning

1 If your client has hyperkalemia, which could be caused by a diminished urinary output, acid-base imbalance, or cellular breakdown, the physician might prescribe sodium polystyrene sulfonate. However, if the client is unable to tolerate it orally because of nausea and vomiting or diminished bowel sounds, it will be necessary to administer it rectally. Assemble the following materials to administer the enema:

☐ prescribed amounts of sodium polystyrene sulfonate and sorbitol

☐ one or more 50-mL piston syringes, depending on the prescribed amounts of the enema solution to be administered

☐ water-soluble lubricant

☐ hemostat or tubing clamp

☐ clean gloves

☐ container for mixing the enema solution

☐ rectal tube with an inflatable balloon

☐ device for inflating the balloon (eg, sphygmomanometer bulb)

☐ kit for administering a cleansing tap water enema after the client has expelled the sodium polystyrene sulfonate

☐ bed-saver pad

☐ bedpan at the bedside (optional) if your client cannot walk to the bathroom

Mix the prescribed amounts of sodium polystyrene sulfonate with the sorbitol and aspirate or pour the solution into the piston syringe(s). If it is too thick for easy administration, dilute it slightly with water.

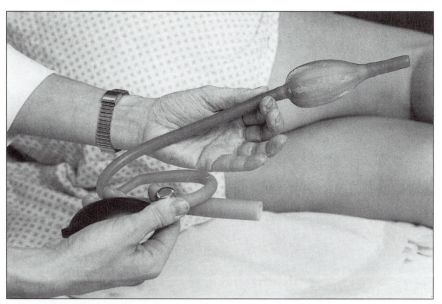

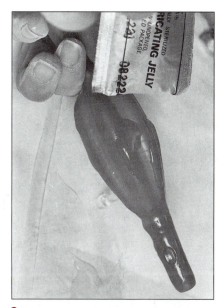

2 Review the procedure in Chapter 5 for administering a retention enema. Wash your hands and explain the procedure to the client. Assist her into a left side-lying (Sims') position, and place a bed-saver pad under the buttocks. Assess the integrity of the balloon at the end of the rectal tube: compress the inflating bulb and count the number of compressions that are needed to inflate the balloon to two-thirds of its capacity (make appropriate modifications for the pediatric population). Make a note of that number. ***Caution:*** *To prevent injury to the rectal tissue, never inflate the balloon more than two-thirds of its capacity once it is in the rectum.*

3 Generously lubricate the tip and balloon of the rectal tube with water-soluble lubricant. Be sure that the balloon is completely collapsed.

Implementing

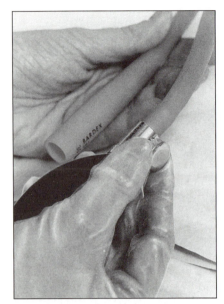

4 Put on a clean glove and insert the deflated balloon into the client's rectum past the external and internal sphincters. Inflate the balloon, compressing the bulb the same number of times required to inflate it to two-thirds of its capacity (see step 2, page 471). Inflating the balloon will help the client retain the solution. Pull back gently on the rectal tube to ensure that the balloon is properly inflated and cannot be pulled past the sphincters.

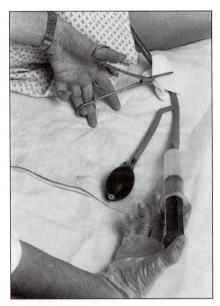

5 Attach the piston syringe containing the solution to the open end of the rectal tube. Position the opened hemostat around the area you will later clamp. Administer the medication in a bolus, clamp the tubing, and remove the empty syringe. Either attach another syringe containing the solution or maintain the clamped tubing for 30–45 minutes, or the prescribed amount of time, until the client is allowed to expel the solution. Be reassuring and periodically advise the client of the time remaining until the solution can be expelled.

Evaluating

6 When the retention time has expired, unclamp the tubing, deflate the balloon, and remove the tube from the client's rectum. The client may then expel the solution. If the client is ambulatory, ask to see the returns in the toilet. Otherwise, assist the client onto the bedpan. After the expulsion, administer cleansing tap water enemas until the returns are clear and no longer brown. Provide materials for cleansing the rectal area and assist the client into a position of comfort. Document the procedure and its results. Continue to assess the client for indications of hyperkalemia: weakness, cramps, twitching, or diarrhea. The physician may prescribe a serum electrolyte test to evaluate the level of serum potassium, and hence the effectiveness of the enema.

PERFORMING CREDÉ'S MANEUVER

Manual pressure applied to the bladder, Credé's maneuver, can be employed to facilitate the removal of urine for clients whose bladders are flaccid—for example, clients with hypotonic neurogenic bladders. The procedure should not be performed without a physician's prescription. It is contraindicated for clients with especially strong sphincter resistance because the high intravesical pressure it produces potentially can result in ureteral reflux and infection. Credé's maneuver is also contraindicated for clients with spinal cord injury at or above T6 because of the potential for autonomic dysreflexia caused by this stimulus.

Assessing and Planning

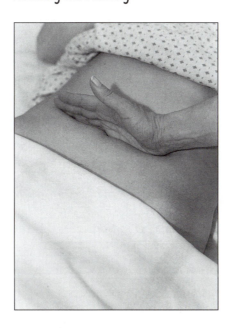

1 Usually the procedure is performed every 4–6 hours to prevent the bladder from becoming overly distended. However, you should periodically assess your client's bladder for distention during the interim periods. When the bladder is full, provide privacy and assist a female client onto a bedpan or provide a urinal for your male client. Clients with arm and hand strength and mobility should be taught to use the maneuver as an alternative to self-catheterization. When the client is in a comfortable position, place the ulnar surface of your hand at the umbilicus.

Implementing

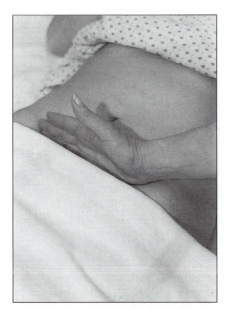

2 Instruct the client to bear down with the abdominal muscles, if possible. Press downward and sweep your hand onto the suprapubic area, using a kneading motion to initiate urination. Continue the maneuver every 30 seconds until urination ceases.

Evaluating

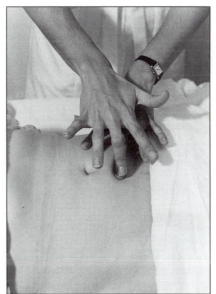

3 Percuss the client's bladder to ensure that all the urine has been removed. If you elicit dull sounds, repeat the procedure until all urine has been expressed. This will help prevent urinary tract infections caused by residual urine. If you elicit tympanic, hollow sounds, assume that the bladder is empty. Remove the urinal or bedpan and assist the client into a comfortable position. Document the procedure.

Caring for Clients Undergoing Dialysis

NURSING GUIDELINES: QUINTON AND PERMCATH DIALYSIS ACCESSES

Description

The Quinton (top in photo) and Permcath (bottom in photo) are large-bore, double-lumen central catheters used for dialysis access. Both have a designated venous side from which blood can be drawn off and an arterial side into which blood can be infused once it has been dialyzed through a dialysis machine.

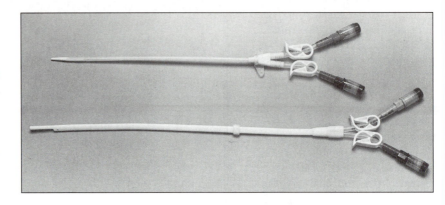

Nursing Considerations

- The Quinton is a shorter, stiffer catheter used for short-term therapy. It can be inserted at the client's bedside like a central line. It is used for short-term dialysis until a more permanent access can be placed.

- The Permcath is a flexible, more pliable catheter that is longer than the Quinton. It has an internal cuff that lies under the skin but outside the vasculature, thereby preventing organisms from passing via the line into the venous system.

- Both catheters are placed into the subclavian vein. Therefore the client must be observed for signs of vena cava syndrome (swelling in the affected extremity; localized discomfort in the shoulder, arm, chest; jugular venous distention secondary to poor drainage of the external jugular vein into the subclavian vein).

- Dressings changes: See procedure "Changing the Exit Site Dressing for a Chronic Central Venous Catheter," page 159.

- Flushing and blood drawing: See procedure "Drawing Blood from a Chronic (Hickman®-type) Central Venous Catheter and Flushing the Catheter Following Blood Withdrawal," page 163.

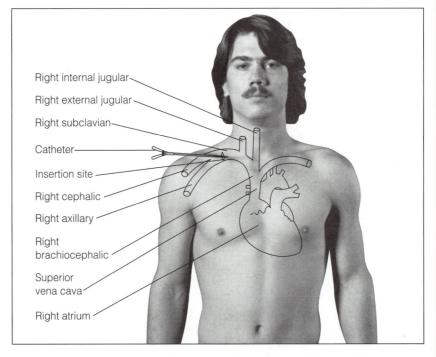

Right internal jugular
Right external jugular
Right subclavian
Catheter
Insertion site
Right cephalic
Right axillary
Right brachiocephalic
Superior vena cava
Right atrium

— To minimize the risk of contamination, wipe the injection cap with a commercially prepared povidone-iodine impregnated pad. Clean off the residual solution with an alcohol sponge.

— The volume of each lumen is printed on the portion of the lumen outside the dressing. Generally, the Quinton is flushed with 2.5 mL of a 1,000 U/mL heparin solution in each port. The Permcath is flushed with 1.2–1.6 mL of a 1,000 U/mL solution of heparin.

ADMINISTERING AN EXCHANGE FOR A CLIENT WITH CHRONIC AMBULATORY PERITONEAL DIALYSIS

Assessing and Planning

Chronic ambulatory peritoneal dialysis (CAPD) removes nitrogenous waste products, chemicals, and fluid from the bloodstream by osmosis, using the client's own peritoneum as a membrane. A concentrated dialysate is instilled into the peritoneal cavity via a special catheter (usually a Tenckhoff). Varying concentrations of glucose are added to the dialysate to enable the drawing or pulling of water and waste products across the membrane and into the peritoneal cavity, from which it is drained as part of the process. The Tenckhoff catheter is inserted into the peritoneum via the abdomen. The wound, when fresh, requires protection with a gauze dressing until it heals in about 8 weeks. After the wound has healed, it is much the same as a pierced ear, and a bandage usually is unnecessary.

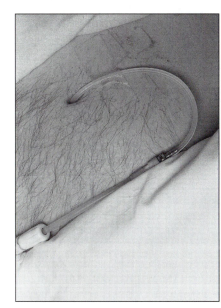

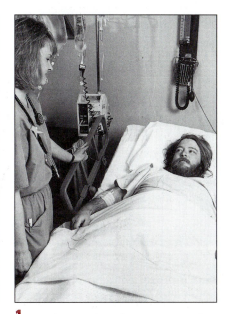

1 Wash your hands. As appropriate, explain which phase of the exchange cycle the client is in and what you are about to do. Position the client for comfort (usually in semi-Fowler's position) and to ensure that there is room for peritoneal expansion.

→

Implementing

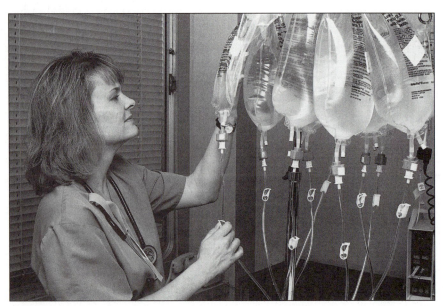

2 This client has dialysate in his peritoneum, and it is ready to be drained. For this phase of the exchange cycle, you will remove the empty bag from the 5-prong pole.

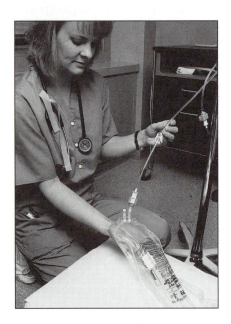

3 Next, place the empty bag on a stool, but *not* on the floor. Be certain that the bag is placed well below the level of the peritoneum to facilitate drainage of the peritoneal fluid into the bag. Usually there are two clamps: one is distal to the client (shown in photo near the nurse's left hand) and the other is proximal. Unclamp the distal tubing leading to the bag to begin the draining of the effluent back into the empty bag. This process will take approximately 20–25 minutes.

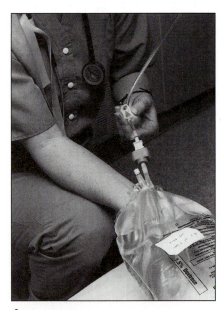

4 When the bag is full, clamp the tubing in preparation for hanging the bag of effluent back on the 5-prong pole.

Evaluating

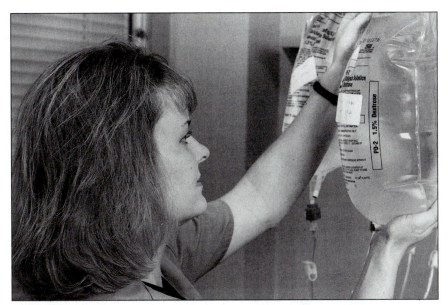

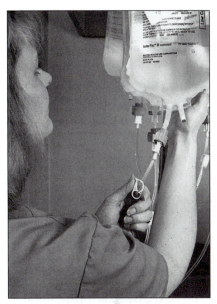

5 Hold the full bag of effluent up to the light. Inspect the fluid. The color should be light to medium yellow or amber in color, and it should be clear. Red-tinged, dark, or cloudy effluent could signal bleeding or infection. Consult the physician immediately if you note these characteristics. The amount of effluent returned may be greater than the amount infused. This is caused by extra fluids being drawn across the peritoneal membrane and is a positive outcome of CAPD. If the amount of the returned effluent is less than the amount instilled, consult the physician promptly because this could mean the client is retaining dialysate fluid due to dehydration, or draining may be ineffective owing to a catheter that is occluded or kinked in the peritoneal cavity. This also could occur if the client is constipated.

6 Select the next bag of dialysate for the exchange. Unclamp the tubing that leads from the bag. The dialysate will take about 15–20 minutes to infuse and will dwell in the peritoneum for approximately 4–5 hours. When this time is up, the process repeats itself (steps 2–5). *Note: The overnight bag of dialysate may remain in the client's peritoneum for up to 8–10 hours.*

Caring for Clients with Urinary Diversions

NURSING GUIDELINES: COMMON TYPES OF URINARY DIVERSIONS

Ileal Conduit (Also Called Ileal Loop, Bricker's Loop, Ileal Bladder)

Description

A 15- to 20-cm (6- to 8-in) segment of the ileum is removed to function as a pipeline for the urine. The ureters are then detached from the bladder, shortened, and anastomosed to the ileum. The ileal segment is brought out through the abdomen, where it forms a stoma. Urine then flows from the kidneys through the ureters and out through the ileal conduit and stoma. The intestine is anastomosed, and it continues to function normally.

Indications

Bladder malignancy, congenital anomalies, intractable incontinence, chronic urinary tract infections, neurogenic bladder.

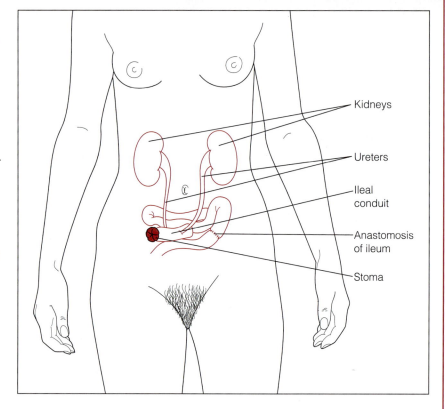

Kidneys

Ureters

Ileal conduit

Anastomosis of ileum

Stoma

Nursing Considerations

Note: *You can also follow these guidelines for clients who have had colon conduits.*

- The continuous flow of urine requires the constant use of an appliance.
- Mucus may be present in the urine because of the nature of the ileal segment that is used.

- If the client has had bladder cancer, a cystectomy also will have been performed, as well as a prostatectomy for the male client.
- An indwelling urethral catheter (drain) might be inserted to drain mucus and to minimize the potential for infection. When the client has had a cystectomy, do *not* irrigate the catheter because doing so could result in peritonitis.

NURSING GUIDELINES: COMMON TYPES OF URINARY DIVERSIONS *(continued)*

- Ureteral stents also might be inserted temporarily to anchor the ureteral-ileal attachment and to prevent the leakage of urine. These stents also drain into the appliance (pouch) and are usually removed on the fifth to seventh post-operative day.

- Inspect the incisional dressing at least every 4 hours, and change it as soon as it is wet, using aseptic technique. Change the dressing carefully to prevent disruption of the drains.

- Assess for indications of a urinary tract infection: chills, increased temperature, flank pain, and hematuria.

- Be alert to the following signs of hyperchloremic metabolic acidosis and hypokalemia caused by the reabsorption of sodium and chloride from the urine in the ileal segment, resulting in compensatory loss of potassium and bicarbonate: nausea, changes in level of consciousness (from sleepy to combative), changes in heart rate, and changes in muscle tone (from convulsions to flaccidity).

- Encourage increased oral intake of fluids as directed and, if the client is hypokalemic, the increased intake of foods high in potassium content, such as bananas, apricots, and cantaloupes.

- Encourage ambulation by the second or third postoperative day to help prevent urinary stasis, which would increase the risk of electrolyte and acid-base imbalance.

- Monitor intake and output, differentiating and recording the total amount of output from all drains, stents, and catheters. Notify the physician if the total urinary output is less than 60 mL over a 2-hour period. In the presence of an adequate intake, this can signal ureteral obstruction, a leak in the urinary diversion, or impending renal failure. Other signs of ureteral obstruction include nausea, vomiting, and flank pain.

- Teach the client the importance of weekly monitoring of urinary pH following hospital discharge to ensure that it is 6.0 or less. Individuals with urinary diversions have a higher rate of urinary tract infection than the general population, and thus it is important to keep their urine acidic to minimize the risk of infection. Encourage clients whose urine tests at a pH greater than 6.0 to increase their fluid intake and, with physician approval, to consume 500–1,000 mg of vitamin C/day to increase their urine acidity.

➔

NURSING GUIDELINES: COMMON TYPES OF URINARY DIVERSIONS (continued)

Cutaneous Ureterostomy

Description

The ureters are resected from the bladder, and one or both then are brought directly through the abdominal wall. Although it is more common for the client to have two stomas requiring the use of two appliances, one ureter might be joined to the other inside the body, resulting in one stoma. Usually the ureters are sutured flush with the skin without a protruding stoma.

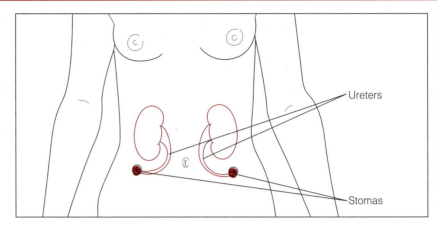

Indications

This is an older method of urinary diversion and one that is employed less frequently than the ileal conduit. It is indicated for clients with intractable incontinence, bladder malignancies, and other urinary conditions in which the more complicated surgeries involving intestinal resections are contraindicated.

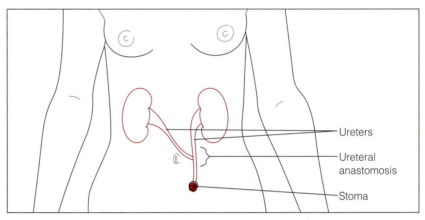

This is often a temporary procedure, for example, for the child for whom later reversal is intended, or it is employed for clients whose life expectancy is minimal.

Nursing Considerations

(Also see the guidelines for the ileal conduit.)

- Because the stoma is small and flush with the skin, fitting the appliance will be challenging. Extra care must be taken to prevent urine leakage and skin breakdown.

- Mucus particles in the collection system are abnormal because an intestinal segment is not used.

- If the client has an indwelling urethral catheter for draining blood and mucus from the diseased bladder, hand irrigate *only* if prescribed.

- Carefully assess the client for these indicators of ureteral and stomal stenosis: oliguria, anuria, and/or a stomal retraction. If stenosis does occur, irreversible damage to the urinary tract may result.

Nursing Guidelines: Common Types of Urinary Diversions (continued)

- Monitor the functioning of the ureteral stents, which exit from the stoma. Their purpose is to maintain patency of the ureters and promote healing of the anastomosis. Each stent can be expected to produce approximately the same amount of urine. Urine draining from these stents should be pink during the first 24 hours, becoming amber-colored by the third postoperative day. Diminished or absent drainage may signal mucus blockage or ureteral problems.

- Monitor intake and output, differentiating and recording the total amount of output from all drains, stents, and catheters. Notify the physician if the total urinary output is less than 60 mL over a 2-hour period. In the presence of an adequate intake, this can signal ureteral obstruction, a leak in the urinary diversion, or impending renal failure. Other signs of ureteral obstruction include nausea, vomiting, and flank pain.

- Teach the client the importance of weekly monitoring of urinary pH following hospital discharge to ensure that it is 6.0 or less. Individuals with urinary diversions have a higher rate of urinary tract infection than the general population, and thus it is important to keep their urine acidic to minimize the risk of infection. For clients whose urine tests at a pH greater than 6.0, encourage them to increase their fluid intake and, with physician approval, to consume 500–1,000 mg of vitamin C/day to increase their urine acidity.

NURSING GUIDELINES: COMMON TYPES OF URINARY DIVERSIONS (continued)

Continent Urinary Diversion

Description

There are several different types of continent urinary diversions, but the two that are most common are the Kock continent urostomy and the Indiana (ileocecal) reservoir. Continent urinary diversions have three components in common: a reservoir, a continence mechanism, and an antireflux mechanism. With the Kock continent urostomy, for example, the reservoir is formed with a 70- to 90-cm (28- to 36-in) segment of ileum, with the center section arranged in a "U" position. The antireflux and continence mechanisms are created via the intussusception of a portion of the bowel segment at each end of the reservoir to form one-way passages. The distal (nipple) valve is in the reservoir, and the proximal (stoma) end is at skin level. The ureters are attached to the proximal, closed end of the ileum. The Indiana reservoir is constructed from the cecum, the ascending colon, and a portion of the ileum. The ileum is decreased in size and brought out to the cutaneous surface to form a stoma. These diversions do not require external appliances for urine collection and are minimally disfiguring to the client.

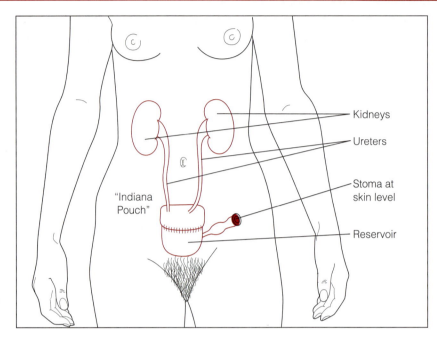

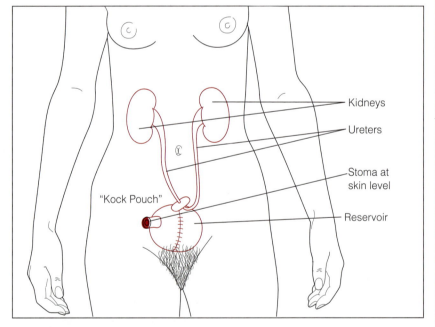

Indications

Urinary tract trauma, congenital birth defects, spinal cord injury, bladder and pelvic malignancies, and for clients with other urinary diversions who desire conversion to a diversion that obviates the need for an external appliance.

Nursing Considerations

- Clients must meet the following selection criteria before surgery: positive prognosis, age and lifestyle needs conducive to the benefits afforded by this procedure, positive motivation toward self-care, strong compliance, physical dexterity with ability to learn and manage self-catheterization every 3–6 hours, and adequate renal functioning.

- Contraindications may include the following: compromised renal functioning, physical or psychologic instability, obesity, extensive preopera-

NURSING GUIDELINES: COMMON TYPES OF URINARY DIVERSIONS *(continued)*

tive radiation therapy, and inability to tolerate a lengthy surgical procedure.

- Be alert to the following early postoperative complications:

    — mucus accumulation with resultant reservoir obstruction.

    — pelvic abscess.

    — fistula formation between the reservoir and cutaneous tissue or adjacent bowel.

    — small-bowel obstruction.

    — pyelonephritis.

- Be alert to the following late complications:

    — incontinence.

    — calculus formation.

    — problems with pouch catheterization.

    — stricture formation at the site of anastomosis of the ureter or bowel.

    — development of hyperchloremic metabolic acidosis (usually mild; see discussion with ileal conduit, page 479).

- No external appliance is used.

- Urine is drained at prescribed intervals by intubating (catheterizing) the reservoir via the external stoma.

- Clients with a Kock continent urostomy usually have urine draining from the reservoir catheter (Medina) and ureteral stents.

- Clients with an Indiana reservoir usually have ureteral stents that exit from the stoma and through which most of their urine drains. In addition, they may have a reservoir catheter that exits from a stab wound and that serves as an overflow catheter.

- Be alert to the following signs of intra-abdominal urine leakage or anastomosis breakdown: flank pain, increased abdominal girth, increased drainage from Penrose drains, and decreased urinary output from the stoma and stents.

- For clients with the Kock continent urostomy, monitor for functioning of the Medina catheter, which is present to prevent reservoir distention and promote healing of the suture lines. Large amounts of mucus will drain from this catheter

in the early postoperative period, necessitating irrigation with 30–50 mL normal saline, which is instilled gently and allowed to drain via gravity drainage. Mucus drainage will continue for several months postoperatively but should lessen in amount.

- Monitor intake and output, differentiating and recording the total amount of output from all drains, stents, and catheters. Notify the physician if the total urinary output is less than 60 mL over a 2-hour period. In the presence of an adequate intake, this can signal ureteral obstruction, a leak in the urinary diversion, or impending renal failure. Other signs of ureteral obstruction include nausea, vomiting, and flank pain.

Following hospital discharge

- Encourage the client to drink 8–10 glasses of water a day (unless contraindicated by an underlying medical condition) to thin the mucus that forms in the reservoir. Thick mucus is often the result of not drinking enough water.

- Teach client to avoid drinking after 7–8 PM and therefore minimize pouch leakage at night.

- Teach client to cut one of the following to the appropriate size and use to cover the stoma: panty liner, sanitary napkin, disposable diaper, bed-saver pad, or an incontinence product.

- Encourage the client to catheterize the pouch on a regularly scheduled basis to ensure steady and progressive enlargement of the pouch.

- Teach the client to relax the abdominal muscles rather than bear down when catheterizing the pouch to facilitate catheter insertion. Changing positions also may help, as will rolling the catheter between the fingers on insertion.

- Teach the client the importance of weekly monitoring of urinary pH following hospital discharge to ensure that it is 6.0 or less. Individuals with urinary diversions have a higher rate of urinary tract infection than the general population, and thus it is important to keep their urine acidic to minimize the risk of infection. For clients whose urine tests at a pH greater than 6.0, encourage them to increase their fluid intake and, with physician approval, to consume 500–1,000 mg of vitamin C/day to increase their urine acidity.

PERFORMING A POSTOPERATIVE ASSESSMENT

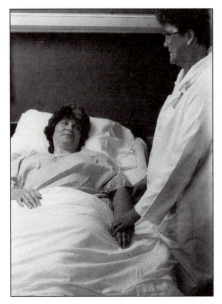

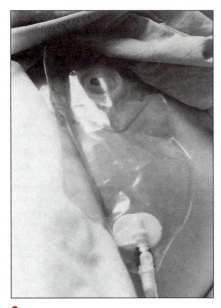

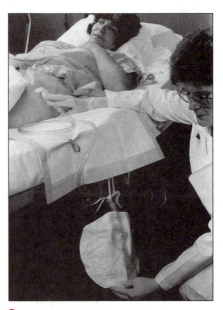

1 Regardless of the type of urinary diversion surgery that was performed, the postoperative assessment of your urostomy client will be basically the same. Explain to the client that you will be assessing her stoma and the area surrounding it (the peristomal area), the amount and character of the urine, and the integrity of the stomal sutures. Remember that your positive and reassuring attitude is crucial to the client's acceptance both of the surgery and of her altered body appearance and function.

2 Apply clean gloves. Then raise the client's gown to expose the pouch, and place a bed-saver pad under the involved flank to protect the bed linen. As you do this, place your hand under the client's back to check for dampness, which could indicate that the pouch is leaking urine. Note that the postoperative pouch angles toward the side of the bed. This makes it accessible to the nurse and enterostomal therapist and facilitates its connection to a urinary drainage bag while the client is on bed rest. Inspect the area around the pouch's attachment to the faceplate to ensure that leakage has not occurred. Ask the client if she is experiencing itching or burning, which are signs of leakage. If either has occurred, the pouch must be changed and replaced with one that fits correctly. Otherwise, your client can continue to wear the same pouch for 3–4 days.

3 Inspect the drainage bag to ensure that urine is flowing adequately and that the output is comparable to the client's intake of fluids. Optimally, the output will be around 1,500 mL/day. A diminished production of urine might be caused by reduced intake, urinary blockage, or kidney failure. An absence of urine can be indicative of a leak in the conduit system or a blockage of the ureters, and could necessitate a return to surgery. Also note the character of the urine. If your client has an ileal conduit, the urine might contain mucus because of the nature of the intestine that was used to form the conduit. This is normal. The urine may be dark in color if the client is taking antibiotics, is dehydrated, or has impaired liver function. Be sure to immediately report abnormal quantities of blood. Some postoperative hematuria is not unusual, but it should decrease gradually.

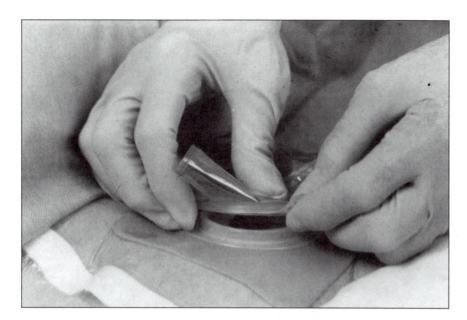

4 To inspect the stoma, position your fingers around the faceplate to anchor it in place, and grasp the tab on the pouch with your other hand. Detach the pouch from the faceplate by lifting up the tab. Be sure to have a clean cloth or gauze pad available to absorb the urine after the pouch has been opened.

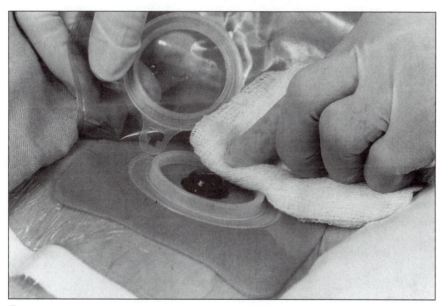

5 To detach the pouch from the faceplate, lift up the tab. When the area has been dried, assess the stoma. It should be pink or red, similar in color to the mucosal lining of the mouth. Slight bleeding may be normal because of the large number of capillaries in the area. Note whether the stoma is flush with the skin or protruding, and assess the degree of edema, if present. Explain to the client that the stoma will continue to decrease in size over the next 6–8 weeks, and this will necessitate frequent stomal measurements to ensure a properly fitting pouch and skin barrier. Make sure the opening in the skin barrier is the exact measurement of the stoma. It should touch the stoma on all sides. Finally, inspect the sutures to make sure they are intact. Replace the pouch, wash your hands, and document your observations.

MANAGING APPLIANCE CARE

APPLYING A POSTOPERATIVE (DISPOSABLE) POUCH

Assessing and Planning

1 A disposable pouch is usually applied on the client's third or fourth postoperative day. The materials used for disposable pouches will vary from agency to agency. The following is a general procedure for pouch application, and it should include these materials or a variation of the same:

☐ stoma measuring guide

☐ disposable pouch

☐ tape (optional)

☐ skin preparation (optional) to protect the skin from a reaction to the tape if it is used

☐ skin barrier such as a pectin wafer

☐ skin cleanser (optional)

☐ scissors

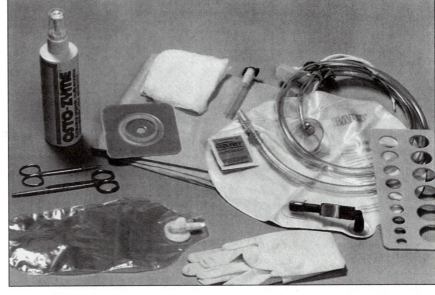

☐ urine collection bag

☐ clean cloths or gauze pads, clean gloves, bed-saver pads for stocking the client's bedside stand

If you will use tape to reinforce the seal of the pouch, cut four strips approximately 10 cm (4 in) in length.

2 Explain the procedure to the client and lower the head of the bed to decrease the angle at the peristomal area, but do encourage the client to inspect the stoma and ask questions during the procedure. This procedure also can be used for client teaching. Place a bed-saver pad under the involved flank to protect the bed linen, and have clean cloths, gauze pads,

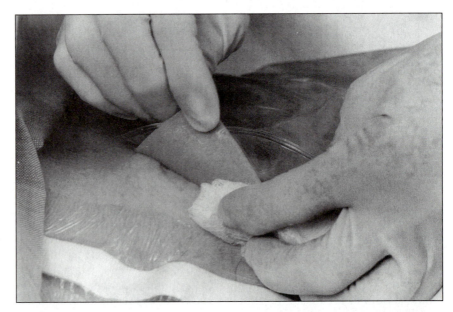

toilet paper, or tampons accessible for absorbing the urine. To remove the pouch, moisten a cloth with warm water and lift up the inside corner of the skin barrier. Place the moist cloth at the loosened corner

and gently depress sections of the skin as you peel back the adhesive material. The moist cloth will help loosen the adhesive and facilitate its removal as quickly and painlessly as possible.

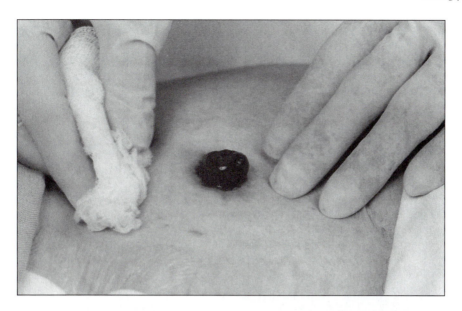

3 When you have removed the skin barrier and pouch, inspect the stoma and peristomal area. Assess for irritation, allergic reactions to the tape or adhesive, weeping, or inflamed hair follicles (folliculitis). If the opening of the skin barrier is too large and allows seepage of urine onto the peristomal area, you might see an alkaline encrustation that consists of white crystalline deposits. Hyperplasia, which is a very tender area of thickened skin, can also result from prolonged exposure to urine, especially if the urine is alkaline.

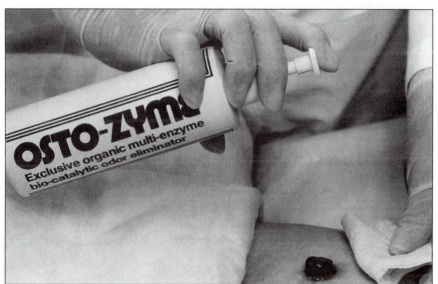

4 Clean the skin with a warm, wet cloth. If you use soap, it must be nonoily because oily soaps will leave a residue, which can prevent the proper adherence of the pouch. Another option is to cleanse the peristomal skin with a skin cleanser/deodorizer (as shown), which also helps remove adhesive residual.

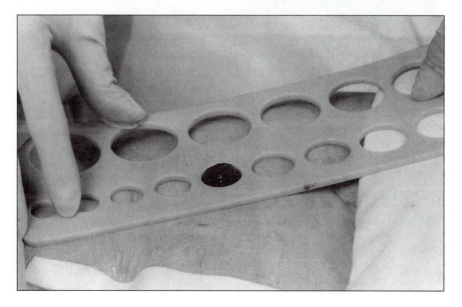

5 Measure the stoma with the measuring guide.

Implementing

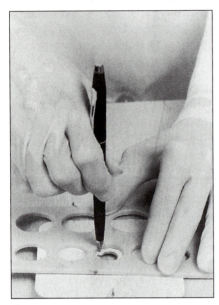

6 Trace the outline of the measured stoma on the back of the pectin wafer skin barrier. If the stoma is irregular in shape, you will need to customize the pattern to fit the shape of the stoma.

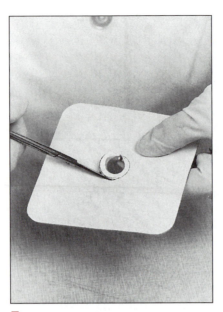

7 Cut out the circle (or shape) you have traced.

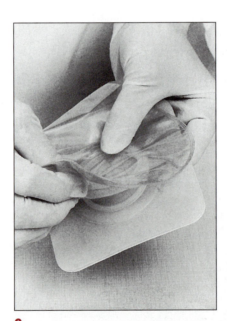

8 Snap the pouch onto the pectin wafer at an angle, as shown.

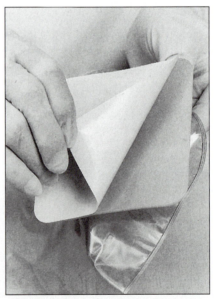

9 Remove the protective paper backing from the pectin wafer. Set the pouch aside, with the adhesive side up.

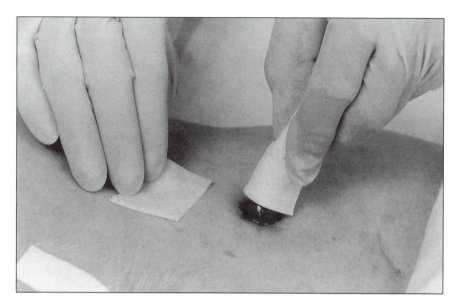

10 If you plan to reinforce the pouch with tape, prepare the periphery of the peristomal skin with a skin preparation before applying the skin barrier and pouch. This will help to prevent a skin reaction to the tape. Be sure to let the skin dry thoroughly before applying the skin barrier and pouch. ***Caution:*** *Do not apply a skin protector to skin that is broken or irritated.* To prevent the client's stoma from draining onto the peristomal area, hold a gauze pad or tampon over the stoma (as shown).

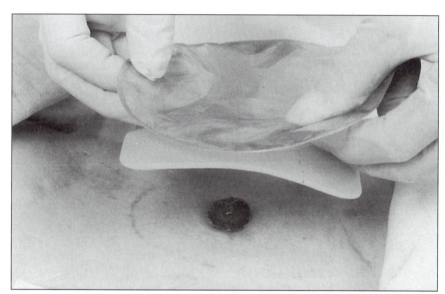

11 Position the pouch so that the opening is directly over the stoma. While the client is on bed rest, angle the tail of the pouch toward the side of the bed (as shown).

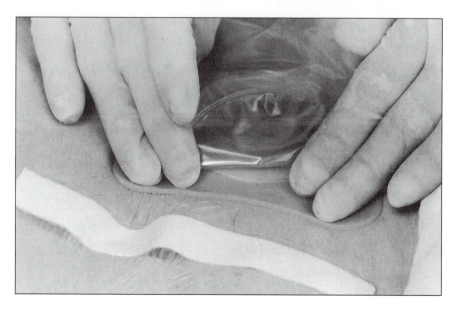

12 Then adhere the barrier and pouch to the client's skin by gently pressing around the periphery with your fingertips. The warmth of your hands will enhance the seal.

Evaluating

13 Document the procedure, noting your assessment of the stoma and peristomal skin, the amount and character of the urine, and the type of equipment and materials you used.

PICTURE FRAMING THE POUCH

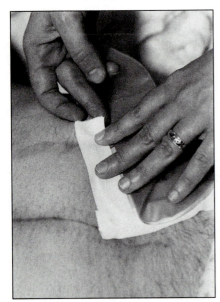

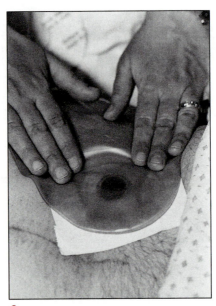

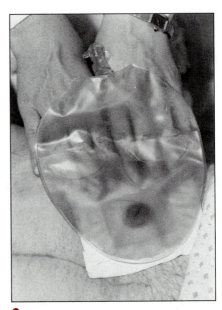

1 If desired, reinforce the seal by "picture framing" the pouch and skin barrier to the client's skin. Attach four strips of tape to form a square around the pouch and skin barrier.

2 Press around the exterior of the pouch.

3 Lift up the tail of the pouch and press along the underside. If you will attach the pouch to a drainage bag at this time, see procedure on page 491. Return the client to a position of comfort, and wash your hands.

CONNECTING THE POUCH TO A URINARY DRAINAGE SYSTEM

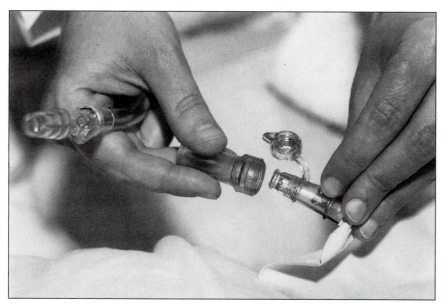

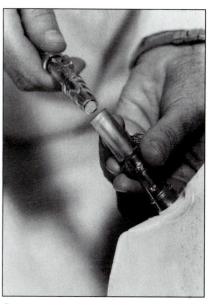

1 During the night, or while your client is on bed rest, ensure that the urinary pouch is attached to a urinary drainage system. A pouch that becomes too full of urine can break the seal of the appliance to the skin. In addition, urine that stagnates in a pouch becomes an excellent medium for bacterial growth, which can lead to urinary tract infections. In the hospital, the client has the option of attaching the pouch to a urinary collection bag and tubing, or to a leg bag (see procedure, pages 463–464). Most pouches are packaged with an adapter (as shown). Remove the plug from the drain on the pouch, and snap on the adapter. *Note: If the urine drainage system is not fresh from its package, wear gloves to prevent contact of your hands with urine.*

2 Insert the drainage system tubing directly into the adapter.

REFERENCES

Bowers AC, Thompson JM: *Clinical Manual of Health Assessment,* ed 4. St Louis: Mosby, 1992.

Horne MM, Jansen PR: Renal-urinary disorders. In Swearingen PL (ed): *Manual of Medical-Surgical Nursing Care,* ed 3. St Louis: Mosby, 1994.

Indiana University Hospitals: *Nursing Procedures and Policies.* Indianapolis, 1994.

Kozier B, Erb G: *Techniques in Clinical Nursing,* ed 4. Redwood City, CA: Addison-Wesley, 1993.

Rice R: *Handbook of Home Health Nursing Procedures.* St Louis: Mosby, 1995.

Sims LK et al: *Health Assessment in Nursing.* Redwood City, CA: Addison-Wesley, 1994.

Spence AP: *Basic Human Anatomy,* ed 3. Redwood City, CA: Addison-Wesley, 1991.

Thompson JM: *Mosby's Manual of Clinical Nursing,* ed 3. St Louis: Mosby, 1993.

Weiskittel P: Renal-urinary dysfunctions. In Swearingen PL, Keen JH (eds): *Manual of Critical Care Nursing,* ed 3. St Louis: Mosby, 1995.

CHAPTER 9

Managing Musculoskeletal Procedures

CHAPTER OUTLINE

ASSESSING THE MUSCULO-SKELETAL SYSTEM

The Musculoskeletal System

Nursing Assessment Guidelines

Performing a General Assessment of the Musculoskeletal System

Inspecting

Palpating the Spine

Evaluating Joint Range of Motion (ROM) and Muscular Strength

Measuring Muscle Girth

Evaluating Activities of Daily Living

Performing Neurovascular Assessments

Evaluating Neurovascular Integrity

Assessing Nerve Function

USING IMMOBILIZATION AND COMFORT DEVICES

Nursing Guidelines: Care of Clients in Immobilization Devices

Soft Cervical Collar

Hard Cervical Collar

Clavicle Splint

Arm/Shoulder Immobilizer

Wrist/Forearm Splint

Abduction Pillow

Knee Immobilizer

Hinged Brace

Denis-Browne Splint

Applying Elastic Bandages

Wrapping a Long, Cylindrical Body Part

Wrapping a Joint

Wrapping a Residual Limb (Stump)

MANAGING ROUTINE CAST CARE

Assisting with Cast Application

Performing Routine Assessments and Interventions for Clients in Casts

Nursing Guidelines: Care of Clients in Casts

Petaling a Cast

MANAGING ROUTINE TRACTION CARE

Making a Bowline Traction Knot

Nursing Guidelines: Care of Clients in Traction

Caring for Clients in Skin Traction

Applying Cervical Traction

Applying a Pelvic Belt

Applying a Buck's Boot for Extension Traction

Caring for Children in Bryant's Traction

Caring for Clients in Skeletal Traction

Performing Routine Care of Clients in Skeletal Traction

Performing Routine Care and Assessments for Clients in Halo Vests

Providing Pin Care

PROVIDING SPECIAL CARE FOR CLIENTS WITH MUSCULO-SKELETAL DISORDERS

Making a Traction Bed

Maintaining a Portable Wound-Drainage System

Applying a Hydroculator Pack (Moist Heat) to Arthritic Joints

Managing the Client with a Blood Reinfusion System

Monitoring the Client Undergoing Continuous Passive Motion (CPM)

Managing the Client Undergoing Cryotherapy via a Knee Compression Dressing

Transferring the Client with a Total Hip Replacement

Assessing the Musculoskeletal System

THE MUSCULOSKELETAL SYSTEM

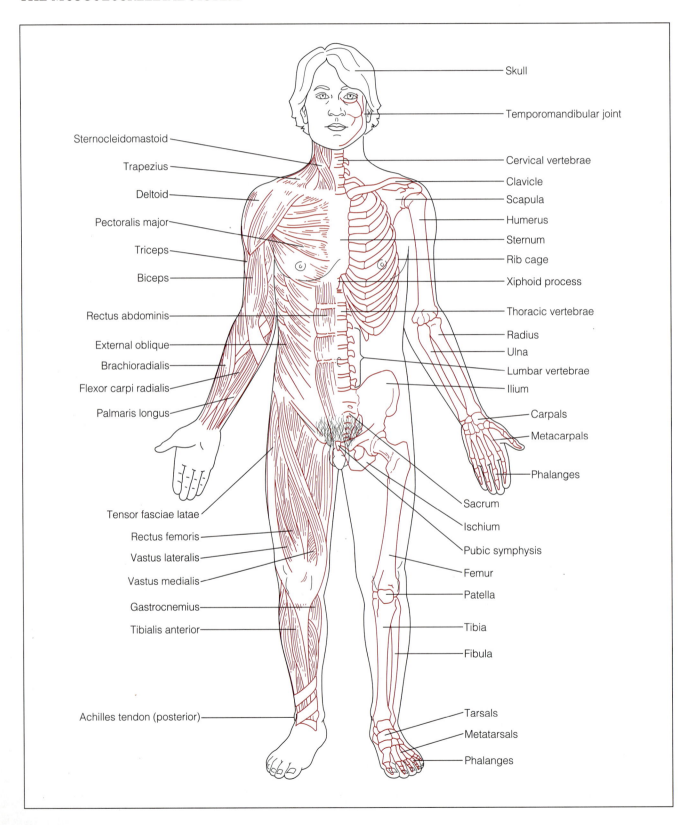

Skull

Temporomandibular joint

Cervical vertebrae

Clavicle

Scapula

Humerus

Sternum

Rib cage

Xiphoid process

Thoracic vertebrae

Radius

Ulna

Lumbar vertebrae

Ilium

Carpals

Metacarpals

Phalanges

Sacrum

Ischium

Pubic symphysis

Femur

Patella

Tibia

Fibula

Tarsals

Metatarsals

Phalanges

Sternocleidomastoid

Trapezius

Deltoid

Pectoralis major

Triceps

Biceps

Rectus abdominis

External oblique

Brachioradialis

Flexor carpi radialis

Palmaris longus

Tensor fasciae latae

Rectus femoris

Vastus lateralis

Vastus medialis

Gastrocnemius

Tibialis anterior

Achilles tendon (posterior)

NURSING ASSESSMENT GUIDELINES

To assess your client's musculo-skeletal system, you need to interview him or her for subjective data; take vital signs; evaluate range of motion (ROM), muscular strength, and activities of daily living; and assess neurovascular integrity. A comprehensive nursing care plan includes a complete evaluation for the following subjective data:

Personal factors: for example, age, marital status, recreational activities; description of home environment—levels, stairways, throw rugs

History or family history of: arthritis, gout, rickets, or other musculoskeletal and joint disorders

Occupation: past and present, type of work, accident potential, safety precautions employed

Activities of daily living: abilities/alterations in the performance of eating, getting dressed, writing, moving, or caring for personal hygiene

Exercise: type, frequency, tolerance/intolerance to

Use of assistive devices: for exam-ple, crutches, cane, walker, wheelchair

History of injuries: what, when, how occurred, degree of recovery

History of musculoskeletal surgery: what, when, results

Medications: for example, use of aspirin and other nonsteroidal anti-inflammatory agents, steroids, antispasmodics

Allergies: for example, to foods, medications, cast materials, adhesives

Pain: location, onset, duration, character, radiation, relieved by, intensified by, effect of weather

Gait disorders: weakness, clumsiness, discomfort, stiffness

Muscular disorders: weakness, fatigue, atrophy, hypertrophy, paralysis, pain, tremors, tics, spasms, aching

Skeletal disorders: history and/or presence of fractures, crepitus, pain, ecchymosis, hematoma

Joint disorders: history or presence or injury, swelling, erythema, enlargement, stiffness, limitation of movement, aching, crepitus

PERFORMING A GENERAL ASSESSMENT OF THE MUSCULOSKELETAL SYSTEM

Provide a warm and private environment for your client, and explain the assessment procedure. For a full inspection, the client should wear only underwear so that you can more accurately assess posture, alignment, and body build.

INSPECTING

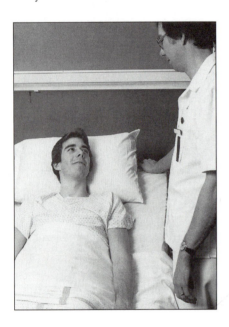

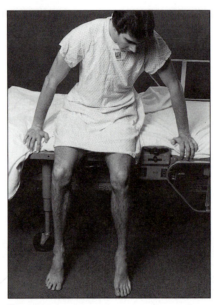

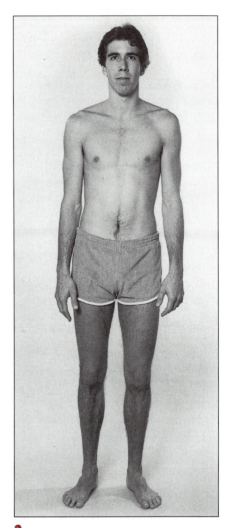

1 If it is not contraindicated, ask the client to get out of bed so that you can evaluate posture, gait, and ROM. Assess his ability to get out of bed. Does he appear to have discomfort, and does he require the use of an assistive device?

2 Once he is out of bed, ask him to stand facing you, with his hands hanging loosely at his sides and his head level. Inspect his body build, and compare one side to the other. Observe for the presence of masses, atrophy, absence of body parts, or gross abnormalities, such as one limb shorter than the other. As a check for scoliosis, assess for asymmetry of the shoulders, the clavicles, and the nipple line.

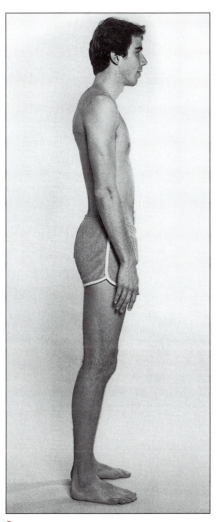 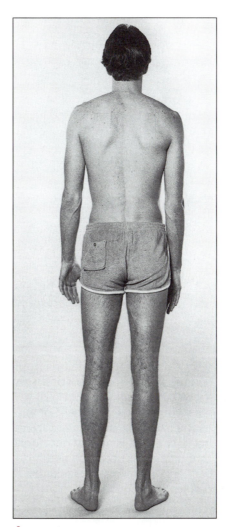 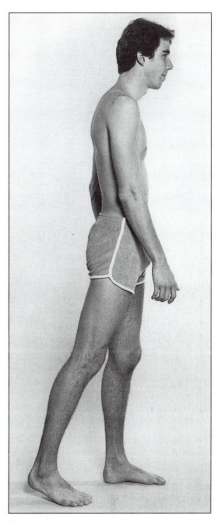

3 Inspect the client laterally to assess spine curvature. Normally in adults, the cervical and lumbar areas will appear moderately concave, whereas the thorax will appear convex. Note an exaggerated inward curve of the lumbar area, called lordosis (swayback), or an abnormal roundness of the thorax, referred to as kyphosis (hunchback). Gibbus is an angular deformity of collapsed vertebrae, which can occur with osteoarthritis or Pott's disease (tuberculosis of the spinal column). Also assess for displacement of the scapulae (winging), which is typically found with scoliosis. A lateral inspection also aids in identifying ankylosing spondylitis because the client will have a stooped appearance.

4 When you inspect the client posteriorly, note the alignment of the spine. If the spine deviates laterally, for example with scoliosis, document the area of deviation; record it as either a "C" or "S" curve. Again, be alert to asymmetry of the shoulders, scapulae, and posterior iliac crests. With advanced structural (nonfunctional) scoliosis, one scapula is usually flattened, whereas the other is elevated. In Sprengel's deformity, the scapula(e) is(are) usually small and located in the lower cervical and upper thoracic area, causing the shoulder(s) to be elevated.

5 If it is not contraindicated, instruct the client to walk; as he does, observe his gait. Are you able to hear dragging, which occurs with spasticity or footdrop? Does he limp, have a distorted gait, or use assistive devices? His weight should be evenly distributed as he steps first onto the heels and then onto the balls of his feet. His toes should point forward, and his arms should swing slightly in opposition to his gait. Be alert to genu varum (bowed legs) or genu valgum (knock-knee). Moderate genu varum is normal in the newborn, possibly due to the intrauterine position. It should become mild by 6 months of age and resolve by 18 months. Mild genu valgum is common between 2 and 3 years of age but should resolve between the ages of 4 and 10. Document your assessment, being certain to note any alterations from the norm.

PALPATING THE SPINE

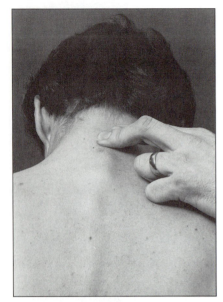 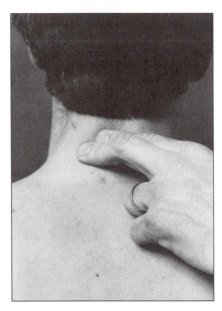 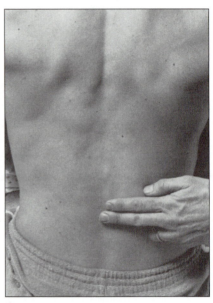

1 *Caution: If the client has a neck injury, all neck movements are contraindicated.* Palpate the cervical spinous processes with the client's neck in a flexed position. Assess the range of motion and question him about the presence of any discomfort. Then instruct the client to return his head to the neutral position (above) so that you can assess for crepitus, a grating sound or sensation that can be heard or felt by the examiner during joint movement. Crepitus is usually not significant unless it is accompanied by pain or compromised circulation.

2 Continue to palpate the entire vertebral column, noting any deviations in alignment, areas of discomfort, or the presence of spasms.

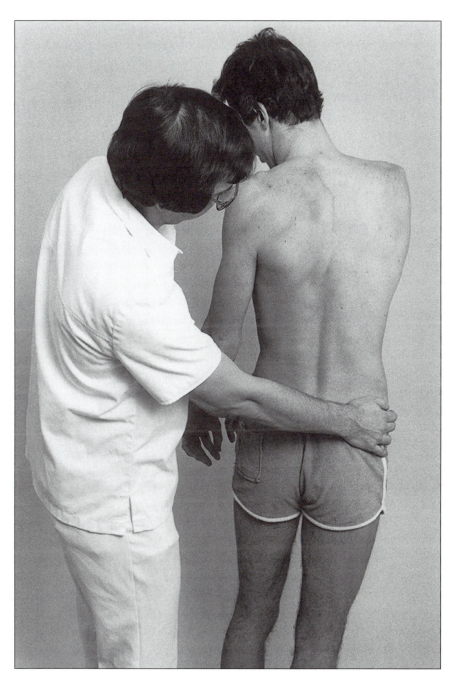

3 To assess the rotation of the lower vertebral column, stabilize the client's hips (as shown) as he rotates his trunk to the right and then to the left. Optimally, the trunk rotation will be bilaterally equal and approximately 30 degrees to either side. Continue to evaluate the client's ROM as he bends forward, backward, and laterally. Clients with some form of muscular dystrophy will exhibit marked weakness of the trunk muscles.

If you suspect that your client has scoliosis, as evidenced by a lateral curvature of the spine, closely observe him as he bends forward at the waist. If the curvature does not resolve as he bends forward, his condition is considered to be nonfunctional. With this type of scoliosis, structural changes occur in the spinal column, making the disorder especially difficult to correct. If your client is an infant, check for congenital hip dislocation by performing Ortolani's click test (see pages 227–228); watch for waddling in the toddler.

EVALUATING JOINT RANGE OF MOTION (ROM) AND MUSCULAR STRENGTH

A general assessment of your client's joints and muscles will involve either one or three phases. In phase one, the examiner demonstrates active ROM on his or her own joints and the client returns the demonstration. Review Chapter 2 to assist you with movement components involved with the ROM of each joint. If the client has independent ROM without discomfort, further assessment is usually unnecessary. However, if the client has limited ROM or ROM with discomfort, it will be necessary for you to perform passive ROM on the involved joints to evaluate the degree of motion (phase two), followed by resistive exercises to assess the strength of the involved muscle groups (phase three). During ROM, assess the joints for bilateral symmetry of motion. Also note any dislocation, subluxation (a partial dislocation), ankylosis, swelling, and crepitus. Assess the muscles for strength, bulk, tone, and bilateral symmetry. Key areas for assessment are presented in the following steps. If you desire greater detail, including the average degrees of motion for each joint, be sure to consult any assessment text. To ensure your client's relaxation and cooperation, assess painful joints and extremities last. *Caution: Never put a fractured extremity through ROM or resistive exercises.*

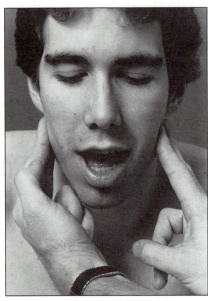

1 Assess your client from head to toe, beginning at the temporo-mandibular joint (TMJ). Place your fingers on the joints (as shown), and instruct the client to move his mandible from side to side and then up and down. Assess for ROM and discomfort or crepitus. *Note: If you have difficulty palpating the joint as depicted here, place your little fingers into the external auditory canals, instead. You should be able to palpate both the mandible and temporal bones as the client performs ROM on the joint.*

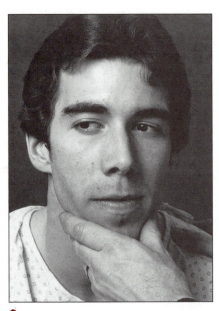

2 If the client experiences either discomfort or limited ROM with the neck movements, perform passive ROM on his cervical joints followed by resistive exercises to evaluate key muscle groups. To evaluate the strength of the neck rotator muscles, restrain the client's head at the mandible as the client attempts to turn his head to each side. *Caution: If the client has a neck injury or a neurologic pathology of the upper extremity, cervical muscle resistive exercises are contraindicated.*

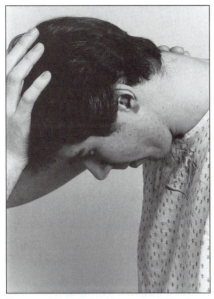

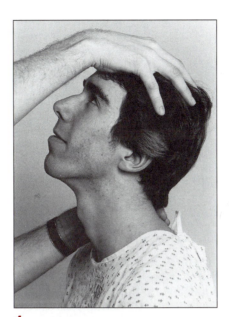

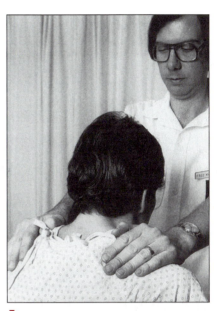

3 To evaluate the neck flexors, ask the client to maintain his neck in a flexed position as you attempt to extend his head.

4 With the client's neck extended, attempt to flex his head toward his chest as he tries to maintain his neck in extension. This will evaluate the strength of the neck extensors.

5 If the client experiences discomfort or limited ROM with the shoulder movements, perform passive ROM on the shoulder joints. Assess the strength of the shoulder elevators by pressing down on the client's acromioclavicular joints as he attempts to raise his shoulders.

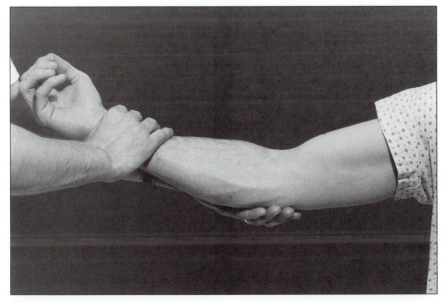

6 Evaluate the client's active ROM of the elbow joints. If he experiences either discomfort or limited ROM, perform passive ROM and then evaluate the strength of the following key muscle groups. Assess the strength of the elbow flexors by holding the client's forearm as he attempts to flex his elbow. Repeat the assessment on the opposite arm. Remember, the dominant arm is normally stronger than the nondominant arm.

➡

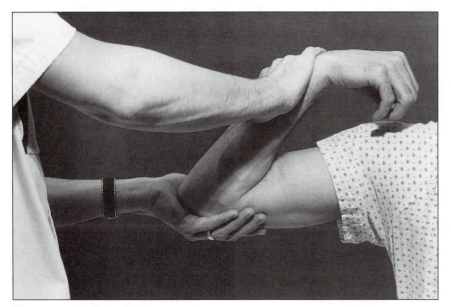

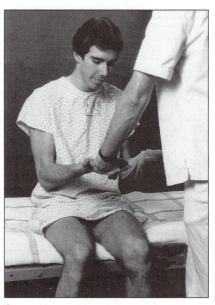

7 Test the strength of the elbow extensors by holding the client's forearm with the elbow in a flexed position as he attempts to extend the elbow. Repeat the assessment on the opposite arm. Again, the dominant arm is normally stronger than the opposite arm.

8 If the client experiences discomfort or limited ROM while performing active ROM on each wrist, perform passive ROM and then evaluate the strength of the wrist flexors. Place your hands against the client's palms and instruct him to push up against your resistance.

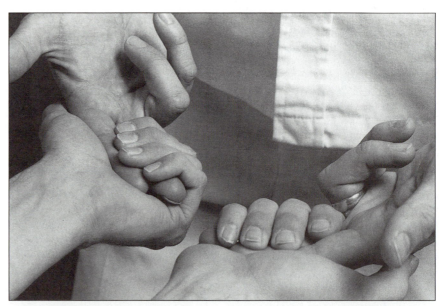

9 Another exercise for evaluating both wrist and hand flexors is to have the client tightly grip your index and middle fingers. Assess the strength of both hands and compare the strength of one to the other. The dominant hand is normally stronger.

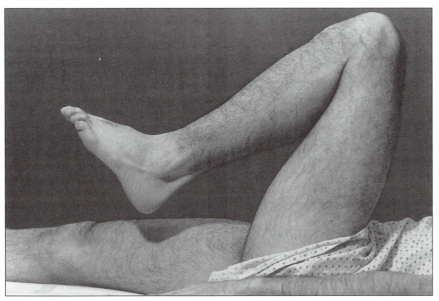

10 When the client has assumed a supine position, closely observe his ability to flex each hip. Instruct him to pull each bent knee alternately in toward his chest. Optimally, the opposite hip will remain extended as the other flexes.

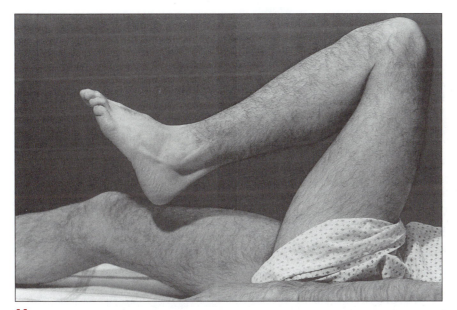

11 If the opposite hip also flexes (as shown) the client has a positive Thomas test, which is indicative of a flexion contracture of that hip. *Note: With the client in this position, you can easily the strength of the* *knee extensors (quadriceps) by holding the client's knee into his chest as he attempts to extend his hip.* Repeat the assessment on the client's opposite side.

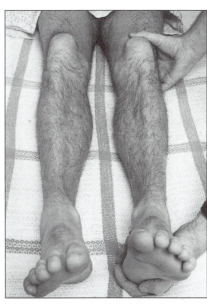

12 If it has been necessary for you to perform passive ROM on the hip joints, evaluate the strength of the hip abductor muscles by holding the client's leg at the midline as he attempts to abduct it.

➡

13 Evaluate the hip adductor muscles by holding the client's leg in the abducted position as he attempts to adduct the leg back to the midline.

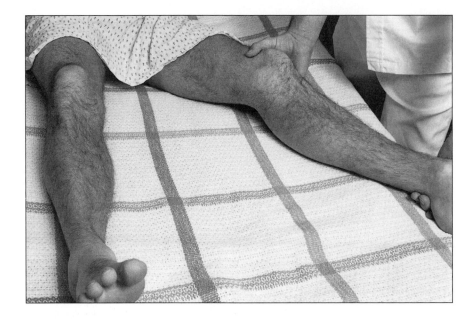

14 If the client has limited ROM or discomfort during the ankle movements, perform passive ROM on both ankles. Then evaluate the strength of the ankle flexors by applying resistance at the dorsum of each foot (as shown) as the client attempts to dorsiflex each foot. Compare the strength bilaterally.

Test the strength of the ankle extensors by pushing against the soles of the feet as the client attempts to plantarflex the feet. Again, compare the strength bilaterally. Document the results of the assessment, being certain to describe in detail any alterations from the norm.

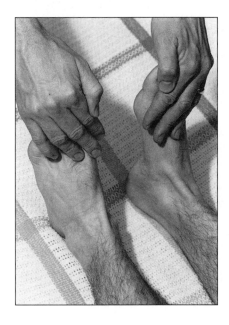

MEASURING MUSCLE GIRTH

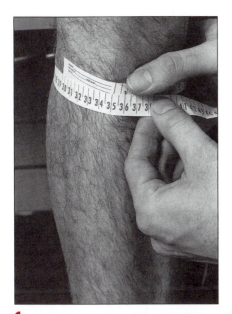

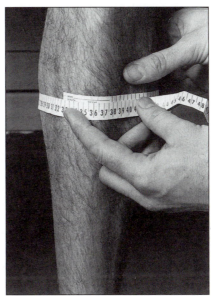

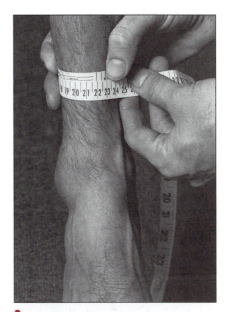

1 When comparing one extremity to the other to assess for unilateral atrophy or hypertrophy, measure the circumference of the proximal, medial, and distal areas of the involved extremity, and compare each measurement to the exact corresponding areas on the opposite extremity. For example, to assess for atrophied or hypertrophied muscles in the lower leg, wrap a nonstretchable tape measure around the leg just below the knee. Measure and document the circumference, and then lightly mark the site you just measured with washable ink.

2 Measure the circumference of the extremity at the area of greatest bulk. After measuring and documenting the circumference, mark the measurement site with the ink.

3 Measure the circumference of the distal end. For example, when measuring the lower leg, position the tape measure just above the medial and lateral malleoli. Mark the circumference site with ink, and then measure the distances between each landmark. Repeat the assessment on the opposite extremity by first measuring and marking the distances from the corresponding landmarks and then measuring the proximal, medial, and distal circumferences. A marked difference in circumference between the extremities often occurs with either disuse atrophy of one extremity or hypertrophy due to overuse of the opposite extremity. When comparing the upper extremities, remember that a slight difference in circumference may be normal because of the preference of the dominant hand.

EVALUATING ACTIVITIES OF DAILY LIVING

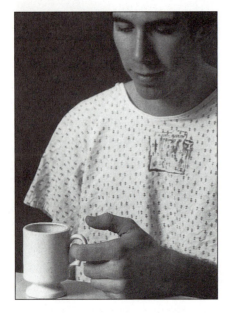

A complete evaluation of the client's musculoskeletal system should include an ongoing assessment of his ability to perform activities of daily living. Observe his ability to eat, write, perform functions of daily hygiene, and get dressed. For example, evaluate his ability to grasp a cup (as shown) or cut his meat, count coins, dial a telephone, write his name, or button or zip his clothing. Determine whether he has full functioning capacity and is therefore independent. If he is slow and tires easily, requires assistance, or is incapable of doing most things for himself, determine the degree of his dependence.

PERFORMING NEUROVASCULAR ASSESSMENTS

EVALUATING NEUROVASCULAR INTEGRITY

Clients with musculoskeletal injuries will require frequent neurovascular assessments of the involved extremities. It is essential that you establish your client's "normal" integrity or baseline prior to the application of an immobilization device because he or she normally may exhibit neurovascular differences when one extremity is compared to the opposite extremity. Therefore, you cannot always rely on a bilateral comparison alone. The areas of assessment should include evaluations for the following: capillary refill, color, temperature, pulse, sensation, numbness/tingling, pain, edema, and motion. Be sure to instruct your clients so that they can recognize these indicators of impairment and alert you immediately should they occur. The figure below is an example of a record for neurovascular and nerve function.

NEUROVASCULAR AND NERVE FUNCTION ASSESSMENT

EXTREMITY ASSESSED:

TIME	COLOR	TEMPERATURE	CAPILLARY REFILL	EDEMA	NUMBNESS/ TINGLING	SENSATION	MOTION	PULSES	PERONEAL NERVE	TIBIAL NERVE	RADIAL NERVE	ULNAR NERVE	MEDIAN NERVE	Initials
									S	S	S	S	S	
									M	M	M	M	M	
									S	S	S	S	S	
									M	M	M	M	M	
									S	S	S	S	S	
									M	M	M	M	M	
									S	S	S	S	S	
									M	M	M	M	M	
									S	S	S	S	S	
									M	M	M	M	M	
									S	S	S	S	S	
									M	M	M	M	M	
									S	S	S	S	S	
									M	M	M	M	M	
									S	S	S	S	S	
									M	M	M	M	M	
									S	S	S	S	S	
									M	M	M	M	M	
									S	S	S	S	S	
									M	M	M	M	M	
									S	S	S	S	S	
									M	M	M	M	M	

S = Sensation   M = Motion

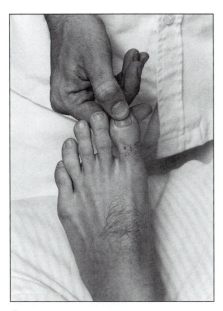

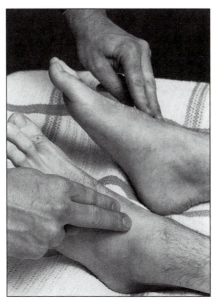

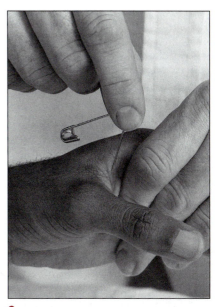

1 *Capillary Refill, Color, and Temperature:* Assess the extremity distal to the injury. Is it warm, cool, or cold? Do the nailbeds of the fingers or toes appear pink, pale, or cyanotic? To assess for adequate circulation, depress the nailbed (as shown) of each toe or finger until it blanches, and then release the pressure. Evaluate the speed at which the blood returns. Is the return sluggish or rapid? Optimally, the color will change from white to pink rapidly (≤2 seconds). If this does not occur, the toes or fingers will require close observation and further evaluation.

2 *Pulsations:* Bilaterally palpate peripheral pulses distal to the injury, and compare the regularity and strength of each. If they are unequal, or if the pulse in the involved extremity does not correspond to the client's baseline, close observation and further assessments are again warranted.

3 *Sensations or Pain:* Touch, lightly pinch, or gently prick the involved extremity with a sterile pin to assess sensation. Question the client about the presence of numbness or tingling. Constant pain with concomitant numbness is significant because it could be caused by a compressed nerve, which if left untreated could result in paralysis of the involved extremity.

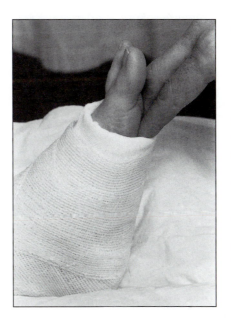

4 *Edema and Motion:* Note any swelling distal to the injury. If the client is wearing a cast, ensure that you can fit two fingertips into the cast opening. Usually, the involved extremity is elevated above the level of the heart immediately after the application of the cast, and it is maintained in this position until edema is no longer a problem. Ice packs can also be applied to the surgical or injury site to help minimize swelling.

Ask the client to move all the involved fingers or toes. Moving all the digits is important because different nerves innervate different digits. Assess for the presence of pain with the movement.

ASSESSING NERVE FUNCTION

The following five assessments of nerve function each have two components. The first element evaluates sensation, and the second evaluates motion. Loss of sensation and movement necessitates an immediate intervention, for example, removing the cast or immobilization device to prevent irreversible damage. Impaired sensation or movement requires an immediate notification of the physician and close observation. Frequently the involved extremity can be elevated higher than its present level to reduce the edema that potentially could be causing the problem.

Assessing the Radial Nerve

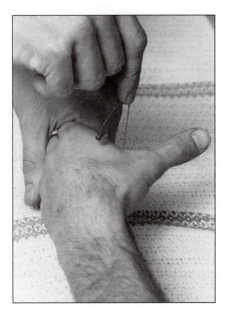 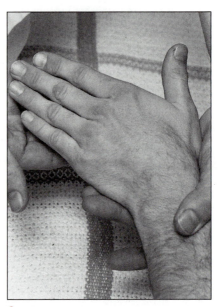

1 Prick the web between the client's thumb and index finger.

2 Instruct the client to hyper-extend his thumb and then to extend all four fingers.

Assessing the Ulnar Nerve

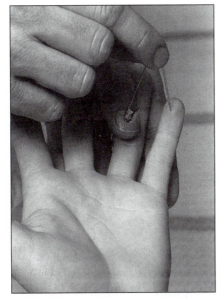

1 Prick the distal fat pad of the small finger.

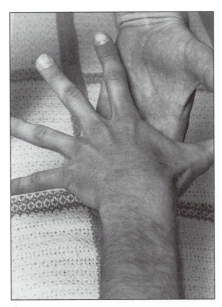

2 Instruct the client to abduct all fingers.

Assessing the Median Nerve

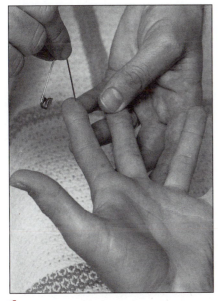

1 Prick the distal fat pad of the index finger.

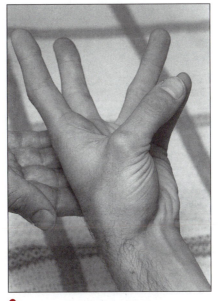

2 Instruct the client to oppose the thumb to the little finger or to flex the wrist.

➡

Assessing the Peroneal Nerve

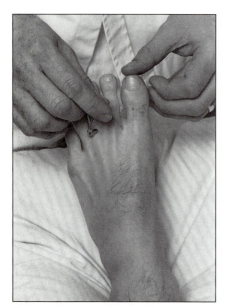

1 Prick the web between the great toe and the second toe.

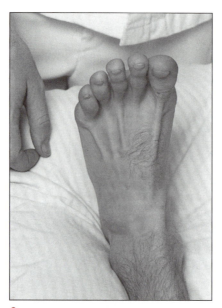

2 Instruct the client to dorsiflex the ankle and extend the toes.

Assessing the Tibial Nerve

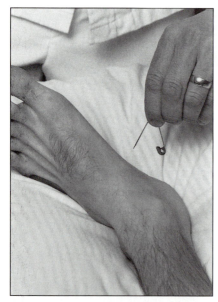

1 Prick both the lateral surface and the medial surface (as shown) on the sole of the foot.

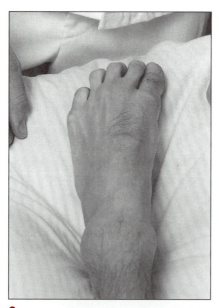

2 Instruct the client to plantarflex the ankle and flex the toes.

Using Immobilization and Comfort Devices

NURSING GUIDELINES: CARE OF CLIENTS IN IMMOBILIZATION DEVICES

Soft Cervical Collar

Description

Felt or foam collar, usually covered with stockinette material. Can be hooked in position or secured in place with Velcro™ strips.

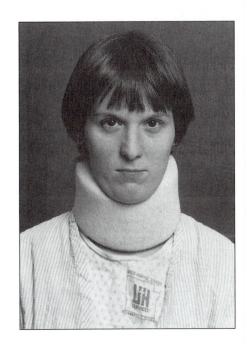

Nursing Considerations

- It is used intermittently or on a short-term basis for the relief of muscle spasms or for cervical immobilization after a cervical injury. Because it provides gentle support only, it should not be used when complete neck immobilization is desired.

- Ensure that the collar fits snugly enough to provide proper immobilization, yet not so tightly that the airway can become obstructed.

- If the physician requests that the neck be kept in slight flexion, position the tapered end of the collar anteriorly.

- If slight extension is desired, place the wide end of the collar anteriorly.

- These collars should be hand-washed and allowed to drip dry.

- Provide the client with oral and written instructions for appliance care, application, and removal.

NURSING GUIDELINES: CARE OF CLIENTS IN IMMOBILIZATION DEVICES (continued)

Hard Cervical Collar

Description

Rigid plastic collar, contoured to fit the chin and neck. Frequently, it is fitted to the client by the orthopedic supply company.

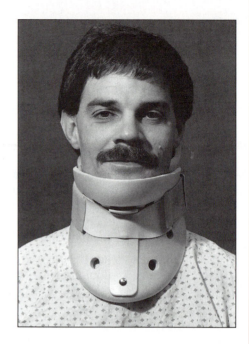

Nursing Considerations

- This type of collar is applied more frequently for long-term use, or in instances when more rigid support is desired, for example after cervical fractures or fusions.

- Ensure that the collar is not so tight that the airway is in danger of obstruction.

- Assess the client for discomfort or skin irritation around the jaw, clavicle, and spinous processes. Pad the bony prominences to prevent this problem.

- Cleanse the collar by sponging it with warm soapy water.

- Provide the client with oral and written instructions prior to discharge regarding appliance care, application, and removal.

NURSING GUIDELINES: CARE OF CLIENTS IN IMMOBILIZATION DEVICES (continued)

Clavicle Splint

Description

Has padded straps that encircle the anterior axillae to provide compression at the clavicular area. Each strap adjusts in size and closes in the back with catch or Velcro™ closures (bottom photo).

Nursing Considerations

- This splint is frequently applied after a clavicular fracture.

- Prior to application, obtain a baseline neurovascular assessment in the upper extremities, and obtain follow-up assessments thereafter, at least every 4 hours.

- Evaluate the tension of the straps with each position change to ensure that the splint provides proper immobilization without excessive pressure at the axillae.

- Assess for discomfort or skin irritation, especially at the axillary areas, and provide skin care as indicated.

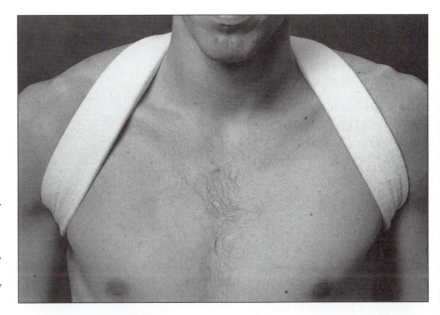

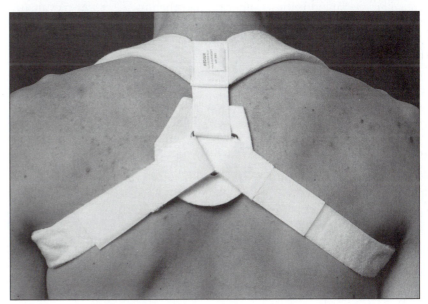

NURSING GUIDELINES: CARE OF CLIENTS IN IMMOBILIZATION DEVICES (continued)

Arm/Shoulder Immobilizer

Description

The polyester and foam fabric has a sling to support the forearm and a strap with Velcro™ on both ends that goes around the chest. The sling provides elbow flexion while supporting the forearm across the abdomen for comfort. The chest strap keeps the shoulder immobilized.

Nursing Considerations

- This device can be used after a shoulder dislocation, clavicular or humeral fracture, shoulder surgery, or acromio-clavicular separation.

- Perform a baseline neurovascular assessment prior to application of the immobilizer, and obtain subsequent assessments thereafter, at least every 4 hours.

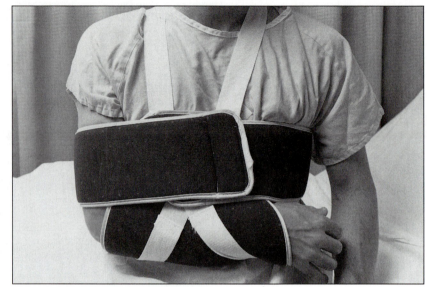

- Also evaluate respiratory status to ensure that the chest band is not too tight.

- Assess for areas of discomfort or skin breakdown, and provide skin care as indicated.

NURSING GUIDELINES: CARE OF CLIENTS IN IMMOBILIZATION DEVICES (continued)

Wrist/Forearm Splint

Description

Foam or vinyl splint with elasticized straps, extending from the palm to the midforearm. It attaches with hooks or Velcro™ strips.

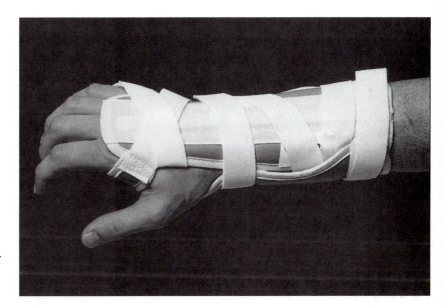

Nursing Considerations

- This splint provides immobilization to the wrist following wrist sprain or wrist surgery, and it prevents ulnar deviation for clients with rheumatoid arthritis.

- Obtain baseline neurovascular status prior to initial application, and at least every 4 hours thereafter.

- Unless it is contraindicated, remove the splint every 8 hours or as prescribed, and assess the skin for breakdown, especially around the splint edges.

NURSING GUIDELINES: CARE OF CLIENTS IN IMMOBILIZATION DEVICES (continued)

Abduction Pillow

Description

An A-shaped pillow, usually of foam construction, with foam straps that wrap around the client's legs.

Nursing Considerations

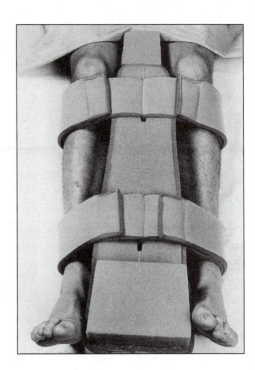

- The pillow keeps the hips in abduction after a surgical hip repair or replacement to help prevent hip dislocation.

- Assess postoperative neurovascular status hourly until stable, and every 4 hours thereafter.

- Ensure that two fingers can fit between the pillow straps and the client's skin.

- Remove the straps every 4 hours and assess the skin for irritation.

- Massage the skin, and sprinkle cornstarch on the client's legs if perspiration is a problem because of the pillow's foam construction.

- When transferring the client to the chair or wheelchair, the physician may request that you keep the pillow in place to prevent hip adduction during the move (see pages 572–581).

- Watch for signs of skin breakdown, especially around the heels and coccyx, and provide skin care as indicated.

- To keep the client's heels off the bed and thus prevent skin breakdown, position a folded towel or narrow pillow just proximal to the client's heels.

NURSING GUIDELINES: CARE OF CLIENTS IN IMMOBILIZATION DEVICES (continued)

Knee Immobilizer

Description

Soft canvas-type fabric that has metal splints along its long axis. It also has adjustable Velcro™ straps to secure it around the client's leg. The appliance prevents knee flexion.

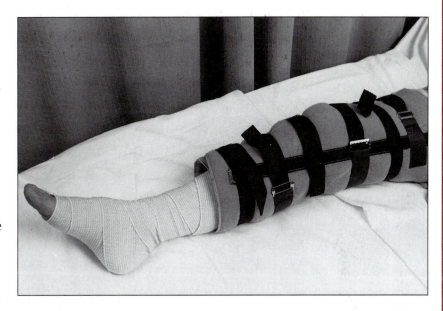

Nursing Considerations

- Generally this device is placed on a client in surgery who has had a total knee replacement.

- The leg may seem bulky to the client because of the bandages underneath. In addition, the client may have a portable wound-drainage system in place (see pages 563–564).

- The immobilizer will remain on the client at all times unless its removal has been prescribed by the physician.

- Perform baseline neurovascular checks on the involved limb upon the client's return from surgery and at least every 4 hours after that. Also, assess the posterior thigh for skin irritation or breakdown caused by pressure of the immobilizer.

- Assess for areas of discomfort, and report increasing pain to the physician.

NURSING GUIDELINES: CARE OF CLIENTS IN IMMOBILIZATION DEVICES (continued)

Hinged Brace

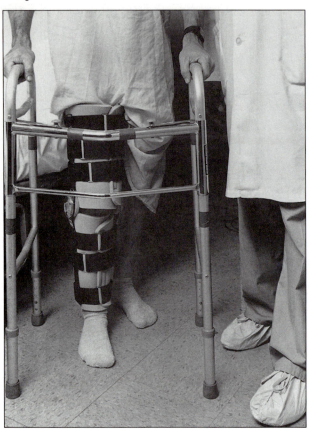

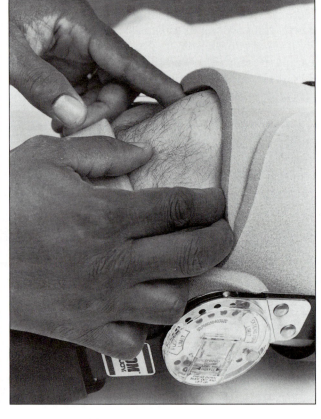

Description

Foam appliance with a metal built-in hinge and dial that are used to set flexion and extension limits for the knee. Velcro™ straps secure the brace around the client's leg. The brace enables the client to ambulate and bend the knee within prescribed limits.

Nursing Considerations

- This device can be used for clients who are being discharged after a total knee replacement. Most clients also will have a walking device (walker or crutches). See photo at left.

- The straps should be snug enough to keep the brace in place but not impede circulation.

- Flexion or extension limits can be set using the dial on the side of the brace. The hinges always should be positioned on the lateral and medial aspects of the patella. See photo at right.

NURSING GUIDELINES: CARE OF CLIENTS IN IMMOBILIZATION DEVICES *(continued)*

Denis-Browne Splint

Description

Two foot plates are attached to a metal crossbar. If oxford-type shoes are not already attached to the crossbar, the feet are strapped to the plates with adhesive tape. The shoes are usually open-toed to accommodate the child's growth.

Nursing Considerations

- This splint is used to apply mild external rotation to the feet for the child with talipes deformities (clubfoot).

- The splint is usually indicated for the infant under 1 year of age, and it is worn at nighttime and during naps.

- Demonstrate removal and application to the parents. Show them skin assessment techniques, especially around the shoe edges. Also show them how to perform neurovascular assessments and observe for impaired circulation in the feet.

- Expect frustration and irritability from an infant who cannot kick her feet in the manner to which she is accustomed. Provide hugs and comfort measures when this splint is worn.

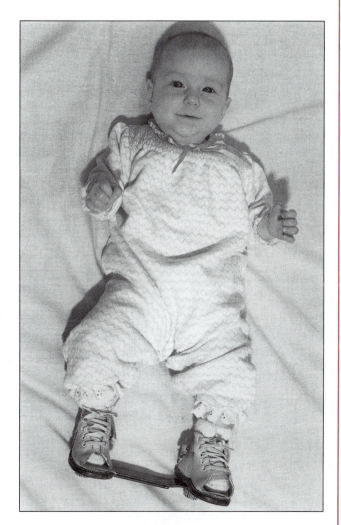

APPLYING ELASTIC BANDAGES

Elastic bandages are applied to provide immobilization and support and to minimize swelling. They are wrapped from the limb's most distal part toward the trunk. Fingers or toes should be left unwrapped to provide access for neurovascular assessments. The bandage should be applied firmly but never tightly, with each turn positioned at equal distances from the others to provide even pressure. Always take baseline neurovascular assessments (see pages 506–507) before wrapping the bandage, and repeat the assessments 15 minutes after the application and every 4 hours thereafter for as long as the bandage is worn. Obtain a bandage of the appropriate width to accommodate the client's affected limb or injured area, for example, a 10 cm (4-in) bandage for the lower leg, a 15 cm (6-in) bandage for the thigh, a 7.5 cm (3-in) bandage for the hand and forearm, and a 5 cm (2-in) bandage for a child. Unless otherwise indicated, remove the bandage at least every 8 hours to assess for excess pressure or irritation and to provide skin care.

WRAPPING A LONG, CYLINDRICAL BODY PART

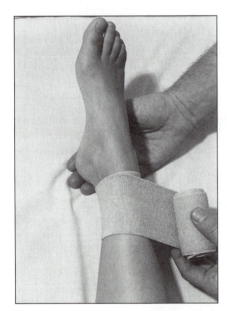 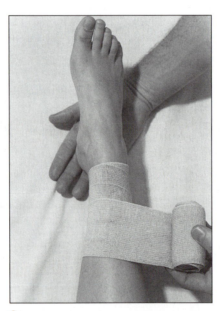 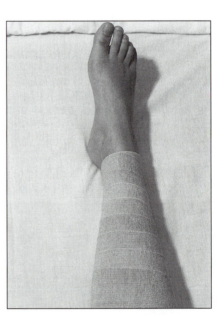

1 A spiral turn is used over a long, cylindrical body part or one of increasing circumference such as the calf. Beginning at the distal end of the limb, make a circular turn by wrapping the bandage once, and then repeating the previous turn to anchor the bandage in place.

2 Spiral turns are made next, overlapping each previous turn by one-half to two-thirds of the width of the roll.

3 Continue to wrap the limb, making sure the completed wrap is evenly spaced and wrinkle-free, and that it is comfortable for the client. Either tape or clip the end of the bandage to secure it in place.

WRAPPING A JOINT

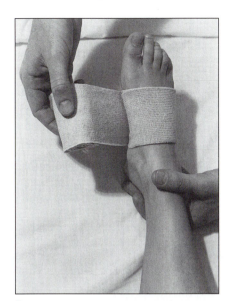

1 Some joints can be properly immobilized or supported with a figure-eight turn. First, anchor the bandage in place by making a double circular turn on the area of the limb distal to the joint.

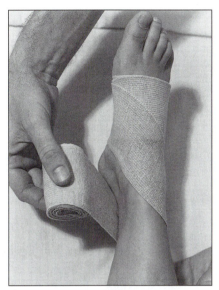

2 Begin a figure-eight turn by making an ascending turn and wrapping the bandage around the joint.

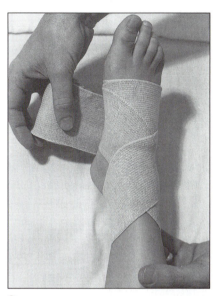

3 Finish the figure-eight turn by making a descending turn.

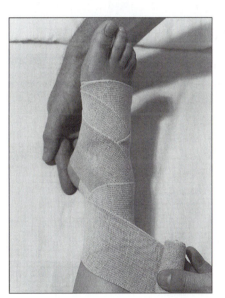

4 Continue the turns by overlapping the bandage in an alternately ascending and descending fashion.

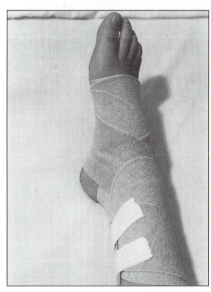

5 When the joint has been wrapped in an even and wrinkle-free manner, secure the end of the bandage to the rest of the wrapped surface with tape or clips. *Caution: If the bandage is to be applied to decrease edema, rather than to support the joint, it is essential that the heel also be wrapped or fluid will collect in the heel, potentially resulting in pressure necrosis.*

WRAPPING A RESIDUAL LIMB (STUMP)

Postoperatively, a residual limb may be wrapped with an elastic bandage or limb shrinker to reduce swelling and to mold the stump for eventual prosthetic fitting. One effective way to wrap a residual limb if an elastic limb shrinker is unavailable is to employ a modified figure-eight turn using an elastic bandage. Be sure to include client teaching in this procedure.

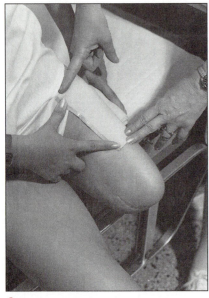

1 It is essential that you position the end of the elastic bandage high on the groin and that this area is properly wrapped without bulging fatty tissue. If the fatty tissue is not contained by the wrapped bandage, the prosthesis will not fit properly.

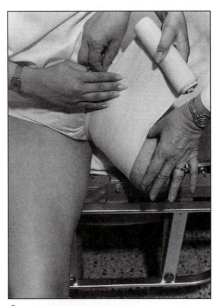

2 Make a circular turn to anchor the bandage in place.

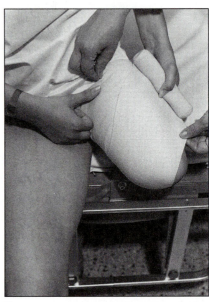

3 Make a spiral turn that overlaps the circular turn, and wrap the distal end of the residual limb.

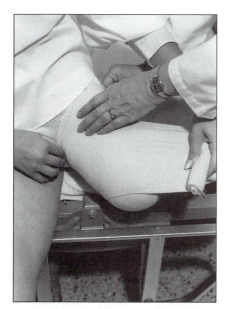

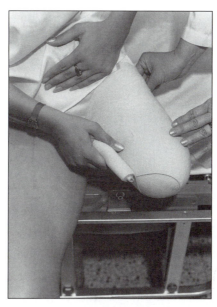

4 Make alternately descending turns (above) and ascending turns until the residual limb has been completely wrapped.

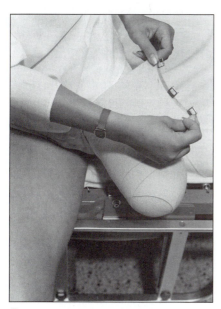

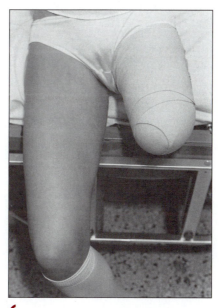

5 Once the residual limb has been wrapped, use tape or clips to secure the end of the bandage to the rest of the wrap.

6 Ensure that the bandage is wrinkle-free and that the client does not complain of discomfort from tightness. Be certain that rolls of fatty tissue do not protrude from the bandage, especially along the groin area. Prior to discharge, your client should be proficient in wrapping the residual limb independently.

Managing Routine Cast Care

ASSISTING WITH CAST APPLICATION

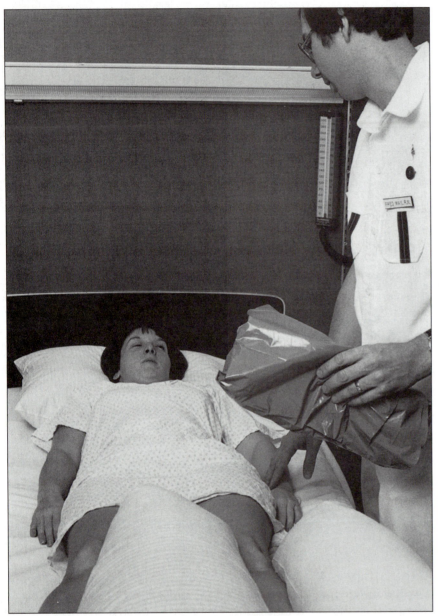

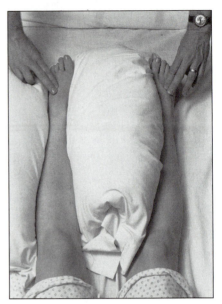

2 Assess the client's neurovascular status by following the procedures, on pages 506–510. Establish the client's baseline in both extremities prior to cast application. Evaluate and record color, temperature, sensation, edema, capillary refill, and pulsations.

1 Prior to cast application, explain the procedure to the client. For example, depending on the type of cast material used, inform her that she might feel heat as the cast is applied and drying, but that the cast might feel cold and damp after that. Assess the skin on the involved extremity (or area to be casted) for impaired vascular supply, abrasions, ecchymotic areas, and lacerations. Any of these conditions should be carefully documented. The client should also be assessed for potential contraindications to casting, such as diabetes mellitus with peripheral vascular disease (PVD), arteriosclerotic vascular disease, or a peripheral neuropathy. Question the client about allergies to any of the cast materials. Use large plastic bags or bed-saver pads to protect the bed linen or cast application site.

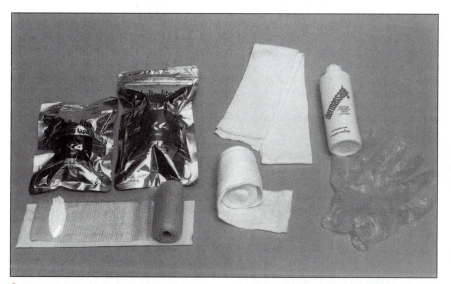

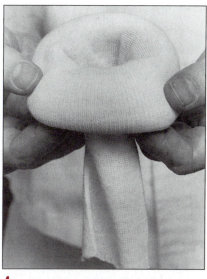

3 The materials used for cast application will vary, depending on whether a plaster or synthetic cast will be applied. The following are materials that are typically used when a synthetic cast is applied:

☐ rolls of cast material

☐ stockinette

☐ padding or sheet wadding

☐ lubricant—either massage cream or one that is water-soluble

☐ two pairs of disposable gloves

In addition, you will need a plastic-lined bucket filled with fresh water. The water temperature will be determined by the brand of synthetic cast material used. Use a water thermometer to assess for the desired temperature. Generally, lukewarm water is used when a plaster cast is applied.

4 After the stockinette has been measured and cut to fit the extremity, ensure that it is rolled to facilitate its application onto the extremity.

➤

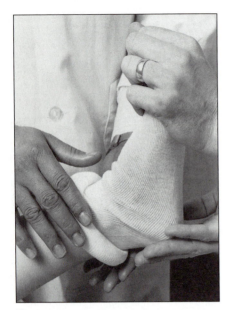

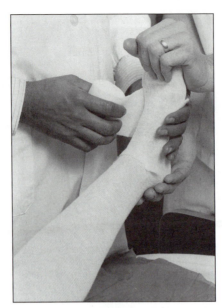

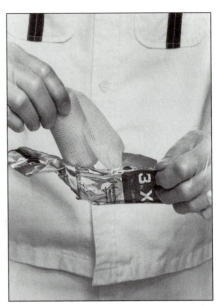

5 Hold the limb erect as the physician applies the stockinette, supporting the extremity in the neutral or prescribed position. The physician will smooth out all the wrinkles after the stockinette has been applied.

6 Continue to support the limb in the neutral or desired position as the physician wraps padding around the extremity. One to three layers of padding will be used, and extra padding may be applied over bony prominences or the injured area. It should not, however, cover the edges of the stockinette. Be certain to maintain the extremity in the same prescribed position throughout the entire procedure. Failure to do so could produce wrinkles inside the cast, potentially resulting in pressure areas that can lead to neurovascular impairment.

7 When a synthetic cast is applied, usually both the physician and the assistant apply gloves, and the synthetic casting material is then removed from its package. Opening the package earlier could affect the chemical composition of the cast material.

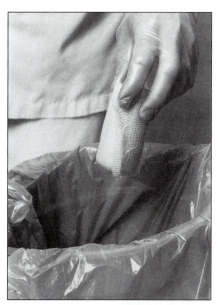

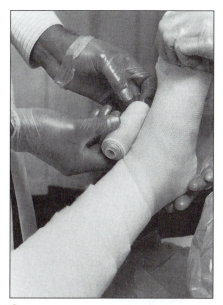

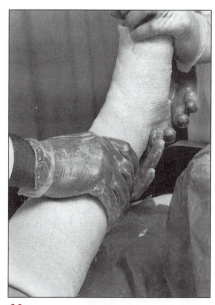

8 The roll of cast material is then immersed in water for the required amount of time, usually 7–12 seconds, but this will vary depending on the type of cast material that is used. Typically, the roll is then gently squeezed to remove the excess water. *Note: Some synthetic cast materials are activated by compression or by special lights and might not require water.*

9 Support the limb by grasping the client's toes (or fingers for arm casts) as the physician applies the cast material. If possible, you should also support the limb in areas on which the physician has not yet applied the cast material. Depending on the size and desired thickness of the cast, one to several rolls of cast material may be applied. The physician takes tucks or twists the cast material to ensure conformity to the limb. The stockinette is then pulled over the cast material to cover proximal and distal opening edges, and it is secured in place by another layer or two of the cast material.

10 To lessen the tack on the gloves and to facilitate the cast molding process, the physician may request that a generous amount of cream or water-soluble lubricant be squeezed onto the gloves. The physician then molds the cast to conform it to the extremity.

➤

Variations with Cast Applications

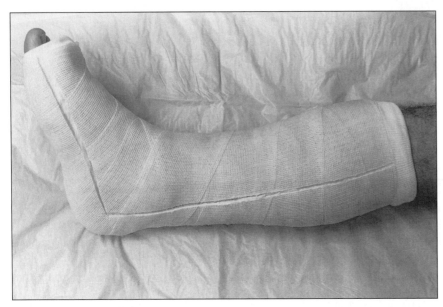

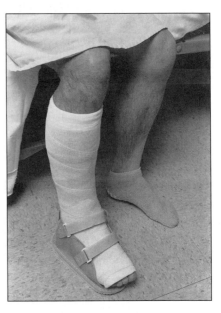

Bivalved cast: A bivalved cast may be applied if the client is expected to experience significant swelling in the casted limb. Initially, the limb is well padded before cast application to prevent injury when the cast is being cut. A cast is applied in the usual manner, and it is then cut on both sides along the long axes (top photo). The cast is then wrapped with an elastic bandage (bottom photo) to stabilize it. If swelling does occur, the elastic bandage can be removed, thereby enabling pressure to be relieved as the cast expands. The elastic bandage may then be reapplied.

Cast shoe: The cast shoe is worn to provide a smoother walking surface for a walking cast and to protect the cast from getting dirty or damaged.

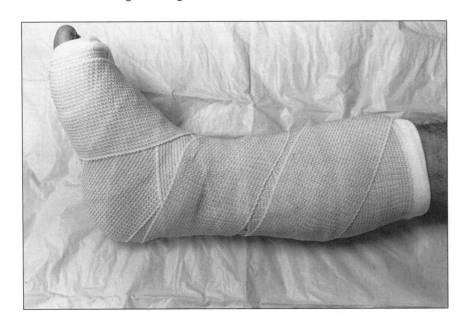

PERFORMING ROUTINE ASSESSMENTS AND INTERVENTIONS FOR CLIENTS IN CASTS

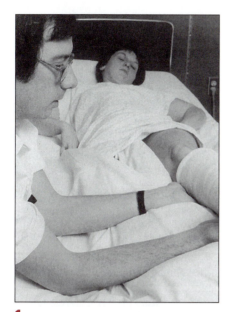

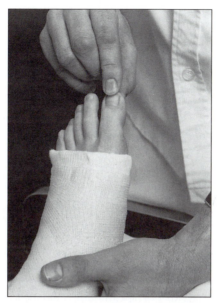

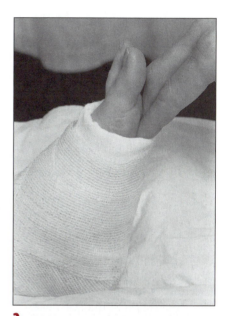

1 After a cast has been applied, elevate the entire extremity above the level of the client's heart by using pillows, suspension, or a Gatch bed. If your client has had surgery or has sustained trauma, place ice packs along the sides of the cast during the first 48 hours to minimize the potential for edema. When handling the cast, extend your fingers and ensure that only your palms come in contact with the cast. Fingerprints on a damp cast could dent or flatten the cast material, causing pressure areas that could result in client discomfort and neurovascular impairment. To enhance drying of the cast, keep sheets and blankets off the cast and reposition the client every 2–3 hours during the first 24–48 hours, the time required for the average-sized plaster cast to dry. A synthetic cast will dry much more quickly. Check under the cast to assess for flattened areas or indentations.

2 Perform neurovascular assessments every 30 minutes for several hours after cast application, and then hourly during the first 24 hours. Compare the assessments to the client's baseline. If they are normal after the first 24 hours, the assessments can be performed every 4 hours during the first few days after cast application. Assess circulation by evaluating the speed of capillary refill, color, and temperature of the toes or fingers. (Review procedures on pages 506–507.)

3 If possible, monitor the pulses distal to the fracture or injury, and assess for edema by inserting two fingers into the proximal and distal cast openings. Review the procedures on pages 508–510, to assist you with your evaluation of your client's nerve function. Describe alterations in neurovascular status to the client so that she can notify you in the event they occur. Explain to the client, significant other, parents, or family members that constant or increasing pain, numbness or tingling, impaired movement of the involved fingers or toes, or pain on passive movement require immediate attention. Any of these signs could signal compartment syndrome, a progressive degeneration of muscle caused by edema in the casted limb, which occludes arterial blood supply. Parents of infants or small children should be shown a basic neurovascular assessment and told to be alert to irritability or constant crying of their child.

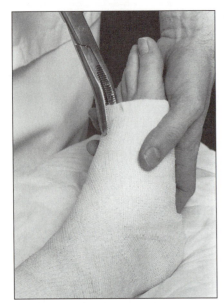

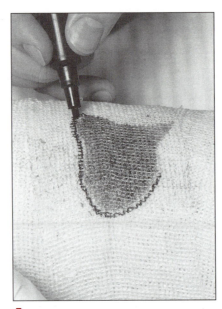

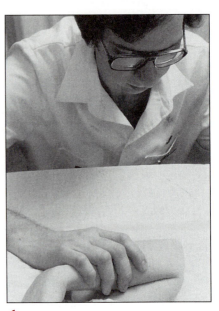

4 Feel along the cast edges to check for rough edges, for plaster crumbs, or for areas that press into the client's skin. It may be necessary to bend the cast edge slightly with a duckbilled cast bender (as shown). Extensive bending and trimming should be done by the physician. When the cast has dried, you can petal the rough edges (see the technique for cast petaling in the next procedure).

5 Monitor postsurgical or post-traumatic drainage by inspecting the entire cast. Encircle—or simply measure—the drainage stain after every shift (depending on agency policy) to provide a baseline for subsequent evaluation of the amount of exudate. Inform the physician of daily amounts and changes. It is also essential that you inspect both the sheet and the underside of the cast to ensure that drainage has not seeped into these areas. A foul-smelling odor from the cast or cast openings should be noted and promptly reported because it can be indicative of an infection. *Caution: Wear gloves if you will come into direct contact with the drainage.*

6 Because your client might be immobilized for several hours or even days, assess the skin integrity on an ongoing basis, especially around bony prominences and cast edges, which have greater potential for skin irritation or breakdown. Massage these sites with alcohol (to toughen the skin) or with a lotion, depending on agency protocol. Before using alcohol, make sure the skin is unbroken.

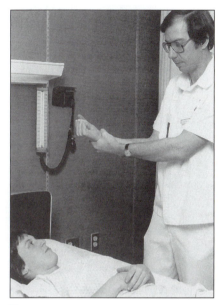

7 Ensure that the client receives full ROM exercises on the unaffected extremities, as well as on the joints distal and proximal to the cast unless it is medically contraindicated. Teach your client active ROM exercises for the unaffected extremities, and assisted ROM for the casted extremity, which can be implemented with physician approval once healing has occurred. Also, explain that moving the fingers or toes of the casted extremity will enhance peripheral circulation to minimize edema and pain. With physician approval, isometric exercises can be taught to the client to minimize muscle atrophy in the affected limb. Teach the isometric (muscle-setting) exercises on the unaffected limb so that the client can adapt the exercise to the casted limb. Demonstrate muscle palpation so that the client can feel the changes that occur with muscle contraction and relaxation.

NURSING GUIDELINES: CARE OF CLIENTS IN CASTS

- Instruct the client not to insert any object into the cast.

- Observe for indicators of pressure areas under the cast: client complaints of burning or pain, drainage on the cast surface, odor from the cast openings.

- If your client has an open wound under the cast, assess for indications of infection: increased temperature and pulse rates; increase in drainage, pain, erythema, and swelling; foul-smelling exudate; restlessness; and an increased white blood cell count.

- Especially during the first 3 days after a fracture, observe the client for indications of a fat embolus (particularly if the client has sustained multiple trauma or a fracture of the hip and femur): increased temperature and pulse rate; precordial chest pain, dyspnea, and cough; and agitation or disorientation. Petechiae at buccal membranes, chest, and hard palate might appear later. Monitor blood gases for respiratory acidosis ($Paco_2$ >40 mm Hg; pH <7.40), and serum and urine values for the presence of fat and lipase. Treatment may include the administration of oxygen, diuretics, and anti-inflammatory agents.

- Be alert to indications of compartment syndrome, which can occur when blood or drainage collect under the tissue of the injured extremity, resulting in swelling and diminished blood flow: client complaints of severe pain, which is usually unrelieved by the usual dosage of analgesic; and neurovascular impairment (increasing circumference of the extremity and capillary return >2 seconds). Later neurovascular findings include *pain* that is increased with pressure applied over the involved compartment and passive movement of the digits, *pallor, polar (coolness), paresthesias, paralysis,* and *pulselessness.* This is a medical emergency: The physician must be notified at once, and the extremity must be elevated above its present position. Typically, the cast is bivalved, and occasionally surgical intervention is required to relieve the problem.

- For comfort and to prevent skin breakdown, a sheepskin pad or pressure-relief mattress should be used under the immobilized client (see Chapter 2).

- A slightly damp cloth with cleanser can be used to clean soiled areas on a plaster cast. Excess moisture must be wiped away after the cleansing. Most synthetic casts can be cleaned with mild soap and water, followed by a thorough rinsing. The synthetic cast should be blotted with towels and then dried with a hand-held hair dryer using a cool setting.

PETALING A CAST

Once the cast has dried and the client's swelling has subsided, rough cast edges can be covered with strips of moleskin or adhesive waterproof tape.

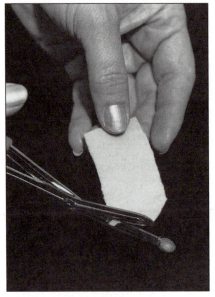

1 Cut several 5.0- to 7.5-cm (2- to 3-in) strips of tape that is 2.5 cm (1 in) in width. The number of strips will be determined by the size of the involved cast area. Then, curve the corners of each strip (as shown).

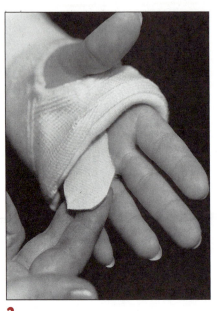

2 Insert the sticky side of the tape into the cast edge. Ensure that the petal is securely adhered and un-wrinkled to prevent unrolling and client discomfort.

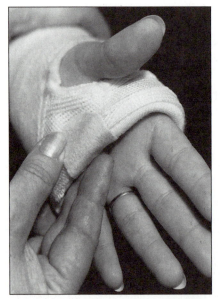

3 Lap the tape over the cast edge and adhere it to the front surface of the cast.

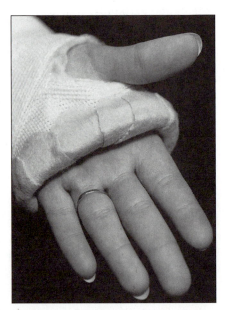

4 Continue the process, overlapping the edges of the tape strips until the rough cast surface has been completely covered by the tape. Teach the procedure to the client so that the tape can be replaced after it becomes soiled or begins to peel.

Managing Routine Traction Care

MAKING A BOWLINE TRACTION KNOT

There are several types of knots that are used for traction. The bowline knot is one that will not slip, and we therefore recommend its use over others.

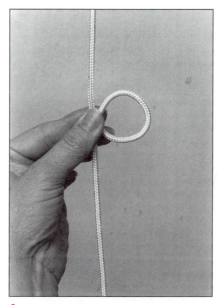

1 Make a loop in a traction rope that is both intact and unfrayed.

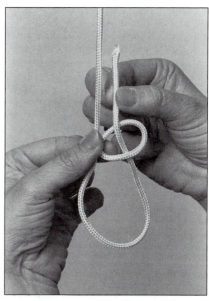

2 Bring the end of the rope up through the loop.

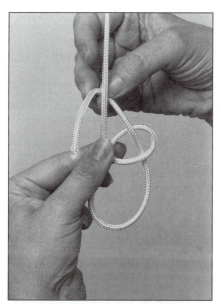

3 Wrap the end behind and around the rope that is proximal to the loop.

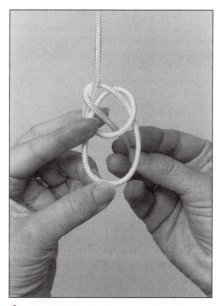

4 Thread the end down through the original loop.

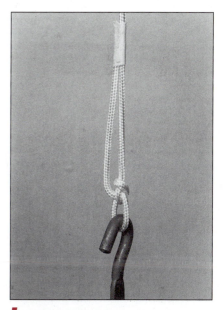

5 Tighten the knot and attach the weight to the loop that is below the knot. To prevent the end from fraying, wrap it with a small strip of tape. it is also a good idea to tape the end to the rope to discourage others from tampering with the knot.

NURSING GUIDELINES: CARE OF CLIENTS IN TRACTION

- Perform and document neurovascular assessments (see pages 506–510) prior to application of the traction apparatus to provide a baseline for subsequent assessments. For nonadhesive skin traction (for example, Buck's boot, cervical collar, or pelvic belt) perform a neurovascular assessment every 4 hours, and 30–45 minutes after every reapplication of the traction. For adhesive skin traction (for example, Buck's with adhesive straps or Bryant's) and skeletal traction, perform the assessments hourly during the first 24 hours, and every 4 hours thereafter if they are normal for the client and remain stable. Assessments should be repeated 30–45 minutes after the extremities are rewrapped with adhesive skin traction.

- Unless the traction involves the neck or upper extremities, provide the client with a trapeze and instruct her or him in its use. *Note: It may be necessary to obtain a physician's prescription for a trapeze for the pediatric population.*

- For clients receiving continuous traction, the use of sheepskin pads or pressure-relief mattresses is essential to the integrity of the skin. Inspect the skin, especially that over bony prominences, and perform skin care at frequent intervals.

- To provide the prescribed line of pull, ensure that the client maintains proper alignment and that the ropes and pulleys are in alignment, as well. Ensure that the weights are hanging freely and that the rope is centered over the pulley track.

- Because the immobilized client is at risk for the development of thrombi secondary to venous stasis, secure a prescription for antiembolic stockings and apply them following the procedure in Chapter 7.

- Make sure the client exercises the uninvolved extremities and joints, using ROM, ankle circling, and isometric (muscle-setting) exercises. Unless contraindicated, isometric exercises should be employed on the involved extremity as well.

- For the immobilized client, monitor and document bowel status and evaluate the diet. Increase roughage and obtain a prescription for a stool softener or cathartic if indicated. Ensure an adequate fluid intake (at least 2–3 L/day) to prevent urinary tract infections, retention, and renal calculi.

- To prevent respiratory complications, encourage coughing and deep-breathing exercises or the use of incentive spirometry; auscultate the chest for lung sounds daily to identify and avert the development of hypostatic pneumonia or atelectasis. For further detail, see Chapter 6.

CARING FOR CLIENTS IN SKIN TRACTION

Skin traction works by exerting a force directly to the body surface, which in turn indirectly affects the underlying muscles and bones. It can be applied to the spine, long bones of the extremities, and pelvis. Unless it is used to stabilize a fracture, skin traction (especially the head halter and pelvic traction) is used intermittently.

APPLYING CERVICAL TRACTION

Cervical traction is applied for clients with cervical spine disorders, "whiplash," muscle spasms in the neck, or neck pain. Generally, nurses can apply cervical traction for the client who does not have a significant fracture or subluxation.

Assessing and Planning

1 Review a traction manual before entering the client's room so that you are familiar with the setup, and then assemble the cervical traction apparatus. Explain the procedure to the client and perform a baseline neurologic assessment on the

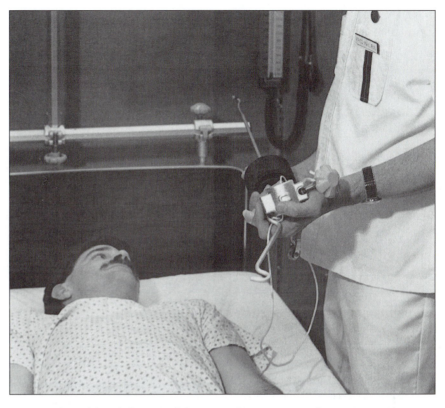

upper extremities. It is essential that the client and family members be informed about the importance of maintaining the prescribed position; avoiding the adjustment or removal of the traction apparatus unless it is approved; and reporting the presence of pressure, pain, paresthesias, or weakness in the neck or upper extremities immediately. The client should remain supine for this therapy, with the shoulders relaxed and level, and the back flattened against the bed.

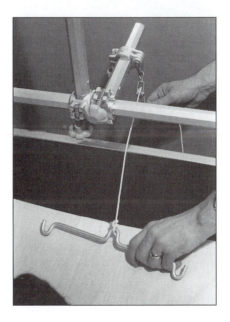

2 Attach the prescribed traction frame to the bed. Ensure that the spreader bar is of an appropriate size. It should be wide enough so that once the cervical collar is attached, the straps will neither touch the sides of the client's head nor pinch his ears. The client should also be positioned far enough down in bed so that there is ample room for the spreader bar and rope. The rope should then be tied to the spreader bar and threaded through the pulley, with the prescribed weight (usually no greater than $2\frac{1}{4}$ kg—5 lb) attached to the opposite end.

Implementing

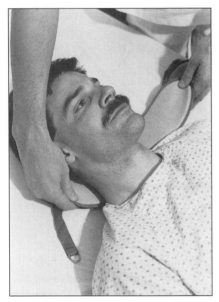
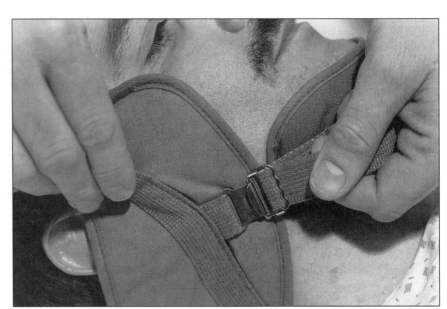

3 Insert the cervical collar carefully under the client's neck; then buckle the straps (right photo).

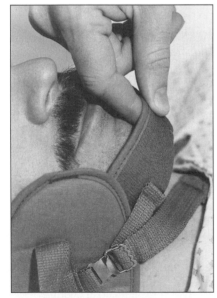
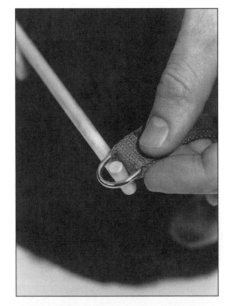

4 Adjust the collar if the strap is not centered over the chin, and make sure that the strap does not touch the client's throat. When the client is comfortable in the collar, attach the ends of the spreader bar through each of the collar rings (right photo). Use slow, even motions to avoid jerking the weights and injuring the client. When the weights are connected, make sure that the traction pull is over the occiput rather than the chin, and that it is bilaterally equal. Ask the client if it pulls more on one side than the other, and adjust it accordingly. Document the procedure.

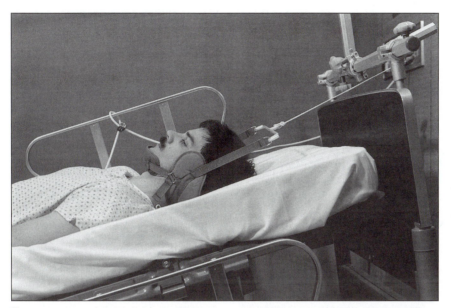

5 The physician may request that the head of the bed be elevated to provide countertraction. If this is the case, ensure that the pulley system can be raised and lowered independent of the bed so that the direction of the traction force can be altered to accommodate the client's position.

Evaluating

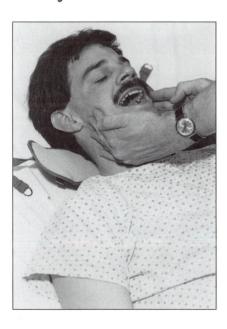

6 If intermittent rather than continuous traction has been prescribed, perform thorough client assessments after removing the collar and discontinuing the traction. Palpate the client's temporo-mandibular joint (see page 500) to assess for discomfort or limited range of motion. Pain in this area, headaches, and neck pain are indications that the weight might be too much for the client's tolerance, and the physician should be informed of the problem. Also, evaluate skin integrity at this time by inspecting the ears, chin, and occipital areas for the presence of skin irritation or pressure from the collar. Inspect and massage the skin over the elbows, heels, sacrum, and other bony prominences as well, to enhance local circulation. Remember to perform neurologic assessments on the upper extremities 30 minutes after the traction has been reapplied.

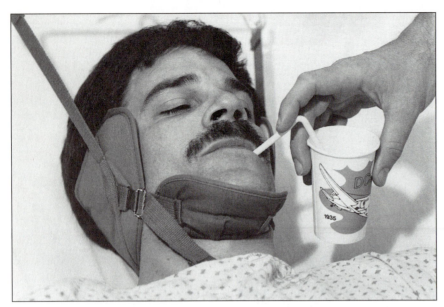

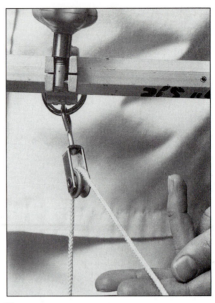

7 Evaluate the client's oral intake. If continuous traction is prescribed, it may be necessary to modify the diet to one that is soft or liquid to facilitate the client's chewing and swallowing. If the client must be immobile for prolonged periods of time, encourage a fluid intake of 2–3 L/day to minimize the potential for a urinary tract infection, retention, and renal calculi. Be sure to keep a glass containing fluids and a straw within the client's reach.

8 During routine assessment of the client, also evaluate the traction apparatus. The weights should hang freely, and the ropes must be unfrayed and centered over the pulley tracks. Check the client's alignment in relation to the traction apparatus to ensure that he receives a direct line of pull.

APPLYING A PELVIC BELT

Pelvic traction is applied for clients with sciatica, low back pain, and muscle spasms in the lower back.

Assessing and Planning

1 Obtain the prescribed traction apparatus and a pelvic belt sized to fit your client. Review a traction manual to assist you with assembling the traction apparatus used by your agency. Explain the procedure to your client, and obtain and record the client's baseline neurologic assessments. In addition, evaluate the strength of both legs by instructing the client to press her feet against both your hands (see step 12, page 542). Explain the importance of maintaining the prescribed position, keeping the traction uninterrupted, and reporting immediately any prolonged discomfort, weakness, or paresthesia of the lower extremities.

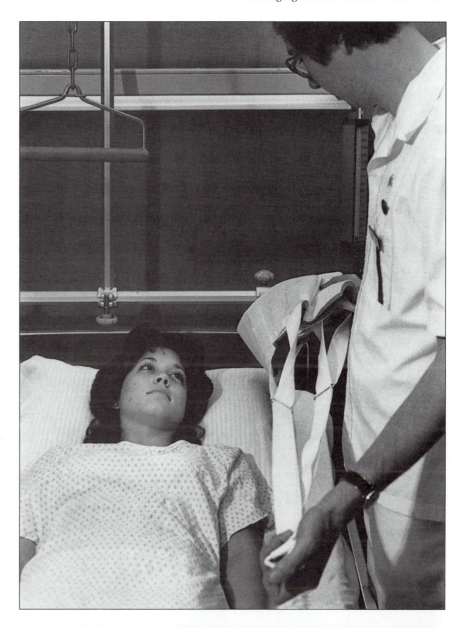

2 For countertraction and comfort, the physician may prescribe the Williams' position in which the client's hips and knees are flexed to approximately 45 degrees and the head of the bed is elevated 20–30 degrees.

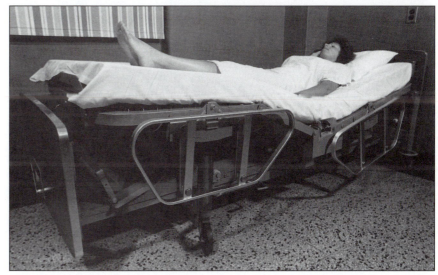

➡

Implementing

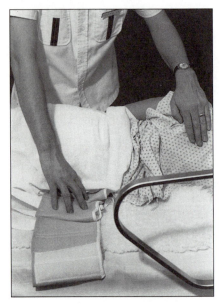

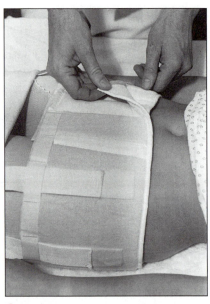

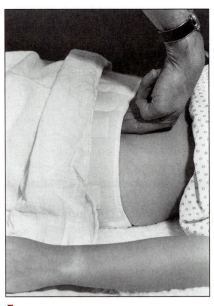

3 To position the belt around the client, assist her into a side-lying position, fan-fold half the belt, and tuck it under her hips. As you assist her onto her other side, pull the fan-folded section from underneath her. As she returns to the supine position, ensure that the belt is evenly centered under her hips.

4 The belt should encircle the pelvis rather than the waistline, with the top of the belt positioned just proximal to the iliac crests. Close the belt by attaching the Velcro™ strips together (as shown).

5 Ensure that the belt is secure enough to accommodate the traction weights without slipping downward. However, it should not be so tight that it causes discomfort and skin irritation or impairs bowel and/or bladder function. You should be able to fit two fingers between the client's skin and the belt.

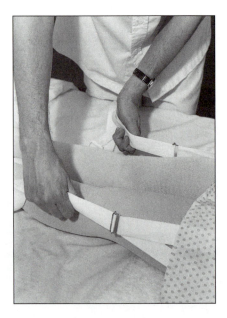

6 Position the straps of the belt along the lower legs, making certain they are equal in length to provide even traction. Adjust the straps if they are not the same length. Attach the prescribed weight, which is usually 8–10 pounds.

Evaluating

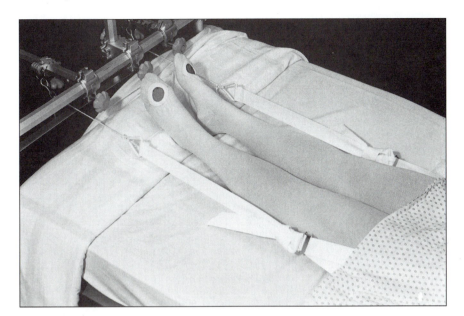

7 Assess the client for proper alignment, and make sure the ropes and pulleys are properly aligned. Ensure that the traction knots are secure and taped at the ends to prevent fraying.

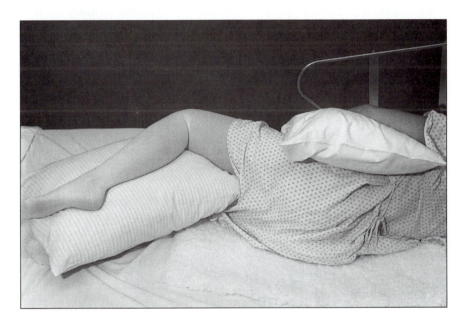

8 If intermittent traction has been prescribed for your client, encourage side-lying positions when she is out of traction. The bed should be flat. Her knees and hips should be flexed; pillows should be placed under the head and upper arm and between the knees to take pressure off the lower back.

➡

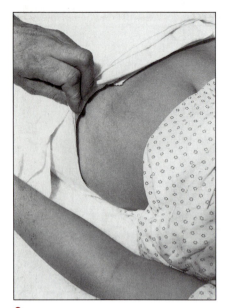

9 At least every 4 hours, assess and massage all skin areas that are prone to breakdown, especially the skin over the iliac crests, sacrum, and greater trochanters.

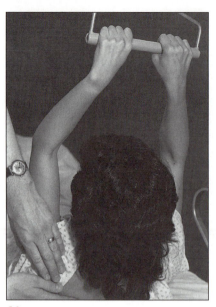

10 Unless it is contraindicated, instruct the client to elevate her upper body by flexing her knees and lifting up on a trapeze. As she does, inspect and massage the back, especially the scapular and sacral areas.

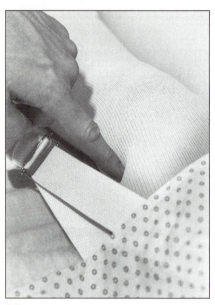

11 Evaluate neurologic status at least every 4 hours, as well as 30–45 minutes after the traction has been reapplied. In addition, be sure to assess for sciatic nerve constriction by evaluating sensation along the lateral thighs, just proximal to the patellas (as shown) as well as the lower legs proximal to the malleoli. Report a lack of sensation or tingling to the physician and remove the client from traction unless otherwise directed.

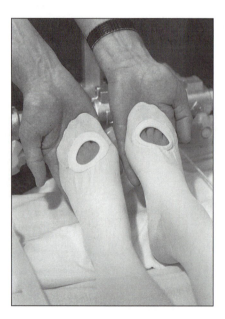

12 Evaluate the strength of both legs by asking the client to press her feet against your hands. Compare this assessment to the baseline assessment you made prior to the initial application of traction.

APPLYING A BUCK'S BOOT FOR EXTENSION TRACTION

Buck's extension is provided for the client either by adhesive straps or by a sponge rubber boot, such as that shown. It is indicated for clients who require presurgical immobilization of a fractured hip, or for clients with fractured femurs, pelvic injuries, sciatica, muscle spasms, degenerative arthritis of the knees, or knee injuries requiring minimal immobilization.

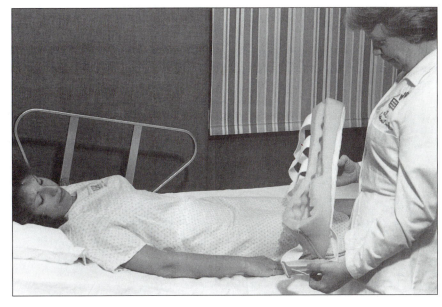

Assessing and Planning

1 Obtain a traction boot of the proper size for your client, as well as the prescribed traction apparatus. Review a traction manual to familiarize yourself with the traction setup prior to entering the client's room. Explain the procedure to the client, and inform the client and family members of the importance of maintaining the prescribed position throughout the therapy; keeping the traction uninterrupted; and immediately reporting prolonged discomfort, weakness, or paresthesias in the lower extremity.

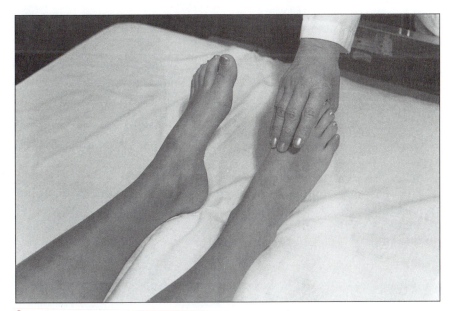

2 Perform and record a baseline neurovascular assessment of the lower extremities prior to applying the traction boot. Also, assess the client's normal ability to dorsiflex her foot because footdrop caused from peroneal nerve compression is an occasional complication of this therapy.

Implementing

3 Gently position the boot under the client's involved foot and calf, and fasten the Velcro™ straps.

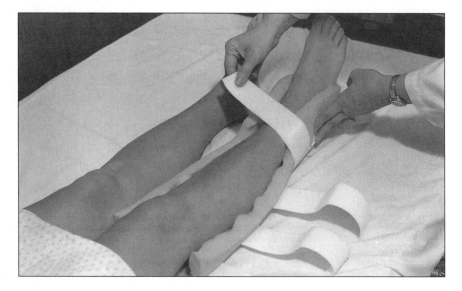

4 Although the boot should fit the client's leg securely, it should not be so tight that it produces pressure areas on the skin. Ensure that two fingertips can fit between the client's leg and each strap. This is especially important for the strap closest to the client's patella. Because it encircles the area in which the peroneal nerve lies close to the fibular head, it can potentially compress the nerve, resulting in peroneal nerve palsy (footdrop).

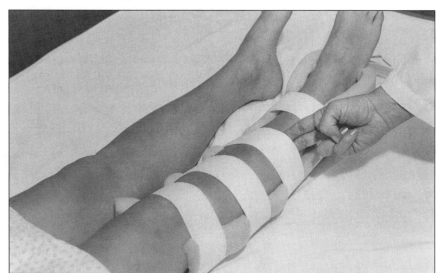

5 Attach the boot to the traction apparatus. Be sure to tape the free end of the knot to prevent it from fraying.

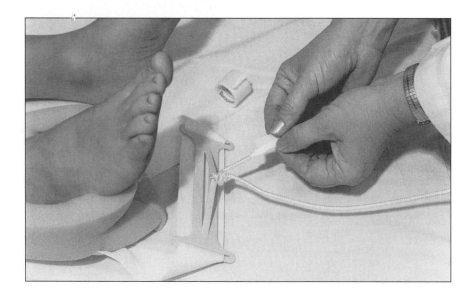

6 If it is prescribed, apply counter-traction by elevating the foot of the bed approximately 15 cm (6 in). *Note: If the physician does not want the foot of the bed elevated, the client's position in bed will require close observation to ensure that she does not slide to the end of the bed.* Attach the prescribed weight, which is usually no greater than 3⅔–4½ kg (8–10 lb).

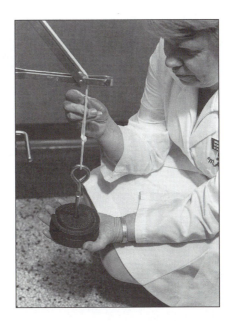

7 Place a narrow pillow or folded blanket under the involved calf to keep the heel off the bed. This will prevent irritation and breakdown caused by mattress pressure on the heel. The pillow should not occlude the popliteal space nor press on the Achilles tendon. Protect the uninvolved heel by applying a heel protector. Document the procedure.

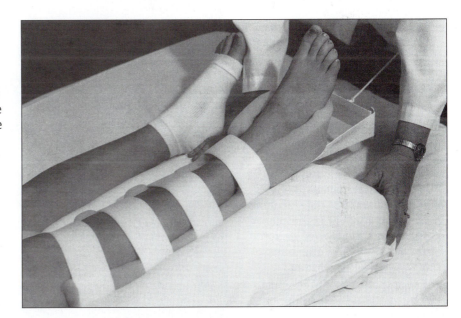

Evaluating

8 Assess the integrity of the client's skin on the involved heel by pulling the boot down and away from the heel (as shown). Remove the heel protector on the uninvolved foot, and inspect and massage the skin. Perform neurovascular assessments every 4 hours, as well as 30–45 minutes after reapplication of the traction boot. Review the procedure on page 510, to assist you in assessing the integrity of the peroneal nerve. Client complaints of tingling on the anterior leg or dorsum of the foot may signal peroneal nerve impairment.

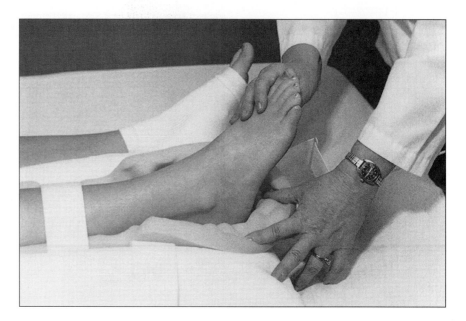

9 Unless it is contraindicated (for example, because of a fracture), remove the traction boot at least every 8 hours and cleanse and dry the leg. The sponge boot can cause increased perspiration, which can lead to skin maceration. Inspect the entire leg at that time to assess for pressure areas or breakdown, especially the dorsum of the foot, both malleoli, Achilles tendon area, anterior tibia, and the fibular head. Encourage the client to exercise her uninvolved extremities actively, as well as the joints distal to the injury if it is not contraindicated. Muscle setting (isometrics) is especially good for the involved leg.

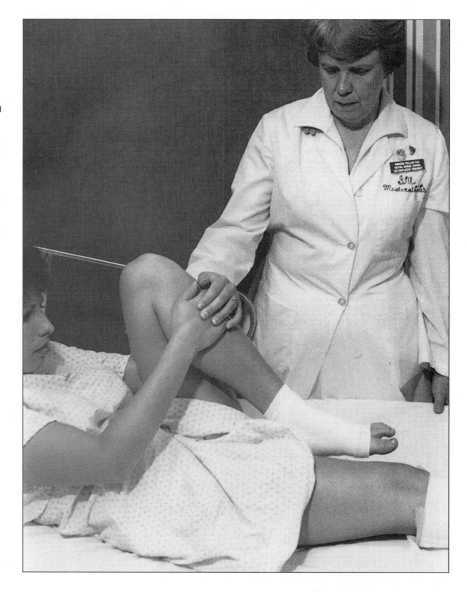

CARING FOR CHILDREN IN BRYANT'S TRACTION

Bryant's traction is employed for infants with fractured femurs, and, in a modified form (as shown in the following photos), for those with congenital dislocated hips (CDH). The traction is always bilateral to provide effective immobilization for both legs. For children with fractured femurs, the hips are flexed at 90 degrees, and the legs and feet are together at the child's midline. Children with CDH begin their treatment in the same position, usually for a period of 3–5 days. After this initial period, the hip abduction process begins, with the degree of abduction gradually increasing over a period of time, to the tolerance of the child.

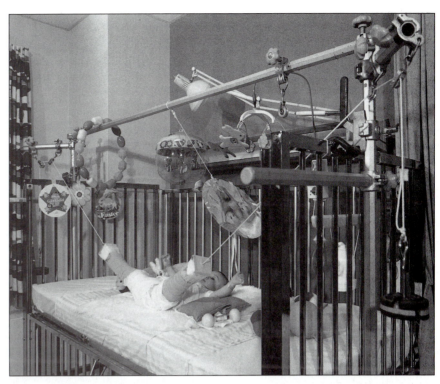

1 Perform neurovascular assessments hourly during the first 24 hours after the initial application of the traction and on a regular basis thereafter once the assessment results prove to be normal for the child. Assessments should also be performed 30 minutes after reapplication of the traction or rewrapping of the elastic bandages (for children with CDH). Review the procedures on pages 506–510 to assist you with neurovascular and nerve function assessments. Be especially alert to indicators of peroneal nerve palsy (footdrop), including the infant's inability to dorsiflex his feet and extend his toes. Make sure the elastic bandages are not too tight around the fibular heads (in the area just distal to the patellas on the lateral legs), and ensure that the child's alignment is correct so that the traction does not promote external rotation. Either situation increases the risk of footdrop or paralysis. Notify the physician immediately if you detect any neurovascular deficit. Also, demonstrate the assessments to the parents or caregivers, stressing their importance. Instruct them to alert you immediately in the event of any compromise, including prolonged irritability of the child.

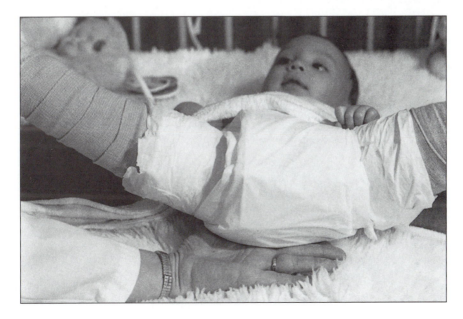

2 Assess the position of the child's buttocks in relationship to the mattress. The traction weight is appropriate if the infant's buttocks just clear the mattress (as shown); you should be able to place a flattened hand under the buttocks. Notify the physician if the buttocks are either too high or too low. He or she may wish to alter the weights.

3 Every 2–4 hours, inspect the infant's skin to evaluate its integrity, especially that over the malleoli, dorsum of the feet, and the groin (as shown).

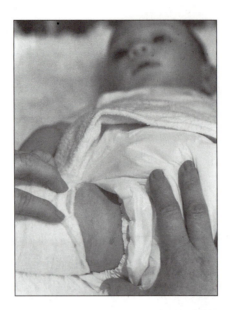

4 For children with CDH who are in modified Bryant's traction, re-wrap the elastic bandages every 8 hours, with physician approval, to enable you to inspect and massage the infant's skin. Then wrap the groin area with waterproof material, such as the plastic from a disposable diaper, to protect the elastic bandages from urine and feces. Ensure that the elastic bandages do not slip down toward the feet because this will alter the traction. *Caution: Do not unwrap the bandages if the child has a fractured femur.*

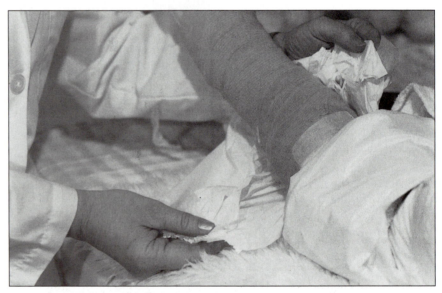

5 To prevent urinary tract infections, you will need to increase the infant's fluid intake. To ensure that the diaper provides total absorption of the urine, you may pad the diaper with a sanitary pad (as shown). This will minimize the potential for saturation of the elastic bandages, which could promote skin maceration. Assess the infant for indications of a urinary tract infection by evaluating the urine for foul-smelling odor and the infant for increased temperature and irritability. Obtain a prescription for urine tests if appropriate.

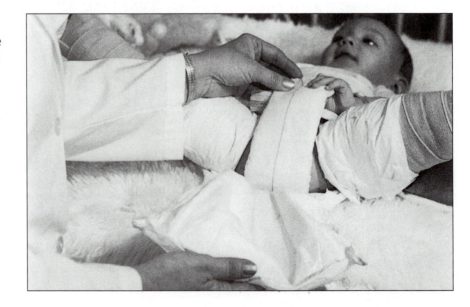

6 Unless the infant has a rash or areas of broken skin, massage the skin over the bony prominences with alcohol (to toughen the skin) or with lotion to minimize the potential for breakdown. Provide a sheepskin or small pressure-alleviation mattress to protect his skin.

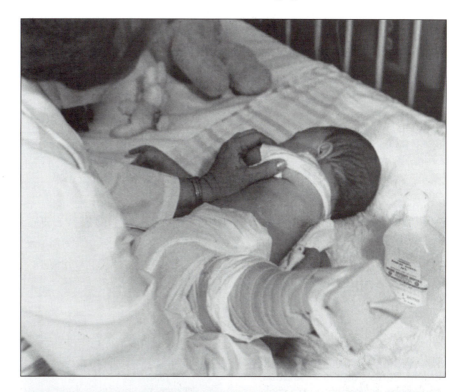

7 For feedings, the infant with CDH can be placed in an infant seat so that his head can be elevated for 30 minutes during and after feedings. This will enhance the passage of the food through the pylorus and minimize the potential for aspiration of vomitus. Make sure the infant seat can accommodate the child's hip abduction without altering the angle or causing excess pressure on the lateral thighs.

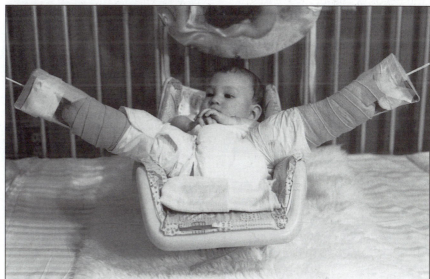

8 Provide the infant with the stimulation of social, emotional, and motor development during his prolonged period of immobility by keeping bright-colored, noise-making toys, mobiles, pictures, and an unbreakable mirror within his eye level. Be sure to put toys within reach, and rearrange the toys daily to provide the infant with a fresh environment. Encourage family members or caretakers to have frequent interaction with the child. Explain that passive ROM exercises on the uninvolved extremities can be incorporated into pat-a-cake and peek-a-boo games.

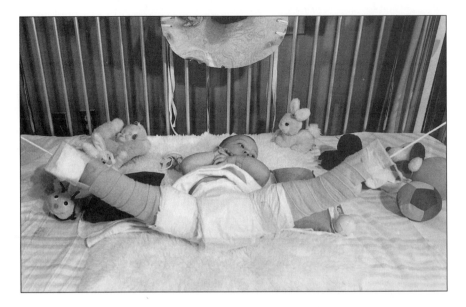

9 Frequent interaction between yourself and the parents or caretakers is essential to ensure that all the needs of the infant are met. Demonstrate procedures such as neurovascular assessments and ROM exercises; assist them as necessary during their first attempts. If possible, provide them with written materials about the care of the infant with a fractured femur or CDH. If a hip spica cast will be applied once the Bryant's traction is removed, do preliminary teaching by demonstrating cast care on a demonstrator doll (as shown).

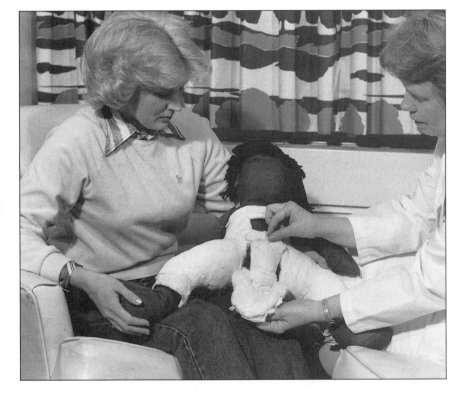

CARING FOR CLIENTS IN SKELETAL TRACTION

PERFORMING ROUTINE CARE OF CLIENTS IN SKELETAL TRACTION

With skeletal traction, pins or wires are inserted directly into or through the bone to provide a direct longitudinal pull as a means of reducing a fracture. Typical sites for skeletal traction on the extremities are the distal femur, the proximal tibia, and the proximal ulna. Casts are occasionally applied to the extremity in conjunction with the skeletal traction to help immobilize the extremity and stabilize the pin. Review and incorporate the Nursing Guidelines for care of clients in traction, page 534.

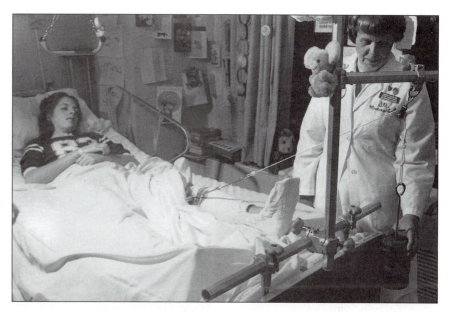

1 At least every 2 hours, inspect the client's alignment with the traction apparatus to ensure that there is a direct line of pull and that it is in a straight line with the fractured bone. Also make sure that the prescribed amount of weight hangs freely and that the rope is intact and centered over the pulley track. Remember that you never should lift or remove the weights. Releasing the traction could result in pain, muscle spasms, and injury to nerves and blood vessels in the involved extremity.

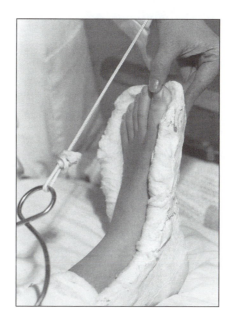

2 Perform neurovascular and nerve function assessments hourly during the first 24 hours after traction application, and at least every 4 hours thereafter as long as the assessment results are normal for the client (review the procedures on pages 506–510).

➤

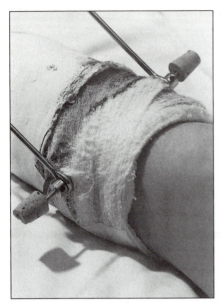

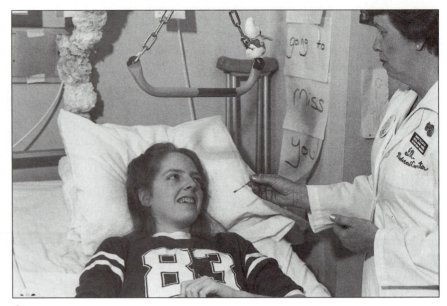

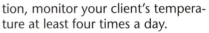

3 Inspect the pin or wire at least once every 4 hours to assess for migration. Monitor the insertion site for indications of infection: erythema; edema; foul-smelling, purulent drainage; or gross bleeding. Report any of these conditions to the physician. Note that the corks are placed on either side of the pin to protect the client and staff members from injury (see page 560 for appropriate pin care).

4 Because an elevated temperature is another indication of infec- tion, monitor your client's tempera- ture at least four times a day.

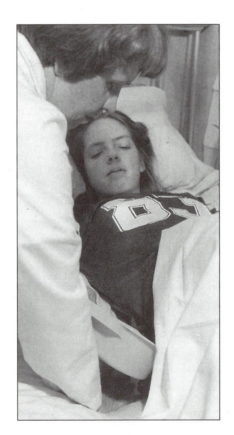

5 Your client in traction might require the use of a fracture bed- pan. To position the fracture bed- pan, instruct the client to flex the uninvolved knee and to press down with the foot to lift the buttocks. A trapeze also can be used to elevate the body. Slide the bedpan under the buttocks from the client's unaf- fected side, with the narrow end inserted first. Be sure to monitor both bowel and urinary function. Immobility can result in constipa- tion, urinary tract infections, and retention. Encourage the intake of foods containing roughage, and ensure an intake of 2–3 L/day of fluid. If indicated, obtain a prescrip- tion for a stool softener.

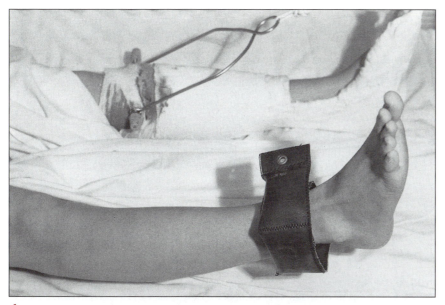

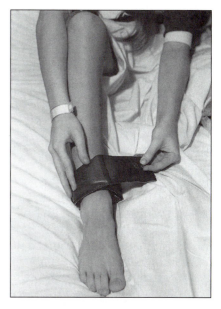

6 Encourage ROM on the uninvolved extremities and isometric (muscle-setting) exercises on both uninvolved and involved extremities. Teach the client how to apply weights (1–2¼ kg—2–5 lb) to the uninvolved ankle (right). Lifting the leg up and down with the resistance of the added weight will enhance the development of the quadriceps muscle in preparation for weight bearing if crutches will be prescribed when the client becomes ambulatory.

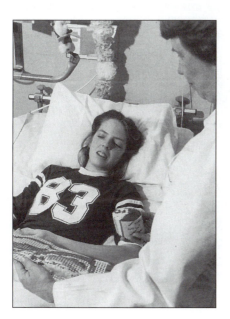

7 Minimizing your client's boredom will require the occasional initiation of bedside projects, as well as provision of newspapers, books, magazines, handicrafts, and puzzles. Always take the time to provide empathy, reassurance, and emotional comfort for the immobilized client.

PERFORMING ROUTINE CARE AND ASSESSMENTS FOR CLIENTS IN HALO VESTS

Halo traction is frequently used for clients with scoliosis, cervical fractures and fusions, torticollus, and rheumatoid arthritis. A metal ring (the halo) surrounding the head attaches to the skull with four pins, each penetrating through the skin and into the skull approximately 30 mm (⅛ in). The traction headpiece attaches to either a plaster or plastic vest to provide head and neck immobilization. The main advantage of halo traction is the early mobility it allows, which reduces the potential for circulatory, respiratory, and neurologic complications.

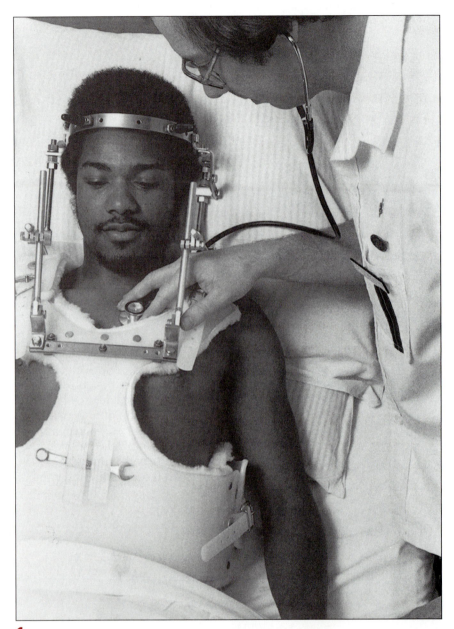

1 Assess the client's respiratory status (see Chapter 6) at least every 4 hours to ensure that the lungs are clear and that the vest does not press on the diaphragm, compromising chest expansion. Pulmonary emboli can occur in clients with spinal cord injuries, yet some clients with neurologic impairment due to a cervical cord injury are unable to feel the pain associated with this disorder. Close assessment of these clients is especially critical. Keep an incentive spirometer at the bedside and instruct the client in its use. Note that an open-ended wrench is taped to the client's vest. This wrench provides immediate release of the bolts to remove the vest in the event the client requires external cardiac compression.

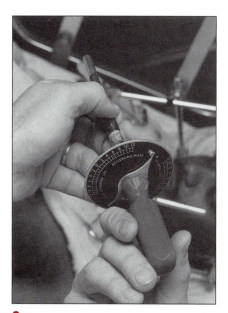

2 In addition, a torque screwdriver should be kept available for the physician for tightening the pins to adjust the degree of tension on the anterior metal bars. The traction is correctly adjusted when there is neither flexion nor extension of the neck. The neck always should be kept in a neutral position.

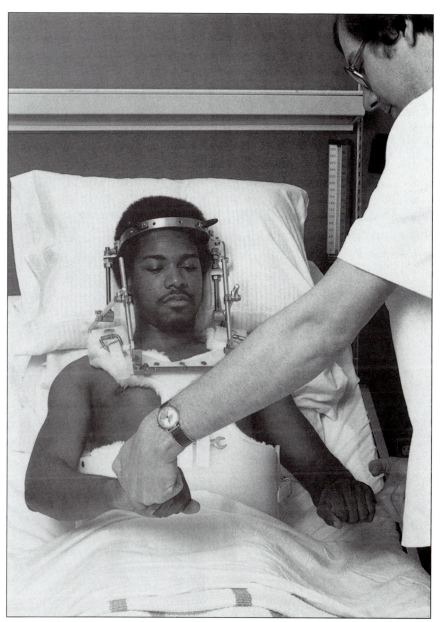

3 After the vest has been applied, assess the client's neurologic status hourly for a minimum of 24 hours until it is stable, and every 4 hours thereafter. Evaluate strength, sensation, and movement of the upper extremities; assess cranial nerve function to ensure that the pins in the skull are not impinging on the cranial nerve (see procedures for assessment in Chapter 10).

➤

4 Instruct the client to perform active or assisted ROM exercises at least three times a day unless it is contraindicated by the client's disorder, for example a cervical fracture.

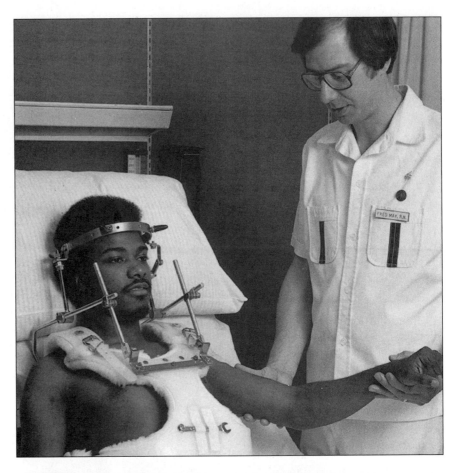

5 Keep careful intake and output records, and encourage fluids to maintain a fluid intake of 2–3 L/day. This will minimize the potential for renal calculi, urinary tract infections, and retention. Evaluate the urine for indications of infection: cloudiness, foul odor, and hematuria. Assess the client for the presence of chills and fever.

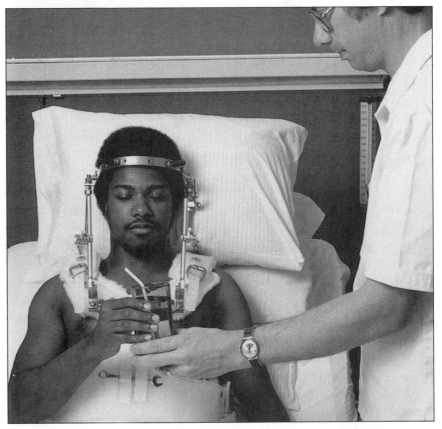

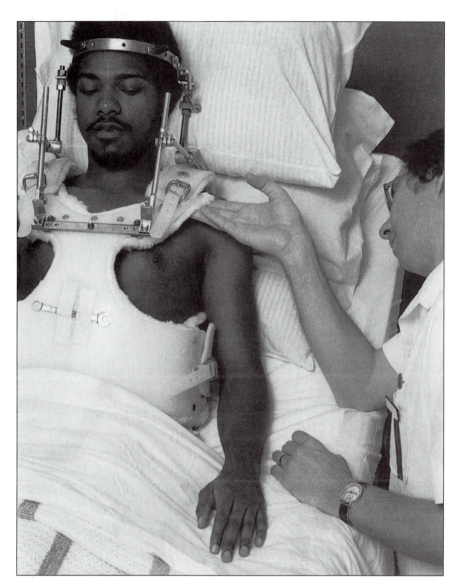

6 At least every 4 hours, inspect and massage the client's skin, especially around the vest edges. Skin irritation and pressure areas are a potential problem of wearing the vest. An air, eggcrate, or water mattress or a sheepskin pad should be used on the bed to help protect the client's skin.

➜

7 Assist the client with position changes every 2 hours to enhance circulation, prevent contractures, and maintain skin integrity. Follow the procedures in Chapter 2 for proper client positioning.

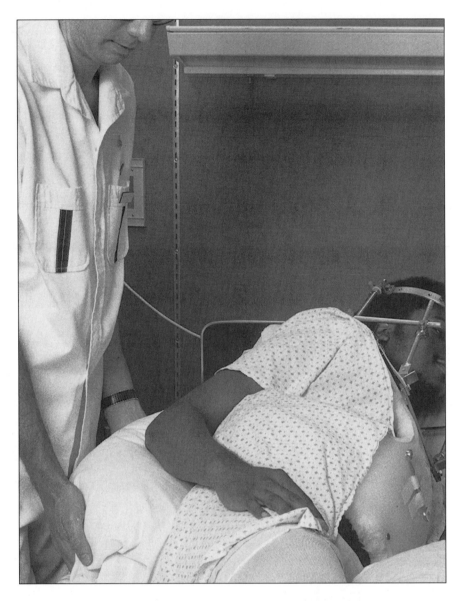

8 The sheepskin that lines the plastic vest should be removed at least weekly for washing and drying. Remove the sheepskin by detaching it from the Velcro™ strips that hold it in place (right). The client's skin should be bathed, rinsed, and dried daily. Specially trained personnel can open the vest at the sides for a more total cleansing and skin inspection.

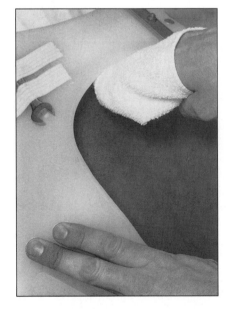
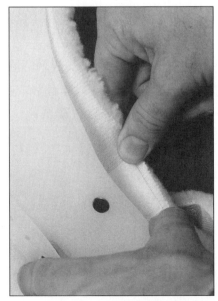

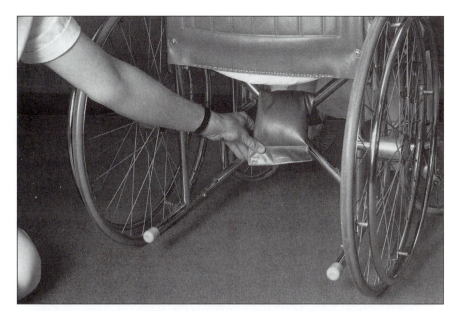

9 At least three times a day, assist the immobile client into a high-backed wheelchair that will support his shoulders. Place a 4½-kg (10-lb) weight at the wheelchair crossbar to prevent the chair from tipping backward (top photo). Be sure to provide the client with a hand mirror or prism glasses because his visual field is greatly impaired by his head and neck immobility.

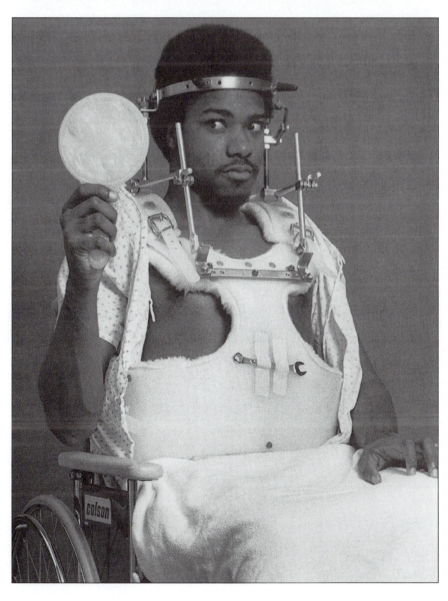

PROVIDING PIN CARE

The frequency and type of pin care will vary according to physician preference. Many experts do agree, however, that iodine solutions should not be used because it is believed that they corrode the pins. If pin care has been prescribed, the site is usually cleansed with hydrogen peroxide, leaving intact any superficial crust; this is followed by application of an antibiotic ointment. Both solutions are applied with sterile cotton-tipped applicators, following aseptic technique. In some instances, sterile 2 X 2 gauze sponges are split to the center and coated with antibiotic ointment, and then centered around the pins.

During pin care, assess for indications of infection: erythema, edema, tenderness, or purulent drainage. In addition, the position of each pin should be evaluated to ensure that it has not migrated. If a pin appears to be loose, the physician should be notified and the client instructed to remain immobile until the pin is secured.

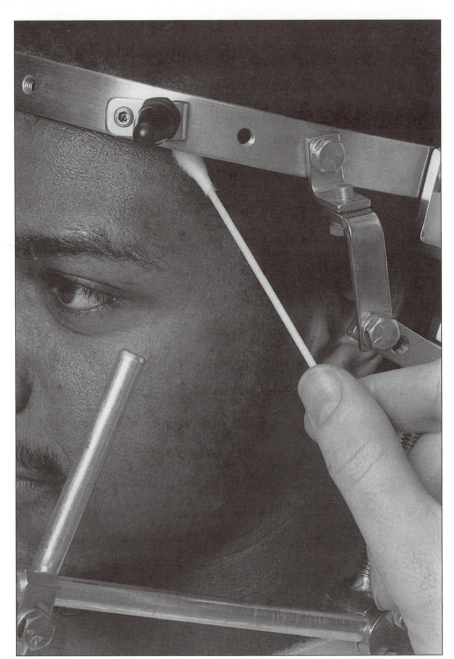

Providing Special Care for Clients with Musculoskeletal Disorders

MAKING A TRACTION BED

If your client is in continuous rather than intermittent traction, it may be necessary for you to change the linen by making the bed from its head to its foot to avoid interfering with the client's alignment and traction apparatus. This procedure is contraindicated for clients in cervical traction, for whom logrolling should be employed instead.

1 Explain the procedure to the client and then raise the bed to an optimal working level. Loosen the linen at the top of the bed.

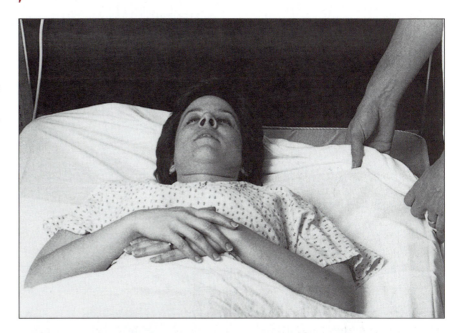

2 Fan-fold and place the fresh linen along the top of the bed.

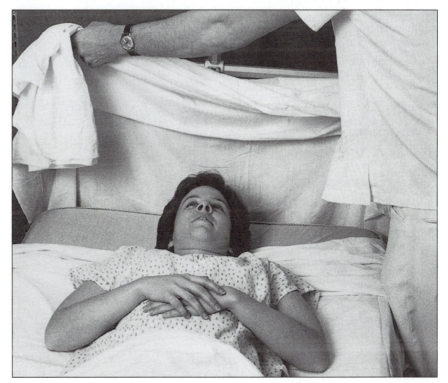

3 Instruct the client to raise her upper body on the trapeze as you begin to remove the used bottom linen. Then, ease the used linen past the client's buttocks.

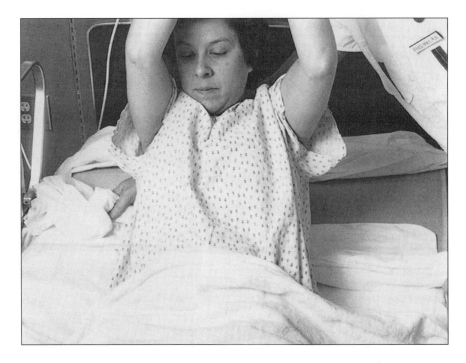

4 Secure the fresh linen to the corners at the head of the bed and pull the linen from the top toward the foot of the bed as the client lifts her upper body on the trapeze. Ease the fresh linen past her buttocks. Complete the bed making after removing the used linen from the bed. Make sure the fresh linen is taut and wrinkle-free.

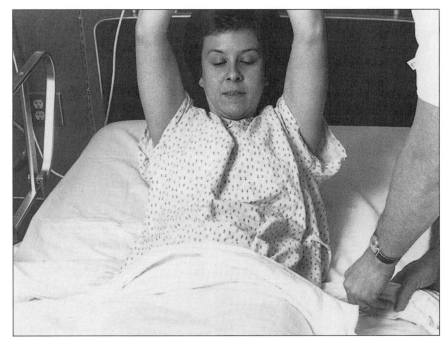

MAINTAINING A PORTABLE WOUND-DRAINAGE SYSTEM

Assessing and Planning

1 If your client has a postsurgical indwelling drain that connects to a portable vacuum container, you will need to inspect the tubing and container for patency; empty the container every shift, or as necessary; and ensure constant suction. When the client is in bed, place the system close to the client's extremity. Use care to avoid tension on the system's tubing. When getting the client out of bed, attach the vacuum container to the client's gown in order to keep the system off the floor and prevent tension at the insertion site.

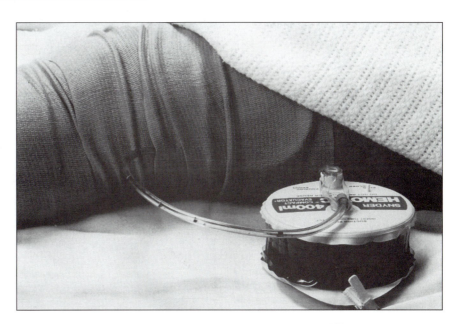

Implementing

2 To empty the vacuum container, obtain the client's measuring container and place a bed-saver pad under your working area to protect the bed linen. Wash your hands, apply gloves, and aseptically pull the drain plug to open the container. Pour the contents into the container without touching the drain port or spout with your hands or the measuring container.

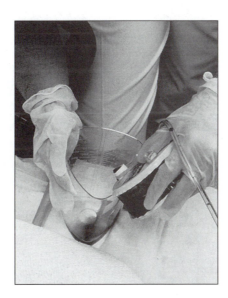

3 When the vacuum container has been emptied, wipe the drain port and plug with an antiseptic wipe.

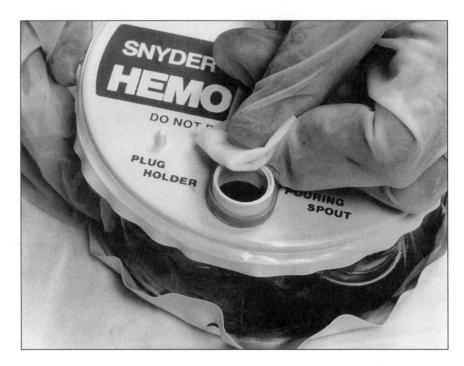

4 Compress the container (as shown), and aseptically reinsert the drain plug as you hold the container compressed. This will reestablish the low-pressure suction. Measure and document the drainage, noting its color, odor, amount, and consistency. Discard the drainage according to agency policy, remove the gloves, and wash your hands again.

Evaluating

5 Continue to monitor the container and tubing for proper drainage and patency, and ensure that suction is maintained. At least every 4 hours, or as necessary, apply gloves, remove the drainage plug, compress the container, and reinsert the plug to reestablish suction.

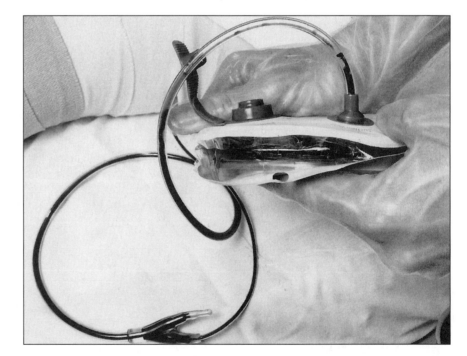

APPLYING A HYDROCULATOR PACK (MOIST HEAT) TO ARTHRITIC JOINTS

A hydroculator pack can be applied to your client's arthritic joints to relieve discomfort and reduce joint stiffness and muscle spasms. Moist heat provides greater relief than dry heat does at the same temperature because it penetrates more deeply and holds the temperature for a longer period of time. Moist heat packs are usually contraindicated for clients with impaired circulation and sensation, skin infections, and prosthetic or reconstructed joints, or complications from previous heat applications, for example blisters or rashes.

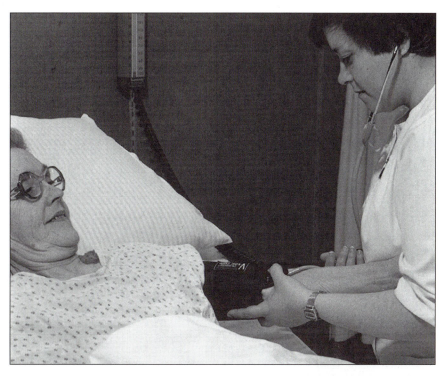

Assessing and Planning

1 Take the client's baseline vital signs. This is especially important with the older adult for whom heat may aggravate an already impaired cardiac condition. Inspect the application site for indications of complications from previous heat applications, and explain the procedure to the client.

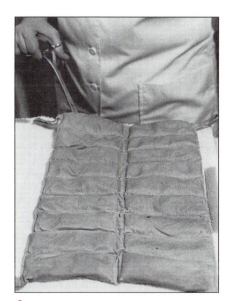

2 Heat the pack in the steam machine or heating device used by your agency. In many agencies, the temperature is controlled so that it never exceeds 48.9 C. Place the heated pack on its terrycloth cover or on a double thickness of terrycloth towels if the cover is unavailable.

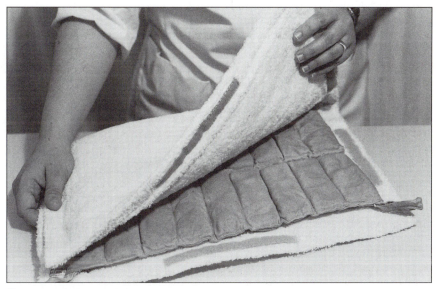

3 Wrap the pack in the double thickness of terrycloth towels or terrycloth hydroculator pack cover.

→

Implementing

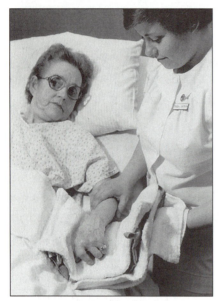

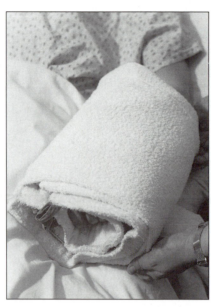

4 Place the covered pack under the client's involved area, and position a folded terrycloth towel under the pack (as shown). The extra towel will protect the bed linen from moisture and help to secure the hydroculator pack in position once it is wrapped around the joints (above). Keep the call light within the client's reach, and instruct her to alert you if the temperature becomes too uncomfortable.

Evaluating

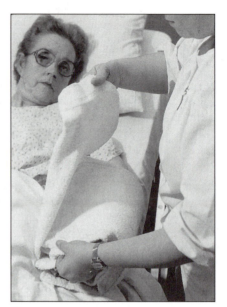

5 Unless the client alerts you sooner, evaluate the temperature of the pack after approximately 10 minutes. Assess the client for potential complications such as diaphoresis, hypotension, and tachycardia. Unwrap the pack and inspect the skin for excess erythema, and then rewrap the pack. Question the client about her comfort level. When the treatment time has elapsed (usually after a total of 20 minutes), remove the pack, evaluate the client's skin, and obtain posttreatment vital signs. Document the procedure and the client's response.

MANAGING THE CLIENT WITH A BLOOD REINFUSION SYSTEM

Assessing and Planning

1 A reinfusion (blood conservation) system, such as the Stryker, is a closed operation that collects, filters, and enables reinfusion of the client's whole blood. Clients who may benefit from this procedure include those with hip and knee replacements, as well as other populations with large draining incisions. The duration of the collection time and reinfusion is established by the physician and system manufacturer's protocol. Because infection is a potential contraindication to reinfusion, monitor the client for the presence of fever: white blood cell count ≥11,000 µl; and signs of local infection, including warmth, erythema, tenderness, and purulent drainage at the wound site.

Monitor the amount of drainage in the reservoir. The shed blood should be reinfused within a 6-hour period of initiating the collection or when drainage accumulates to approximately 400 mL, whichever comes first (Standards Committee, American Association of Blood Banks, 1994). If the client does not already have an IV infusion of normal saline, establish one at this time (see section "Administering Blood and Blood Components," page 145, for details) with 500 mL normal saline, if it is prescribed. Obtain a standard blood administration set with a 40-micron microaggregate filter and tubing with a three-way stopcock.

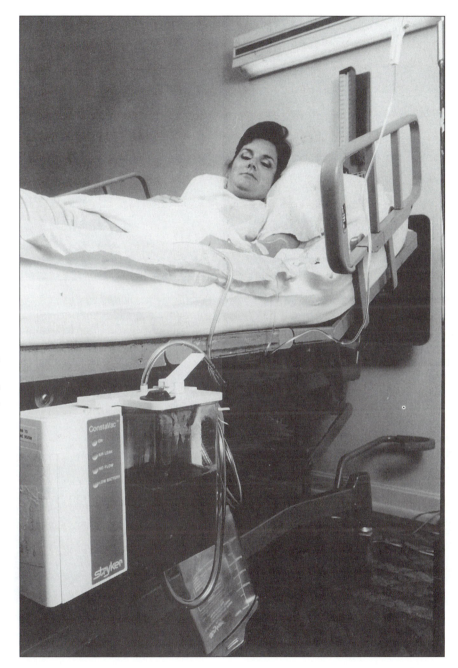

Implementing

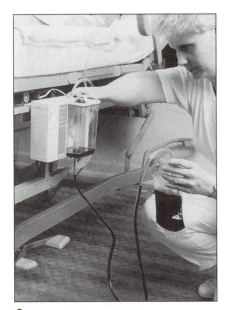

2 When it is time to reinfuse the blood, uncoil the blood bag tubing (this will facilitate blood flow), and press the valve lever on top of the reservoir to transfer the blood from the reservoir to the blood bag. Approximately 250–300 mL of blood will be reinfused to the client, and another 100 mL will remain at the bottom of the reservoir. Some manufacturers recommend that this remaining fluid not be reinfused because it may contain fats that have risen to the top of the collected fluid. When the blood has been transferred to the blood bag, clamp off the blood bag tubing as close to the blood bag as possible.

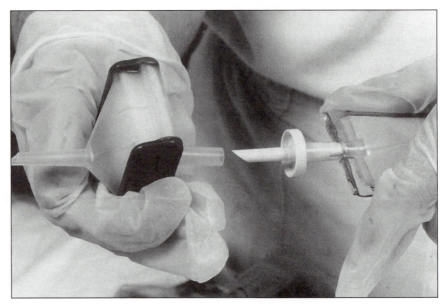

3 Put on clean gloves to prevent contact with the client's blood. Attach the 40-micron filter to the spiked end of the standard blood infusion tubing.

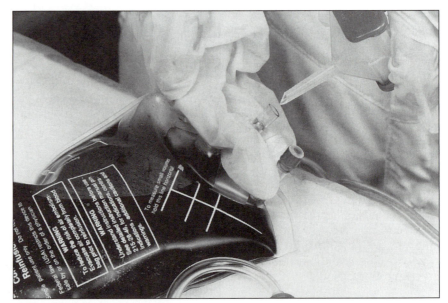

4 Next, remove the protective cover from the port of entry into the blood bag and insert the blood filter into the blood bag (as shown).

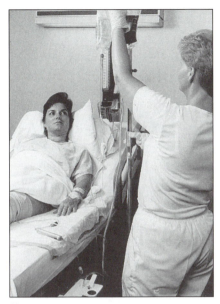

5 Hang the blood bag as shown and prime the tubing to ensure that all air has been expelled from the tubing.

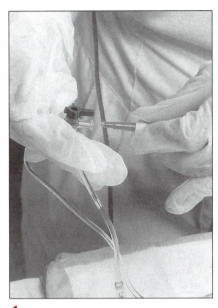

6 Using a twisting motion, attach the distal end of the primed blood infusion set to the three-way stopcock that is attached to the saline infusion.

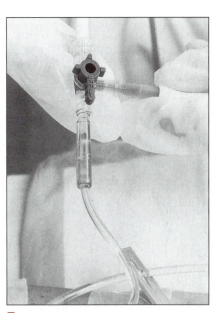

7 Turn the stopcock so that it is off to the saline and open to the blood.

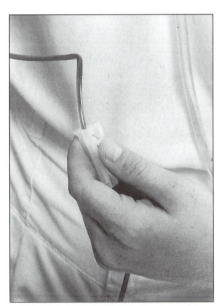

8 Unclamp the blood and let it run in over a 1- to 2-hour period or as prescribed.

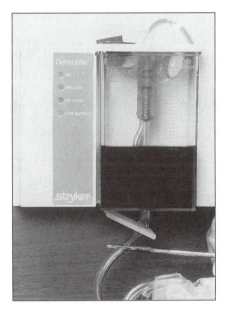

Evaluating

9 Monitor the client at frequent intervals to ensure that the blood is infusing appropriately. When the blood has infused into the client, clamp the tubing between the reinfusion system and the blood bag. After the initial collection period has been started, a total of two infusions may be administered within an 8-hour period. If this is the last infusion, you may snip off the blood bag tubing (as shown) if desired. Wipe the exposed tubing with a dry gauze pad to prevent blood from dripping onto the floor, or cap the tubing with a cap supplied by the manufacturer.

MONITORING THE CLIENT UNDERGOING CONTINUOUS PASSIVE MOTION (CPM)

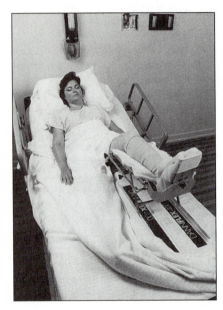 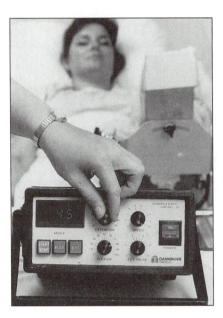

Clients with the following disorders or surgeries may benefit from CPM: total knee or hip replacement, synovectomy, tibial plateau fracture, open menisectomy, hip fracture, or femoral shaft fracture fixation. Benefits of CPM include more flexion, which results in greater joint range of motion, and less postoperative pain and joint swelling.

The following are nursing considerations when managing the client in knee CPM:

- Ensure that the machine is anchored securely to the bedframe.

- Place a pillowcase over the sheepskin (under the client's lower leg) to keep it clean.

- Adjust the machine so that it is in a flat (0-degree) position when putting the client on and taking the client off the machine.

- Set the foot pedal in a neutral position and make sure it touches the bottom of the client's foot lightly.

- Position the client's knee over the point at which the machine bends.

- Stay with the client through one complete cycle when first putting her on the machine to ensure that she can tolerate the movement.

- Keep the hand control for the machine within the client's reach, and teach her how to turn the machine on and off.

- For optimal results, try to keep the machine in continuous motion for at least 20 hours/day.

- Remove ace bandages or elastic stockings every 8 hours (or as policy permits) for skin care and assessment of tissue and skin integrity.

- The goal of therapy is 90-degree knee flexion prior to the client's hospital discharge.

The physician prescribes the amount of flexion, usually 45 degrees. Adjust as prescribed.

MANAGING THE CLIENT UNDERGOING CRYOTHERAPY VIA A KNEE COMPRESSION DRESSING

Clients who have undergone arthroscopic surgery may benefit from cryotherapy with a knee compression dressing to minimize swelling. This device has a nylon cuff that fits securely around the knee. The cooler is filled with ice and water, and the tube leading from the cooler to the cuff enables up to 8 hours of cryotherapy.

The following are nursing considerations for managing the client undergoing cryotherapy via a knee compression dressing.

- Cryotherapy is contraindicated for individuals with Raynaud's disease or other vasospastic processes and for those who have hypersensitivity to the cold or compromised peripheral circulation.

- The cooler is filled with ice and water. After applying the empty cuff to the client's knee, attach the distal end of the drain hose to the cuff, open the air vent (at the top of the cooler), and raise the cooler, which will enable the cold water to flow into the cuff. After the water has flowed into the cuff and been sealed off (this will vary according to manufacturer), the cooler may be placed on the floor.

- Avoid elevating the cooler above the cuff higher than 37.5 cm (15 in) to prevent compression pressures >30 mm Hg.

- The recommended period of time for application of this device is 20–30 minutes, repeated 3–4 times per day.

- If possible, avoid use of this compression device in conjunction with elastic bandages, since the pressure effects may be cumulative.

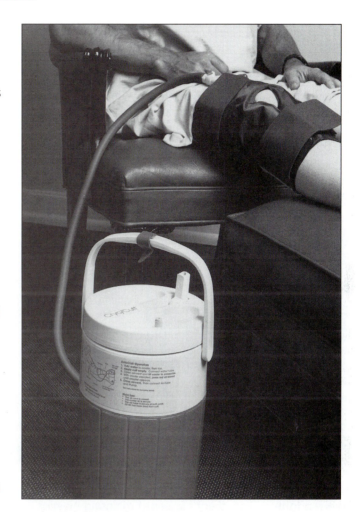

- Apply the compression dressing directly to the bare knee when possible because any under-wrappings may insulate the knee from the cryotherapy.

- Secure the straps of the cuff so that they are snug but not constrictive. This will facilitate the application of cold compression to the knee when the cuff fills with water.

TRANSFERRING THE CLIENT WITH A TOTAL HIP REPLACEMENT

When hip adduction and hip flexion are contraindicated, for example for a client with a total hip replacement, follow these steps to transfer the client from the bed to the wheelchair. Be sure that the client has enough upper body strength and mobility in the uninvolved leg to assist you with this procedure. If this is the client's first transfer, you may need a second person to help. Explain the procedure to the client and ensure that he understands each step and his role during the transfer.

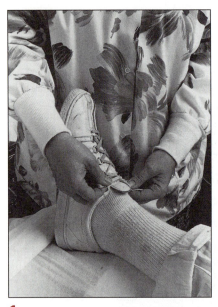

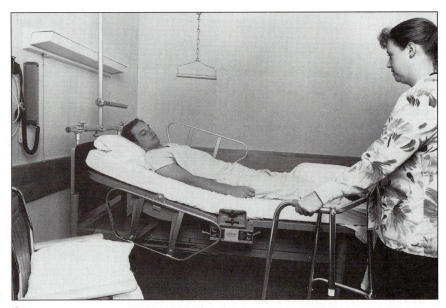

1 Put a sturdy rubber-soled shoe on the client's uninvolved foot so that he can safely pivot during the transfer. Footies with rubber gripper soles also would be appropriate.

2 Place a pillow between the client's knees to maintain his hips in abduction. Position a wheelchair at a 45-degree angle to the head of the bed on the side opposite the client's involved hip. Lock both the wheelchair and the bed to keep them stable during the move. Either swing away or remove the footrests so that they will not obstruct the move. If the wheelchair has an adjustable backrest, tilt it back to minimize the hip flexion for the client once he sits in the chair. However, if the chairback does not recline, place a pillow in the seat to help keep the client's hip in as much extension as possible. Then, place a walker close to the bed on the same side as the wheelchair so that the client can grasp it once he is in a sitting position.

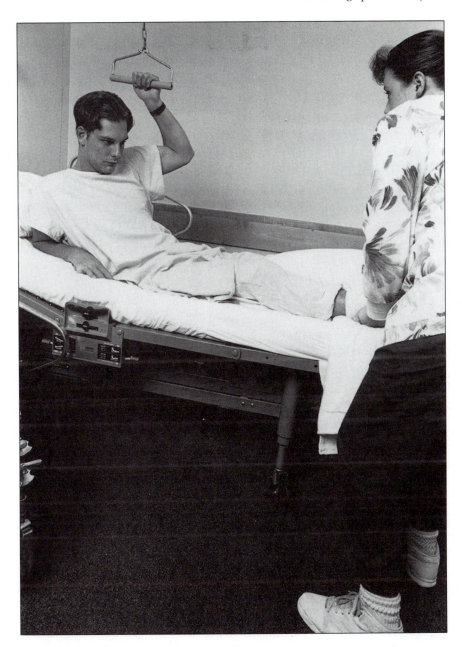

3 Raise the head of the bed to a level the client can tolerate, but no greater than 45 degrees. Remember to keep the client's hips in minimal flexion to prevent dislocation of the involved hip. Although it is not possible to keep the client's hips in full extension during this procedure, by keeping them constantly abducted with a pillow the potential for dislocation is minimized.

4 To begin the transfer, grasp both the client's legs (with the pillow between them), and ask the client to lift his upper body into a slight sitting position as you do. Remember to bend your knees, keep your back straight, and separate your feet to provide a wide base of support.

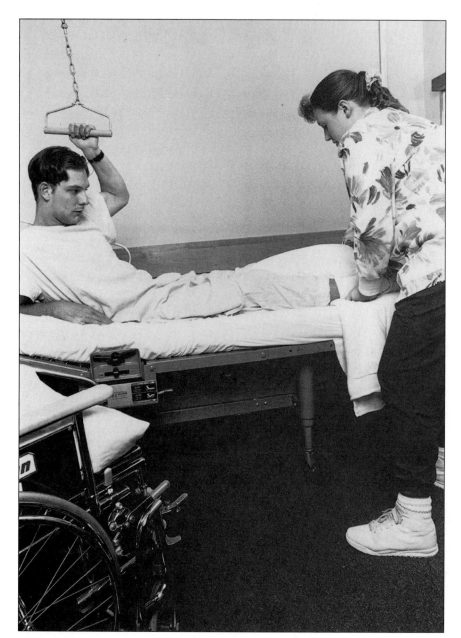

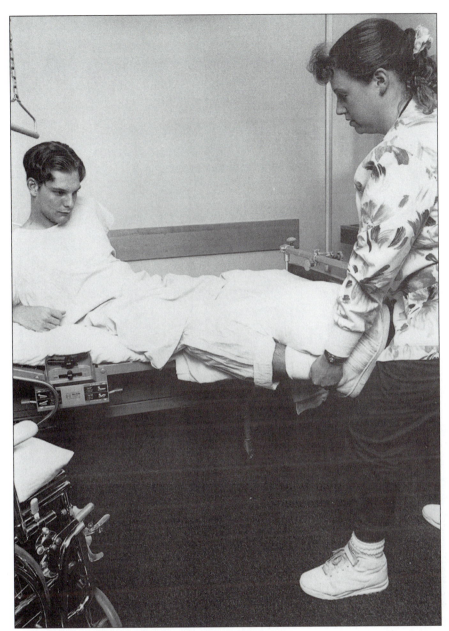

5 Pivot onto your forward foot as you move the client's legs to the side of the bed. Remember to keep your back straight and feet separated to provide a wide base of support. The client's operative leg should remain in extension to prevent hip flexion.

6 Once the client is sitting comfortably on the side of the bed with his operative leg extended, place the walker in front of him. Stand close to the client and separate your feet to provide a broad base of support. Guard him as he prepares to stand.

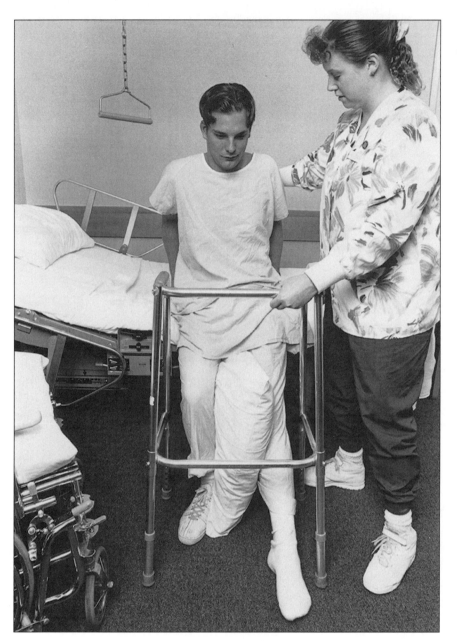

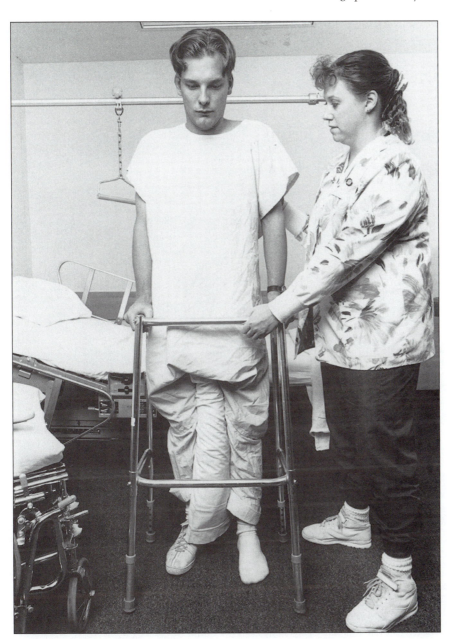

7 Once your client's legs are off the bed, instruct him to grasp the sidearms of the walker with both hands and bear weight on his non-operative leg unless the physician has allowed weightbearing on both legs. Instruct the client to keep his shoulder on the affected side back and the operative hip extended. The client will then push off and lift himself off the bed to stand at the walker. Continue guarding him, standing close and remaining in the wide stance.

8 When the client is standing, instruct him to push down on the walker and pivot on his nonoperative foot until the backs of his legs are positioned against the seat of the wheelchair. *Note: You will need to remove the pillow from between his knees for this pivot and replace it before he sits.*

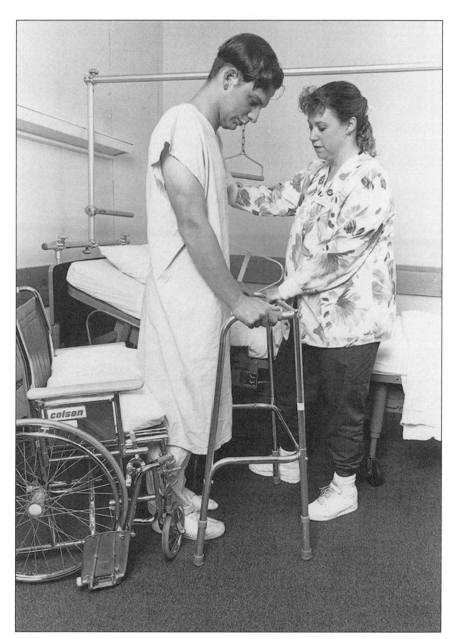

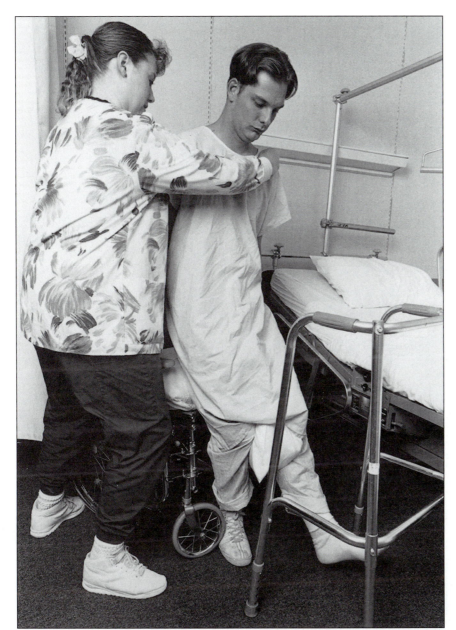

9 When the client attains the position described on the facing page, instruct him to grasp both armrests and prepare to sit, avoiding bending at the waist. Guard the client as shown, and keep your body close to his, maintaining a wide base of support with your feet.

10 As the client lowers his body into the wheelchair, bend your knees and lower your body as you continue to guide him.

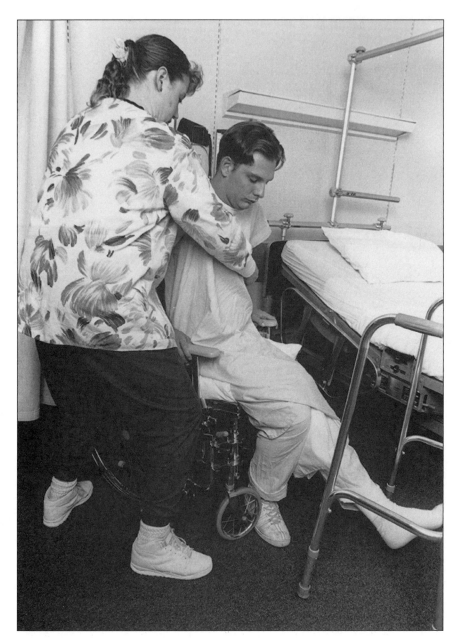

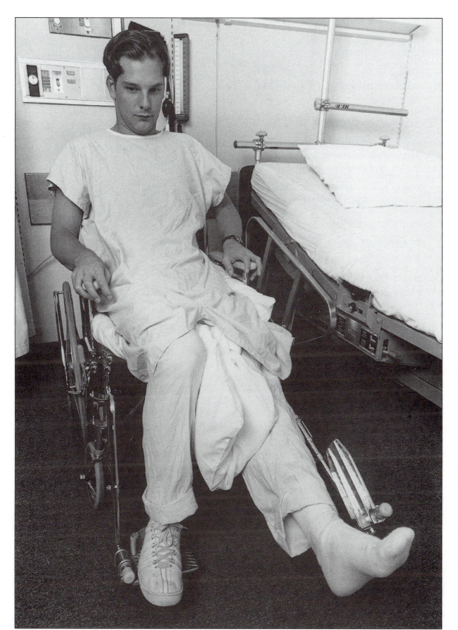

11 Support the client's involved leg with his knee in slight flexion by repositioning the legrest and replacing the pillow between his knees. Ensure that his hips are minimally flexed and that they remain in abduction. To return the client to the bed, reverse these steps.

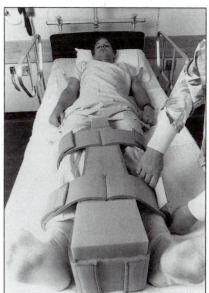

Some physicians request that their clients use an abduction pillow in place of a regular pillow to maintain their hips in abduction. Use of this device does not change the procedure as written.

REFERENCES

Bowers AC, Thompson JM: *Clinical Manual of Health Assessment,* ed 4. St Louis: Mosby, 1992.

Gluchacki B: Recognizing compartment syndrome. *Nursing 91* 21(10):33, 1991.

Hertling D: *Management of Common Musculoskeletal Disorders,* ed 2. Philadelphia: Lippincott, 1990.

Indiana University Hospitals: *Nursing Procedures and Policies.* Indianapolis, 1994.

Kozier B, Erb G: *Techniques in Clinical Nursing,* ed 4. Redwood City, CA: Addison-Wesley, 1993.

Maher AB, Salmond SW, Pellino TA: *Orthopaedic Nursing.* Philadelphia: Saunders, 1994.

Mourad LA: *The Nursing Process in the Care of Adults with Orthopaedic Conditions,* ed 3. Albany, NY: Delmar, 1993.

Rice R: *Handbook of Home Health Nursing Procedures.* St Louis: Mosby, 1995.

Ross D: Ischemic myositis. In Swearingen PL, Keen JH (eds): *Manual of Critical Care Nursing,* ed 3. St Louis: Mosby, 1995.

Ross D: Musculoskeletal disorders. In Swearingen PL (ed): *Manual of Medical-Surgical Nursing Care,* ed 3. St Louis: Mosby, 1994.

Sims LK et al: *Health Assessment in Nursing.* Redwood City, CA: Addison-Wesley, 1994.

Slye DA: Orthopedic complications: Compartment syndrome, fat embolism syndrome, and venous thromboembolism. *Nurs Clins North Am* 26(1):113–132, 1991.

Spence AP: *Basic Human Anatomy,* ed 3. Redwood City, CA: Addison-Wesley, 1991.

Standards Committee, American Association of Blood Banks: *Standards for Blood Banks and Transfusion Services,* ed 16. Bethesda, MD: American Association of Blood Banks, 1994.

Styrcula L: Traction basics, part I. *Orthopaedic Nurs* 13(2):71–74, 1994.

Styrcula L: Traction basics, part II. *Orthopaedic Nurs* 13(3):55–59, 1994.

Styrcula L: Traction basics, part III. *Orthopaedic Nurs* 13(4):34–44, 1994.

Thompson JM: *Mosby's Manual of Clinical Nursing,* ed 3. St Louis: Mosby, 1993.

Webber-Jones J et al: Managing traction: Do you know Carol P. Smith? *Nursing 94* 24(7):66–70, 1994.

Managing Neurosensory Procedures

CHAPTER OUTLINE

ASSESSING THE NEUROLOGIC SYSTEM

The Neurologic System

Nursing Assessment Guidelines

Monitoring the Status of a Neurologically Impaired Client

Performing a Neurologic Check

Testing Cerebellar and Motor Function

Assessing Sensory Function Using a Dermatome Chart

Evaluating Deep Tendon Reflexes

Assessing Cranial Drainage for the Presence of Cerebrospinal Fluid

CARING FOR CLIENTS WITH NEUROLOGIC DISORDERS

Assisting the Client with a Transcutaneous Electrical Nerve Stimulator Device

Providing Care During a Seizure

Using a Hyperthermia or Hypothermia System

Assessing Clients with Subarachnoid Drains

Nursing Guidelines: Care of Clients on Special Beds and Frames

 Roto Rest Kinetic Treatment Table

 Clinitron Air Fluidized Therapy

 Therapulse Pulsating Air Suspension Therapy

CARING FOR CLIENTS WITH DISORDERS OF THE SENSORY SYSTEM

Assessing Auditory Function

Performing the Watch Test

Performing the Weber and Rinne Tests

Irrigating the External Auditory Canal

Irrigating the Eye

Assessing the Neurologic System

THE NEUROLOGIC SYSTEM

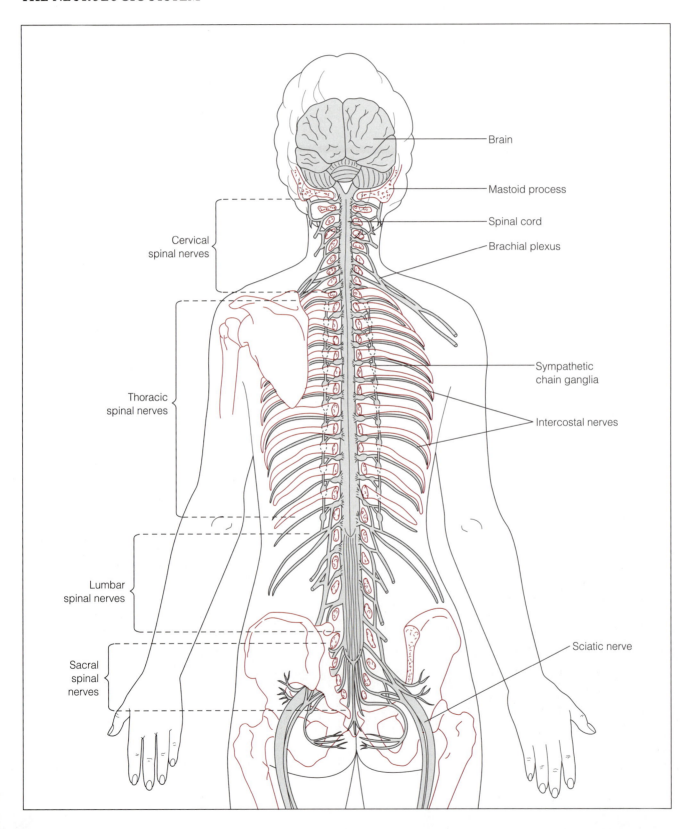

Brain

Mastoid process

Spinal cord

Brachial plexus

Cervical spinal nerves

Thoracic spinal nerves

Sympathetic chain ganglia

Intercostal nerves

Lumbar spinal nerves

Sacral spinal nerves

Sciatic nerve

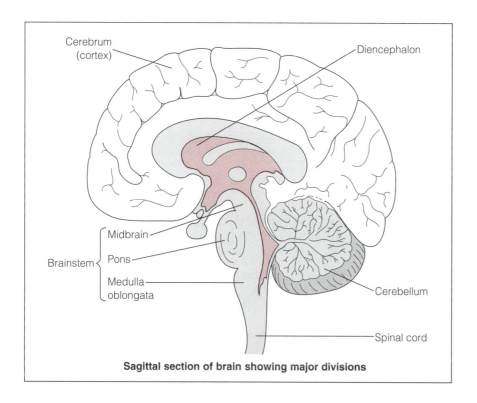

Sagittal section of brain showing major divisions

Nursing Assessment Guidelines

To assess your client's neurologic system, you need to interview the client, family members, or significant others for subjective data; take vital signs; and perform a basic assessment of neurologic function. A comprehensive nursing care plan includes a complete evaluation for the following subjective data:

Personal factors: for example, age, marital status, educational level, environmental/employment description, amounts of alcoholic beverages consumed, exercise patterns, leisure activities, stress level

History or family history of: diabetes mellitus, hypertension, seizures, neurologic disorders, cardiac disease

History of: fainting, weakness, paralysis, tics, tremors, coordination impairment, nervousness, dizziness, neurologic trauma or surgery

Integrity of integration: periods of confusion or loss of memory; impairment of emotions, judgment, speech

Activities of daily living: independent, requires assistance, dependent

Use of assistive devices: for example, cane, walker, wheelchair

Medications: for example, antispasmodics, antiepilepsy drugs, sedatives, depressants, antidepressants, anti-inflammatory agents, antiemetics, over-the-counter drugs; history of medication allergies

Balance problems: frequency, precipitating factors, position, time of day, relation to activity

Pain: location, onset, duration, character, radiation, relieved/intensified by, paresthesias, anesthesia (loss of sensation)

Headaches: history, frequency, onset, duration, character, precipitating factors, location, presence of photophobia, relieved/intensified by

Seizures: frequency, presence of aura or other prodomal symptoms, duration, clinical presentation during and after, necessity for oxygen or medication during or after (for example, with status epilepticus)

MONITORING THE STATUS OF A NEUROLOGICALLY IMPAIRED CLIENT

PERFORMING A NEUROLOGIC CHECK

A neurologic check is a part of an ongoing assessment of the neurologically impaired client. It should be performed at specific intervals to evaluate the client's level of consciousness, pupillary reflexes, and motor and sensory function. A neurologic check is not as extensive as a complete neurologic examination, and we suggest that you consult an assessment text if you desire greater detail. The components of a neurologic check may vary, depending on agency protocol or the client's condition, so be sure to follow the guidelines established by your agency or those prescribed by the physician.

Once a complete baseline check has been performed, the neurologic check should then be performed every 1–2 hours, or as frequently as every 15 minutes for clients who are unstable. Document each assessment, comparing the results to previous checks, and notify the physician of changes in the client's condition. Even subtle deterioration is significant, and it can alert you to the need for immediate medical intervention.

Familiarize yourself with the following terms and definitions for levels of consciousness. Terminology may vary from agency to agency.

Alert/Awake:	responds promptly and appropriately to verbal and tactile stimuli
Lethargic:	drowsy, responds slowly yet appropriately
Obtunded:	somnolent, may be disoriented when awake
Stuporous:	arouses with difficulty, may be combative, might respond to simple commands
Semicomatose:	responds to painful stimuli only
Comatose:	unresponsive even to painful stimuli, hypotonic

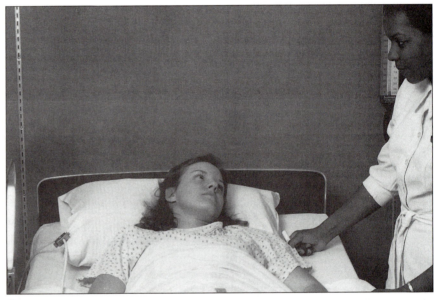

1 Evaluate your client's level of consciousness using the Glasgow Coma Scale (see Table 10.1) or some other objective means for the rapid evaluation of consciousness and detection of changes and trends. Take vital signs and assess the client for a slowed or rapid pulse rate, a rising systolic blood pressure, and a widening pulse pressure, which can occur with increasing intracranial pressure. Count the respirations, noting the rate, depth, and rhythm. Be especially alert to Cheyne-Stokes respirations, which are distinguished by periods of hyperventilation followed by periods of apnea. This is one type of breathing pattern that can occur with a brain dysfunction. Biot's is another type of respiration pattern that can occur with neurologic impairment, such as increased intracranial pressure and meningitis. Biot's respirations are characterized by slow and deep or rapid and shallow breaths, followed by periods of apnea. For more information, see Table 10.2, "Assessing Respiratory Patterns." Because wide fluctuations in temperature can occur with the neurologically impaired client, monitor the client's temperature closely.

Table 10.1   Glasgow Coma Scale

Assessment of	Client response	Score
Best eye-opening response (Record "C" if eyes are closed due to swelling.)	Spontaneously	4
	To speech	3
	To pain	2
	No response	1
Best motor response (Record best upper-limb response to painful stimuli.)	Obeys verbal command	6
	Localizes pain	5
	Flexion—withdrawal	4
	Flexion—abnormal	3
	Extension—abnormal	2
	No response	1
Best verbal response (Record "E" if endotracheal tube is in place or "T" if tracheostomy tube is in place.)	Conversation—oriented x 3	5
	Conversation—confused	4
	Speech—inappropriate	3
	Sounds—incomprehensible	2
	No response	1
Total score:	15 = normal	
	13–15 = minor head injury	
	9–12 = moderate head injury	
	3–8 = severe head injury	
	≤7 = coma	
	3 = deep coma or brain death	

Source: Swift CM: Neurologic disorders. In Swearingen PL: *Manual of Medical-Surgical Nursing Care,* ed 3. St Louis: Mosby, 1994. Used with permission by Mosby-Year Book.

If your client does not awaken easily to your voice or touch, press on the nailbeds, of if this is ineffective, *cautiously* apply painful stimuli. For example, exert pressure with your knuckles on the sternum or pinch the sternocleidomastoid muscle, being certain to avoid causing any harm to the client. Either stimulus should elicit a response. If the client is comatose, observe the posture after a painful stimulus has been applied. Posturing can be indicative of neurologic damage or disease. *Decerebrate* posturing (left photo), which can occur with upper brainstem injury, is the extension of the extremities after a stimulus. *Decorticate* posturing (right photo) is upper extremity flexion with lower extremity extension, and it can occur with an injury to the cortex.

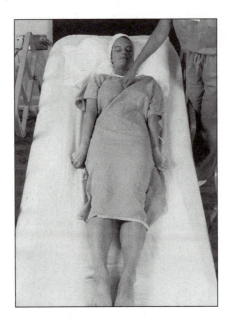
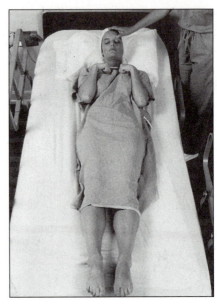

Table 10.2 Assessing Respiratory Patterns

Type	Waveform	Characteristics	Possible clinical condition
Eupnea		Normal rate and rhythm for adults and teenagers (12–20 breaths/min).	Normal pattern when awake.
Bradypnea		Decreased rate (<12 breaths/min); regular rhythm.	Normal sleep pattern, opiate or alcohol use, tumor, metabolic disorder.
Tachypnea		Rapid rate (>20 breaths/min); hypoventilation or hyperventilation.	Fever, restrictive respiratory disorders, pulmonary emboli.
Hyperpnea		Depth of respirations greater than normal.	Meeting increased metabolic demand (eg, sepsis, MODS, SIRS, and exercise).
Apnea		Cessation of breathing; may be intermittent.	Intermittent with CNS disturbances or drug intoxication; obstructed airway; respiratory arrest if it persists.
Kussmaul's		Deep, rapid (>20 breaths/min), sighing, labored.	Renal failure, DKA, sepsis, shock.

Table 10.2   Assessing Respiratory Patterns *(continued)*

Type	Waveform	Characteristics	Possible clinical condition
Cheyne-Stokes		Alternating patterns of apnea (10–20 sec) with periods of deep and rapid breathing. Lesions located bilaterally and deep within cerebral hemispheres.	CHF, opiate or hypnotic overdose, thyrotoxicosis, dissecting aneurysm, subarachnoid hemorrhage, IICP, aortic valve disorders; may be normal in older adults during sleep.
Central neurogenic hyperventilation		Rapid (>20 breaths/min), deep, regular. Lesions of midbrain or upper pons thought to be source of pattern.	Primary injury (ischemia, infarction, space-occupying lesion); secondary injury (IICP, metabolic disorders, drug overdose).
Apneustic		Deep, prolonged inspiration, followed by 20–30 sec pause and short expiration. Lesion located in lower pons.	Anoxia, meningitis, basilar artery occlusion.
Cluster		Irregular breaths occurring in clusters with periods of apnea. Overall pattern irregular. Lesion located in lower pons or upper medulla.	Primary and secondary injury as above may produce this respiratory pattern.
Ataxic (Biot's)		Irregular deep or shallow breaths. No discernible pattern. Lesion located in medulla.	Primary and secondary injury as above may produce this respiratory pattern.

MODS = multiple organ dysfunction syndrome

SIRS = systemic inflammatory response syndrome

CNS = central nervous system

DKA = diabetic ketoacidosis

CHF = congestive heart failure

IICP = increased intracranial pressure

Source: Stowe AC, Swearingen PL: Heart and breath sounds. In Swearingen PL and Keen JH eds: *Manual of Critical Care Nursing,* ed 3. St Louis: Mosby, 1995. Used with permission by Mosby-Year Book.

Observe and test the client's orientation to time, place, and person; behavior; mood; knowledge; memory; and speech patterns. Are the responses prompt and appropriate to the questions asked, and does she respond correctly to simple commands? Note her facial expression and the ability to maintain eye contact with you, and assess whether her mood is appropriate to the situation. One way to test abstract reasoning is to ask the client to interpret a simple proverb. Long-term and short-term memory can be evaluated during a health history. Finally, note whether the client's speech patterns are appropriate for her educational, socioeconomic, and ethnic background. It is wise to avoid asking questions that can be responded to with "yes" or "no" answers.

As you evaluate mental status, inspect the client's eyes. They should open spontaneously, and both eyes should move together in unison. Evaluate the size and shape of the pupils and note whether they are bilaterally equal. Use a pupil gauge (at right) to assist you with documenting their size. Be alert to dilatation of one pupil, which occurs with head injuries resulting in epidural and subdural hematoma or uncal herniation. Dilatation of the pupil on the affected (injured) side is termed *ipsilateral dilatation*. Dilatation of the pupil on the opposite side is termed *contralateral dilatation*. Table 10.3 describes the functions and dysfunctions of the cranial nerves.

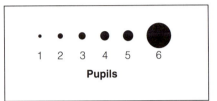

Pupils

Table 10.3 Functions and Dysfunctions of the Cranial Nerves

Cranial nerve	Type	Functions	Dysfunctions
I Olfactory	Sensory	Smell	Anosmia

II Optic	Sensory	Sight
		    Visual acuity
		    Visual fields
		Fundus
			Blindness
			Visual field deficits

III Oculomotor	Motor	Pupillary constriction Elevation of upper eyelid Extraocular movements	Ptosis, diplopia, pupillary dilatation, strabismus
IV Trochlear	Motor	Downward and inward movement of eye	Eye will not move downward or inward
V Trigeminal	Sensory and motor	*Motor:* Temporal and masseter muscles (jaw clenching and lateral movement for mastication) *Sensory:* Facial, scalp, anterior two-thirds of tongue, lips, teeth, proprioception for mastication, corneal reflex	Paresis or paralysis of muscles of mastication, decreased facial sensation Loss of corneal reflex
VI Abducens	Motor	Lateral eye movement	Eye will not move laterally
VII Facial	Sensory and motor	*Sensory:* Taste in anterior two-thirds of tongue, proprioception for face and scalp *Motor:* Facial expression, lacrimal and salivary glands	Loss of taste in anterior two-thirds of tongue Paresis or paralysis of facial muscles; facial droop; loss of secretion of submandibular, sublingual, and lacrimal glands
VIII Acoustic	Sensory	*Cochlear division:* Hearing *Vestibular division:* Balance	Tinnitus, deafness Vertigo, nystagmus

Table 10.3 Functions and Dysfunctions of the Cranial Nerves *(continued)*

Cranial nerve	Type	Functions	Dysfunctions
IX Glossopharyngeal	Sensory and motor	*Sensory:* Taste in posterior one-third of tongue; pain, touch, heat, cold in tongue, tonsils, soft palate, and pharynx *Motor:* Elevation of the soft palate, movement of pharynx, secretion and vasodilatation of parotid glands for saliva; gag reflex	Loss of taste, pain, touch, heat, and cold in posterior one-third of tongue, tonsils, and soft palate. Paresis or paralysis of soft palate and pharynx, dysphagia, dysarthria, hoarseness, loss of gag reflex
X Vagus	Sensory and motor	*Sensory:* Muscles of pharynx, larynx, esophagus, and thoracic and abdominal viscera; external ear, mucous membranes of larynx, trachea, esophagus, thoracic and abdominal viscera; lungs (stretch receptors), aortic bodies (chemoreceptors), respiratory/GI tract (pain receptors) *Motor:* Muscles of pharynx, larynx, esophagus, thoracic and abdominal viscera; respiratory/GI tract (smooth muscle), pacemaker and cardiac atrial muscle	Similar to dysfunction of glossopharyngeal Loss of gag reflex and difficulty swallowing
XI Spinal accessory	Motor	Sternocleidomastoid and trapezius muscles	Paresis or paralysis of sternocleidomastoid and trapezius muscles Inability to turn head or shrug shoulders
XII Hypoglossal	Motor	Tongue movement	Paresis or paralysis of the tongue

Source: Stowe AC: Cranial nerves: Functions and dysfunctions. In Swearingen PL, Keen JH eds: *Manual of Critical Care Nursing,* ed 3. St Louis: Mosby, 1995. Used with permission by Mosby-Year Book.

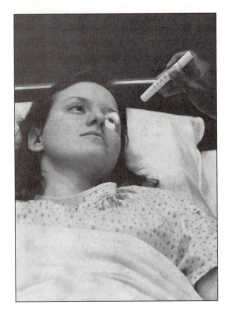

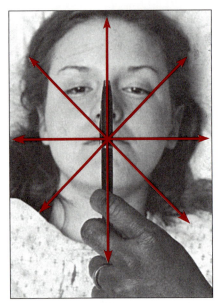

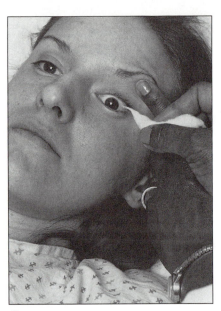

2 Check the pupillary response to light. Dim the lights and instruct the client to focus her gaze on an object in her direct line of vision. Move your penlight from outside the client's field of vision toward the pupil and shine the light into the left eye, observing for a pupillary reaction. Repeat the test on the right eye. Optimally, both pupils will react equally (and at the same rapid rate) and constrict to the same size. Evaluate the client's consensual light reflex by observing each pupil as the light is shined into the opposite eye. The right pupil should constrict as the light is shined into the left eye, and vice versa. If this response does not occur, the client might have brain-stem dysfunction.

3 In some clinical situations, the physician may request that you test the client's extraocular eye movements during the neurologic check. To do this, position a pen 30–37.5 cm (12–15 in) from the client's nose. Instruct the client to focus her eyes on the pen but to avoid moving her head. Slowly move the pen up and down, to each side, and then on the diagonals, as depicted by the arrows in the photo. If her third (oculomotor), fourth (trochlear), and sixth (abducens) cranial nerves are intact, she should be able to follow the movements of the pen with her eyes moving in unison. Describe any deficit, if present. Observe for involuntary, rapid movements of the eyeball (nystagmus), which can occur with neurologic impairments such as a cerebrovascular accident (CVA), cerebellar tumor, or multiple sclerosis. Nystagmus also can occur with phenytoin (Dilantin) toxicity.

4 To assess the alert client's blink (corneal) reflex, lightly brush your fingertips across the eyelashes. If this reflex is normal, the client will respond by blinking. If the client is not alert, gently touch the outer aspect of each cornea with a wisp of cotton (as shown). If the client neither blinks nor tears, the fifth cranial (trigeminal) nerve might be compromised. *Note: If the client is a contact lens wearer, a diminished reflex might occur normally.*

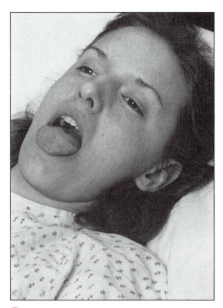 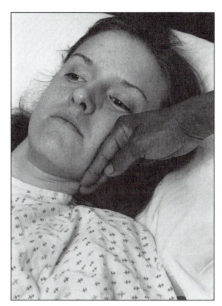 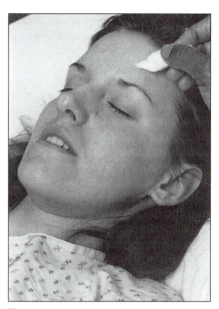

5 Evaluate the ability of the client to extend her tongue. Note whether the tongue quivers excessively or deviates to one side, and document accordingly. Your client's inability to perform this task, or excessive quivering on one side of the tongue, suggests an impairment of the 12th cranial (hypoglossal) nerve, which can occur with a CVA.

6 The 11th cranial (spinal accessory) nerve mediates the sternocleidomastoid and upper trapezius muscles. To test its integrity, place your hand against the client's cheek and instruct her to turn her head toward your hand. Repeat the assessment on the opposite side. With a neurologic impairment, such as a CVA or a brain tumor, the client may have a unilateral deficit in strength.

7 Test the client's nerve sensory function next. Explain that she is to describe both the sensation and the location of the sensation while her eyes are closed. Be sure to show her the cotton wisp so that she does not become alarmed, expecting a painful process. Touch the client's forehead.

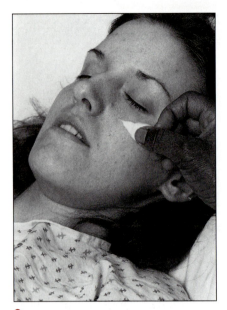
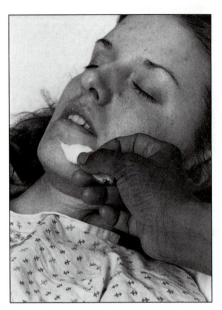
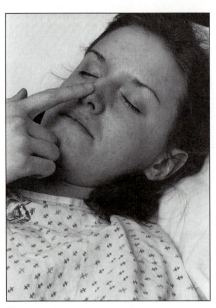

8   Touch her cheek and then her chin (center photo). Repeat the test on the opposite side of the client's face. She should describe a tickling sensation on all three areas of the face, and the sensations should be felt equally on both sides. If the response is abnormal, you can use a sterile pin to assess other areas of the body. However, a pin should be used judiciously, and never on the face. See the procedure on pages 598–599, for assessing sensory function using a dermatome chart.

9   To test coordination (cerebellar function), instruct the client to close her eyes and to touch her nose alternately with the index fingers of her right hand and then her left hand, gradually increasing the speed of the movements. With a normal response, the movements will be smooth and accurate.

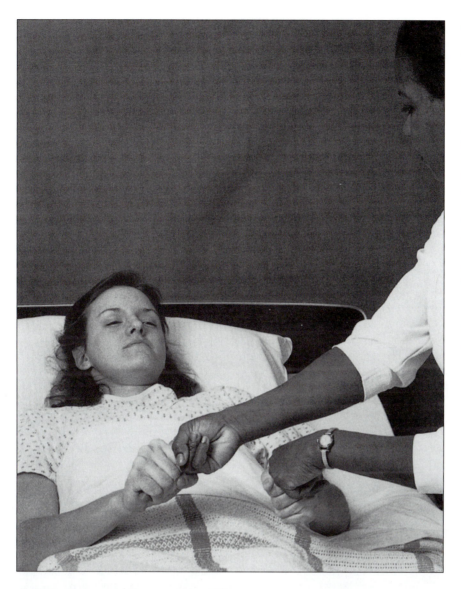

10 To evaluate the motor function of the client's upper extremities, ask her to grip and squeeze your index and middle fingers. Document the strength of each hand, noting whether the grip is bilaterally equal or unequal. Remember, however, that the client's dominant hand normally may be stronger than the nondominant hand.
Note: To recall quickly which of the client's hands is stronger, cross your hands so that your right hand is grasped by the client's right hand and your left hand by the client's left hand. By recalling which of your hands was gripped more tightly, you can readily document which of your client's hands is stronger. Other tests for upper extremity motor function are found in Chapter 9.

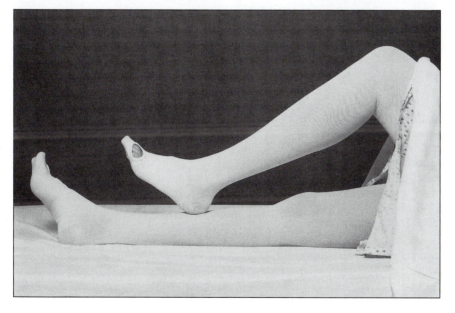

11 To evaluate the coordination (cerebellar function) of the lower extremities, instruct the client to slide her left heel down her right shin and to repeat the procedure on her left shin using her right heel. She should be able to do this smoothly and accurately. Document any deficit.

12 To evaluate the motor function of the lower extremities, push your hands against the soles of the client's feet. Instruct her to resist the pressure. Document the response, noting whether it is bilaterally equal or unequal. Note also whether the tone of the muscles is normal, hypotonic, or hypertonic. Other tests for lower extremity motor function are found in Chapter 9.

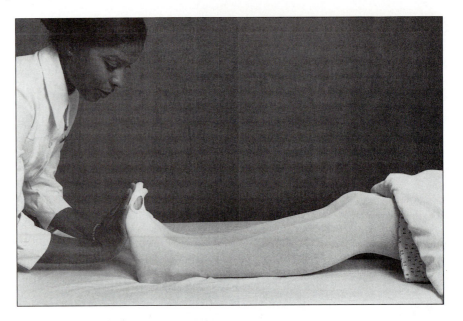

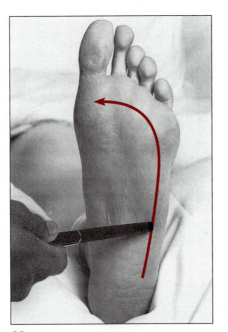

13 To test the client's plantar reflex, stroke along the lateral surface of the sole of each foot, as shown by the arrow on the photograph. If the toes curl downward, her response is normal. However, if the small toes fan apart and the large toe dorsiflexes toward the client's head, this is called Babinski's reflex. A positive Babinski's reflex is considered normal in the infant under 12–18 months, but it is a sign of motor nerve dysfunction in the adult.

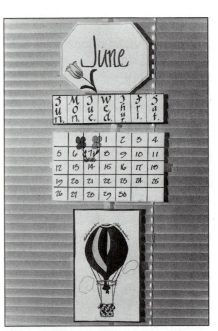

14 To help orient the neurologically impaired client to the month and date, keep a brightly colored calendar within sight. Also, photographs of family and friends are important constants in the client's life and should be used in the hospital environment whenever possible.

TESTING CEREBELLAR AND MOTOR FUNCTION

If your client is ambulatory, you can perform gross motor and balance testing to evaluate cerebellar function. See steps 9–12 in the preceding procedure for motor and cerebellar testing for the client who is on bed rest.

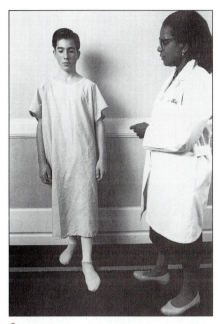

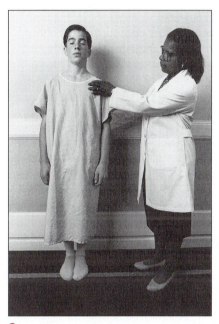

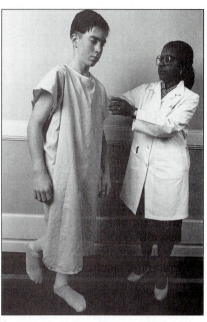

1 Instruct the client to walk across the room in a straight line. Observe the gait and posture. Normally, movements will be smooth and even, and the arms will swing slightly in opposition to the gait. Be alert to an unsteady gait, rigid or flaccid arm movements, and swaying, which can occur with a cerebellar dysfunction.

2 Evaluate the client for a positive Romberg's sign. Instruct him to stand still, with his arms at his sides and his feet together. He should first perform the test with his eyes shut, maintaining the stance for a full minute, and then repeat the test with his eyes open. Without touching him, guard him with your hands as you observe him in this position. Normally, you can expect to see slight swaying. Excessive swaying or an inability to maintain the stance without widening his foot base (whether the client's eyes are open or shut) occurs with a positive Romberg's sign. If he has trouble maintaining his balance only when his eyes are shut, he has a loss of position sense referred to as *sensory ataxia*. If he cannot maintain his balance whether or not his eyes are open or shut, the condition is referred to as *cerebellar ataxia*.

3 Instruct the client to stand first on one foot and then on the other. Guard him as you observe his stance. Normally, the stance can be maintained for at least 5 seconds. An inability to maintain the stance occurs when equilibrium is disturbed. Document the results of the testing.

ASSESSING SENSORY FUNCTION USING A DERMATOME CHART

If you are assessing a neurologically impaired client who is alert and cooperative, you can evaluate sensory function by testing dermatome zones. Dermatome zones, which are divided into segmental skin bands as depicted by these overlays, compare anatomically to the innervation by a dorsal root to a cutaneous nerve. These nerves

deliver the sensations of pain, temperature, touch, and vibration to the spinal cord and, ultimately, to the brain. The *spinothalamic* tract transmits the sensations of pain, temperature, and crude touch; the *dorsal column* tract transmits the perceptions of light touch and vibrations. Even though there is usually a great deal of overlap in

nerve distribution, a knowledge of the dermatome zones can help you locate the approximate level of the neurologic lesion or injury. For example, a diminished or heightened response at the client's thumb can alert you to a potential disorder at level C6 of the spinal cord.

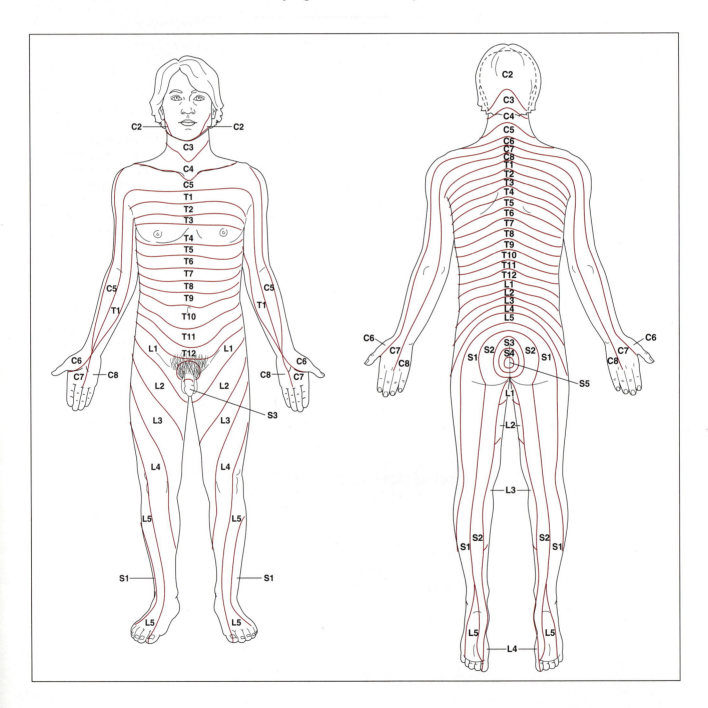

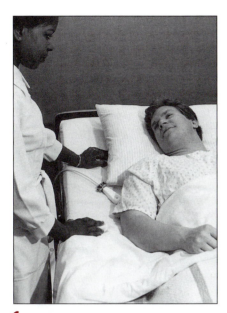

1 Explain the procedure to the client, and display the instruments that will be used during the assessment. A sterile safety pin and cotton wisp are commonly used to test sensation.

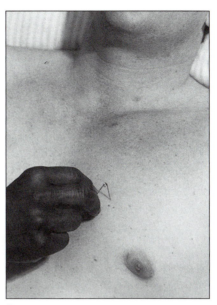

2 To test the spinothalamic tract, you can use both the pointed (above) and blunt (right) ends of a safety pin. Instruct the client to keep his eyes closed, and then stimulate anatomic locations at random, using both ends of the pin. Ask the client whether he feels a sharp or dull sensation. An abnormal response necessitates a more thorough assessment. Record the

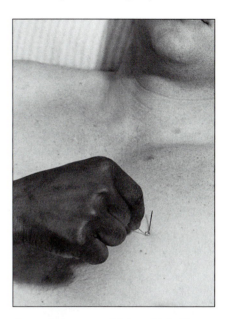

dermatome zone(s) in which the client has a diminished, heightened, or absent sensation. *Note: Because the spinothalamic tract transmits both pain and temperature, you can assess sensory function with warmth and coolness, for example, by using test tubes filled with warm and cool water. The use of both testing modalities is rarely necessary, however.*

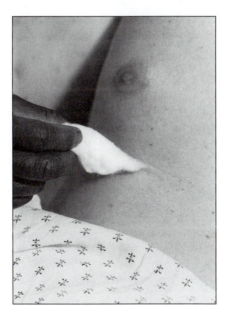

3 The dorsal column tract is assessed for light touch perception by brushing a cotton wisp against the client's skin. Again, test random areas and ask the client to alert you as soon as the sensation is felt. Record the dermatome zone(s) in which the client has diminished, heightened, or absent sensations.

EVALUATING DEEP TENDON REFLEXES

Deep tendon reflexes (DTRs) are present in all normal adults. An absence of or heightened reflexes denote a pathology associated with an interruption of an impulse at the associated anatomic site in the spinal cord. Evaluate your client's DTRs according to the following scale:

0   Nonreflexive

1+ Hyporeflexive—diminished response, can occur normally in the older client

2+ Normal

3+ Brisk—not always associated with a pathology

4+ Hyperreflexive

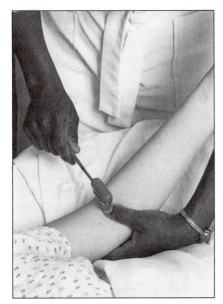 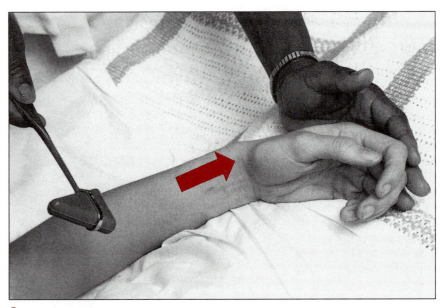

1 To test the biceps reflex (C5–C6 innervation), place your thumb over the client's biceps tendon at the antecubital fossa. Flex the client's elbow slightly, and then percuss your thumb with the pointed end of the reflex hammer. In a normal response, the client's elbow will flex and you should feel the tendon contract. Repeat the test on the tendon in the opposite extremity, noting the tone and symmetry of the reflex.

2 To test the brachioradialis (supinator) reflex (C5–C6 innervation), rest the client's forearm on a flat surface such as the bed or the client's lap, maintaining the hand in a moderate curve. Using the blunt end of the reflex hammer, percuss the brachioradialis tendon, which is located 2.5–5.0 cm (1–2 in) above the wrist over the radius (see arrow). In a normal response, the client's elbow will flex and the forearm will rotate laterally. Test the reflex of the tendon in the opposite extremity, noting the tone and symmetry of the response.

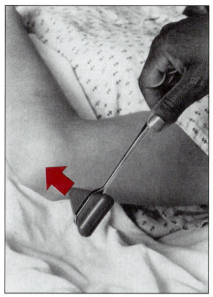

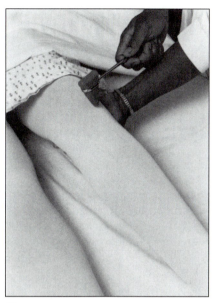

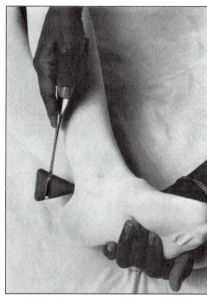

3 To test the triceps reflex (C6–C7–C8 innervation), flex the client's elbow. Using the pointed end of the reflex hammer, percuss the triceps tendon just proximal to the olecranon between the epi-condyles (see arrow). The elbow should extend as the triceps tendon contracts. Repeat the test on the tendon in the opposite extremity, noting the tone and symmetry of the reflex.

4 To test the patellar reflex (L2–L3–L4 innervation), have the client sit on the edge of the bed. If the client is unable to sit, flex and support the knee at the popliteal space (as shown) and percuss the patellar tendon just distal to the patella. Use the pointed end of the reflex hammer and tap the site lightly. The knee should extend, and the quadriceps muscle should contract. Test the reflex on the tendon in the opposite extremity, noting the tone and symmetry of the reflex. *Note: In the older adult, the response may be normally hyporeflexive.*

5 To test the ankle reflex (S1–S2 innervation), place the knee in slight flexion and then externally rotate and dorsiflex the ankle. Percuss the Achilles tendon with the pointed end of the reflex hammer. The client's ankle should plantarflex as the tendon contracts. Repeat the test on the tendon in the opposite extremity, noting the tone and symmetry of the reflex. Document the results of the assessment procedure.

ASSESSING CRANIAL DRAINAGE FOR THE PRESENCE OF CEREBROSPINAL FLUID

If your client has sustained a craniocerebral injury or is recovering from a craniotomy, careful observation of any drainage from the eyes, ears, nose, or traumatic area is critical. Cerebrospinal fluid is colorless and generally nonpurulent, and its presence is indicative of a serious breach of cranial integrity. Because the risk of bacteria entering into the brain is very high if a tract exists, *any* suspicious drainage should be reported immediately. Because cerebrospinal fluid contains glucose, you can test clear, nonsanguineous drainage with a glucose reagent stick and compare the results to the back of the reagent container. The test results will be positive for the presence of glucose if the drainage contains cerebrospinal fluid.

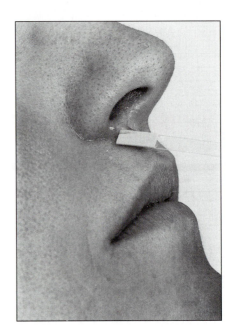

Caring for Clients with Neurologic Disorders

ASSISTING THE CLIENT WITH A TRANSCUTANEOUS ELECTRICAL NERVE STIMULATOR DEVICE

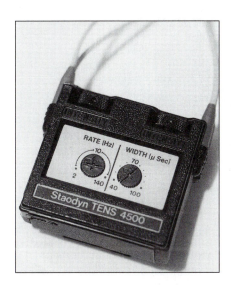

A transcutaneous electrical nerve stimulator (TENS) device is battery operated, and it is used to deliver electrical impulses to the body to relieve pain. A client experiencing acute or chronic pain, for whom narcotics are contraindicated or ineffective, will especially benefit from this device. It is used most frequently for chronic back pain or headaches. It should not be used, however, for clients with cardiac pacemakers because the electrical impulses it generates can interrupt pacing. In addition, it should be avoided for clients who are pregnant, or who have dysrhythmias or myocardial ischemia.

Assessing and Planning

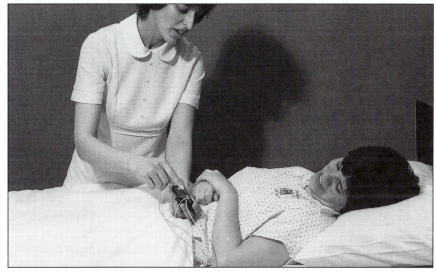

1 If your client has been using a TENS device, chances are she has already been trained in its use and application by a TENS specialist.

Consult with the TENS specialist or read the manufacturer's instructions for operating the device before explaining it to your client.

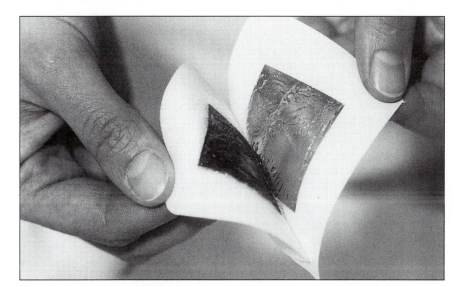

2 The electrodes are either reusable or disposable. Either they require the use of a conducting gel, or they are water conductive and will need moistening with water. Many disposable electrodes, such as that in the photo, already contain the conducting gel and are self-adhering.

➡

Implementing

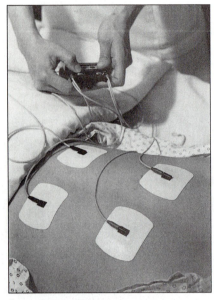

3 Attach the electrodes to the client's skin according to the pattern designed for your client. For example, for postoperative clients, place the electrodes on both sides of the incision. For clients with radiating pain, place the electrodes over the involved nerve roots along the spine. Attach the lead wires, making sure they are securely connected at both ends.

Evaluating

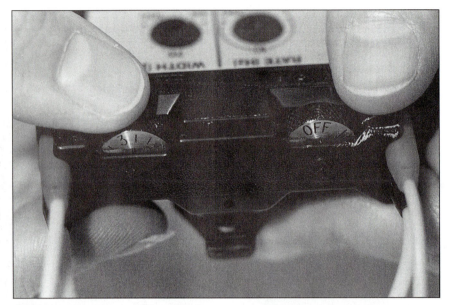

4 Many TENS devices have two dials that are labeled "intensity," "energy," or "amplitude," and each operates a set of two electrodes. In addition, most devices have a rate (frequency) dial that can be adjusted to deliver the desired number of electrical impulses per second, as well as a pulse-width dial that adjusts the impulse duration. Newer devices may have a pulse button that is selected for rate or width. Arrow buttons are then used to increase or decrease the type of pulse selected. A mode setting also may be present that allows a conventional (constant) stimulation or a modulated variable setting. The client can select the most comfortable and effective mode for pain relief. If the client experiences a burning or itching sensation, lower the pulse-width dial. If the sensation is too intense, lower both the amplitude dial and the pulse-width dial and adjust the rate accordingly. A mild to moderate sensation is the goal with this therapy. A sensation that is too intense can result in muscle spasms caused by overstimulation of the nerve.

PROVIDING CARE DURING A SEIZURE

Assessing and Planning

Implementing

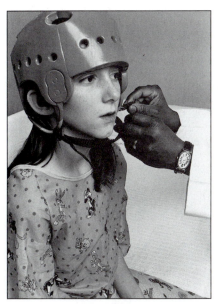

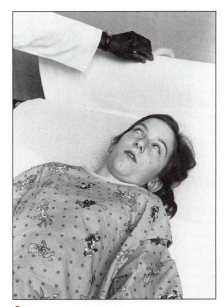

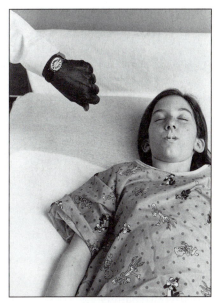

1 A client history of seizure disorders or the potential for a seizure should alert you to the need for protective measures. These include an oral airway of an appropriate size at the bedside table or taped to the headboard, raised and padded side rails, and a padded headboard. Children with seizure disorders can wear soft seizure helmets (as shown) when they are ambulatory.

2 If your client has a seizure, remove her pillow and, if possible, position her head to the side to promote drainage of secretions and prevent aspiration into the lungs. If your client's tongue is obstructing her airway, remove the oral airway from the bedside table or headboard and insert it cautiously (see procedure, Chapter 6).

3 A single seizure can last from 2 to 5 minutes. Always stay with the client, noting the onset, duration, and type of seizure. Do not attempt to restrain her, since this can increase the risk of injury. Observe the client's posture, pupillary changes, skin color, and the extremities involved. When the seizure has ceased, comfort and reorient the client, noting any cyanosis or difficult respiratory patterns. If the cyanosis persists, be sure to have oxygen available.

Evaluating

Document the seizure carefully, using descriptive terminology. Note the time of onset and duration, and any information about possible precipitating events.

USING A HYPERTHERMIA OR HYPOTHERMIA SYSTEM

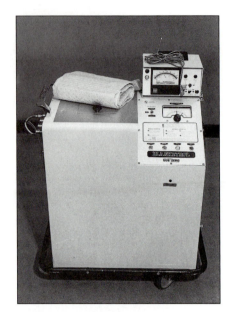

Many neurologic disorders involve the hypothalamus, the part of the brain that regulates body temperature. When vast fluctuations in body temperature occur, a hyperthermia or hypothermia system such as the Blanketrol® in these photos can be used to help keep your client's temperature within normal range, thereby minimizing the risk of irreversible brain damage.

Assessing and Planning

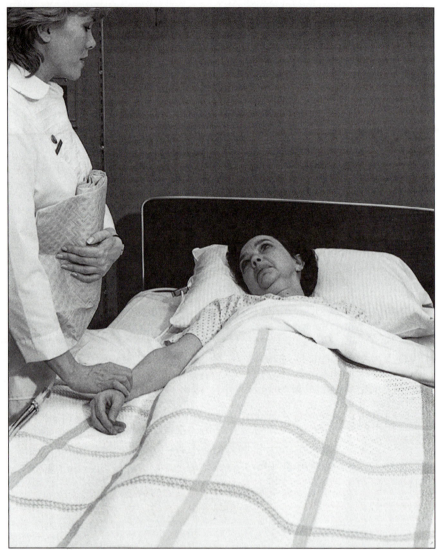

1 Explain the procedure to the client and inform her that she will feel either warmth or coolness. Instruct her to alert you if the temperature becomes too extreme. Perform and record baseline assessments of the client's vital signs and neurologic status. Note the integrity of the skin and document its condition before initiating the treatment. *Note: If the client's temperature will be greatly decreased, coat the skin with a thin layer of lanolin ointment to help prevent cold burns.*

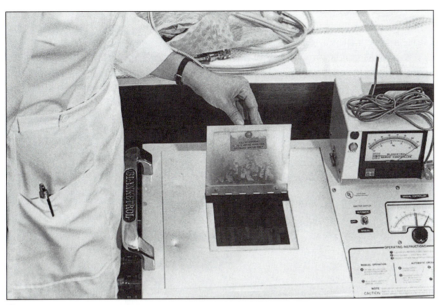

2 Ensure that the fluid level in the Blanketrol® unit is at least 1.25–2.50 cm (½–1 in) above the coils in the reservoir. Add distilled water if necessary.

Implementing

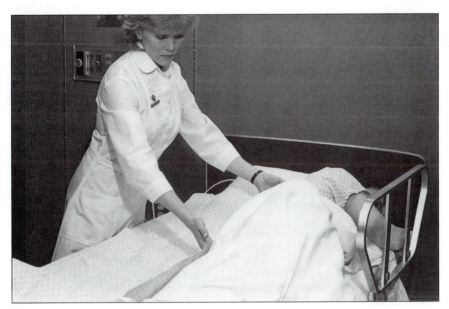

3 Cover the blanket with either a blanket cover or a sheet. With the client in a side-lying position, fan-fold and lay the blanket along the client's side, with the hose end of the blanket at the foot of the bed. Tuck the blanket under the client's buttocks and shoulders.

➡

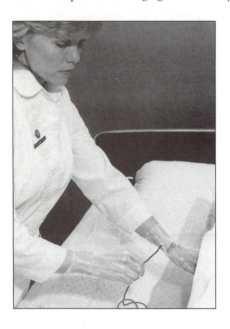

4 While the client is still on her side, apply a glove, coat the rectal probe (thermometer) with a water-soluble lubricant, and insert it approximately 7.5–10 cm (3–4 in) into the rectum (adjust the insertion length accordingly for the pediatric population). Tape it to the buttocks with hypoallergenic tape (for the neonate, tape the unlubricated probe to a fleshy area, such as the abdomen). Then assist her onto the opposite side so that you can straighten the blanket, and return her to her back so that the maximum amount of skin surface is in contact with the blanket. *Note: If a rapid increase or decrease in your client's temperature is needed, a second blanket can be used to cover the client.*

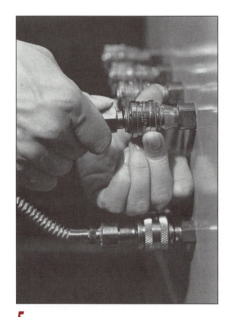

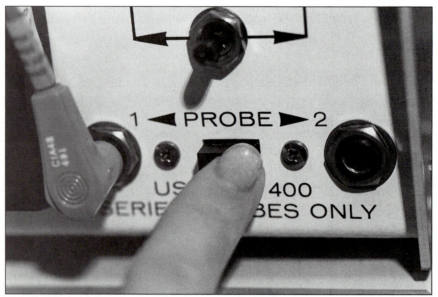

5 To connect the blanket hose to the Blanketrol®, locate the connectors on the side of the machine. Grasp the collar on the female connector that is directly above the attached hose. Push the collar back and insert the male fitting. Release the collar and push the male fitting until it locks in place. Make sure the master switch is in the "off" position, and connect the three-pronged plug to the outlet. Ensure that the servo-controller is plugged into the receptacle on the Blanketrol®.

6 Insert the rectal probe plug (shown on the left in the above photo) into one of the probe receptacles. Then turn the probe selector toward the corresponding receptacle (as shown).

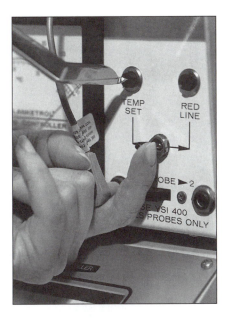

7 Set the prescribed temperature by pushing the temperature set switch to the left and turning the temperature set control screw with your scissors to the prescribed temperature (as shown). When the switch is released, the needle pointer will show the core temperature. This is the same switch you will push to check the calibrations by adjusting the needle to the red line.

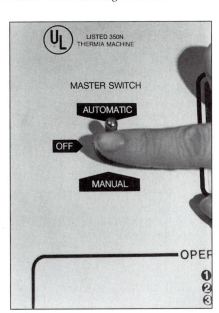

8 Move the master control switch on the Blanketrol® to "automatic." Document the procedure, the client's baseline assessment, and the response and tolerance to the treatment.

Evaluating

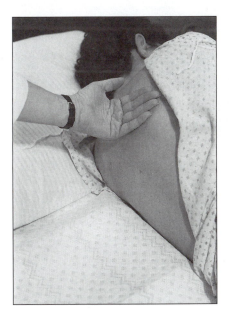

9 Perform and document neurologic checks and vital signs, and compare them to the client's baseline. Assess the client's skin integrity and temperature, and be alert to alterations such as swelling or color changes that could indicate frostbite or burns. Check the servo-controller reading to ensure that the client's temperature is reaching the desired level.

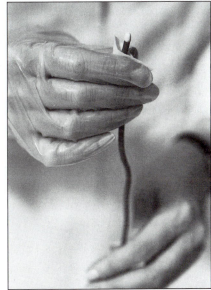

10 Periodically remove the rectal probe and assess the client's body temperature with a rectal thermometer to ensure that the probe is accurately recording the client's actual body temperature. Clean and reinsert the probe.

ASSESSING CLIENTS WITH SUBARACHNOID DRAINS

Subarachnoid/lumbar drains are small catheters that are placed in the lumbar cistern of the spinal column via lumbar puncture. Most often, these drains are placed after cranial or ear, nose, or throat (ENT) surgery in which there is the risk of cerebrospinal fluid (CSF) leak. By having a means to drain off a specific amount of CSF, thus reducing the circulating CSF, pressure on the dural incision is minimized.

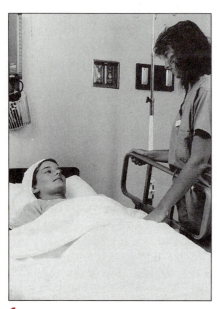

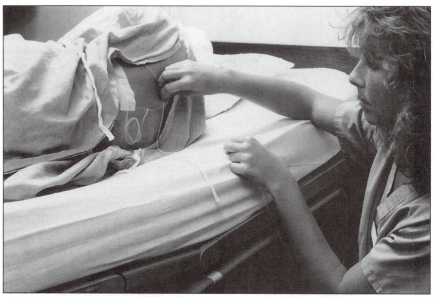

1 Monitor the client to ensure that the head of the bed is in the correct prescribed position with the zero point of the drainage pressure scale, which is attached to a support such as an IV pole. Usually, the zero point of the subarachnoid/lumbar drainage system is positioned on the same plane as the client's earlobe.

2 Assess the insertion site for the presence of infection, including erythema, warmth, purulent drainage; cerebrospinal fluid leakage, which would appear as a clear fluid; and the integrity of the attachment of the subarachnoid catheter to the drainage tubing.

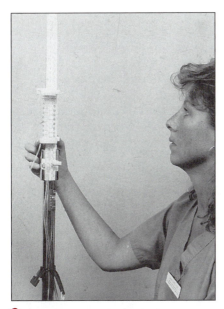 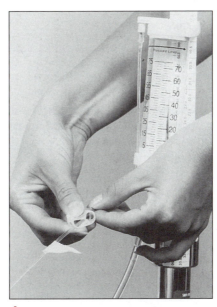 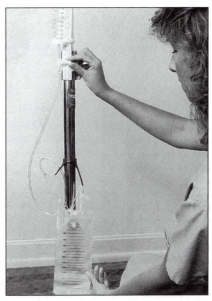

3 The position of the drip chamber on the IV pole is determined by the amount of cerebrospinal fluid drainage: the greater the amount of drainage, the higher the prescribed position of the drip chamber to slow the release of the CSF. Monitor the client for severe headache and nausea, early signs of too rapid drainage of the CSF. If this condition were allowed to continue, signs of neurologic deterioration would occur owing to downward shifting of intracranial contents: decreased LOC, irritability, confusion, weakness, paresis, and changes in pupillary reactivity and size (see pages 586–590). The grid along the pole is measured in centimeters. The physician will specify the amount in centimeters to move the drip chamber in relationship to the client's clinical condition.

4 Be aware that if you must change the client's position, clamp the drain first (unless otherwise directed) to prevent a rapid change in the circulating volume of CSF that could result in a change in the client's neurologic status. Ensure that a tape tab is positioned between the tubing clamp and the drip chamber (and as close to the drip chamber as possible) to keep the clamp out of contact with the client. This will prevent the client from inadvertently rolling over onto the clamp and stopping the flow of CSF.

5 Every 2–4 hours (or as prescribed), note and document the amount of drainage in the drip chamber, and adjust the stopcock to empty the CSF into the drainage bag. Change the drainage bag every 24 hours (or per agency protocol), using sterile technique. Be sure to clamp the drainage tubing first to prevent rapid outflow of large amounts of CSF.

NURSING GUIDELINES: CARE OF CLIENTS ON SPECIAL BEDS AND FRAMES

Complications of immobility such as atelectasis, pneumonia, decubitus ulcers, and renal calculi are frequent occurrences in clients with neurologic disorders. Because many of these clients are unable to participate actively in their own turning, and yet may require frequent turning without the interruption of their alignment, special beds are often indicated to facilitate nursing care and to prevent or minimize the complications of prolonged bed rest. The Roto Rest Kinetic Treatment Table, Clinitron Air Fluidized Therapy, and Therapulse Pulsating Air Suspension Therapy are three types of beds or frames that may be used by your agency. Follow manufacturer's instructions carefully to ensure the proper care and safe turning for your clients.

Roto Rest Kinetic Treatment Table

The Roto Rest is an automatic turning table that continuously rotates the client from side to side every 3.5 minutes, achieving a 62-degree lateral angle. This continuous lateral rotation can enhance the distribution of pulmonary blood flow. The client is secured to the table via closely fitting pads that conform to the extremities and trunk. When the table achieves its most lateral position, the padded knee and shoulder braces give added security. Safety straps are also available for confused or combative clients. In addition to cervical traction, the table also allows the application of traction to all extremities.

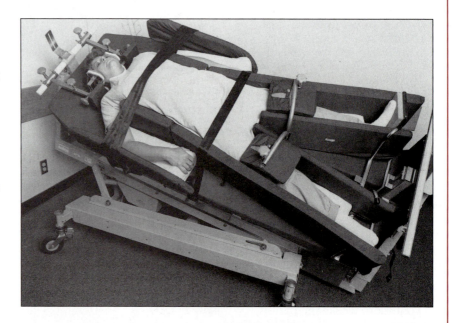

- To minimize the risk of skin irritation or inhibited chest excursion, ensure that a hand's breadth can comfortably fit between the client and the padded side packs. Adjust the packs if the space is greater than a hand's breadth because skin irritation can result from the client sliding against the side packs during the table's lateral rotation.

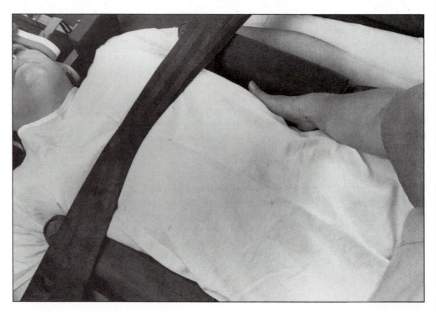

NURSING GUIDELINES: CARE OF CLIENTS ON SPECIAL BEDS AND FRAMES (continued)

• The foot pedal is used to provide constant pressure, thereby preventing foot drop. Because of the constant pressure applied by the pedal, it is important that you alternate the pedal from the right to left foot every 2 hours to provide relief to your client.

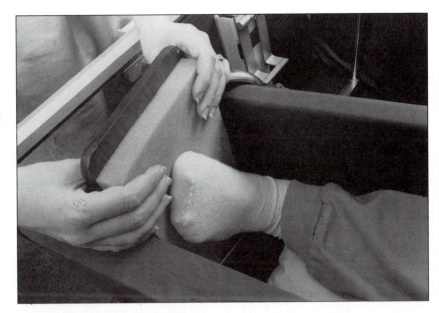

• The Roto Rest can be changed from automatic to manual by raising the lever at the posterior end of the table (as shown). In addition, a constant horizontal surface or lesser turning angles can be achieved with the degree-adjustment dial, which is also at the posterior end of the table.

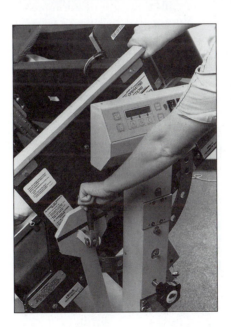

NURSING GUIDELINES: CARE OF CLIENTS ON SPECIAL BEDS AND FRAMES (continued)

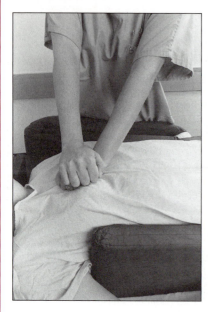 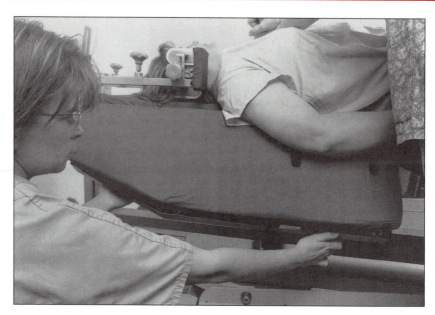

- In an emergency situation in which your client requires chest compressions for cardiopulmonary resuscitation (CPR), level the table's surface, and begin to deliver the compressions (left). Because of the table's firm surface, it is not necessary to use a cardiac board. When help arrives, one of you can then lower the siderails and remove the padded thoracic side packs (right).

- In nonemergency situations, the lowered side arm also allows you access to the client's upper extremities for full range of motion exercises.

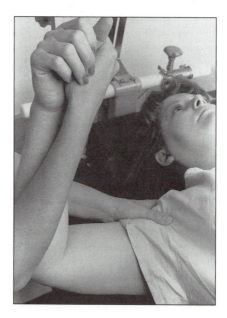

NURSING GUIDELINES: CARE OF CLIENTS ON SPECIAL BEDS AND FRAMES (continued)

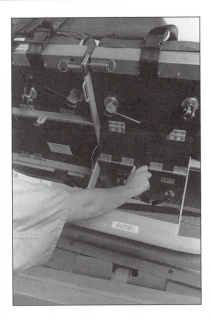 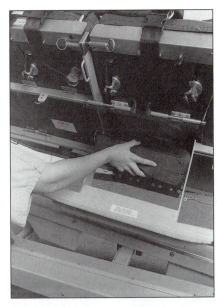 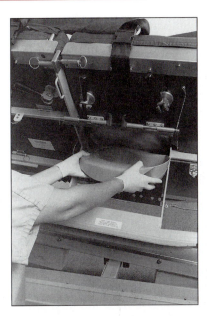

- When the client needs to use a bedpan, first lock the table in its most lateral position, and then open the rectal hatch (left). Remove the rectal pack (center).

Insert a full-sized bedpan (right), close the rectal hatch, place the client in a horizontal position, and lock the table in that position.

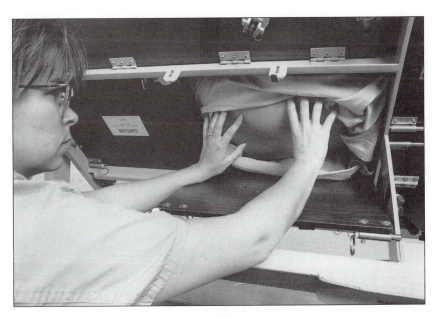

- Other openings such as the cervical and thoracic hatches allow accessibility to the client for bathing, skin care, and inspection.

➤

NURSING GUIDELINES: CARE OF CLIENTS ON SPECIAL BEDS AND FRAMES (continued)

Clinitron Air Fluidized Therapy

Clients with altered tissue and skin integrity (eg, those with burns, grafts, or pressure ulcers) and those at risk for pressure ulcers (eg, clients on strict bed rest or with impaired sensation or limited mobility) may benefit from air fluidized therapy, which gives the benefits of flotation and yet achieves this end in a completely dry environment. When the system is turned on, room air is drawn into the system, filtered, cooled or heated, and forced upward through the "beads," which sets them in motion and creates the effect of fluid and flotation.

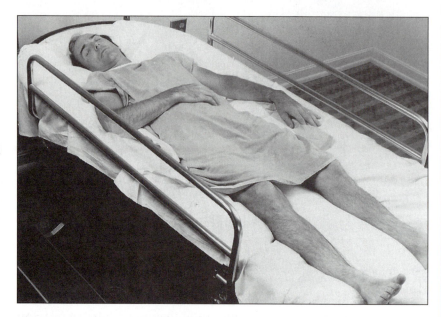

- To turn the client into a side-lying position, first have him cross his arms. Then roll the sheet toward his body, with your hands positioned at his hips and shoulder. Pull him toward you and turn him to the side as you lift up on the sheet.

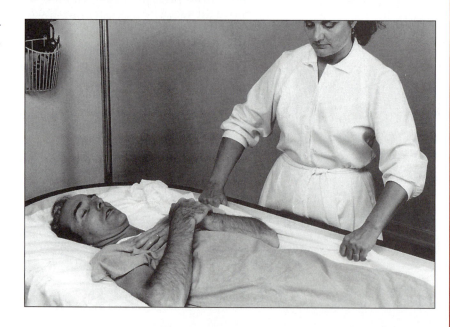

NURSING GUIDELINES: CARE OF CLIENTS ON SPECIAL BEDS AND FRAMES (continued)

- If you have turned the client into a side-lying position to perform a procedure that necessitates the client's being still, such as a dressing change, turn the bed off (see page 619) before implementing the procedure to ensure client immobilization.

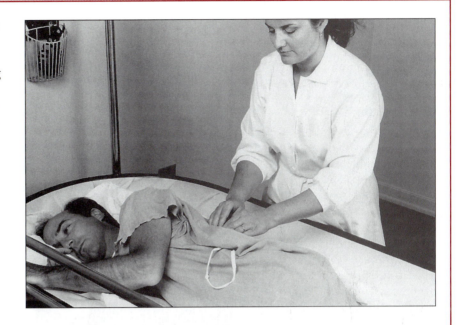

- To raise the head of the bed, for example, for meals or insertion of a nasogastric (NG) tube, it will be necessary to insert a foam wedge. To do this, position the foam wedge contoured side out at the head of the bed. Then wrap a sheet around the client's head and shoulders and ask him to grasp a trapeze (or get a helper if the bed is not equipped with a trapeze).

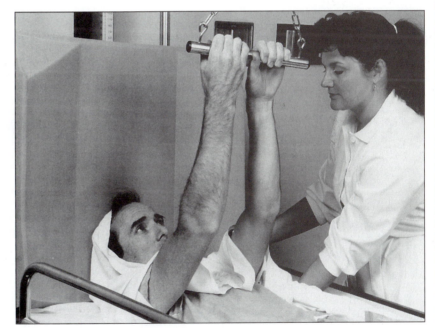

NURSING GUIDELINES: CARE OF CLIENTS ON SPECIAL BEDS AND FRAMES (continued)

As the client raises his upper body, slide the wedge down and under his upper body.

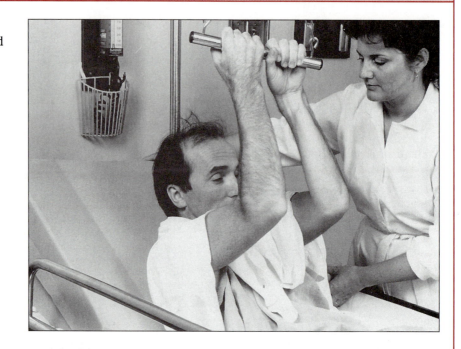

Then, straighten the sheet around the foam wedge.

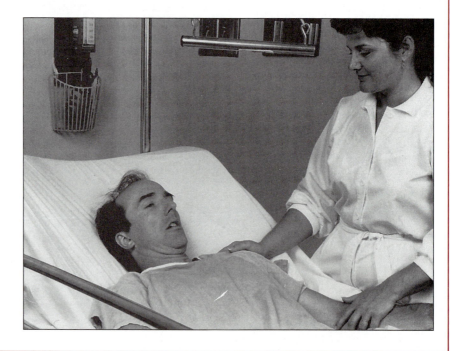

NURSING GUIDELINES: CARE OF CLIENTS ON SPECIAL BEDS AND FRAMES (continued)

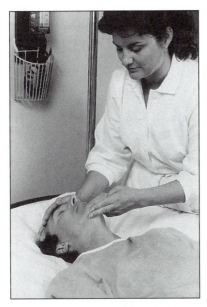

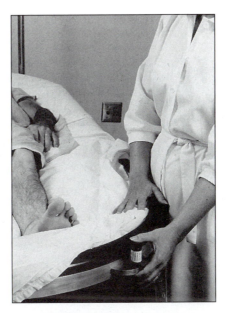

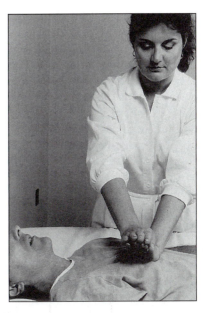

Note: If the client requires CPR, it will be necessary to perform the head tilt maneuver before turning the system off. Turning the system off before tilting the client's head back would make it difficult to position the head in the hardened bed surface.

After performing the head tilt maneuver, turn the system off by pressing the button at the end of the bed (as shown).

Once you have turned off the system, you then can perform chest compressions on the hardened surface (as shown).

NURSING GUIDELINES: CARE OF CLIENTS ON SPECIAL BEDS AND FRAMES (continued)

Therapulse Pulsating Air Suspension Therapy

The Therapulse system adds continuous pulsating action to the benefits of a static low-air-loss system for clients with the same needs as those on an air fluidized system. Suspension on the air cushions, which alternate inflation with deflation, helps keep skin pressure below the point of capillary closure and thus helps minimize the risk of tissue breakdown. The system also provides a temperature-controlled, dry environment.

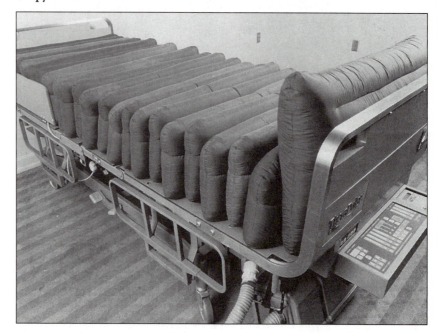

- Cover the cushions only with the cover sheet provided by the manufacturer. If your client is incontinent, use special pads under the client's buttocks (as shown) to protect the cover sheet and help keep the client dry and comfortable. To ensure that the client is getting maximum pressure relief to all tissue, inspect the client's degree of sinking into the cushions when in the supine position. Optimally, the client sinks approximately 40% into the cushions. If this is not occurring, check with the manufacturer's representative for adjustment.

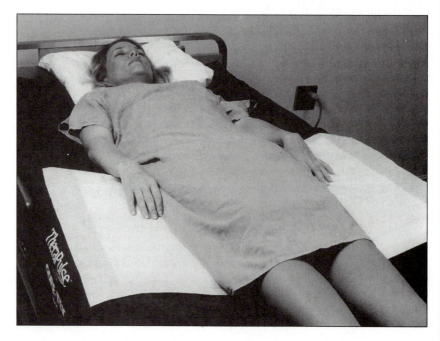

NURSING GUIDELINES: CARE OF CLIENTS ON SPECIAL BEDS AND FRAMES (continued)

- To turn the client from side to side and perform other nursing procedures, turn the adjuster dial to "instaflate," which will stop the pulsations from occurring and provide a firm surface for client care. To return the client to the pulsation mode following completion of nursing care, turn the dial back to "memory return."

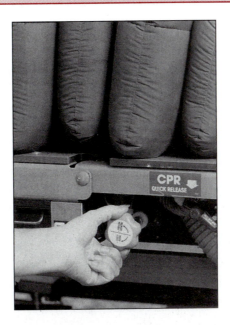

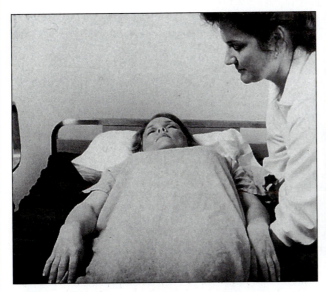

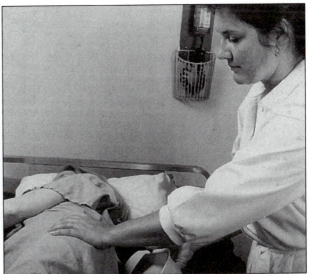

- Post a turning schedule and turn the client from side to side to help prevent respiratory problems caused by immobility. After turning the adjuster dial to "instaflate," position your arms under the client's trunk and turn her onto her side (see Chapter 2 for turning guidelines).

- Once the client is on her side, you can perform routine assessment and nursing care, such as providing a bedpan. To position the bedpan, you must first press the seat deflation button. Then slide the bedpan under the client's hips, as shown, and press the button again to reinflate that area of the bed. If it is not contraindicated, raise the head of the bed.

➡

NURSING GUIDELINES: CARE OF CLIENTS ON SPECIAL BEDS AND FRAMES (continued)

- If CPR is indicated, depress the CPR quick-release lever. This will deflate the bed in seconds.

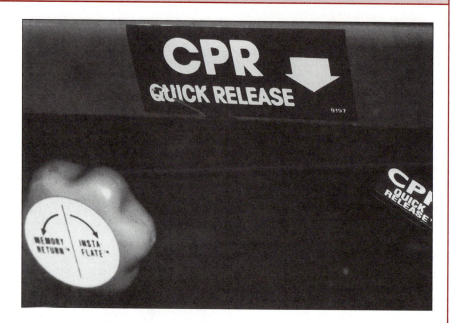

- Deflating the bed will enable you to initiate CPR promptly, without the necessity of a crashboard.

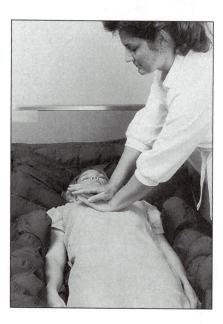

Caring for Clients with Disorders of the Sensory System

ASSESSING AUDITORY FUNCTION

There are several methods for assessing your client's hearing for acuity. The simplest method is to stand approximately 60 cm (2 ft) from the client and out of his or her vision. Instruct the client to cover her ear as your whisper two-syllable words such as *baseball* or *armchair*. With normal hearing, the client should be able to hear and repeat at least 50% of your words at this distance. If the client is unable to hear the whispered word, gradually increase the intensity of your voice until your words are heard and repeated. Perform the same test on the client's opposite ear, using different words.

PERFORMING THE WATCH TEST

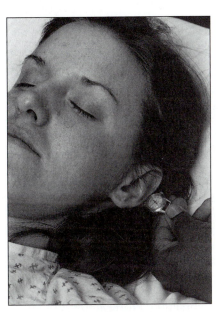

Another method for testing hearing acuity is the watch test, whereby the client covers one ear as you position a ticking watch approximately 2.5–5.0 cm (1–2 in) from her uncovered ear. Instruct the client to alert you when she no longer can hear the watch, and slowly move the watch away from the ear. With normal hearing, the client should be able to hear the ticking 5 cm from her ear, provided she is in a quiet room. Repeat the test on the opposite ear, and record the farthest distance at which the client was able to hear the ticking for both ears.

PERFORMING THE WEBER AND RINNE TESTS

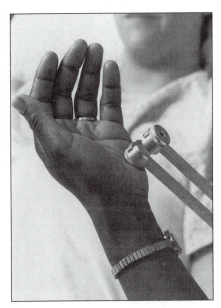

1 The Weber and Rinne tests are more sophisticated assessments of your client's auditory function. A combination of the two tests can help categorize an auditory dysfunction as either conductive or sensorineural (perceptive). With conductive hearing loss, there is a physical obstruction of the sound, such as a fusion of the stapes or a foreign body in the external canal. With a sensorineural hearing loss, the dysfunction can occur with the eighth cranial nerve, or in the cortex itself. To perform either the Weber or the Rinne test, first activate a tuning fork by holding it by its base and gently striking the prongs against the palmar surface of your hand (as shown). This will cause the prongs to vibrate.

➡

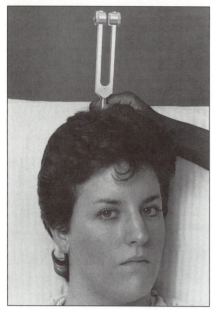

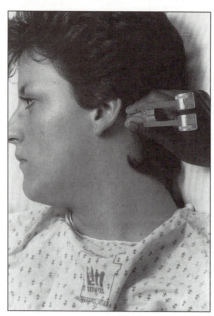

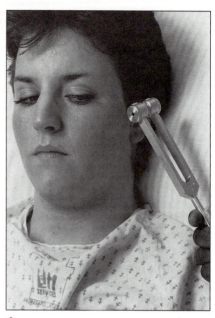

2 To perform the Weber test, activate the tuning fork, and position the base of the fork on the top of the client's head (as shown) or at the top of the forehead. Normally, the client will hear the sound equally in both ears. This is recorded as Weber negative. With conductive loss the sound will lateralize to the poorer ear. This occurs because the normal ear is penetrated by ordinary room noise, masking hearing in that ear. The poorer ear, on the other hand, is not penetrated by ordinary room noise and thus can hear the bone-conducted sound. Document the results as either "Weber negative" or "Lateralization Right" (or "Left").

3 To perform the Rinne test, instruct the client to cover one ear. After activating the tuning fork, position its base on the mastoid process of the uncovered ear. Instruct the client to alert you once she no longer can hear the sound. As soon as she alerts you, make a mental note of the amount of time during which she heard the sound.

4 Immediately move the prongs of the tuning fork in front of the uncovered ear, approximately 1.25–2.5 cm ($\frac{1}{2}$–1 in). Because air conduction lasts at least twice as long as bone conduction, the client should be able to hear the sound twice as long in this position. The reverse is true if the client has conductive hearing loss. Repeat the test in the opposite ear. Document the results as positive if the client has normal hearing, or negative if the results are reversed.

IRRIGATING THE EXTERNAL AUDITORY CANAL

Assessing

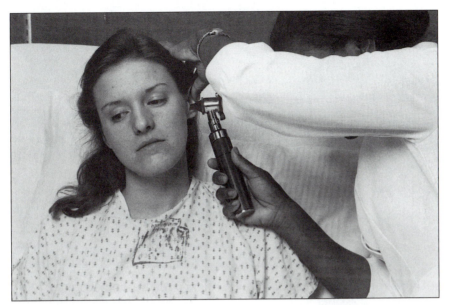

1 The physician may prescribe external auditory canal irrigation to remove cerumen or debris. Before irrigating the ear, explain the procedure to the client. Inspect the pinna of the ear and the meatus of the external auditory canal for signs of redness, abrasions, or discharge. An otoscope may be used to assess the location and amount of cerumen or debris and to ensure that the tympanic membrane is intact. For an adult, lift the pinna up and back to straighten the canal; for a child, pull the earlobe down and back. Instruct the client to tilt her head toward the unaffected ear. Insert the speculum of the otoscope slowly and carefully. Be sure that you have selected a speculum that will comfortably fit in the external canal. Smaller specula have a greater potential for damaging the ear. *Caution: If the tympanic membrane is not intact, do not proceed with the irrigation.*

Planning

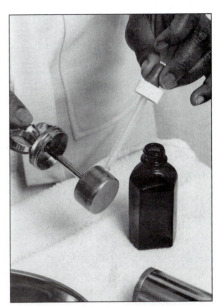

2 After inspecting the client's ear, prepare the prescribed irrigating solution, making sure it is warmed to room temperature. For an adult, use either a 50-mL rubber bulb (asepto) or a Pomeroy ear syringe. For a child, obtain a 20- to 30-mL syringe with a rubber tip. If you use a Pomeroy syringe, first oil the plunger with one to two drops of lubricant (as shown) to minimize the friction of the plunger against the barrel.

Implementing

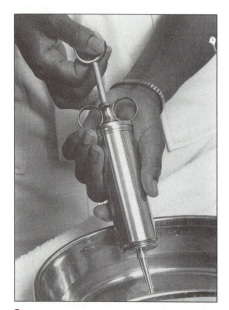

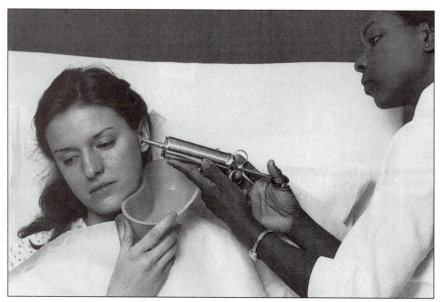

3 Aspirate approximately 50 mL of the irrigant into the syringe.

4 Drape the client with a bed-saver pad, and ask her to hold an emesis basin under her affected ear. Position the tip of the syringe very carefully into the external canal so that it angles either up-ward (as shown) or toward the wall of the canal to avoid injecting the irrigant onto the tympanic mem-brane. Make sure the client tilts her head toward the unaffected ear.

After correctly positioning the syringe, lift the pinna up and back and slowly inject the irrigant until you have administered the pre-scribed amount. ***Caution:*** *Stop the procedure immediately and notify the physician if the client complains of a sudden pain in her ear. This is an indication that the tympanic mem-brane may have been perforated.*

Evaluating

5 Observe the return as it drains into the emesis basin. When the procedure has been completed, dry the outer ear with cotton balls and inspect the external auditory canal once more with the otoscope to evaluate the effectiveness of the irrigation. Document the proce-dure, noting the amount and type of irrigant, the character of the return, and your final evaluation of the external auditory canal.

IRRIGATING THE EYE

Assessing and Planning	Implementing	Evaluating

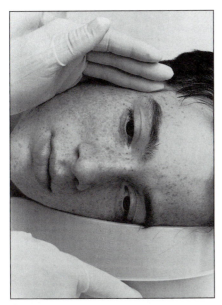

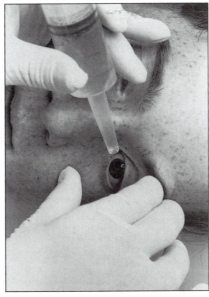

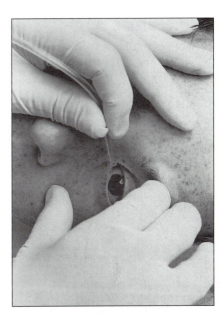

1 If an eye irrigation has been prescribed for your client, assemble the following supplies:

- ☐ sterile irrigating solution warmed to room temperature
- ☐ sterile 50-mL syringe (or sterile infusion tubing if larger amounts of irrigant are to be used)
- ☐ sterile gauze pads
- ☐ bed-saver pads
- ☐ emesis basin
- ☐ clean gloves

Fill the syringe with the irrigant. Explain the procedure to your client and position him so that he is on his side with his affected eye lowermost. Position the emesis basin underneath the affected eye, and drape the client's gown and bed with the bed-saver pads. Then wash your hands, and apply clean gloves.

2 Retract the upper and lower eyelids with your thumb and index finger, and administer the irrigant so that it flows from the inner to the outer canthus.

Note: Follow the same procedure if you are using infusion tubing to deliver the irrigant.

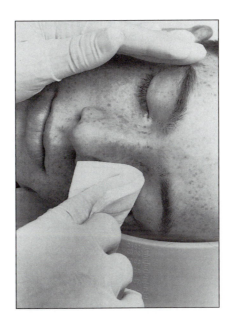

3 After completing the procedure, blot the client's eye gently with a sterile gauze pad, wiping from the inner to the outer canthus. Document the procedure, noting the type and amount of irrigant and the client's tolerance to the procedure.

REFERENCES

Bay-Monk H, Steinmetz CG: *Nursing Care of the Eye.* Norwalk, CT: Appleton-Lange, 1988.

Birdsall C, Greif L: How do I manage extraventricular drainage? *Am J Nurs* 90(11):47–49, 1990.

Bowers AC, Thompson JM: *Clinical Manual of Health Assessment,* ed 4. St Louis: Mosby, 1992.

Callanan M, Stowe AC: Neurologic dysfunctions. In Swearingen PL, Keen JH (eds): *Manual of Critical Care Nursing,* ed 3. St Louis: Mosby, 1995.

Clochesy J, Breu C, Cardin S, et al: *Critical Care Nursing.* Philadelphia: Saunders, 1993.

Deveau B: Sensory disorders. In Swearingen PL: *Manual of Medical-Surgical Nursing Care,* ed 3. St Louis: Mosby, 1994.

Eden-Kilgour S, Miller B: Understanding neurovascular assessment. *Nursing 93* 23(8)56–57, 1993.

Hudak CM, Gallo BM: *Critical Care Nursing: A Holistic Approach.* Philadelphia: Lippincott, 1994.

Indiana University Hospitals: *Nursing Procedures and Policies.* Indianapolis, 1994.

Kozier B, Erb G: *Techniques in Clinical Nursing,* ed 4. Redwood City, CA: Addison-Wesley, 1993.

Newell F: *Ophthalmology: Principles and Concepts.* St Louis: Mosby, 1992.

O'Brien K: Managing the seizure patient. *Nursing 91* 21(1):63–65, 1991.

Potter PA, Perry AG: *Fundamentals of Nursing: Concepts, Process, and Practice.* St Louis: Mosby, 1993.

Rice R: *Handbook of Home Health Nursing Procedures.* St Louis: Mosby, 1995.

Sims LK et al: *Health Assessment in Nursing.* Redwood City, CA: Addison-Wesley, 1994.

Spence AP: *Basic Human Anatomy,* ed 3. Redwood City, CA: Addison-Wesley, 1991.

Stevens SA, Becker KL: A simple, step-by-step approach to neurologic assessment, *Nursing 88* 18(9):53–61, 1988.

Stowe AC: Cranial nerves: functions and dysfunctions. In Swearingen PL, Keen JH (eds): *Manual of Critical Care Nursing,* ed 3. St Louis: Mosby, 1995.

Swearingen PL, Stowe AC: Assessing respiratory patterns. In Swearingen PL, Keen JH (eds): *Manual of Critical Care Nursing,* ed 3. St Louis: Mosby, 1995.

Swift CM: Neurologic disorders. In Swearingen PL (ed): *Manual of Medical-Surgical Nursing Care,* ed 3. St Louis: Mosby, 1994.

Thompson JM: *Mosby's Manual of Clinical Nursing,* ed 3. St Louis: Mosby, 1993.

Index

(Note: page numbers followed by *t* indicate tabular material)

A/B ratio (ankle-brachial ratio), 401–402
Abbott pump, 149–153
Abdominal examination
  auscultating, 240
  of children, 239, 242
  girth measurement, 242
  inspecting, 239
  of neonates, 225, 239
  palpating, 241–242
  percussing, 241
  postpartum, 205
  prenatal, 194–200
Abduction pillow, 516, 572–581
ABG (arterial blood gas) analysis, 354
Activities of daily living, 506
Admission procedures, newborn, 215–220
Adventitious breath sounds, 318, 319*t*
Aerosol therapy, 351, 352, 361–362
Air bubbles, injection, 98, 106
Air embolism, 154, 155, 176
Air fluidized therapy beds, 616–619
Air lock, injection, 106
Air mattress, 54–55
Airborne pathogens, 12, 13
  CDC precautions, 7, 8–11*t*
Airways, 320–341
  endotracheal tube, 322
  inserting artificial, 325–328
  mouth-to-mask ventilation, 329
  nasopharyngeal tube, 321, 327–328
  nursing guidelines, 320–324
  oral, during seizures, 605
  oropharyngeal tube, 320, 325–326
  tracheostomy
    buttons, 324
    cuffs, 335–336
    hygiene, 337–340
    replacing cannulas, 341
    suctioning, 330–334
    tubes, 323
Allergic reactions
  blood transfusions, 145, 146, 147–148*t*
  IV medications, 133, 135

Allergy testing, 95
Alternating pressure mattress, 55
Amniotic fluid assessment, 201
Analgesia, patient-controlled, 149–153
Anaphylactic reactions, 96, 148*t*
Ankle-brachial ratio (A/B ratio), 401–402
Ankles
  assessment, 504, 601
  exercises, 47–48
  reflex, 601
Antiembolic stockings, 417–419, 534
Antimicrobial agents, 4, 21
Antiseptic agents, 4, 4–5*t*
Apical lung expansion exercises, 362
Apical pulse, 226, 393
Aprons, protective, 12
Arm exercises, postmastectomy, 187–189
Arm/shoulder immobilizer, 514
Armboard, for venipuncture site, 127–129
Arterial blood gas (ABG) analysis, 354
Arterial pulse, 394–395, 395*t*
Auditory function tests, 623–624

Babinski's reflex, 596
Back pain, 202
Balance testing, 597
Bandages, elastic, 520–523
Basal lung expansion exercises, 363
Bathing
  clients on air mattress, 55
  sitz bath, 191, 207
Bed scale, for weighing clients, 436
Beds
  changing linens on traction, 561–562
  special, 612–622
Biceps reflex, 600
Biot's (ataxic) respirations, 586, 589*t*
Bivalved cast, 528
Bladder
  assessing, 433–434

continuous irrigation of, 465–466
  Credé's maneuver, 473
  postpartum, 205
Blakemore gastric tube, 246
Blanketrol® system, 606–609
Blankets, hyper/hypothermia, 606–609
Blink (corneal) reflex, 592
Blood glucose monitoring
  in neonates, 218
  self-monitoring, 142–144
Blood pressure, 397–400
  children, 399
  classification chart, 400*t*
  neonates, 230
Blood reinfusion system, 567–569
Blood samples
  neonatal, 218
  vacuum collection systems, 140–141
  venipuncture for, 117–119, 126
  via Hickman® catheters, 163–165
  via subcutaneous ports, 173–174
Blood transfusions, 144–148
  adverse reactions to, 145, 146, 147–148*t*
  hemolysis prevention, 144
  incompatible IV solutions with, 144
  nursing guidelines for safe, 144
  preparing for, 145–146
  saline/heparin lock after, 146
  venipuncture for, 146
Bloodborne pathogens, 7, 11*t*
Body mechanics
  in moving and lifting clients, 64
  for performing ROM exercises, 34–35
Body temperature assessment
  in neonates, 222
  in neurologic impairment, 586
  hyper/hypothermia blanket, 606–609
Boot, Buck's traction, 543–546
Brace, hinged knee, 518

Brachial pulse
  ankle-brachial ratio (A/B ratio), 401–402
  neonatal, 226
Brachioradialis (supinator) reflex, 600
Breast pumps, 212–214
Breastfeeding, 207–211
  comfort measures, 204, 209, 214
  milk expression, 211–214
Breasts
  engorgement, 204
  postpartum assessment, 204
  self-examination (BSE), 183–186
Breath sounds, 318, 319*t*
Breathing exercises, 362–363, 365
Bricker's loop, 478–479
Bronchodialator aerosols, 86, 87, 366
Broviac® catheters, 166
Bruits, 197, 240
Bryant's traction, 547–550
BSE (breast self-examination), 183–186
Buck's traction boot, 543–546
Buerger-Allen exercises, 425–427
Bulb syringe, 231
Burns, cold, 606, 609
Burping infants, 210
Butterfly (wing-tipped) needle
  for children, 118
  injecting medications into, 133
  inserting and taping, 120–121

Canes, 62
CAPD (chronic ambulatory peritoneal dialysis), 475–477
Capillary refill assessment, 507
Capillary tubes, 218
Cardiac catheterization, 411–413
Cardiopulmonary resuscitation. *See* CPR
Cardiovascular procedures, 385–428
  ankle-brachial ratio (A/B ratio), 401–402

continued

Cardiovascular procedures (continued)
arterial pulses, 394–395, 395*t*
blood pressure, 397–400, 400*t*
central venous pressure (CVP), 414–416
EKG electrodes, 409–410
jugular vein, 396
monitoring cardiac patients, 396–416
paradoxical pulse, 403
postcardiac catheterization, 411–413
telemetry electrodes, 405–408
telemetry lead sites, 404
for vascular disorders, 417–427
Cardiovascular system assessment, 388–393
anatomical landmarks, 386, 388–390, 394
assessment guidelines, 387
heart sounds, 390–393, 390–391*t*, 393*t*
inspecting and palpating, 389
Casts
application of, 524–528
bivalved, 528
care for clients with, 529–532
edema assessment, 507
exercises for clients in, 531
neurovascular assessments, 529
nursing guidelines, 531
petaling, 530, 532
postsurgical/trauma drainage, 530
shoe for, 528
Catheterization (cardiac), 411–413
Catheterization (urinary)
home care, 443
indwelling (Foley), 446–460
intermittent (Robinson), 437–445
Catheters
central venous
assessing for infection, 160
blood samples via, 163–165
Broviac®, 166
changing solution and tubing, 167
dressing changes, 159–162
Groshong™, 166
Hickman®, 159–167
irrigating, 166
long-term (chronic), 154, 159–167
nursing guidelines, 154–156
repairing, 154, 168–169
for dialysis, 474–477
exdwelling, 461–464
for insulin pumps, 112
lumbar, 610–611
over-the-needle, 121–125
Permcath, 474

Quinton, 474
softset, 112
Tenckhoff, 475
urinary
condom (exdwelling), 461–464
exdwelling, 461–464
Foley (indwelling), 446–460
Robinson (straight), 437–445
suprapubic, 467
Texas (exdwelling), 461–464
See also Implantable subcutaneous ports
CBI (continuous bladder irrigation), 465–466
CDC. *See* Centers for Disease Control and Prevention
CDH (congenital dislocated hips), 547–550
Centers for Disease Control and Prevention (CDC)
handwashing protocols, 7
precautions, 7, 8–11*t*
recommended cleaning agents, 4–5*t*
Central venous catheters. *See under Catheters*
Central venous pressure (CVP), 155, 156, 414–416
Cerebellar function tests, 594–597
Cerebrospinal fluid (CSF) drainage, 602, 610–611
Cervical collars, 511, 512, 535–538
Cervical traction, 535–538
Cervical vertebrae assessment, 498
Cervical/uterine radiation implants, 193
Cesarean birth, postpartum assessment, 207
Chest physiotherapy, 368–376
Chest tubes, 377–383
monitoring, 379–381
nursing guidelines, 377–378
removing, 382–383
Cheyne-Stokes respirations, 586, 589*t*
Chickenpox, 12, 13
Children
Bryant's traction, 547–550
with casts, 529
chest physiotherapy, 374–376
colostomies, 290
Denis-Browne splints, 519
ear irrigation, 625
enemas, 279
ileostomies, 293
injections for, 101, 106, 107
IV therapy, 117, 118, 128, 132, 138
seizure care, 605
traction care, 547–550
trapezes (bed), 534
Chronic ambulatory peritoneal dialysis (CAPD), 475–477

Circulatory overload, 144, 148*t*
Clavicle splint, 513
Cleansing agents, 4, 4–5*t*
Client transport, CDC precautions, 10*t*
Client-controlled analgesia, 149–153
Clinitron bed, 616–619
Closed-glove technique, 22–23
Cold burns, 606
Collars, cervical, 511–512, 535–538
Colon conduits, 478–479
Colostomies, 286–291, 304–306
pediatric, 290
Coma
assessing for, 586–587
Glasgow Coma Scale, 587*t*
Compartment syndrome, 529, 531
Congenital dislocated hips (CDH), 547–550
Consciousness
assessing level of, 586–587
Glasgow Coma Scale, 587*t*
Constant positive airway pressure (CPAP) mask, 347
Continent ileostomy, 294, 307–309
Continent urinary diversion, 482–483
Continuous bladder irrigation (CBI), 465–466
Continuous passive motion (CPM), 570
Coordination tests, 594–597
Corneal (blink) reflex, 592
Coughing, assisted, 364
CPAP (constant positive airway pressure) mask, 347
CPM (continuous passive motion), 570
CPR protocols
on air mattress, 55
on alternating pressure mattress, 55
on Clinitron bed, 619
on Roto rest turning table, 614
on Therapulse bed, 622
Cranial nerves
assessment, 590, 592–593
functions/dysfunctions, 590–591*t*
Credé's maneuver, 473
Crepitation, 316, 379
Crepitus, 498
Crutches, 61, 63
Cryotherapy, 571
CSF (cerebrospinal fluid) drainage, 602, 610–611
Cuffs
pneumatic sequential pressure, 420–422
tracheostomy, 335–336
Cut-down, venous, 154
Cutaneous ureterostomy, 480–481
CVP (central venous pressure) catheters, 155, 156
measurement, 414–416

Dacron cuff, 154
Deep tendon reflexes (DTRs), 600–601
Deep-breathing exercises, 362–363
Dehydration, 435, 436
Deltoid injection site, 105, 106
Demerol (meperidine), 149, 153
Denis-Browne splint, 519
Dermatome zones, 598–599
Diabetes management
blood glucose monitoring, 142–144
insulin pumps, 110–112
insulin shock, 112
Diagonal-movement exercises, 49–52
Dialysis
catheters for, 474, 475
chronic ambulatory peritoneal, 475–477
Diaphragmatic breathing exercises, 363
Dilantin (phenytoin), 592
Dilating veins, for venipuncture, 119
Doppler auscultation, 197, 230
Doppler probe, 395
Dorsal column tract test, 598–599
Dorsal gluteal injection site, 101–102, 106
Douche (vaginal irrigation), 92–93
Drainage, cranial, 602
Drainage bags, urinary
connecting pouches to, 491
emptying, 454
leg drainage system, 461–464
Dressing changes, 25–30
for catheters, 156, 157, 159–162
on clients in Clinitron beds, 617
disposing of, 26
establishing sterile field for, 18–20
home care considerations, 28
irrigating a wound, 29–30
packing a wound, 25–28
pouring sterile solutions for, 20
standard precautions during, 7–11
tracheostomy, 339
Dressings
compression, cryotherapy via, 571
gauze, 126, 156
for IV insertion sites, 126, 134
for neonates, 126
transparent, 126, 156

Ear drops, 84
Ear irrigation, 625–626
Eggcrate mattress, 53
Elastic bandages, 520–523
Elastic stockings, 417–419
Elbow
assessment, 501–502
exercises, 40

Electrocardiogram electrodes, 409–410
Electronic fetal monitoring, 198–200
Embolism
air, 154, 155, 176
fat, 531
Endotracheal tube, 322
Enemas
Kayexalate, 470–472
nonretention, 277–279
retention, 280–282
Engorgement, breast, 204, 229
Erythromycin, ophthalmic, 216
Esophageal-nasogastric (Blakemore) tube, 246
Exdwelling catheters, 461–464
Exercises
ankle, 47–48
breathing, 362–363, 365
Buerger-Allen, 425–427
diagonal movement, 49–52
elbow, 40
finger, 41–43
hip, 44–46
isometric, 531, 534, 546, 553
knee, 44–46
lower extremity, 52
lung inflation, 362–367
mastectomy, postsurgical, 187–189
neck, 35–37, 49
proprioceptive neuromuscular facilitation, 49–52
range of motion (ROM), 34–48, 187, 531
shoulder, 37–39
toe, 47–48
upper extremity, 50–51
wrist, 41–43
External urinary devices, 461–464
Extremities
dangling from bedside, 67–68
exercises for, 50–52
Eye drops, 83–84
neonatal, 216
Eye shields, 13, 21
Eyes
assessing movements of, 592
blink (corneal) reflex, 592
irrigating, 627
protection of, 9t, 13, 21
pupillary response, 592

Face masks. *See* Masks
Face shields, CDC precautions, 8t
Fat embolism, 531
Feeding pumps, 267
Feedings, tube, 264–270
Fetal status assessment
electronic monitoring, 198–200
estimating gestational age, 194
fundal height measurement, 194
heart tones (FHTs), 196–197
Leopold's maneuvers, 195
McDonald's rule, 194

palpating fetal parts, 194–195
ultrasonic (Doppler) auscultation, 197
uterine activity, 198–200
FHTs (fetal heart tones), 196–197
Fingers
exercises for, 41–43
nailbed assessment, 507
Flotation pads, 54
Fluid-resistive aprons or gowns, 12
Foley (indwelling) catheters, 446–460
emptying drainage bag, 454
home care considerations, 448
inserting, 446–448
irrigating, 457–459
nursing guidelines, 449
removing, 460
strap anchors for, 450–451
urine meters, 455–456
urine specimens, 452–453
Fontanelles, 222
Foot pedals, on turning tables, 613
Foot pumps, 423–424
Foot supports, 59
Footprints, neonatal, 215
Forearm/wrist splint, 515
Frames, immobilization, 612–622
Fremitus, 316, 379
Fundal height
postpartum, 205
prenatal, 194
Fundal massage, 205

Gait assessment, 497
Gastric lavage, 271–272
Gastric tubes, 244–273
aspirating stomach contents, 91, 256, 273
double-lumen, 245
esophageal-nasogastric (Blakemore), 246
feedings through, 264–270
four-lumen (Minnesota sump), 247
gastrostomy, 248, 268–270
gastrostomy button, 250–251
home care considerations, 248
inserting, 252–260
irrigating, 261
lavage for, 271–272
nasogastric tube, 252–257
nursing guidelines, 244–251
orogastric tube, 260
PEG tube, 249
removing, 262–263
single-lumen, 244
small-bore feeding tube, 258–259
Gastrointestinal procedures, 235–309
enemas, 277–282
gastric tubes, 244–273
intestinal tubes, 274–276

rectal tubes, 283–284
stoma care, 286–309
stool tests, 285
Gastrointestinal system assessment, 235–243
abdomen, 239–242
anatomical landmarks, 236
assessment guidelines, 237
oral cavity, 238
rectum, 243
Gastrostomy button, 250–251
Gastrostomy tube, 248, 268–270
Gatch bed, 529
Gauze restraints, 129
Gestational age estimation, 194
Glasgow Coma Scale, 586, 587t
Gloves
CDC precautions, 8t
putting on, 13, 16–17, 21–23
removing, 14
sterile, 16–17, 21–23
Glucose levels
in cranial drainage fluid, 602
in neonates, 218
self-monitoring of, 142–144
Gluteal injection site, 101–103, 106, 108
Goggles, 13, 21
Gowns
CDC precautions, 9t
putting on, 12, 21–24
removing, 14–15
sterile, 21–24
Grasp reflex, 225
Groshong catheters, 166
Gynecologic procedures, 182–214
anatomical landmarks, 182
assessment guidelines, 182
breast self-examination (BSE), 183–186
cancer risk assessment, 182
mastectomy exercises, 187–189
perineal care, 190–192
radiation implant cautions, 193

Halo vest traction, 554–560
pin care, 560
Hand rolls, cones, splints, 60
Handwashing, 4–7, 8t
cleansing agents, 4, 4–5t
procedure, 6–7
sterile gloves and, 21
Hearing tests, 623–624
Heart sounds, 390–393, 390–391t
murmurs, 392, 393t
Heimlich valve, 381
Hematocrit, in neonates, 218
Hemi canes, 62
Hemolysis prevention, 144
Heparin
flushing lines with, 156, 158, 163, 165, 170, 173–174, 474
injections, 97, 99, 100
locks, 134–135, 175
Hickman® catheters, 159–167

blood samples from, 163–165
High-flow oxygen delivery system, 342
Hinged brace (knee), 518
Hip
abduction pillow, 516, 572–581
assessment, 503–504
congenital dislocation (CDH) traction, 547–550
exercises, 44–46
replacement, moving clients with, 572–581
Hip spica cast, 550
Hollister® male urinary collection system, 461
Home care considerations
central venous catheters, 162
crutches, canes, walkers, 63
disposing of syringes, needles, 99
dressing changes, 28
Foley catheters, 433, 448
gastric tubes, 90, 248, 266
infection control, 6, 28, 99
injections, 99
mattresses/pads, 54
nasogastric tubes, 90, 266
needles/syringes, 90, 99
occult blood in stools, 285
oxygen tanks, 342
postmastectomy exercises, 188
suctioning, 333
tracheostomies, 333, 337
urinary catheters, 443, 448
wound care, 28
Hoyer lifts, 78–79
Huber needle, 158, 170
Humidified oxygen, 351, 352, 358–360
Hydroculator (moist heat) pack, 565–566
Hyperglycemia/hypoglycemia, 112
neonatal, 218
Hyperthermia/hypothermia blanket, 606–609

Ileal conduit (bladder/loop) diversion, 478–479
Ileoanal reservoir, 295–296
Ileocecal (Indiana) reservoir, 482–483
Ileostomy, 292–294, 307–309
pediatric, 293
IM (intramuscular) injections, 101–109
Immobilization devices
nursing guidelines, 511–519
special beds and frames, 612–622
Implantable subcutaneous ports
accessing, 170–172
blood samples from, 173–174
establishing heparin lock, 175

continued

Implantable subcutaneous ports (continued)
nursing guidelines, 158
Incubators (isolettes), 349
Indiana (ileocecal) reservoir, 482–483
Indwelling urinary catheters. See Foley (indwelling) catheters
Infant feeding, 207–211
bottle feeding, 209
breastfeeding, 207–211
burping after, 210
positioning for, 208–209
postcesarean, 209
Infants
in Bryant's traction, 547–550
chest physiotherapy, 374–376
in Denis-Browne splints, 519
incubators (isolettes), 349
oxygen hood for, 348
Infection control, 3–31
CDC precautions, 7, 8–11t
cleansing agents, 4–7, 4–5t
handwashing, 4–7, 4–5t
home care considerations, 6, 28
isolation, 7, 8–11t
protective attire, 12–15
sterile procedures, 16–24
throat cultures, 24
tubercular clients, 7
wound care, 25–30
Infusion pumps, 137
Infusion sets, 113–116
for intermittent therapy, 134–135
piggyback, 136–137
priming, 116, 136
Inhalers
metered-dose, 86
nebulizers, 87
Injectable medications, 95–109
Injections
disposing of needles, sharps, 110
intradermal, 95–96
intramuscular (IM), 101–109
neonatal, 217
subcutaneous, 97–100
Z-track technique, 108–109
Insulin
pumps, 110–112
rotating injection sites, 97
shock, 112
Intermittent positive pressure breathing (IPPB), 335, 366–367
Intestinal tubes, 274–276
Intradermal injections, 95–96
Intramuscular (IM) injections, 101–109
air locks, 106
muscle sites for, 101–105
Z-track technique, 108–109
Intravenous (IV) fluids, 113–139
armboards or splints for, 127–129
infusion sets and solutions, 113–116

medications, 130–139
by hanging container, 130–131
by intermittent infusion, 134–135
by IV bolus, 132–133
by piggyback container, 136–137
by volume-control set, 138–139
preparing for, 113–129
venipuncture for, 117–126
wrist restraints for, 128–129
IPPB (intermittent positive pressure breathing), 335, 366–367
Irrigation
catheter, 166
ear, 625–626
eye, 627
vaginal, 92–93
wound, 29–30
Isolation precautions, 7, 8–11t
Isolettes (incubators), 349
Isometric exercise, 531, 534, 546, 553
IV fluids. See under Intravenous

Jejunostomy tube, 276
Joints
moist heat for, 565–566
range of motion assessment, 500–504
wrapping with elastic bandages, 521
Jugular vein inspection, 396

Kayexalate (sodium polystyrene sulfonate) enema, 470–472
Kidneys
dialysis, 474–477
palpating, 435
procedures. See under Renal
Knee joint
continuous passive motion for, 570
cryotherapy, 571
exercises, 44–46
hinged brace, 518
immobilizer splint, 517
Knots, bowline traction, 533
Kock continent urostomy, 482–483

Lactation, 211, 212–214
Leg cramps, 202
Leg drainage systems, 461–464
Leopold's maneuvers, 195, 198
Lifting clients
body mechanics of, 64
for dangling extremities, 67–68
from stretcher to bed, 69–75
from wheelchair to bed, 76–77
immobile clients, 66, 68, 72–75
mechanical devices for, 78–79
mobile clients, 65, 67
moving up in bed, 65–66

nursing guidelines, 64
Limb shrinker, elastic, 522
Linen
CDC precautions, 9t
changes, on traction beds, 561–562
Lochia assessment, 206
Logroll transfer technique, 74–75, 561
Lumbar catheters, 610–611
Lung inflation techniques, 362–367

McDonald's rule, 194
Mantoux tuberculin skin test, 95
Marshall Kaneson breast pump, 212
Masks
aerosol, 351
CPAP, 347
oxygen, 342–362
protective
airborne pathogens and, 7, 13
CDC precautions, 9t
putting on, 13
removing, 15
Venturi, 346, 356–357
Mastectomy exercises, 187–189
Mattresses and pads
air, 54–55
alternating pressure, 55
CPR with special, 55, 614, 619, 622
eggcrate, 53
flotation, 54
pressure-relief, 53–55, 531
sheepskin, 53, 531, 557, 558
Measurements, neonatal, 229
Mechanical lifting devices, 78–79
Medela electric breast pump, 213–214
Median nerve assessment, 509
Medications
injectable, 95–109
insulin pumps, 110–112
intradermal, 95–96
intramuscular, 101–109
subcutaneous, 97–100
intravenous, 130–139
piggy-back, 136–137
patient-controlled analgesia, 149–153
topical, 83–94
eye, ear, nose drops, 83–85
inhalants, 86–87, 351, 361–362
nitroglycerin, 88–89
rectal, 94
vaginal (douche), 92–93
via nasogastric tube, 90–91
Mental status assessment, 590
Meperidine (Demerol), 149, 153
Metaproterenol, 87, 366
Metered-dose inhaler, 86
Mid-deltoid injection site, 105, 106
Midline catheter (MLC), 157

Minnesota sump gastric tube, 247
Mitt restraints, 129
MLC (midline catheter), 157
Mobilization of clients, 34–63
canes, crutches, walkers, 61–63
dangling extremities, 67–68
exercises
proprioceptive neuromuscular facilitation, 49–52
range of motion, 34–48
Moist heat (hydroculator) packs, 565–566
Morphine, 149, 153
Motor function tests, 595–596
Mouth, examination of, 238
Mouth-to-mask ventilation, 329
Moving clients, 64–79, 561, 572–581
Murmurs, heart, 392, 393t
Muscle-setting (isometric) exercise, 531, 534, 546, 553
Muscles
atrophy/hypertrophy assessment, 505
girth measurement, 505
injection sites, 101–105
strength assessment, 500–504
Musculoskeletal procedures, 493–582
blood reinfusion systems, 567–569
continuous passive motion (CPM), 570
cryotherapy compression dressing, 571
hip replacement clients, 572–581
hydroculator packs (moist heat), 565–566
immobilization devices, 511–532
abduction pillow, 516, 572–581
arm/shoulder immobilizer, 514
cast care, 524–532
cervical collar, 511–512
clavicle splint, 513
Denis-Browne splint, 519
elastic bandage, 520–523
hinged brace, 518
knee immobilizer, 517
nursing guidelines, 511–519, 531
wrist/forearm splint, 515
traction care, 533–560
bowline knots, 533
making traction beds, 561–562
skeletal traction, 551–560
skin traction, 535–550
wound-drainage systems, 563–564
Musculoskeletal system assessment, 494–510
anatomical landmarks, 494
assessment guidelines, 495
in children, infants, 497, 499

daily living activities, 506
inspecting, 496–497
joint range of motion, 500–504
muscle girth, 505
muscular strength, 500–504
nerve function, 508–510
neurovascular integrity, 506–507
spine, 498–499

Nailbed assessment, 507
Nasal oxygen cannula, 343
Nasogastric tube
aspirating for stomach contents, 91, 256, 273
for clients on Clinitron beds, 617
feeding through, 264–267
home care considerations, 90, 266
inserting, 252–259
irrigating, 262–263
large-bore, 91
medications via, 90–91
removing, 261
small-bore, 90, 91, 258–259
tests for correct placement of, 256
Nasopharyngeal tube, 321, 327–328
Nebulizers, 87
pneumatic (jet), 351, 361–362
Neck
assessment, 498, 501
cervical collar, 511–512
exercises, 35–37, 49
traction, 535–538
Needleless injection port, 15, 134, 164, 170
Needles, disposing of, 110
Neonatal assessment, 220–230
abdomen, 225
auscultation, 221
axillary temperature, 222
blood pressure, 230
blood samples, 218
breath sounds, 221
eyes, ears, nose, mouth, 221–224
general inspection, 220
genitalia, 226
head, 222–224
heart sounds, 221
hips, 227–228
lower extremities, 227–228
measurements, 229
Ortolani's click, 227–228, 449
palpation, 222–228
pulse rates, 226
rectum, 227
reflexes, 223–224
umbilical cord, 225
upper extremities, 225
urine specimen, 219–220
weight, 229
Neonatal care, 215–233
admitting to nursery, 215–220
eye drops, 216
feeding, 207–111

footprinting, 215
IV therapy dressings, 126
oxygen hood therapy, 348
phototherapy, 233
suctioning, 231–232
umbilical cord, 231
vitamin K injection, 217
Nephrostomy tube, 468–469
Nerve function assessment, 508–510
cranial, 590, 590–591t
Neurologic system assessment, 584–602
anatomical landmarks, 584–585
assessment guidelines, 585
auditory function, 623–624
cerebellar function, 594–597
consciousness levels, 586–587, 587t
cranial drainage, 602
deep tendon reflexes, 600–601
motor function, 597
neurologic status check, 586–596
neurovascular assessments, 506–510
respiratory patterns, 586, 588–589t
sensory function, 598–599
Neurosensory procedures, 583–628
ear irrigation, 625–626
eye irrigation, 627
hyperthermia/hypothermia, 606–609
seizure care, 605
in special beds or frames, 612–622
subarachnoid/lumbar drains, 610–611
TENS devices, 603–604
Neurovascular assessment, 506–510
for children in Bryant's traction, 547
for clients in casts, 529
for clients in skeletal traction, 551
elastic bandages and, 520
Newborn. *See under* Neonatal
Nitrazine test strips, 201
Nitroglycerin ointment, disks, 88–89
Nosocomial infections. *See* Infection control
Nose drops, 85
Numbness, 507
Nursery admission procedures, 215–220
Nursing guidelines
for assessment
breast cancer risks, 182
cardiovascular system, 387
gastrointestinal system, 237
musculoskeletal system, 495
neurologic system, 585
renal-urinary system, 432
respiratory system, 313

for procedures
aerosol therapy, 351, 352
artificial airways, 320–324
blood administration, 144
cast care, 531
catheters, central venous, 154–157
chest tubes, 377–378
continuous bladder irrigation, 466
Foley catheter, 449–459
gastric tubes, 244–251
immobilization devices, 511–519
implantable subcutaneous port, 158
incubators, 349
insulin pump, 110–112
intestinal tubes, 274–276
lifting/moving clients, 64
nephrostomy tube, 468–469
ostomies, 286–296
oxygen delivery devices, 342–350
Permcath catheter, 474
positioning clients, 56–60
pressure-relief mattresses/pads, 53–55
Quinton catheter, 474
special beds/frames, 612–622
suprapubic catheter, 467
telemetry lead sites, 404
traction, 534
transferring clients, 64
ureteral stents, 468–469
urinary diversions, 478–483
venous access devices, 154–158

Occult blood stool testing, 285
Occupational Safety and Health Administration (OSHA), 7
bloodborne pathogens standard, 11t
Open-glove technique, 22
Ophthalmic medications, 83–84
for neonates, 216
Oral cavity examination, 238
Orientation to time/place/person, 590
Orogastric tube, 260
Oropharyngeal tube, 320, 325–326
Ortolani's click test, 227–228, 499
OSHA (Occupational Safety and Health Administration), 7
bloodborne pathogens standard, 11t
Ostomies. *See* Stoma care
Over-the-needle catheters, 121–125
Oxygen delivery, 342–350, 354

Packing wounds, 25–28
Pads. *See* Mattresses and pads
Palm prints, neonate, 215

Paradoxical pulse, 403
Particulate respirators (PRs), 7
Patch tests, skin, 296
Patellar reflex, 601
Patient-controlled analgesia (PCA), 149–153
Peau d'orange, 183
Peg (percutaneous endoscopic gastrostomy) tube, 249
Pelvic belt traction, 539–542
Percussion, chest physiotherapy, 368–376
Percutaneous endoscopic gastrostomy (PEG) tube, 249
Perineal care, 190–192
Peripheral vascular access devices, 117–126
Peritoneal dialysis, 475–477
Permcath catheters, 474
Peroneal nerve assessment, 510
Petaling casts, 530, 532
Pharynx, examination of, 238
Phenytoin (Dilantin), 592
Phototherapy, 233
Piggyback infusion sets, 136–137
Pin (traction) care, 552, 560
Plantar reflex, 596
Pneumatic jet nebulizer, 351, 361–362
Pneumatic sequential compression devices, 420–422
Pneumothorax, 379–381, 383
Positioning
for assisted exercises, 34–52
body mechanics for, 34–35
of crutches, 61–63
for dangling extremities, 67–68
for halo traction clients, 558
for infant feeding, 209
nursing guidelines, 56–60
of pressure-relief pads, 53–55
prone, 58
semi-Fowler's, 57
side-lying, 57
on special beds or frames, 612–622
supine, 56–57
Positioning aids
foot cradles, 59
foot supports, 59
hand rolls, cones, splints, 60
sandbags, 59
trochanter rolls, 58–59
Postpartum procedures, 203–214
assessment, 203–207
breast pumps, 212–214
fundal massage, 205
infant feeding, 207–211
perineal care, 207
Posturing (neurosensory) assessment, 588
Pouches
for fecal drainage, 297–301
Indiana, 482–483
Kock, 482–483
urinary, disposable, 486–491
urostomy, 484–491

Precordium. *See under Cardiovascular*
Prenatal procedures, 194–202
    abdomen assessment, 194–200
    amniotic fluid assessment, 201
    back pain relief, 202
    comfort measures, 202
    Doppler auscultation, 197
    electronic fetal monitoring, 198–200
    estimating gestational age, 194
    fetal heart tones (FHTs), 196–197
    fundal height measurement, 194
    leg cramp relief, 202
    Leopold's maneuvers, 195, 198
    McDonald's rule, 194
    palpating fetal parts, 194–195
    tocodynamometers, 198–200
    ultrasonic transducers, 198–200
    uterine activity assessment, 198–200
Pressure-relief mattresses/pads, 53–55, 531
Prone positioning, 58
Proprioceptive neuromuscular facilitation exercises, 49–52
Protective clothing, 12–15
PRs (particulate respirators), 7
Pulsating air suspension therapy (Therapulse) bed, 620–622
Pulse oximetry, 354
Pulse rates
    ankle-brachial ratio (A/B ratio), 401–402
    apical, 226, 393
    arterial, 394–395, 395*t*
    brachial, 226, 401–402
    Doppler ultrasonic probe for, 395
    neonatal, 226
    paradoxical, 403
    peripheral, 507
    scale for evaluating, 395*t*
Pupils, assessing, 590, 592

Quad canes, 62
Quinton catheters, 474

Radial nerve assessment, 508
Radiation implants, 193
Range of motion (ROM)
    assessment, 500–504
        trunk rotation, 499
    exercises, 34–48
        alternatives to, 49–52
        body mechanics for, 34–35
        contraindications, 34
        IV-restrained clients, 128, 129
        postmastectomy clients, 187–189
        terminology of, 34

traction clients, 534, 550, 553, 556
turning table clients, 614
when to initiate, 34
Reagent strips/sticks, 142–144, 602
Rectal examination, 243
Rectal medications, 94
Rectal tubes, inserting, 283–284
Reflexes
    ankle, 601
    Babinski's, 596
    biceps, 600
    blink, 592
    Brachioradialis (supinator), 600
    deep tendon (DTRs), 600–601
    grasp, 225
    patellar, 601
    plantar, 596
    rooting, 223
    startle, 224
    sucking, 224
Reinfusion (blood) system, 567–569
Renal-urinary procedures, 429–492
    catheterization, 437–460
    continuous bladder irrigation, 465–469
    Credé's maneuver, 473
    dialysis, 474–477
    external urinary devices, 461–464
    Kayexalate enema, 470–472
    nephrostomy tube, 468–469
    postoperative pouches, 486–491
    suprapubic catheter, 467
    ureteral stents, 468–469, 479, 481, 483
    urinary diversions, 478–491
Renal-urinary system assessment, 430–436
    anatomical landmarks, 430–431
    bladder, 433–434
    kidneys, 435
    nursing assessment guidelines, 432
    postoperative, 484–485
    skin turgor, 435
    timed urine specimen, 436
    weighing client, on bed scale, 436
Residual limbs (stumps), wrapping, 522–523
Respiratory procedures, 311–384
    artificial airways, 320–341
        nursing guidelines, 320–324
    chest tubes, 377–383
    respiratory therapy, 342–376
Respiratory system assessment, 312–319
    anatomical landmarks, 312
    assessment guidelines, 313
    breath sounds, 318
    examining the thorax, 314–319

respiratory patterns, 586, 588–589*t*
Respiratory therapy, 342–376
    aerosol masks, 351–352, 361–362
    breathing exercises, 362–363, 365
    chest physiotherapy, 368–376
    converting masks, 355
    humidification, 351, 352, 358–360
    incentive spirometer, 365
    for infants, 348–349
    lung inflation exercises, 362–367
    nebulizers, 351, 361–362
    nursing guidelines, 342–353
    oxygen, 342–350, 354
    Venturi mask, 346, 356–357
Restraints, 128–129
Resuscitator, manual, 330–334
Rinne test, 623–624
Robinson (straight) catheters, 437–445
ROM. *See* Range of motion
Romberg's sign, 597
Rooting reflex, 208, 223
Roto rest kinetic treatment table, 612–615

Saline/heparin lock, 134–135
    after blood transfusions, 146
Sandbags, 59
Scoliosis, 497, 499
Segmental transfer technique, 69–71
Seizures, care during, 605
Self-monitoring, blood glucose, 142–143
Sensory system procedures, 623–627
    auditory function tests, 623–624
    coordination tests, 594–597
    dermatome zones testing, 598–599
    ear irrigation, 625–626
    eye irrigation, 627
    neurovascular assessment, 506–510
    sensory function tests, 593–594, 598–599
Sepsis, during blood transfusions, 148*t*
Sequential pressure cuffs, 420–422
Sharps, disposing of, 110
Sheepskin pads, 53, 531, 557, 558
Shingles, 12
Shoulder joint
    assessment, 501
    exercises, 37–39, 187–189
    immobilizer slings, 514
Side-lying positioning, 57, 209
Sigh maneuver, 331, 332
Sitz bath, 191, 207
Skin patch-testing, 296
Skin turgor assessment, 435
Soap, 4, 4–5*t*

Sodium polystyrene sulfonate (Kayexalate) enema, 470–472
Softset catheter, 112
Sorbitol, 470
Souffle, 196, 197
Speech pattern assessment, 590
Spine, assessment of, 496–499
Spinothalamic tract tests, 598–599
Spirometer, incentive, 365
Splints
    clavicle, 513
    Denis-Browne, 519
    forearm/wrist, 515
    knee immobilizer, 517
    as positioning aids, 60
    for venipuncture sites, 127–129
Startle reflex, 224
Stents, ureteral, 468–469, 479, 481, 483
Sterile attire/gloves, putting on, 21–24
Sterile fields, establishing, 18–20
Sterile packs, opening, 18
Sterile procedures, 16–24
    establishing sterile field, 18–20
    putting on sterile attire, 16–17, 21–24
Sterile solutions, pouring, 20
Stockings, elastic, 417–419
Stoma care, 286–309
    applying drainable pouch, 297–301
    colostomies, 286–291
        irrigation of, 304–306
    cutaneous ureterostomy, 480–481
    dilation of, 302–303
    ileoanal reservoir, 295–296
    ileostomy, 292–293
        continent, 294, 307–309
    Indiana pouches, 482–483
    Kock pouches, 482–483
    nursing guidelines, 286–296
    skin patch-testing, 296
    tracheostomy hygiene, 337–340
    urostomies, 484–491
Stomach contents, aspirating for, 91, 256, 273
Stool testing, for occult blood, 285
Stretcher transfers, 69–75
Stryker reinfusion system, 567–569
Stumps (residual limbs), wrapping, 522–523
Subarachnoid/lumbar drains, 610–611
Subcutaneous injections, 97–100
Subcutaneous ports, implantable, 158, 170–172
Sucking reflex, 224
Suctioning, bulb (nasal/oral), 231–232

Supinator (brachioradialis) reflex, 600
Supine positioning, 56–57
Suppositories, rectal, 94
Suprapubic catheters, 467
Surgi-gator, 192
Sutures, neonatal, 222
Syringes, home care considerations, 90

T-piece, respiratory, 353
Telemetry monitoring
  applying electrodes, 405–408
  identifying lead sites, 404
Temperature, body. *See* Body temperature
Temporomandibular joint, 500, 537
Tenckhoff catheter, 475
Tendon reflexes, deep (DTRs), 600–601
TENS (transcutaneous electrical nerve stimulator) devices, 603–604
Therapulse bed, 620–622
Thoracic examination, 312–319
Throat cultures, 24
Thrombolytic therapy, 155
Tibial nerve assessment, 510
Tingling, 507
Tocodynamometers, 190–200
Toe exercises, 47–48
Tongue assessment, 238, 593
Topical medications, 83–94
  eye, ear, nose drops, 83–85
  inhalants, 86–87, 366
  nitroglycerin, 88–89
  rectal, 94
  vaginal, 92–93
  via nasogastric tube, 90–91
Total hip replacement clients, transferring, 572–581
Tracheostomy button, 324
Tracheostomy care
  hygiene, 337–340
  replacing cannulas, 341
  suctioning, 330–334
Tracheostomy collar, 352
Tracheostomy cuffs, 335–336
Tracheostomy ties, 339–340
Tracheostomy tube, 323
Traction boot (Buck's), 543–546
Traction care, 533–560
  bowline knots, 533

linen changes, 561–562
  nursing guidelines, 534
  skeletal traction, 551–560
    care of clients in, 551–553
    halo vests, 554–560
  skin traction, 535–550
    Bryant's traction, 547–550
    buck's boot, 543–546
    cervical traction, 535–538
    pelvic belt, 539–542
Transcutaneous electrical nerve stimulator (TENS) devices, 603–604
Transferring (moving) clients, 64–79
  from crutches to chair, 63
  from stretcher to bed, 69–75
  from wheelchair to bed, 76–77
  immobile clients, 66, 68, 72–75
  logroll technique, 74–75, 561
  mechanical lifting devices, 78–79
  moving up in bed, 65–66
  nursing guidelines, 64
  segmental transfer technique, 69–71
  to dangle extremities, 67–68
  with total hip replacement, 572–581
Transportation of clients, CDC precautions, 10*t*
Trapezes, 65, 534
Trochanter rolls, 58–59
Tuberculosis, 7, 95
Turning immobile clients, 66, 68, 72–75
  on special beds or frames, 612–622
Turning tables, 612–615

Ulnar nerve assessment, 509
Ultrasonic auscultation, 197, 230
Ultrasonic probe, 395
Ultrasonic transducers, 198–200
Umbilical cord care, 225, 231
Ureteral stents, 468–469, 479, 481, 483
Ureterostomy, cutaneous, 480–481
Urinary diversions, 478–491

continent, 482–483
  cutaneous ureterostomy, 480–481
  ileal conduit, 478–479
  nursing guidelines, 478
Urinary system. *See* Renal-urinary system
Urine specimens
  catheterization for, 437–460
  neonatal, 219–220
  timed, 436
  via Foley catheters, 452–453
Urokinase, 155
Urostomy, Kock continent, 482–483
Uterine tone assessment, 205
Uterine/cervical radiation implants, 193

VADs. *See* Venous access devices
Vaginal irrigation (douche), 92–93
Valsalva's maneuver, 383, 459
Vascular procedures, 417–427
  Buerger-Allen exercises, 425–427
  elastic stockings, 417–419
  foot pump, 423–424
  pneumatic sequential compression cuffs, 420–422
Vastus lateralis injection site, 104, 106
  in neonates, 217
Venipuncture, 117–126
  antimicrobial ointments, 126
  armboards/splints, 127–129
  for blood samples, 140–141
  for blood transfusions, 146
  choosing/preparing site, 118–119
  dilating the vein, 119
  dressings for, 126
  immobilizing extremity for, 127–129
  over-the-needle catheter insertion, 121–125
  taping needle or catheter, 121, 125
  wing-tipped (butterfly) needle insertion, 120–121
Venous access devices (VADs), 154–176
  central venous catheters, 154, 155, 159–167

implantable subcutaneous ports, 158
  midline catheters, 157
  nursing guidelines, 154–158
  peripherally inserted central catheters, 156
Ventilation, mouth-to-mask, 329
Ventrogluteal injection site, 103, 106
Venturi mask, 346, 356–357
Vibration, chest physiotherapy, 368–376
Vitamin K injections, 217
Volume-control IV set, 138–139

Walkers, 62
Watch test, 623
Weber test, 623–624
Weight determination
  of neonates, 229
  via bed scale, 436
Wheelchairs
  for halo traction clients, 559
  transferring client from, 76–77
Wing-tipped (butterfly) needle
  for children, 118
  injecting medications into, 133
  inserting and taping, 120–121
Wound care, 25–30
  dressing changes, 25–28
  establishing sterile field for, 18–20
  home care considerations, 28
  indwelling drains for, 563–564
  irrigating, 29–30
  packing, 25–28
  portable wound-drainage, 563–564
  standard precautions during, 7–11
Wound-drainage systems, 563–564
Wrist
  assessment, 502
  exercises, 41–43
  restraints, 128–129
  splints for, 515

Z-track injections, 108–109